Drug Discovery and Antiaging Approaches for Human Longevity

Jen-Tsung Chen
National University of Kaohsiung, Taiwan

IGI Global
Scientific Publishing
Publishing Tomorrow's Research Today

Vice President of Editorial	Melissa Wagner
Director of Acquisitions	Mikaela Felty
Director of Book Development	Jocelynn Hessler
Production Manager	Mike Brehm
Cover Design	Jose Rosado

Published in the United States of America by
IGI Global Scientific Publishing
701 East Chocolate Avenue
Hershey, PA, 17033, USA
Tel: 717-533-8845
Fax: 717-533-7115
Website: https://www.igi-global.com E-mail: cust@igi-global.com

Library of Congress Cataloging-in-Publication Data

Names: Chen, Jen-Tsung editor
Title: Drug discovery and antiaging approaches for human longevity / edited by Jen-Tsung Chen.
Description: Hershey, PA : Medical Information Science Reference, [2025] | Includes bibliographical references and index. | Summary: "This book aims to summarize antiaging biology and technological advancements in drug development to extend the human lifespan"-- Provided by publisher.
Identifiers: LCCN 2025005828 (print) | LCCN 2025005829 (ebook) | ISBN 9798369397305 hardcover | ISBN 9798369397312 paperback | ISBN 9798369397329 ebook
Subjects: LCSH: Aging--Prevention | Drug development
Classification: LCC RA776.75 .D783 2026 (print) | LCC RA776.75 (ebook)
LC record available at https://lccn.loc.gov/2025005828
LC ebook record available at https://lccn.loc.gov/2025005829

British Cataloguing in Publication Data
A Cataloguing in Publication record for this book is available from the British Library.

Table of Contents

Detailed Table of Contents

Reactive oxygen species (ROS) can cause oxidative stress which plays a prominent role in the pathophysiology of several health conditions, such as cardiovascular disorders, neurodegenerative diseases, importantly cancer prevention and aging/longevity. Many medicinal and food plants, spices and beverages contain phenolics, polyphenols, carotenoids, isothiocyanates, allicin, even chlorophyll and other secondary metabolites (PSM) with substantial antioxidant properties. Therefore, the supplementation of our diet with plant-derived antioxidants is regarded as a potential strategy to delay or even prevent the onset of age-related diseases and to promote longevity. In order to understand the underlaying biochemical and pharmacological mechanisms, scientists have employed the nematode Caenorhabditis elegans as a model, which can easily be maintained in the laboratory. C. elegans has been used for over the last 25 years to explore the antioxidant and anti-aging properties of isolated PSM and complex plant extracts. In this chapter, recent studies on the antioxidant, longevity-promoting and neuroprotective activities of plant extracts and isolated PSM in C. elegans were reviewed.

Aging is a complicated process influenced by various factors that disturb cellular function and alter organism equilibrium over time. This chapter provides an updated overview, focusing on mechanisms like genomic instability, telomere attrition, mitochondrial failure, and DNA damage buildup. Cellular senescence is addressed in age-related illnesses, highlighting irreversible cell cycle arrest and pro-inflammatory aspects. Epigenetic processes, specifically DNA methylation and inherited histone modifications, contribute to age-related phenotypes. Longevity research covers factors like FOXO, SIRT, and autophagy. Nutrient-sensing pathways and the microbiome's role in aging are explored, along with therapeutic interventions targeting these pathways. This synthesis of recent discoveries in genetics, molecular biology, and translational research provides a comprehensive perspective on aging biology and future clinical applications. By integrating insights from various fields, this chapter aims to develop innovative strategies to promote healthy aging and longevity.

Aging is an inevitable biological process that affects every living organism. It is influenced by a complex interplay of factors like genetics, environment, and lifestyle. These factors gradually lead to changes in an individual's body's physiological functions over a period of time. With modern society's increased workload and bustling lifestyles, many individuals are gradually neglecting their health, which accelerates the aging process and contributes to the development of critical health conditions. This chapter will explore two of the key biological mechanisms associated with aging—telomere shortening and elevated homocysteine levels—and examine potential interventions to mitigate their effects.

The field of anti-aging pharmacology has seen remarkable advancements over recent years, driven by the growing understanding of the molecular and genetic mechanisms underlying aging. This chapter explores the latest developments in anti-aging pharmacological interventions, including senolytics, caloric restriction mimetics, and autophagy enhancers. We delve into the role of molecular pathways such as mTOR, sirtuins, and AMPK in aging, and discuss how drugs targeting these pathways hold promise for extending lifespan and improving healthspan. The chapter also examines the challenges of translating these interventions from preclinical models to human applications, considering both efficacy and safety. Ethical considerations and regulatory frameworks will be discussed, along with prospects for future research and clinical implementation in the quest to combat aging and age-related diseases.

Aging is a natural process characterized by the gradual decline of cellular function and increased susceptibility to diseases. Gene therapy offers a promising approach to combat age-related diseases by targeting and modifying specific longevity-associated genes with aging processes such as mitochondrial dysfunction and telomere shortening. Recent advancements have shown that modifying specific genes can slow down or reverse certain aspects of aging, potentially extending healthy lifespan. Gene-editing technologies like CRISPR and AAV-based antiaging gene therapies have shown success in treating conditions such as cardiovascular disease, neurodegeneration, and metabolic disorders. Experimental research indicates that improving DNA repair pathways and lowering oxidative stress may be able to reverse aging characteristics. This chapter explores the current advancements, challenges, and future prospects of gene therapy as a therapeutic strategy for age-related diseases.

Tharani Sureshkumar, PSGR Krishnammal College for Women, India
Krishnasreya Mohandas, PSGR Krishnammal College for Women, India
Elakkiya Maruthamuthu Rathinam, PSGR Krishnammal College for Women, India
Chitra Devi Balasundaram Saraswathy, PSGR Krishnammal College for Women, India
Sarmad Moin, Suresh Gyan Vihar University, India

Stem-cell therapy is a promising approach to combating aging by targeting cellular degeneration and tissue repair. This chapter provides a comprehensive overview of advancements in stem-cell therapy for anti-aging, examining how stem cells can reverse or slow age-related changes at molecular and tissue levels. We explore various stem cell types used in anti-aging therapies, including mesenchymal stem cells (MSCs), induced pluripotent stem cells (iPSCs), and embryonic stem cells (ESCs), highlighting their roles in tissue regeneration, immune enhancement, and cellular rejuvenation. Additionally, this chapter discusses recent clinical trials, potential applications for age-related diseases, and key ethical and safety considerations in stem-cell-based anti-aging treatments. As the field progresses, we examine emerging trends and challenges, including regulatory hurdles and the need for robust clinical evidence. This chapter provides a balanced, up-to-date perspective on stem-cell therapy's potential to revolutionize anti-aging interventions and enhance longevity.

Tejasvini Ramesh, Amity Institute of Biotechnology, Amity University, Mumbai, India
Rajshri Singh, Amity Institute of Biotechnology, Amity University, Mumbai, India
Sagar H. Barage, Amity Institute of Biotechnology, Amity University, Mumbai, India

Aging is a complex process characterized by various biological, morphological, and anatomical changes. The epigenetic modifications include DNA methylation, histone modifications, and the action of non-coding RNA play essential roles in genes function as we age. With age, the cascade of epigenetic alterations can lead to genetic mutations and altered gene expression, contributing to a range of age-related diseases. Recent studies suggest that external factors such as climate change and environmental stressors disrupt these epigenetic mechanisms and trigger harmful epigenetic changes that lead to earlier onset of aging-related conditions. Further, this modification contributes to development of cardiovascular disease, neurodegenerative diseases, and metabolic syndromes, underscoring the importance for understanding the epigenetic aspects of these health issues. We have shed light on role of epigenetic factors and mechanisms involved in aging and the development of related diseases.

Aging is a complex process influenced by biological mechanisms, lifestyle choices, environmental factors, and genetic predispositions. Key biological hallmarks include genomic instability, mitochondrial dysfunction, and OS, which contribute to age-related diseases such as CVD, NDD and sarcopenia. Lifestyle factors like diet, physical activity, and sleep quality significantly impact health. Genetic variations and epigenetic modifications further modulate individual aging trajectories. OS driven by reactive oxygen species, plays a central role in aging, with antioxidants from natural sources offering protective benefits. This chapter deliberates the overview of the aging process with special emphases on OS and methods for mitigating its effects; it further highlights the necessity for individualized techniques like nutrigenomics and examines treatment approaches. Future studies should prioritize large-scale investigations and include genetic, environmental, and lifestyle factors to promote healthy aging and enhance quality of life.

This chapter delves into the realm of traditional medicine to uncover natural compounds with potential anti-ageing properties. It examines the historical context and foundational principles of traditional medical systems, emphasising their holistic approaches to health and longevity. The chapter identifies key herbal compounds renowned for their anti-ageing effects, exploring their mechanisms of action, including antioxidant activity, anti-inflammatory properties, and modulation of cellular pathways. Furthermore, it evaluates the scientific evidence supporting these claims, discusses the integration of these herbal solutions into modern healthcare, and addresses safety considerations. The chapter concludes by highlighting future research directions and the importance of a balanced approach to incorporating traditional herbal remedies into contemporary anti-ageing strategies.

Over the last decade, the revolution in ageing science has propelled advancements in therapies aimed at extending lifespan. The analysis of the traditional indicators of ageing has yielded reliable evidence to establish the existence of at least three new indicators, therefore creating opportunities for the advancement of innovative methods aimed at promoting lifespan. The pursuit of geroprotectors is highly intriguing, as it aims to identify the alchemical substance that promotes successful ageing and extends lifespan. Natural origin geroprotectors, including metformin, resveratrol, aspirin, and spermidine, are widely acknowledged as valuable agents that enhance longevity. Ongoing research is predominantly investigating the potential of plant secondary metabolites as pharmacological modulators of healthspan and lifespan. Therefore, this chapter rigorously evaluate the existing activities and significant findings in the area of longevity research.

This chapter explores the role of natural compounds in mitigating age-related challenges such as loneliness, elder abuse, dehydration, falls risk, and incontinence. As ageing progresses, physiological and psychological vulnerabilities increase, necessitating targeted nutritional interventions to enhance overall well-being. The chapter examines bioactive compounds, including antioxidants, omega-3 fatty acids, and polyphenols, which support cognitive health, emotional resilience, and physical function. It also discusses hydration strategies, muscle-strengthening nutrients, and bladder-supportive diets that reduce common geriatric risks. Additionally, ethical considerations, socioeconomic barriers, and policy implications are examined to ensure equitable access to nutritional support. By bridging traditional knowledge with contemporary research, this chapter advocates for an evidence-based, multidimensional approach to improving the quality of life in older adults through dietary optimisation.

Protein glycation, or simply glycation, is the process by which sugar binds to amino acids, producing reactive oxygen species (ROS) and free radicals. These chemicals generated by glycation play a role in oxidative stress and the formation of Advanced Glycation End Products (AGEs), further leading to disorders such as diabetes and cardiovascular disease. Synthetic substances have been studied for their ability to reverse glycation. However, the adverse effects they cause lead to the search for natural glycation inhibitors. Medicinal plants and compounds derived from them, including polyphenols, polysaccharides, terpenoids, vitamins, alkaloids, and peptides, have been studied and have demonstrated encouraging potential in reducing glycation-induced damage through early-stage inhibitory effects, chelating metal ions, reducing reactive oxygen species (ROS) and reactive carbonyl species (RCS), and blocking other important glycation pathway sites. Nevertheless, more study and an integrated approach are recommended to fully comprehend the molecular mechanism and processes behind this.

Kinases are essential for signaling pathways that affects biological processes. The kinase inhibitors potential as therapeutic medicines to prolong lifespan has been brought to light by recent research which includes aging and longevity, one is mTOR modulation. For instance, it has demonstrated that mTOR inhibition mimics the effects of caloric restriction, a tried-and-true strategy for increasing lifespan in animals. These inhibitors can control pathways related to inflammation, stress reactions, and DNA repair—essential to the aging. Preclinical research on small-molecule inhibitors that target kinases, including PI3K, JNK, and IGF-1 has shown promise. These substances can decrease build-up of cellular damage, alleviate illnesses, and increase longevity. Though these are encouraging, the intricacy of kinase networks and off-target consequences make it difficult to translate insights into safe and efficient. To optimize kinase inhibitors for anti-aging therapies, more study is required, with a particular emphasis on safety, effectiveness, and avoiding adverse effects.

Recent advances in understanding epigenetic mechanisms have revealed promising therapeutic strategies for addressing skin aging and maintaining dermal homeostasis. This comprehensive review examines the convergence of nutritional interventions and pharmaceutical approaches in modulating epigenetic pathways critical to skin health. We analyze emerging evidence on key dietary compounds, including polyphenols, vitamins, and minerals, and their roles in DNA methylation, histone modifications, and chromatin remodeling within dermal tissues.

This chapter critically examines the ethical and social implications of anti-aging therapies and lifespan-extending interventions. It explores the tension between individual benefits and societal good, addressing issues such as equity, access, and the commercialization of these treatments. Key topics include the potential exacerbation of health disparities, the redefinition of aging, and the societal impacts of extending life. Drawing from bioethics, sociology, and public policy, the chapter analyzes case studies and proposes ethical frameworks to guide future research and policy, aiming to provide a balanced perspective on the benefits and risks of anti-aging technologies.

Preface

INTRODUCTION

In recent years, the quest for prolonged human healthspan and lifespan has intensified as aging populations grow across the globe. While aging is a natural and inevitable process, science is rapidly advancing in its understanding of the molecular, genetic, and environmental factors that influence how we age. This book, *Drug Discovery and Antiaging Approaches for Human Longevity*, presents a multidisciplinary exploration of strategies that address aging at its root—through pharmacological, nutritional, genomic, and technological innovations.

Our contributors—scientists, pharmacologists, biotechnologists, and clinicians—provide diverse perspectives on the mechanisms and interventions related to aging. The chapters span a wide range of topics, including plant-based antioxidants, telomere biology, AI-assisted drug development, gene and stem-cell therapies, epigenetics, and natural compounds with geroprotective properties. This breadth of content ensures a comprehensive overview of both fundamental insights and applied therapeutic approaches designed to delay or reverse the aging process.

The volume begins with a focus on natural products and biological mechanisms, transitions into technological and pharmacological strategies, and closes with innovative perspectives on nutrition, herbal medicine, and targeted molecular interventions. Each chapter has been carefully selected to reflect both the complexity of aging and the creativity of emerging anti-aging science. Together, they provide an essential resource for researchers, healthcare professionals, and policy-makers engaged in promoting healthy longevity.

CHAPTER OVERVIEW

Chapter 1: Plant Natural Products with Anti-Aging, Antioxidative and Neuroprotective Properties

This chapter investigates the potential of plant-derived secondary metabolites—such as phenolics, carotenoids, and isothiocyanates—as natural antioxidants with anti-aging and neuroprotective effects. Using *Caenorhabditis elegans* as a model organism, the chapter reviews recent studies on the efficacy of isolated compounds and complex plant extracts in delaying oxidative stress and age-related degeneration, proposing dietary supplementation as a strategy for promoting longevity.

Chapter 2: Biology, Genetics and Molecular Aspects of Aging: An Update

Providing a comprehensive update on the biology of aging, this chapter explores genomic instability, telomere shortening, mitochondrial dysfunction, and cellular senescence. It delves into the roles of epigenetics, nutrient-sensing pathways, and the microbiome in aging, while also addressing therapeutic strategies that leverage genetic and molecular insights to foster healthy aging and extended lifespan.

Chapter 3: Exploring the Role of Telomere Dynamics and Homocysteine Levels in Aging and Potential Intervention Strategies

This chapter focuses on two crucial biological indicators of aging—telomere shortening and elevated homocysteine levels. It examines how these factors contribute to age-related decline and highlights possible lifestyle and pharmacological interventions aimed at mitigating their effects, especially in the context of modern, high-stress living.

Chapter 4: Anti-Aging Pharmacology: Advances and Prospects

Highlighting recent developments in anti-aging pharmacology, this chapter examines interventions such as senolytics, caloric restriction mimetics, and autophagy enhancers. It discusses the therapeutic targeting of aging-related pathways like mTOR, sirtuins, and AMPK, while also addressing translational challenges, ethical issues, and future prospects for clinical application.

Chapter 5: Gene Therapy Against Age-Related Diseases

Focusing on the potential of gene therapy to treat age-related conditions, this chapter discusses how gene editing tools like CRISPR and AAV vectors can target aging mechanisms such as telomere attrition and mitochondrial dysfunction. It outlines promising preclinical results and highlights the therapeutic potential and challenges of applying gene therapy to extend healthy lifespan.

Chapter 6: Stem-Cell Therapy for Anti-Aging

This chapter presents a comprehensive overview of stem-cell therapies for reversing age-related cellular degeneration. It details the therapeutic potential of mesenchymal, embryonic, and induced pluripotent stem cells in tissue regeneration and immune support, while also exploring clinical applications, ethical concerns, and future research directions in regenerative aging medicine.

Chapter 7: Epigenetics of Aging and Epigenetic Modifications of Aging-Associated Diseases

Examining the epigenetic landscape of aging, this chapter reviews mechanisms such as DNA methylation and histone modifications that influence gene expression over time. It highlights how these changes contribute to aging and related diseases and considers environmental factors and external stressors that exacerbate harmful epigenetic alterations.

Chapter 8: Natural Antioxidants and Their Impacts on Aging: Insights into Mechanisms for Extending Life Span

Focusing on oxidative stress as a central driver of aging, this chapter investigates natural antioxidants and their protective effects on cellular and systemic aging processes. It integrates insights from nutrigenomics and lifestyle interventions, advocating for personalized strategies that combine genetics, nutrition, and environmental factors to promote healthy aging.

Chapter 9: Herbal Solutions for Longevity: Anti-Ageing Compounds from Traditional Medicine

This chapter explores traditional medicine systems to uncover herbal remedies with scientifically supported anti-aging properties. It discusses key compounds, their mechanisms of action, and the integration of traditional knowledge into modern healthcare, while emphasizing the importance of safety, regulation, and future research in herbal longevity solutions.

Chapter 10: Lifespan-Extending Natural Compounds

Investigating natural geroprotectors like metformin, resveratrol, and spermidine, this chapter reviews their role in extending lifespan and promoting healthy aging. It highlights recent findings on plant secondary metabolites and evaluates their pharmacological potential in longevity research, while proposing new biomarkers and intervention strategies.

Chapter 11: Nutritional Powerhouses: Exploring Natural Compounds for Anti-Ageing

This chapter focuses on bioactive nutritional compounds that support aging populations by improving cognitive, emotional, and physical resilience. It discusses the role of antioxidants, omega-3s, and hydration strategies in managing geriatric risks, while addressing ethical and policy challenges in ensuring equitable nutritional support for older adults.

Chapter 12: Addressing Glycation in Aging: Natural Remedies, Synthetic Approaches, and Clinical Applications

Exploring the damaging effects of glycation and the formation of advanced glycation end products (AGEs), this chapter evaluates both synthetic and natural inhibitors. It emphasizes plant-based compounds with antioxidative and chelating properties that may reduce glycation-related aging damage, while calling for further molecular research and integrated treatment strategies.

Chapter 13: The Role of Kinase Inhibitors in Healthy Aging: Potential Pathways and Challenges

This chapter explores the therapeutic potential of kinase inhibitors in modulating aging-related pathways such as mTOR, PI3K, JNK, and IGF-1. By mimicking caloric restriction and regulating inflammation, DNA repair, and cellular stress responses, these inhibitors show promise in delaying aging and extending lifespan. The chapter highlights encouraging preclinical results while addressing the complexity of kinase networks and the need for further research to ensure safety, efficacy, and precision in anti-aging applications.

Chapter 14: Integrative Pharmaceutical and Nutritional Approaches to Epigenetic Modulation in Skin Aging

Focusing on the interplay between nutrition, pharmaceuticals, and epigenetics, this chapter reviews strategies for managing skin aging at the molecular level. It analyzes how dietary components like polyphenols and essential micronutrients influence DNA methylation, histone modification, and chromatin remodeling, offering a multi-targeted approach to preserving dermal health and promoting skin longevity.

Chapter 15: Ethical and Social Issues in Anti-Aging Medicines: Balancing Scientific Innovations with Societal Values

This chapter examines the ethical, social, and policy challenges surrounding anti-aging interventions. It addresses concerns over equitable access, commercialization, and the societal implications of extended lifespans. Drawing from interdisciplinary perspectives, the chapter proposes ethical frameworks to balance innovation with fairness, ensuring that anti-aging technologies serve both individual and collective well-being.

CONCLUSION

As editor of this volume, I am struck by the shared vision among contributors: that aging is not merely a passive decline, but a biological journey that can be influenced—perhaps even redirected—through intentional, evidence-based interventions. Whether through plant-derived compounds, gene editing, or artificial intelligence in drug discovery, the contributors present compelling evidence that aging can be better understood and more effectively managed.

Equally important are the ethical, societal, and translational considerations that accompany these advancements. Longevity should not be a privilege of the few, but a benefit made accessible through equitable healthcare, thoughtful regulation, and interdisciplinary collaboration. By bridging traditional medicine with modern biotechnology, and merging basic research with clinical potential, this book underscores the importance of holistic and inclusive approaches to human longevity.

I sincerely thank all the authors for their rigorous work and insightful contributions. It is my hope that this collection will inspire further research, spark new collaborations, and ultimately contribute to strategies that improve the quality and length of human life. Let this book serve as both a foundation and a springboard for the future of anti-aging science.

Jen-Tsung Chen
National University of Kaohsiung, Taiwan

Chapter 1
Plant Natural Products With Anti-Aging, Antioxidative, and Neuroprotective Properties

Michael Wink
https://orcid.org/0000-0002-7875-4510
Heidelberg University, Germany

ABSTRACT

Reactive oxygen species (ROS) can cause oxidative stress which plays a prominent role in the pathophysiology of several health conditions, such as cardiovascular disorders, neurodegenerative diseases, importantly cancer prevention and aging/longevity. Many medicinal and food plants, spices and beverages contain phenolics, polyphenols, carotenoids, isothiocyanates, allicin, even chlorophyll and other secondary metabolites (PSM) with substantial antioxidant properties. Therefore, the supplementation of our diet with plant-derived antioxidants is regarded as a potential strategy to delay or even prevent the onset of age-related diseases and to promote longevity. In order to understand the underlaying biochemical and pharmacological mechanisms, scientists have employed the nematode Caenorhabditis elegans as a model, which can easily be maintained in the laboratory. C. elegans has been used for over the last 25 years to explore the antioxidant and anti-aging properties of isolated PSM and complex plant extracts. In this chapter, recent studies on the antioxidant, longevity-promoting and neuroprotective activities of plant extracts and isolated PSM in C. elegans were reviewed.

1 INTRODUCTION

In this chapter, the focus is on plant secondary metabolites (PSM) with antioxidant and anti-aging properties. After an introduction in the evolution and function of PSM and thus their usefulness in the treatment of various diseases and health conditions (so-called phytotherapy), we focus on health conditions caused by reactive oxygen species (ROS). The role and function of ROS in physiology is briefly explained. Since ROS are an important mediator of several health conditions and crucial in the aging process, PSM with antioxidant and protein-modifying properties are a key for therapy and antiaging strategies. Next, the important animal model system *Caenorhabditis elegans* is introduced, which allows the *in vivo* investigation of antioxidant and longevity promoting effects of PSM and also of synthetic

DOI: 10.4018/979-8-3693-9730-5.ch001

drugs. The main part of the chapter is a tabulation of relevant studies in *C. elegans* with extracts or isolated PSM from food and medicinal plants with antioxidant, neuroprotective and longevity promoting properties. Several of these plants are already used in medicine or as nutraceuticals or could be interesting candidates for application as anti-aging drugs.

1.1 Evolution and Function of Plant Secondary Metabolites (PSM)

A common trait of plants is the production of a wide diversity of small organic molecules, termed plant secondary metabolites (PSM) or specialized metabolites. Over 100,000 chemically different structures are known, but more are to be expected when all plants have been phytochemically analyzed one day (Wink 2003, 2008, 2010a,b, 2015; van Wyk and Wink 2017).

We can distinguish between PSM containing a nitrogen atom in their molecule structure and those without. Among nitrogen-containing PSM, the heterogenous class of alkaloids include more than 27000 structures, mostly derived from amino acids as biosynthetic precursors. Important groups of alkaloids include tropane, pyrrolizidine, quinolizidine, morphinane, isoquinoline, quinoline, simple indole, monoterpene indole, diterpene and steroidal alkaloids. Most alkaloids are quite toxic with pronounced activities on the nervous system, cell viability and DNA (intercalation, alkylation). Other nitrogen-containing PSM include cyanogenic glucosides (releasing the toxic HCN after activation), the glucosinolates (releasing the isothiocyanates with pungent taste), several non-protein amino acids and simple amines (Wink 2003, 2008, 2010a,b, 2015; van Wyk and Wink 2017).

PSM without nitrogen are more numerous: The main classes are the terpenoids and phenolics. Most terpenoids, consisting of mono-, sesqui-, di-, tri-, tetra and polyterpenes, are lipophilic and most of them can disturb the fluidity of biomembranes. Among triterpenes and C27 steroids, many of them occur as conjugates with sugar chains (so-called saponins), making them amphiphilic; they can complex cholesterol in biomembranes and make them leaky (Wink 2003, 2010a,b, 2015; van Wyk and Wink 2017). Phenolic PSM consist at least of one aromatic ring, which is substituted with one or several phenolic OH groups. An important physicochemical characteristic of phenolics is that the hydroxyl groups can dissociate under physiological conditions; they form negatively charged phenolate ions. Phenolics and especially polyphenols with several phenolic OH groups can strongly interact with all proteins by forming ion bonds in addition to hydrogen bonds. As a consequence, phenolics can modulate the 3D structure of proteins and can inhibit receptors, enzymes, ion channels and importantly modulate the activity of transcription factors thus influencing gene transcription. In addition, phenolics and polyphenols are strong antioxidants which can scavenge oxygen radicals (see below) (Wink 2003, 2010a,b, 2015; van Wyk and Wink 2017).

PSM have evolved over 500 million years as defense and signal compounds (Figure 1). Plants are sessile organisms which cannot run away when attacked by a plant-eating animal, a herbivore. Instead, plants started to produce PSM with deterrent or toxic properties. Plants also needed defense against bacteria, fungi and viruses, which are abundant in their environment. Again, plants which do not have an adaptive immune system, evolved PSM with antimicrobial activities. In addition, plants compete with other plants for water, nutrient and light; they also use PSM to inhibit germination and growth of other plants (a strategy called allelopathy). In addition, plants use PSM as antioxidants and as signal compounds to attract pollinating and fruit-dispersing animals, or in other plant-plant, plant-animal and plant-microbe interactions (Wink 2003, 2010a,b, 2015; van Wyk and Wink 2017).

Plants usually produce and store mixtures of PSM which contain PSM of different chemical classes. Often, a main PSM is accompanied by derivatives differing in various functional groups. Thus, an individual plant can store hundreds of different PSM, whose composition can differ between plant organs, developmental stages and within populations. This variability appears to be a strategy against enemies which have overcome the chemical defense barrier (Wink 2003, 2010a,b, 2015; van Wyk and Wink 2017).

As a consequence of a long evolution period with natural selection, PSM have been shaped as bioactive molecules which can interfere or modulate molecular targets in animals and microbes. This is the reason, why humans have used and still use plants to improve health, combat infections and diseases. In the context of this book, it is important that some PSM can counteract oxidative stress and the aging process (Wink 2003, 2010a,b, 2015; van Wyk and Wink 2017).

Figure 1. Functions of secondary or specialized metabolites (PSM) in plants and in plant-plant, plant-animal and plant-microbe interactions

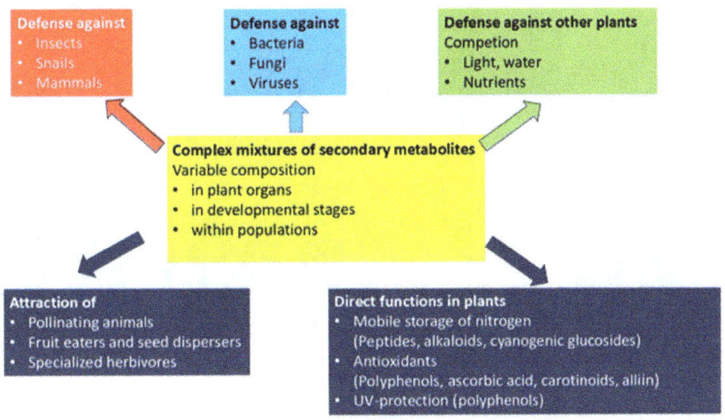

1.2 ROS and ROS Related Diseases

Reactive oxygen species (ROS) are naturally occurring molecules in all cells. They represent a variety of highly reactive substances derived from oxygen, hydrogen and water. Important ROS include hydroperoxide (H_2O_2), hydroxyl radical ($OH^{\bullet}$), hydroxyl ion (OH^-), superoxide (O_2^-), and singlet oxygen ($^1O_2$) (Figure 2) (Alberts et al. 2015; Sies and Jones, 2020).

ROS are important molecules with positive and negative properties. They play a positive role in basal physiological processes, such as inflammation, fight against microbes and cancer cells, immune response, cell signaling, and cell differentiation (Sies and Jones, 2020). Several mechanisms regulate the intracellular redox homeostasis, including antioxidant enzymes such as catalase, superoxide dismutase and the redox mediator glutathione. ROS can be overproduced under stress conditions caused by UV light, radioactive irradiation, air pollution, pain, inflammation and psychological problems (Figure 2) causing oxidative stress.

ROS and oxidative stress can exert negative effects in cells as ROS can oxidize cellular macromolecules, such as proteins, lipids and importantly DNA. The interaction with DNA can cause mutations: The DNA base guanosine can be oxidized by ROS to 8-oxoguanosine (8oxoG). 8oxoG no longer pairs with cytosine (C) (as would guanosine) but with adenosine (A). In DNA this can lead to point mutations, which can have influence on protein properties and gene transcription (Wink 2015; van Wyk and Wink 2017). In consequence, mutated cells no longer exert their original duties or can even develop into tumor cells. ROS-related health disorders include cancer, cardiovascular and neurodegenerative diseases (Franceschi et al. 2018).

Figure 2. Schematic view of Reactive Oxygen Species (ROS), their synthesis and interactions with molecular targets, causing diseases and aging. In addition, major plant derived antioxidants are highlighted.

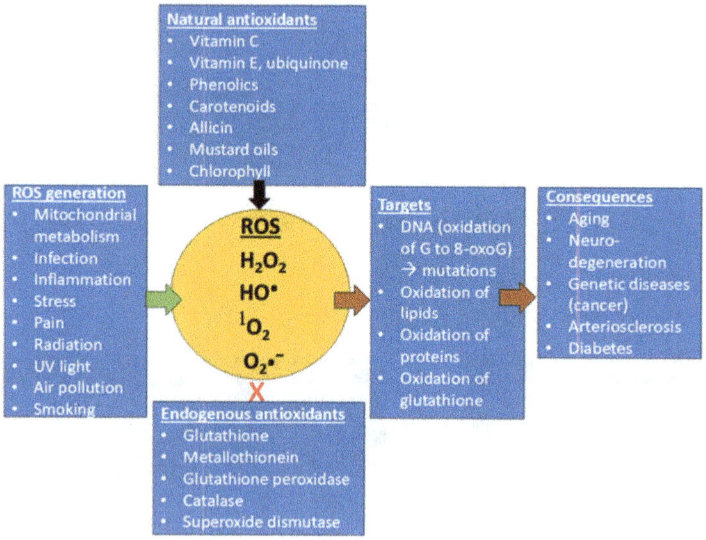

1.3 ROS and Aging

The ROS-mediated health conditions are often collectively termed "age-related diseases" because they increase during the aging process. ROS are continuously generated during respiration in mitochondria. As mitochondria also contain DNA, coding for important proteins of the respiratory chain, the mitochondrial genes can become mutated by ROS over time (Ösz et al. 2025). As a consequence, the metabolic activity of mitochondria can decrease, causing a decline of vigor and resilience of the aging body. Therefore, the influence of ROS on mitochondria has been discussed as a cause of aging, in addition to the shortening of telomeres of chromosomes in each round of cell division (Alberts et al. 2015).

Life-expectancy in humans has increased worldwide, because of better medical therapies, hygiene and living conditions during the last 100 years. As a consequence of a higher longevity, the incidence of age-related diseases and conditions has increased and will further increase in the future (WHO 2015). This conclusion asks for the development and application of nutritional and medicinal interventions to slow down the aging process and age-related health disorders. Apparently, the regular consumption of antioxidative PSM in food, beverages and nutraceuticals, could be such a useful intervention (Sies and Jones, 2020; Wink 2022, 2024). A beneficial effect of a nutrition rich in antioxidants for the prevention and treatment of aging and age-related health conditions has been documented in several epidemiological, observational and clinical studies (Cesari et al. 2004; Scalbert et al. 2005; Wang et al. 2011; Mursu et al. 2014; Devore et al. 2012; Kotecha et al. 2016;).

1.4 Investigations of PSM With Antioxidant Properties

Compounds with antioxidant properties can inactivate ROS and oxygen radicals which can be measured *in vitro* in a variety of chemical assays (DPPH, ABTS and FRAP). Widely known natural antioxidants include vitamin C and vitamin E, which are added to many health drinks and nutraceuticals (Wink 2022, 2024). Among PSM, the most important class of antioxidants are phenolics and polyphenols, such as flavonoids, stilbenes, catechins and tannins. Also, carotenoids and other terpenoids, mustard oils, allicins (from garlic) and some polysaccharides exert antioxidant activities (Figure 2).

As mentioned above, PSM evolved as bioactive molecules which can interfere with several targets in cells and the body; they constitute typical multi-target drugs (Wink 2008, 2015). The activity of antioxidant PSM is not restricted to a simple scavenging of free radicals (Wink 2015) because they can modulate the activity of highly conserved signaling pathways governing stress resistance and aging in humans and many other animals. Of particular importance in this context is the insulin/IGF (insulin-like growth factor)-like signaling (IIS) pathway (Lee and Johnson 2004; Kampkötter et al. 2007; Chiang et al. 2012; Chen et al. 2013a,b,c; de Freitas Bonomo et al. 2014; Peixoto et al. 2019a,b; Guerrero-Rubio et al. 2020; Kenyon 2011; Conte et al. 2015; Zheng et al. 2018; Sural et al. 2019; Adedara et al. 2025) (Figure 3).

Figure 3. Importance of the transcription factors DAF-16, SKN-1, HSF-1 for the expression of genes regulating oxidative and thermal stress, longevity, mitophagy and autophagy in C. elegans.

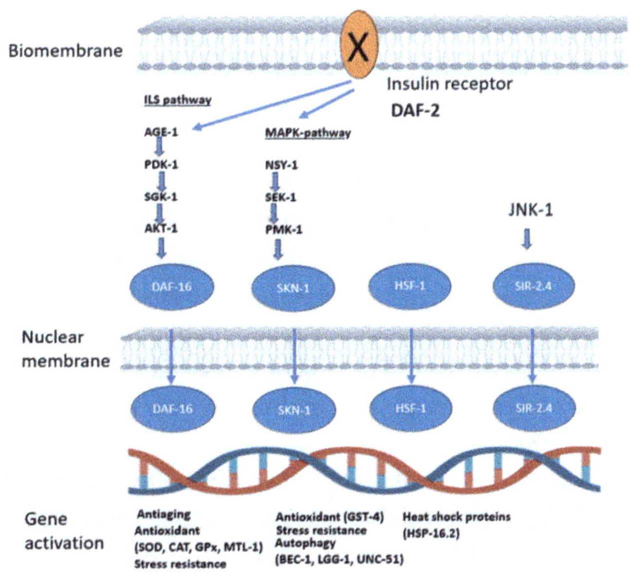

Intervention studies with humans are expensive and in the case of age-rated health conditions require long time-periods before a clear conclusion can be reached. Therefore, animals with a short life expectancy are favored in nutritional and pharmacological research. Among vertebrates, mice, rats and fish (e.g. zebra fish) are important model systems. However, also some invertebrates such as fruit flies (*Drosophila melanogaster*) and the nematode *Caenorhabditis elegans*, have been established as powerful model systems in longevity research (McIntyre et al. 2022; Mishra et al. 2022; Bhatt and Tiwari 2023; Loo et al. 2023; Yasuda et al. 2023; Ösz et al. 2025) They have a short life span, can be raised in large numbers, can be genetically modified and most importantly, many of their central signaling pathways are homologues to those in humans.

In this review, the focus lies on *C. elegans*, which is widely recognized as model of choice to study and screen the properties of plant extracts, beverages and isolated PSM in the context of antioxidants, longevity, aging and aging-related health conditions (Kenyon 2011; Lublin and Link 2013; Leonov et al. 2015; Barardo et al. 2017).

1.5 The Usefulness of C. Elegans to Study Antioxidant and Lifespan Promoting Effects of PSM

C. elegans is an unsegmented small, slender and tubular nematode, consisting of about 1000 cells whose functions have been described in detail (Corsi et al. 2015). The body is characterized by a transparent cuticle, muscles, nervous system, digestive apparatus with pharynx and intestines and reproductive organs. This nematode mostly reproduces as a hermaphrodite, i.e. such a nematode has both female and male sex organs (Meyer 1997; Strange 2006). In the laboratory, mostly hermaphrodite strains are cultivated. *C. elegans* is a short-lived animal with a life-span of 2-4 weeks, thus an optimal model for longevity studies: The development from egg to adult is short and usually completed in three days. After hatching, the larva undergoes four larval stages (L1 to L4) leading to an adult nematode of 1 mm length. Adult nematodes produce about 300 eggs during a fertile period of five days. Thus, *C. elegans* can be easily produced in quantities in a short time. When living conditions become difficult during larval development, L1-larva can stop their development and enter the non-growing "dauer" stage, which can last several months, until conditions improve (Roxo and Wink, 2022).

As mentioned before, *C. elegans* is a versatile model, which can easily be grown under controlled conditions in the laboratory in large numbers. Another advantage: Since the nematodes are simple invertebrates, regulatory issues are much easier than for studies involving vertebrates. The nematodes are usually kept on agar plates with Nematode growth media and fed with *Escherichia coli* OP50, a strain auxotrophic for uracil. *C. elegans* has the advantage that several genetically modified mutants have been developed by chemical or radiation mutagenesis, in addition to RNA interference and CRISP-Cas9 modifications, which allow the study of several diseases and signaling pathways (available from WormBase, an open-access repository for *C. elegans* biology, genetics and genomics). Especially important are strains which allow the investigation of gene expression and the *in vivo* localization of proteins (labeled with fluorescent markers, such as GFP or GLP) (Roxo and Wink, 2022).

The *C. elegans* genome comprises about 100 Mega bases coding for roughly 20,000 protein-coding genes, of which more than 40% have human homologues, among them genes regulating aging and longevity (Markaki and Tavernarakis 2010; Kim et al. 2018). The aging process in *C. elegans* is quite similar to that in vertebrates, as the underlying pathways are evolutionary old and conserved (Figure 3). Also *C. elegans* gets old and dies after 2-4 weeks. The markers and signs of aging (lipofuscin accumulation, decreased rates and coordination of pharyngeal and body movements, mitochondrial dysfunctions, in addition to a degradation of internal organs) can be investigated using a dissecting or fluorescence microscope (Roxo and Wink, 2022).

An important signaling pathway in the context of oxidative stress, temperature stress and aging is the Insulin/IGF-1 pathway (Figure 3). When insulin-like peptides bind to the insulin-like transmembrane receptor DAF-2, the next signal protein AGE-1 and other kinases (among them AKT-1/AKT-2) become phosphorylated (Table 1). Finally, the transcription factors DAF-16 and SKN-1 will be phosphorylated. In their phosphorylated form, both transcription factors cannot enter the nucleus and thus they remain inactive. When *C. elegans* suffers from starvation, oxidative or heat stress via ROS, IIS- signaling is reduced or inhibited. In consequence, the proteins of the signal chain become dephosphorylated and the non-phosphorylated transcription factors DAF-16 and SKN-1 can enter the nucleus and regulate the gene responsible for stress resistance and longevity (Roxo and Wink, 2022).

Table 1. Components of the IIS pathway in C. elegans and respective mammalian/human homologues (from Roxo and Wink 2022)

Gene	Homologue
daf-2	Mammalian insulin and insulin-like growth factor (IGF-1) transmembrane receptor (IGFR)
age-1	Catalytic subunit p110 of the mammalian phosphatidylinositol-3-kinase (PI3K)
pdk-1	Mammalian Akt/PKB kinase PDK1
akt-1/2	Mammalian serine/threonine kinase AKT/PKB
sgk-1	Serum and glucocorticoid inducible kinase SGK
pptr-1	Mammalian PP2A regulatory subunit B56â
daf-16	Human forkhead box-O (FoxO) transcription factors FoxO1, FoxO3 and FoxO4
skn-1	Mammalian nuclear factor erythroid-2-related factor (Nrf)
hsf-1	Human heat shock factor HSF1

DAF-16 is a key transcription factor of the IIS pathway, but also regulates the expression of other genes in the mTOR (mechanistic target of rapamycin) and sirtuin (SIRT) signaling pathways (Lin et al. 2001; Wolff et al. 2006; Robida-Stubbs et al. 2012; Seo et al. 2013; Sen et al. 2020). DAF-16 is responsible for the transcriptional regulation of genes relevant for stress response, including the catalase isoforms CTL-1 and CTL-2 (Murphy et al. 2003), the mitochondrial MnSOD isoform SOD-3 (Barsyte et al. 2001), and the metal-binding protein metallothionein 1 (MTL-1) (Barsyte et al. 2001), Together with HSF-1, DAF-16 is a transcriptional modulator of genes regulating protein turnover, namely *hsp-16.2* coding for the heat shock protein 16.2 (HSP-16.2) (Lee et al. 2003; Landis and Murphy 2010). SKN-1 regulates the transcription of detoxification genes, such as *gst-4* (phase II detoxification enzyme glutathione *S*-transferase 4; GST-4), and of autophagy-related genes (Tullet et al. 2008; Blackwell et al. 2015).

2 ANTIOXIDANT, LIFESPAN-PROMOTING AND NEUROPROTECTIVE EFFECTS: INVESTIGATIONS OF PLANT EXTRACTS AND ISOLATED PSM IN C. ELEGANS

2.1. Assay Systems

The *C. elegans* model has been used during the last 25 years to discover antioxidant and longevity promoting effects of isolated PSM and of plant extracts and the underlying molecular mechanisms (Figure 3). To determine **intracellular ROS levels**, the accumulation of a fluorescent dye H_2DCFDA (2',7'-dichlorofluorescein diacetate) in cells was often determined. After deacetylation in the cell, 2',7'-dichlorofluorescein (DCF) is a target for ROS; when oxidized the fluorescent signal is reduced and can be quantified by fluorescence microscopy (Labuschagne and Brenkman 2013).

Stress resistance can also be determined in so-called **survival assays**, in which the nematodes are pretreated with an extract or PSM and then exposed to oxidative, heat or osmotic stress. After 24 to 72 h post treatment, the number of surviving nematodes is counted. In order to induce oxidative stress, the nematodes are treated with a high concentration of **pro-oxidant compounds**, such paraquat, a commercially available herbicide, hydrogen peroxide (H_2O_2) or tert-butyl hydroperoxide (t-BOOH) or with juglone, a naphthoquinone from walnut tree (*Juglans regia* L.) (Senchuk et al. 2017).

Another simple and low-cost assay can be used to investigate the effect of PSM and of neurodegeneration or stress conditions on longevity: After single or multiple treatment doses, the number of worms is determined over the lifecycle of the nematodes until all worms have died. Results of survival assays are typically illustrated in Kaplan-Meier curves. Several genetically modified *C. elegans* strain can help to elucidate the pathways of a potential lifespan extending effector.

The investigation of the activity and cellular localization of potential protein mediators is facilitated by the use of genetically modified *C. elegans* strains. The respective proteins carry two types of fluorescent reporters (GFP – green fluorescent protein; YFP -yellow fluorescent protein). For transcriptional reporters, a fluorescent reporter is fused to the promotor of the gene of interest. When the promotor is activated, the fluorescent reporter protein is expressed revealing its concentration and cellular localization. The strains CF1553 (Libina et al. 2003), TJ375 (Link et al. 1999) and CL2166 (Link and Johnson 2002), expressing *sod-3p*::GFP, *hsp-16.2p*::GFP and *gst-4p*::GFP, respectively, are typical examples for this experimental approach. In a different strategy, the fluorescent reporter gene is fused in-frame in the gene of interest so that the function of the respective gene is not disturbed. Examples for translational reporters are the strains TJ356 (Henderson and Johnson 2001), LD1 (Leiers et al. 2003) and OG497 (Morton and Lamitina 2013) allowing the intracellular localization of the transcription factors DAF-16::GFP, SKN-1::GFP and HSF-1::GFP in the cytosol or in the nucleus (Roxo and Wink, 2022). The strains CF1038, EU1 and PS3551 are knock-out mutants for the transcription factors DAF-16, SKN-1 and HSF-1 and are often employed in such assays (Roxo and Wink, 2022).

C. elegans has not only been used as a model for antioxidant or lifespan extending compounds, but also for aging related neurodegenerative diseases such as Alzheimer (AD), Huntington (HD) and Parkinsons disease (PD) (Link et al. 2003; Giunti etal. 2021; Hayden et al. 2022; Uphayay et al. 2023; Wang et al. 2024b). Strains used to study these diseases carry genes which may be connected with the corresponding diseases and potential interventions should inhibit or slowing down the expression of the corresponding and their symptoms (Roxo and Wink, 2022).

To study **Alzheimer's disease** (AD), the nematodes are engineered to express amyloid beta (Aβ) in muscles or neuronal cells; it has been assumed that Aβ peptides of 1-42 amino acids in length ($A\beta_{1-42}$) are the most toxic for the development of AD (Franceschi et al. 2018; Lublin and Link 2013; Selkoe and Hardy 2016; Regitz et al. 2016). In the strain CL4176, the human $A\beta_{1-42}$ is expressed in body wall muscles; when Aβ oligomers develop, a loss of motor function can be determined, indicated by progressive paralysis of the nematodes (Link et al. 2003). *C. elegans* strains such as CL2355, express human $A\beta_{1-42}$ in neurons under the control of the synaptobrevin gene (*snb-1*) promotor (Link 2006; Wu et al. 2006). A progressive accumulation of Aβ in the neurons can be investigated by studying chemotaxis and other neuronally affected behaviors (Dosanjh et al. 2010). PSM or extracts which inhibit the aggregation of Aβ can delay the paralysis phenotype and enhance a chemotactic response (Dostal and Link 2010).

Huntington's disease (HD) is apparently caused by the aggregation of huntingtin carrying polyglutamine (polyQ) residues (Brignull et al. 2006). In the transgenic strain AM141 (Morley et al. 2002) a peptide with 40 polyQ repeats is connected to a YFP reporter. The expression is under control of the *unc-54* promotor, which encodes a major myosin heavy chain protein. The *unc-54* promotor helps to localize Q40::YFP in the body wall muscle cells, where it its expression can be investigated by fluorescence microscopy. The number of polyQ aggregates is taken as a measure for the expression of polyQ40::YFP aggregates (Roxo and Wink, 2022).

Parkinsons Disease (PD) is a neurodegenerative disorder caused by a destruction of dopaminergic neurons. When *C. elegans* is treated with N-methyl-4-phenylpyridinium (MPP+) and 6-hydroxydopamine (6-OHDA), the nematodes develop signs of neurotoxicity which appear to be related to those in PD. In strain BZ555 GFP is expressed, so that the number of dopaminergic neurons can be quantified. In addition, the accumulation and aggregation of the small peptide α-synuclein in the substantia nigra has been associated with neurodegeneration. In NL5901, α-synuclein::YFP is overproduced; its expression or its inhibition can be studied by fluorescence microscopy (Roxo and Wink, 2022).

2.2 Effects of PSM and Plant Extracts on Oxidative Stress, Longevity and Neurodegeneration

During the last 25 years, a number of studies have been published which used the different mutant strains of *C. elegans* to study the effect of PSM and plant extracts on resistance to oxidative stress, longevity or age-related neurodegenerative diseases, such as AD, PD and HD (Reviews in Giunti etal. 2021; Hayden et al. 2022; Roxo and Wink, 2022; Zhu et al. 2022; Wink 2022, 2024; Uphayay et al. 2023; Gao et al. 2023; Kirschweger et al. 2023; Song and Zhang 2023; Park 2024; Chen et al. 2024b; Proshkina et al. 2024; Wang et al. 2024b).

The review does not include synthetic drugs or human intervention or cross-disciplinary studies nor clinical research; it also leaves out questions of bioavailability, formulations, regulatory issues and a deep discussion of all pathways, protein targets and molecular mechanisms which have been discussed in the field of aging biology.

Many plant extracts which were found to be active in this context, contain higher concentrations of phenolics and polyphenols. But also other PSM, such as carotenoids, isothiocyanates, terpenoids, saponins, polysaccharides and even the ubiquitous chlorophyll, can exhibit antioxidant, antiaging and neuroprotective properties (Table 2 and 3). The tables are based on our previous revies (Roxo and Wink, 2022; Wink 2022, 2024) and a new literature search in Web of Science which was limited to newer peer-reviewed publications in the time period 2022-2025; for earlier work consult published reviews (Giunti etal. 2021; Hayden et al. 2022; Roxo and Wink, 2022; Zhu et al. 2022; Wink 2022, 2024; Uphayay et al. 2023; Gao et al. 2023; Kirschweger et al. 2023; Song and Zhang 2023; Park 2024; Chen et al. 2024b; Proshkina et al. 2024; Wang et al. 2024b).

Table 2. A selection of plant extracts or isolated PSM with antioxidant and lifespan enhancing properties in C. elegans.(largely extended version of Roxo & Wink 2022; new data mostly from 2022 - 2025)

Plant species (family)	Main PSM	Bioactivity in *C. elegans*	References
Acanthopanax senticosus (Araliaceae)	Polysaccharide CQ-1	- Increased survival during acute oxidative stress - increased expression of *sod-3, cat, daf-16* - Reduction of MDA - Reduced accumulation of lipofuscin - Prolonged lifespan of wild-type worms	Bai et al. 2025
Acer truncatum (Sapindaceae)	Flavonoids	- Reduction of acute oxidative stress - Increase in CAT and Sod - Reduction of ROS and MDA - Reduced accumulation of lipofuscin - Prolonged lifespan	Zhang et al. 2023
Agrimonia procera (Rosaceae)	Phenolic acids, flavonoids, ellagitannins, and procyanidins	- Increased survival during acute oxidative stress in a DAF-16-dependent manner - Reduced ROS levels under thermal stress - Prolonged lifespan of wild-type worms under basal and under thermal stress conditions in a DAF-16-dependent manner.	Saier et al. 2018
Albizia lebbeck (Fabaceae)	Quercetin-3â-D-glucoside, robinetin, vitexin, kaempferol, kuromanin, daidzein, tanshinon I, nootkatone, rutin, and luteolin	- Increased survival during acute oxidative stress - Increase of the expression of *sod-3* - Prolonged lifespan of wild-type worms under basal stress conditions	Phoraksa et al. 2023, 2025
Alnus rugosa (Betulaceae)	Baicalein- 5,6-dimethylether	- Increased survival under acute oxidative stress - Reduced ROS levels under basal stress conditions - Translocation of DAF-16 to the nucleus - Increased expression of *sod-3* - Reduced accumulation of lipofuscin	Ayoub et al. 2024
Alpinia oxyphylla (Zingiberaceae)	6-Gingerol, nootkatone, alpha-cyperone, germacrone	- Decrease of ROS and MDA - Increase of SOD and CAT - Increased survival under acute oxidative stress - Improved pharyngeal pumping and motility - Reduced accumulation of lipofuscin - Translocation od DAF-16 and SKN-1 to the nucleus - Upregulation of *sod-3, gst-4, daf-16,* and *skn-1* genes - Downregulation of *daf-2* and *age-1* genes - Lifespan prolongation, depending on DAF-16 and SKN-1	Xiao et al. 2022

continued on following page

Table 2. Continued

Plant species (family)	Main PSM	Bioactivity in *C. elegans*	References
Anacardium occidentale (Anacardiaceae)	MeOH extract: flavonoid glycosides Hexane extract: palmitic acid, á-linolenic acid, and â-caryophyllene	- Increased survival under acute oxidative stress - Reduced ROS levels under basal stress conditions in a DAF-16- and SKN-1-dependent manner; - Decreased expression of *hsp-16.2* under oxidative stress and increased expression of *gst-4* and of *sod-3* - Translocation of DAF-16 to the nucleus - Reduced accumulation of lipofuscin and improved pharyngeal pumping rate - Lifespan elongation of wild-type worms but not of *mev-1* mutants	Duangjan et al. 2019a
Anoectochilus roxburghii (Orchidaceae)	Kinsenoside	- Increased survival under acute oxidative stress - Reduced ROS levels under basal stress conditions - Increased the expression of *sod-3, sir-2.1, hsp-16.2, cat, sek-1, skn-1, hsf-1,* and *gst-4* -Translocation of SKN-1 and HSF-1 to the nucleus - SKN-1 and HSF-1 main signaling pathway - Lifespan elongation of wild-type worms but not in DAF-16, SKN-1 and HSF-1 mutants - Reduced accumulation of lipofuscin and improved pharyngeal pumping rate	Yuan et al. 2025
Aronia melanocarpa (Rosaceae)	Anthocyanins, proanthocyanins, chlorogenic acid, quercetin derivatives, polysaccharides	- Enhancement of resistance to oxidative stress - Reduction of ROS level - Increase of pharyngeal pumping - Reduction of lipofuscin accumulation - Increase of SOD and CAT - Increase of lifepan via PMK-1 pathway	Zhang et al. 2024a
Artemisia argyi (Asteraceae)	Flavonoids: kaempferol, L-epicatechin, apigenin, catechin, quercetin, luteolin, formononetin, and naringenin;	- Increased survival under acute oxidative stress - Translocation of DAF-16 to the nucleus - Increased expression of *sod-3, hsp-16.2, daf-16* - Reduced accumulation of lipofuscin and improved pharyngeal pumping rate - Lifespan elongation of wild-type worms -not in daf-2 (e1370), age-1(hx546), sgk-1 (ok538), daf-16 (mu86), skn-1 (zu67) hsf-1 (sy441) mutants	Wang et al. 2024a

continued on following page

Table 2. Continued

Plant species (family)	Main PSM	Bioactivity in *C. elegans*	References
Artemisia selengensis (Asteraceae)	Caffeoylquinic acids	- Reduction of ROS - Increased survival under acute oxidative stress - Improved pharyngeal pumping and motility - Reduction of lipofuscin accumulation - Upregulation of *sod-3, ctl-1, hsp-16.2, hsp-12.3, skn-1, gst-4* and *gcs-1* genes - Activation of DAF-16 and SKN-1 by SIR-2.1 signaling and and mitochondrial dysfunction pathways, - Life span elongation	Li et al. 2022a
Aspalathus linearis; (Fabaceae)	Aspalathin (dihydrochalcone), isoorientin, orientin, nothofagin, quercetin-3-O-robinobioside	Aspalathin and leaf extract: - Increased survival to acute oxidative stress - Reduced ROS levels under normal conditions - Decreased the expression of *hsp-16.2* under mild oxidative stress - Extend the life span under glucose-induced oxidative stress	Chen et al. 2013a
Brassica chinensis **&** other Brassicaceae	Sulphoraphane (isothiocyanate)	- Increased survival under acute oxidative stress - Reduced ROS levels under basal stress conditions in a DAF-16-dependent manner - Increased the expression of *sod-3, mlt-1* and *gst-4* - Translocation of DAF-16 to the nucleus - DAF-16-dependent lifespan elongation of wild-type worms - Reduced accumulation of lipofuscin and improved pharyngeal pumping rate	Qi et al. 2021
Caesalpinia mimosoides (Fabaceae)	3-O-methylgallate, 4-aminomethylindole, emmotin A, theogallin and gallic acid	- Increased survival against acute oxidative stress - Reduction of ROS levels under basal stress conditions in a DAF-16-dependent manner; - Increased expression of *sod-3* under basal conditions and decreased expression of *hsp-16.2* under mild oxidative stress - Nuclear translocation of DAF-16 - Slightly prolonged the lifespan of wild-type worms - Reduced the accumulation of lipofuscin	Rangsinth et al. 2019
Calycophyllum spruceanum ((Rubiaceae)	Gardenoside, 5-hydroxymorin, cyanidin, taxifolin, and 5-hydroxy-6-methoxycoumarin-7-glucoside.	- Increased survival under oxidative stress; DAF-16 dependent - Reduced ROS levels under basal stress conditions - Decreased expression of *hsp-16.2* and increased expression of *sod-3* - DAF-16- dependent longevity increase - Improved pharyngeal pumping rate	Peixoto et al. 2018

continued on following page

Table 2. Continued

Plant species (family)	**Main PSM**	**Bioactivity in *C. elegans***	**References**
Camelia sinensis (Theaceae)	Catechins (catechin, epicatechin, gallocatechin, epigallocatechin, epicatechin gallate, epigallocatechin gallate); Oolonghomobisflavan A andoolonghomobisflavan B; theanine	- Increased survival under oxidative stress - Reduced ROS levels under basal stress conditions in a DAF-16-dependent manner - Decreased the expression of *hsp-16.2* and *gst-4* under mild oxidative stress - Nuclear translocation of DAF-16 - Reduction of lipofuscin accumulation - Prolonged lifespan of wild-type worms in N2 and *fem-1(hc17)* strains, **Theanine:** - Correction of mtDNA damage from UVC damage - Upregulation of *bec-1* (autophagy), *dct-1* (mitophagy), and *hsp-60* - Lifespan elongation by activating autophagy, mitophagy, and UPRmt	Abbas and Wink 2009, 2010, 2014; Zhang et al. 2020, 2022, Chen et al. 2024a
Campomanesia adamantium (Myrtaceae)	Ellagic acid and derivatives, procyanidins, flavonoids (quercetin derivatives), antioxidant lipophilic pigments and ascorbic acid	- Increased survival under acute oxidative and thermal stress - Improved mobility - Upregulation of SOD-3 and GST-4 -Translocation of DAF-16 to the nucleus -Increased lifespan	de Araújo et al. 2023
Canna coccinea (Cannaceae)	Rosmarinic acid, caffeic acid, isorhamnetin	- Increased survival under oxidative stress - Reduced ROS levels under basal stress conditions	Spotorno et al. 2025
Carlina acaulis (Asteraceae)	Polyacetylene: Carlina oxide, root extract: curcumene	- Increased survival to acute oxidative stress - Decreased expression of *hsp-16.2* - Nuclear localization of DAF-16	Link et al. 2016
Capsicum annuum (Solanaceae)	Capsaicin glucoside, dihydro-capsaicin glucoside	- Reduction of ROS - Protection against acute oxidative and heat stress - Upregulation of *daf-16*, *skn-1* and related downstream t genes (*sod-3, hsp-16.2, gst-4* and *gcs-1*) - Improved pharyngeal pumping and chemotaxis	Elkhedir et al. 2022

continued on following page

Table 2. Continued

Plant species (family)	Main PSM	Bioactivity in *C. elegans*	References
Caryocar villosum (Caryocaraceae)	Phenolic acids (gallic acid, ellagic acid), hydrolysable tannins and triterpenoid saponins (caryocarosides)	- Increased survival under acute oxidative stress - Reduction of ROS levels under basal conditions, independently of DAF-16, SKN-1 and HSP-16.2 - Increased expression of *sod-3* under both basal and oxidative stress conditions. - Decreased expression of *gst-4* and *hsp-16.2* under mild oxidative stress - Nuclear translocation of DAF-16 - DAF-16- and SKN-1-dependent longevity	Roxo et al. 2020
Cassia abbreviata (Fabaceae)	Proanthocyanidins	- Increased survival to acute oxidative stress - Reduced ROS levels under basal stress; - Decreased the expression of *hsp-16.2* under mild oxidative stress - Nuclear translocation of DAF-16.	Sobeh et al. 2018
Cassia fistula (Fabaceae)	Flavonols (quercetin derivatives, kaempferol glycosides), anthraquinones (emodin, rhein) and procyanidin derivatives	- Increased survival to acute oxidative stress - Reduced ROS levels under basal stress - Increase of expression of *sod-3* under basal conditions, and decrease of *hsp-16.2* and *gst-4* gene expression under mild oxidative stress - Nuclear localization of DAF-16	Thabit et al. 2018
Cirsium japonicum (Asteraceae)	Chlorogenic acid, linarin, pectolinarin, silychristin, silydianin, and taxifolin	- Reduced ROS levels - Increased survival under acute oxidative stress - DAF-16 and SKN-1 dependent increase of lifespan	Cho et al. 2023; Yen et al. 2023
***Citrus* species** (Rutaceae)	Hesperitin (flavonoid)	- Decreased ROS accumulation - Increased survival under acute oxidative stress - Increase of body bending and pharyngeal pumping frequency, - Upregulation of *daf-18*, *daf-16*, *gst-2*, *gst-3*, *gst-4*, *gst-39*, *hsp-16.11*, *sip-1*, *clpp-1*, and *dve-1* in stressed *C. elegans* - Downregulation of *ist-1* and *kgb-1* in stressed *C. elegans.* - Prolongation of lifespan - Involvement of IIS, HSP, mtUPR, and JNK pathways.	Wang et al. 2024b

continued on following page

Table 2. Continued

Plant species (family)	Main PSM	Bioactivity in *C. elegans*	References
Clerodendrum speciosum, C. spicatus (Lamiaceae)	Phenolic acids and derivatives; tiliroside, rhamnazin-3*O*-rutinoside, quercetin methyl galloyl-hexoside, acacetin trioside, rhamnazin-3-*O*-rutinoside; rosmarinic acid	- Increased survival to acute oxidative stress - Reduced ROS levels under basal stress - Upregulation of SOD and CAT - Nuclear localization of DAF-16 - Reduction of lipofuscin accumulation - Reduction of fat accumulation - Improvement of pharyngeal pumping and motility - Increase of lifespan - Involvement of DAF-16, HSF-1 and NHR-49 pathways	Youssef et al. 2022; Xiao et al. 2024
Coffea arabica (Rubiaceae)	Chlorogenic acid	- Lifespan extension - Importance of DAF-16a, *ddb-1* and SKN-1	Siswanto et al. 2022
Crataegus pinnatifida and related species (Rosaceae)	Vitexin, isovitexin	- Increased survival to acute oxidative and heat stress - Reduction of ROS and MDA level - Reduction of lipofuscin - Improved motility and pumping activity - Upregulation of *sod-1, gst-4, gcs-1, hsp-16.1* - DAF-16 and SKN-1 activation and nuclear translocation - Increase of longevity depending on *daf-2, age-1, akt-1, daf-16, skn-1,* and *hsf-1* but not *eat-2*	Wang et al. 2022a; Tao et al. 2023
Curcuma longa (Zingiberaceae)	Curcumin	- Model for obesity treatment - Improved chemotaxis and movement - SKN-1 dependent suppression of glucose-associated lipid accumulation - Increased expression of *skn-1, sod-3, sod-1, sod-2, sod-3, gst-4* - Down-regulation of MAPK signaling pathway-related genes *(sek-1, pmk-1, nsy-1).* - Improved resistance to heat and oxidative stress - Nuclear translocation of SKN-1 - Increase of longevity (N2)	Xu et al. 2023; Savova et al. 2024
Daucus carota (Apiaceae)	Polyacetylenes: isofalcarinol	- Improved motility and oxidative stress resistance - AMPK activation - Enhanced mitochondrial biogenesis - Increased ATP production - Extension of lifespan	Thomas et al. 2023

continued on following page

Table 2. Continued

Plant species (family)	Main PSM	Bioactivity in *C. elegans*	References
Endopleura uchi (Humiriaceae)	Bergenin (polyphenol)	- Increased survival to acute oxidative stress - Reduced ROS levels under basal stress - Increased expression of *sod-3* under basal conditions, and decreased expression of *hsp-16.2* under mild oxidative stress - DAF-16-dependent longevity - Improved pharyngeal pumping rate	Peixoto et al. 2019b
***Epimedium* spec.** (Berberidaceae)	Flavonoids: Icariin	- Improved resistance to heat and oxidative stress (DAF-2 dependent) - Reduction of lipid accumulation - DAF-2 dependent increase in motility and chemotaxis - Nuclear translocation of DAF-16. - Upregulation of *daf-2*, *daf-16*, *sir-2.4*, *sir-2.1*, *skn-1*, *hsf-1*, *jnk-1* and *mtl-1* - Extension of lifespan via modulation of the DAF-2 pathway	Todorova et al. 2024
Euclea divinorum (Ebenaceae)	Catechins, gallocatechins, myricetin, polyphenols, tannins, saponins, sterols, terpenoids, and triterpenoids	- Increased survival to acute oxidative stress	Bogari et al. 2022
Eucommia ulmoides (Eucommiaceae)	Iridoid glucosides: aucubin, geniposide, geniposidic acid, and asperuloside	- Nuclear translocation of DAF-16 - Improved pharyngeal pumping, mobility, muscle morphology - Reduction of lipofuscin accumulation - Improved resistance to oxidative and heat stress - Activation of LGG-1 and SOD3 - Stimulation of mitochondrial fission and mitophagy - Transcriptional regulation of *daf-16, drp-1, eat-3, lgg-1,* and *dct-1* -Enhanced DAF-16 dependent longevity	Chen et al. 2023a
***Eugenia uniflora* L.** (Myrtaceae)	Anthocyanins (cyanidin 3-O-glucoside, delphinidin 3-O-glucoside) and flavonols (myricetin and quercetin derivatives)	- Increased survival to acute oxidative and heat stress - Reduced ROS and protein carbonyl levels - Increased the expression of *sod-3* and reduction of *hsp-16.2* - Nuclear translocation of DAF-16. - DAF-16-dependent longevity	Tambara et al. 2018

continued on following page

Table 2. Continued

Plant species (family)	Main PSM	Bioactivity in *C. elegans*	References
Euterpe precatoria (Arecaceae)	Anthocyanins (cyanidin-3-rutinoside, cyanidin-3-glucoside and peonidin-3-rutinoside)	- Increased survival under oxidative stress in a DAF-16-dependent manner - Reduced ROS and protein carbonyl levels under basal stress - Increased expression of *sod-3* under basal conditions, and decreased expression of *hsp-16.2* under mild oxidative stress - Nuclear translocation of DAF-16 - Reduced the accumulation of lipofuscin and improved pharyngeal pumping rate	Peixoto et al. 2016 a,b
Fragaria × ananassa (Rosaceae)	Anthocyanins: Pelargonidin-3-glucoside (Pg3G)	- Pg3G counteracts negative effects of oleic acid on learning, chemotaxis and behavior - Reduced ROS levels under basal conditions - Increased expression of *sod-3, hsp5, hsp-6* under basal conditions - Upregulation of *gab-1, ace-1, dop-1, mod-1*, and *eat-4* - Role of UPRmt in reducing OA-induced neurotoxicity by Pg3G	Han et al. 2025
Gardenia jasminoides (Rubiaceae)	Iridoid glucosides: Geniposide	- Inhibition of IIS and activation of SKN-1 pathway - Improvement of pharyngeal pumping, muscle quality, and motility - Reduction of lipofuscin content - Reduction of ROS accumulation - Nuclear translocation of SKN-1 - Increased the life span -Neuroprotective effect against â1–42 toxicity in GRU102	Choi et al. 2023
Glochidion zeylanicum (Phyllanthaceae)	Gallic acid and catechins	- Increased survival to oxidative stress in a DAF-16 and SKN-1 dependent manner - Reduced ROS levels under basal conditions - Increased expression of *sod-3* under basal conditions - Increased expression of *gst-4* and decreased expression of *hsp-16.2* under mild oxidative stress - Nuclear translocation of DAF-16 and SKN-1 - Reduced the accumulation of lipofuscin and improved pharyngeal pumping rate - Lifespan increase of wild-type worms	Duangjan et al. 2019, 2021

continued on following page

Table 2. Continued

Plant species (family)	Main PSM	Bioactivity in *C. elegans*	References
Glycyrrhiza glabra; G. uralensis (Fabaceae)	Isoliquiritigenin, liquiritigenin, glycyrrhizic acid, and glycyrrhetinic acid	- Increased survival to acute oxidative stress - Reduced ROS levels under basal stress - Decreased the expression of *hsp-16.2* under mild oxidative stress - Nuclear translocation of DAF-16 and SKN-1	Link et al. 2015; Link and Wink, 2019; Chen et al. 2023b
Hibiscus sabdariffa (Malvaceae)	Anthocyanins (delphinidin-3-sambubioside and cyanidin-3-sambubioside) and flavonoids	- Induced nuclear localization of DAF-16 and SKN-1 - Prevention of age-related decline of locomotion - Reduced accumulation of lipofuscin - Prolongation of lifespan of wild-type worms in a DAF-16- and SKN-1-dependent manner	Koch et al. 2020
Hippophae rhamnoides	Flavonol glycosides (Isorhamnetin glycosides, quercetin glycosides and kaempferol glycosides)	- Increased survival under oxidative and heat stress - Reduction of ROS and MDA - Stimulation of SOD and CAT expression - Involvement of DAF-16, and HSF-1 pathways - Upregulation of *sod-3*, *ctl-1*, *hsp16.2*, and *hsp12.6* - Lifespan extension AD - Inhibition of AChE and MAO-A in CL4176 - Delay of paralysis	Wang et al. 2022b; Zhao et al. 2024a
Houttuynia cordata (Saururaceae)	Flavonoids: quercitrin, kaempferol; cyanidins	- Increased survival under oxidative and heat stress - Reduction of ROS - Increased the activity of CAT, SOD-3, SIR-2 - Nuclear translocation of DAF-16 - Reduced accumulation of lipofuscin - Lifespan elongation of wild-type worms	Kim et al. 2024
Ilex paraguariensis (Aquifoliaceae)	Polyphenols and methylxanthines	- Increased survival under oxidative stress - Reduced ROS levels - Nuclear translocation of DAF-16 - Lifespan elongation of wild-type worms.	Lima et al. 2014
Lonicera japonica (Caprifoliaceae)	Polysaccharides	- Increased motility and pharyngeal pumping - Reduction of lipofuscin accumulation - Increased survival under oxidative and stress - Upregulation of *daf-16, sod-3*, *gst-4* and *hsp-16.2* genes - Translocation of DAF-16 to the nucleus - DAF-16 dependent prolongation of lifespan	Zhu et al. 2023

continued on following page

Table 2. Continued

Plant species (family)	Main PSM	Bioactivity in *C. elegans*	References
Lycium ruthenicum, Lycium barbarum (Solanaceae)	Flavonoids: rutin, chlorogenic acid, and kaempferol; anthocyanins: petunidin-3-*O*-glucoside	- Reduction of ROS and MDA - Increased the activity of CAT and SOD - Involvement of JNK-1, SKN-1 and DAF-16 pathways - Reduced accumulation of lipofuscin - Upregulation of *daf-16, dod-3, ama-1, sod-2, gcs-1* and *skn-1* g - Prolongation of the mean lifespan - Improved locomotion, pharyngeal pumping rate and stress resistance	Niu et al. 2022; Zhang et al. 2024b; Xu et al. 2025a
Momordica charantia (Cucurbitaceae)	Saponins: Cucurbitacins	- Improved motility and muscle morphology - ROS reduction - Activation of SOD and CAT - Lifespan prolongation in N2 and CL2006 (AD model) - Upregulation of *akt-1*, *cat-1*, *hsf-1*, *sir-2.1*, *hlh-30*, and *lgg-1*,genes - Downregulation of *age-1* gene - Involvement of IIS pathway with *sir-2.1* and *hlh-30*	Zhang et al. 2022b
Moringa oleifera (Moringaceae)	Glucosinolates, isothiocyanates (moringin)	- Upregulation of *gst-4, sod-1, skn-1* expression and other glutathione-related genes - Translocation of SKN-1 to nucleus - Increase of life span via SKN-1 pathway	Farias-Pereira et al. 2024
Olea europaea (Oleaceae)	Polyphenols	- Increased survival to heat stress - Reduced ROS and MDA levels under heat stress - Reduced expression of *hsp-16.2* under stress - Increased the activity of CAT, GSH-Px and SOD - Nuclear translocation of DAF-16	Luo et al. 2019
Oryza sativa (Poaceae)	Anthocyanins	- Enhanced resistance to acute oxidative stress - Reduction of lipofuscin accumulation - Down regulation of *age-1* and *daf-2*, - Upregulation of *sir-2.1*, *ctl-1*, *ctl-2*, *gst-4* and *sod-3* and *daf-16* - Nuclear translocation of DAF-16 - Activation of SOD-3, CAT, and GST-4 - Reduction of ROS, and MDA accumulation - Extension of lifespan HD: Reduction of polyQ40 aggregation in AM141, AD: reduction of paralysis in CL4176 - Improved chemotaxis t in CL2355	Li et al. 2023

continued on following page

Table 2. Continued

Plant species (family)	Main PSM	Bioactivity in *C. elegans*	References
Paeonia suffruticosa (Paeoniaceae)	Polyphenols: paeonol	-Improvement of motility, pharyngeal pumping and body size - Increased survival to heat and oxidative stress - SOD expression and GSH content - Upregulation of *sod-2, sod3, daf-16, skn-1, gst-4, hsp-16.2* and *ctl-1* genes - Nuclear translocation of DAF-16 and SKN-1 - Reduction of lipofuscin accumulation - Participation of DAF-16, SKN-1, and HSF-1 - Lifespan prolongation	Li et al. 2024a
Paullinia cupana (Sapindaceae)	Methylxanthines (caffeine, theobromine and theophylline), polyphenols (catechins and epicatechin)	- Increased survival to heat and oxidative stress in a DAF-16-dependent manner - Reduced accumulation of ROS in wild-type and Aâ-expressing worms; - Increased expression of *sod-3* under basal stress conditions, and decreased expression of *hsp-16.2* both under basal and mild oxidative stress - Lifespan prolongation of wild-type worms - Improved mobility and pharyngeal pumping rate; - Increased proteasomal and lysosomal degradation. **Caffeine and methylxanthines:** - Increased survival under oxidative stress - Translocation of DAF-16 and SKN-1 - Upregulation of sod-3, gst-4, gcs-1p; and downregulation of hsp-16.2p under oxidative stress - Lifespan prolongation of wild-type worms, independent of DAF-16 and SKN-1	Boasquivis et al. 2018, Peixoto et al. 2017; Li et al. 2019
Pelargonium sidoides (Geraniaceae)	Oxygenated coumarins, various phenolics and polyphenols EPs7630®	- Increased survival to oxidative stress - Decreased the expression of *hsp-16.2* under mild oxidative stress - Nuclear translocation of DAF-16.	Rezaizadehnajafi and Wink, 2014

continued on following page

Table 2. Continued

Plant species (family)	Main PSM	Bioactivity in *C. elegans*	References
Phyllanthus emblica (Phyllanthaceae)	Coniferaldehyde	- Increased survival under oxidative stress - Reduced ROS levels under basal stress - Increased expression of *aak-2, skn-, gst-4* and *par-4* gene but not *daf-16* - Nuclear translocation of SKN-1 -Improved pharyngeal pumping rate and mobility - Activation of PAR-4/LKB-1-AAK-2/AMPK-SKN-1/NRF-2 pathway and induction of autophagy - Reduced accumulation of lipofuscin - Lifespan prolongation of wild-type worms	Ramatchandirane et al. 2024
Pogostemon cablin (Lamiaceae)	Essential oil: Patchouli alcohol (a sesquiterpene)	- Improved survival under acute oxidative stress and motility - Reduction of spawning, lipid accumulation and ROS levels - Nuclear translocation of DAF-16 - Increase of *jnk-1, jkk-1, ist-1, pha-4, sod-3, lipl-4, mtl-1, kgb-2, hsp-16.2* and *fat-6* expression - Reduction of lipofuscin accumulation - Prolongation of lifespan and health span via JNK-1/DAF-16 signaling pathway - Amelioration of senescence	Xu et al. 2024b
Prunus avium (Rosaceae)	Anthocyanins: Cyanidin-3-*O*-glucoside; Cyanidin-3-*O*-rutinioside	- Increased survival rate under heat stress	Filaferro et al. 2022
Punica granatum and many other plants (Lythraceae)	Pentagalloyl glucose (gallotannin)	- Reduction of ROS in normal and high-fat nematodes - Increase of antioxidant enzymes - Regulation of decrease of fat accumulation via SKN-1 pathway - Upregulation of *mdt-15, pod-2, elo-2, fat-6,* and *fat-7* genes - Down-regulation of *fat-5, acs-2, vit-2* and *lipl-4*	Luo et al. 2024
Rehmannia glutinosa (Orobanchaceae)	Oligosaccharides (stachyose raffinose, melibiose, mannotriose); catalpol (iridoid glucoside)	- Enhancement of antioxidant enzyme system (SOD, CAT, GSH-Px) - Reduction of lipofuscin accumulation - Reduction of ROS under normal conditions and oxidative stress - Upregulation of *daf-16, skn-1, age-1,* and their downstream genes, *sod-3*, and *gcs-1* - Down-regulation of *age-1* expression - Prolongation of lifespan - Effects on microbiome and metabolome	Liang et al. 2023

continued on following page

Table 2. Continued

Plant species (family)	Main PSM	Bioactivity in *C. elegans*	References
***Salvia rosmarinus* (syn. *Rosmarinus officinalis*)** (Lamiaceae)	Flavonoids (quercetin, rutin and kaempferol) and phenolic acids (chlorogenic, caffeic, rosmarinic and carnosic acids)	- Increased survival under oxidative and heat stress in a DAF-16-, HSF-1- and SKN-1-dependent manner; - Decreased the levels of ROS under oxidative stress independently of DAF-16, HSF-1 and SKN-1 - Prolonged lifespan in a HSF-1- and SKN-1-dependent manner	Zamberlan et al. 2016
Schotia brachypetala (Fabaceae)	Flavonoid glycosides, procyanidins, anthocyanins, dihydrochalcones, and hydroxy benzoic acid derivatives	- Increased survival to oxidative stress - Reduced ROS levels under basal stress - Decreased the expression of *hsp-16.2* under mild oxidative stress - Nuclear translocation of DAF-16	Sobeh et al. 2016
Scutellaria baicalensis (Lamiaceae)	Flavonoids. baicalin	- Downregulation of Wnt ligands *mom-2* and *cwn-2* - Upregulation of ELT-3 and antiaging gene Klotho (*C50F7.10* and *E02H9.5)* - Reduction of acute oxidative stress via SKN-1 and DAF-16 - DAF16 dependent reduction of lipofuscin and ROS - DAF-16 translocation to nucleus - Improved pharyngeal pumping and motility - Lifespan elongation via ELT-3 and SKN-1	Mohanti et al. 2023
Sideritis scardica (Lamiaceae)	Caffeoylquinic acids, acteoside, and flavonoids	- Increased survival under heat stress independent of DAF-16; - Increased the expression of *hsp-16.2* under heat stress - Prolonged lifespan of wild-type worms	Heiner et al. 2018; Nishioka et al. 2020
Spinacea oleracea (Amaranthaceae)	Chlorophyll	- Increased survival to acute oxidative stress - Upregulation of sod-3, and downregulation of hsp-16.2 under oxidative stress - HSP-16 translocation to nucleus - Improved pharyngeal pumping rate - Extension of lifespan in wildtype nematode	Wang and Wink 2016
Styphnolobium japonicum (Fabaceae)	Fruit extract: Phenolic acids, flavonoids, flavan-3-ols, and proanthocyanidins	- Increased survival to acute oxidative stress - Reduced ROS levels under basal stress - Increased expression of *sod-3* under basal conditions, and decreased expression of *gst-4* and *hsp-16.2* under mild oxidative stress - Translocation of DAF-16 and SKN-1 into nucleus	Thabit et al. 2023

continued on following page

Table 2. Continued

Plant species (family)	Main PSM	Bioactivity in *C. elegans*	References
Syzygium nervosum (syn. *Cleistocalyx nervosum* var. *paniala*) (Myrtaceae)	Anthocyanins	- Reduced the levels of ROS under UV-A-induced oxidative stress - Increase of SOD activity - Upregulation of the expression of *daf-16*, *skn-1* and *sir-2.1*, and down-regulation of the expression of *daf-2*, *age-1*, and *utx-1* - Prolonged lifespan independently of DAF-16 - Reduced the accumulation of lipofuscin	Pransanth et al. 2019
Thesium chinense (Santalaceae)	Astragalin (isoflavone)	- ROS reduction - Upregulating of *daf-16* through inhibition of *daf-2* - Activation of AMPK and MAPK pathways - Upregulation of *sir-2.1*, *sir-2.4*, *aak-2*, *daf-16*, *sod-3*, and *skn-1* - Extension of lifespan	Wang et al. 2024c
Terminalia catappa (Combretaceae)	Flavonoids and phenolics: gallic acid, orientin, vitexin, ellagic acid, arjungenin, arjunolic acid, betulinic acid.	- Increased survival to acute oxidative stress - Reduction of lipid and ROS accumulation under normal conditions and 2% glucose treatment, dependent on DAF-16 and SKN-1 - Prolongation of lifespan under normal conditions and 2% glucose treatment depending on DAF-16, SKN-1 and ATGL-1 - Regulation by aak-1 pathway	Kim et al. 2023
Triticum aestivum (Poaceae)	Purple wheat: Anthocyanins (cyanidin-3-glucoside, peonidin-3-glucoside and malvidin-3-galactoside)	- Reduced the levels of ROS under basal conditions - Decreased the expression of *hsp-16.2* under mild oxidative stress - Translocation of DAF-16 to the nucleus - Prolonged lifespan of wild-type and *mev-1* mutants in a DAF-16- dependent manner.	Chen et al. 2013c
Uncaria tomentosa (Rubiaceae)	Oxoindole alkaloids: Mitraphylline, isomitraphylline; organic acids, proanthocyanidins, sterols, and triterpenes	- A leaf extract (not the alkaloids) reduced ROS levels under normal conditions independent on DAF-16 but depending on SKN-1 - Increased survival under oxidative stress - Expression of *sod-3*, *gst-4*, and *hsp-16.2* under oxidative stress	Azevedo et al. 2019
Vaccinium vitis-idaea (Ericaceae)	Anthocyanins and other flavonoids	- Induced nuclear translocation of DAF-16 and HSF-1 - Extended lifespan in DAF-16-dependent manner; - Improved mechanosensation and axon branching in posterior touch receptor neurons in a DAF-16 dependent manner	Scerbak et al. 2018

continued on following page

Table 2. Continued

Plant species (family)	Main PSM	Bioactivity in *C. elegans*	References
Vitis vinifera (Vitaceae)	Resveratrol; leaf extract: flavonoids, catechins, gallic acid	**Resveratrol:** - Increased survival under oxidative stress - Reduced ROS levels under basal stress -Decreased the expression of *hsp-16.2* under mild oxidative stress - Extension of life span under glucose-induced oxidative stress but not under normal conditions **Leaf extract:** - Increased survival under oxidative stress - Reduced ROS levels under basal stress - Translocation of DAF-16 to the nucleus - Upregulation of the expression of stress-response genes *gst-4* and *sod-3* and downregulation of the expression of *hsp-16.2* - Reduced accumulation of lipofuscin but no lifespan extension under normal conditions (resveratrol)	Chen et al. 2013b; Duangjan et al. 2021
Warburgia salutaris (Canellaceae)	Catechin, 11á-hydroxy muzigadiolide, mukaadial, pereniporin B, and 11á-hydroxycinnamosmolide	- Increased survival under oxidative stress - Reduced ROS levels under basal stress - Decreased the expression of *hsp-16.2* under oxidative stress - Translocation of DAF-16 to the nucleus	Abdelfatta et al 2022
Ximenia americana* var. *caffra (Oleaceae)	Condensed tannins, flavonol glycosides, flavone glycosides, and flavonol diglycosides.	- Increased survival under oxidative stress - Reduced ROS levels under basal stress - Decreased the expression of *hsp-16.2* under mild oxidative stress - Translocation of DAF-16 to the nucleus	Bakrim et al. 2022
Ziziphus jujuba (Rhamnaceae)	Polysaccharides, zizybeoside I and II, rutin, saponins, oleanonic acid, and ursolic acid	- Increase of body length and width, head thrashes, body bends, and brood size - Increase of pharyngeal pumping - Reduction of ROS - Resistance to oxidative and heat stress - Increase of SOD-3, CAT, and GSH. - Nuclear translocation of DAF-16 - Upregulation of *daf-16*, *skn-1*, *sod-3*, and *gcs-1* expression - Reduced lipofuscin accumulation - Prolonged lifespan of wild-type via DAF-16 and SKN-1	Han et al. 2024; Zhang et al. 2024b

Table 3. Plant extracts with neuroprotective properties in C. elegans. (extended version of Roxo & Wink 2022; new data mostly from 2022-2025) Abbreviations: AD = Alzheimer Model; PD = Parkinson Model, HD = Huntington Model

Plant species Type of extract	Main PSM	Bioactivity in *C. elegans*	References
Acanthopanax senticosus (Araliaceae)	Hyperoside	**AD** - Reduction of ROS level in CL4176 - Delayed Aâ-induced paralysis in CL4176	Wang et al. 2023a
Alnus rugosa ((Betulaceae)	Baicalein- 5,6-dimethylether	**AD** - Delayed Aâ-induced paralysis in CL4176 **HD** - Reduced the number of polyQ40 aggregates in AM141	Ayoub et al. 2024
Anoectochilus roxburghii (Orchidaceae)	Kinsenoside	**AD** - Delay of the progression of temperature-mediated paralysis in CL4176 - Improved chemotaxis	Yuan et al. 2025
Astragalus membranaceus (Fabaceae)	Formononetin	**PD** PD models NL5901 and BZ555 strains - Mitigation of dopaminergic neuron degeneration - Amelioration of dyskinesia - Reduction of ROS - Reduced alpha-synuclein formation - Upregulation of *gst-4, gcs-1, sod-3,* and *daf-16* under MPP(+) treatment	Wang et al. 2024c
Bacopa monnieri (Plantaginaceae)	Flavonoids, triterpene saponins, bacoside	- Reduction of ROS in N2 - Reduces juglone induced hsp-16 expression **AD** - Reduction of the number of Aâ aggregates - Delayed Aâ-induced paralysis in CL4176 -Improved chemotaxis **PD** - Reduced alpha-synuclein formation - Reduction of 6-OHDA induced neurotoxicity in BZ555 **HD** - Reduced the number of polyQ40 aggregates - Reduction of polyQ mediated neurotoxicity	Heiner 2017
Beta vulgaris (Ammaranthaceae)	Betalains: betanin and isobetanin	**AD** - Reduction of Aâ-deposits and aggregate formation (A*â*40 and A*â*42) - Delayed Aâ-induced paralysis in CL2006	Imamura et al. 2022

continued on following page

Table 3. Continued

Plant species **Type of extract**	**Main PSM**	**Bioactivity in *C. elegans***	**References**
Caesalpinia bonduc (Fabaceae)	Diterpenes: Caesalmin C	**AD** - Delayed Aâ-induced paralysis in CL4176 depending on DAF-16, but not of SKN-1 or HSF-1 - Reduction of Aâ-deposits and aggregate formation - Upregulation of *sod-3*, *gst-4*, and *rpt-3* genes and proteasome activity - Down-regulation of *ace-1* - Inhibition of AchE	Zhang et al. 2022b
Camelia sinensis (Theaceae)	Catechins (catechin, epicatechin, gallocatechin, epigallocatechin, epicatechin gallate, epigallocatechin gallate); Oolonghomobisflavan A and oolonghomobisflavan B	**AD** - EGCG reduced Aâ-deposits and aggregate formation in CL2006 - Delayed Aâ-induced paralysis in CL4176 - Improved chemotaxis in CL2122 and CL2355 **HD** - Reduced the number of polyQ40 aggregates	Abbas and Wink 2010; Zhang et al. 2020
Canna coccinea (Cannaceae)	Rosmarinic acid, caffeic acid, isorhamnetin	**PD** - Reduced alpha-synuclein formation	Spotorno et al. 2025
Cannabis sativa (Cannabaceae)	Cannabidiol	**AD** - Reduction of A*â* aggregation - Delayed Aâ-induced paralysis and improved motility and pumping - Phenolic OH group of CBD is important for activity **PD** - Reduction of DA neuron damage and ROS induced by 6-OHDA - Improving food-sensing behavior in BZ555 - Reduction of á-Syn aggregate formation - Lifespan extension - Stimulation of ubiquitin-like proteasomes	Muhammad et al. 2022; Zhang et al. 2022c
Carlina acaulis (Asterceae)	Carlina oxide, root extract: curcumene	**AD** - Delayed Aâ-induced paralysis	Link et al. 2016
Cassia fistula (Fabaceae)	Flavonols (quercetin derivatives, kaempferol glycosides), anthraquinones (emodin, rhein) and procyanidin derivatives	**AD** - Delayed Aâ-induced paralysis; **HD** - Reduced the number of polyQ40 aggregates.	Thabit et al. 2018

continued on following page

Table 3. Continued

Plant species Type of extract	Main PSM	Bioactivity in *C. elegans*	References
***Citrus* species** (Rutaceae)	Seed extract with flavonoids; limonin, hesperitin (flavonoid)	- Lifespan extension in N2 - Reduction of lipofuscin accumulation - Improved pharyngeal pumping and motility in N2 **AD** - Prevention of the formation of Aâ aggregates (effect on 3D structure) - Reduction of Aâ -mediated cytotoxicity and oxidative stress - Extension of lifespan in CL4176 - Higher motility and reduced lipofuscin accumulation - Upregulation of *acr-16* and p*myo-3* - Increase of autophagy genes *lgg-1 & bec-1* - Improvement of health span and lifespan. **PD** Reduction of á-synuclein accumulation and 6-OHDA- mediated neurotoxicity via autophagy induction **HD** -Reduction of polyQ40-induced neurotoxicity via autophagy induction	Long et al. 2022; Kumar et al 2023; Dong et al. 2024
Coptis japonica **(but also *Berberis* and *Phellodendron spec.*)** (Ranunculaceae, Rutaceae)	Isoquinoline alkaloids: berberine	- Generation of ROS (pro-oxidant) - Extension of healthy lifespan in wild type strains, higher motility and reduced lipofuscin accumulation - Life span extension via PMK-1/SKN-1 pathway **HD** - Reduction of polyQ accumulation **AD** - Delay of paralysis - Improvement of AD and HD via PMK-1/SKN-1pathway	Xiao et al. 2025
Endopleura uchi (Humiriaceae)	Bergenin (polyphenol)	**HD** - Reduced the number of polyQ40 aggregates	Peixoto et al. 2019b
Euterpe precatoria (Arecaceae)	Anthocyanins (cyanidin-3-rutinoside, cyanidin-3-glucoside and peonidin-3-rutinoside)	**AD** - Improved chemotactic response under Aâ-induced neurotoxicity; **HD** - Decreased the number of polyQ40 aggregates.	Peixoto et al. 2016 a,b

continued on following page

Table 3. Continued

Plant species **Type of extract**	**Main PSM**	**Bioactivity in** *C. elegans*	**References**
Fragaria × ananassa (Rosaceae)	Fisetin	- Reduction of ROS levels - Resistance to acute oxidative stress - Upregulation of *skn-1, ctl-1, sod-3, gst-4, bec-1, lgg-1* genes - Lifespan extension **AD** - Reduction of Aâ-induced neurotoxicity, dependent on DAF-16 and SKN-1 in CL4176 **PD** - Improvement of dopaminergic neurons	Park et al. 2022
***Fraxinus chinensis* and related species** (Oleaceae)	Coumarins: aesculin	**AD** - Improved survival under acute oxidative stress in N2 - Reduction of ROS - Activation of SOD, HSP-16 and CAT and reduction of MDA in N2 - Lifespan prolongation in CL2006 - Improved paralysis effects and chemotaxis - Antioxidative effects via DAF-16 and HSF-1 - Transcriptome analysis	Wang et al. 2022c
Garcinia mangostana (Clusiaceae)	á-Mangostin, ã-mangostin, gartanin, garcinone	**AD** - Inhibition of Aâ42 oligomer aggregation - Reduced paralysis **PD** - Neuroprotection against 6-OHDA induced PD - Lifespan prolongation in 6-OHDA-treated N2	Estrada-Valencia et al. 2022; Thew et al. 2024
Gastrodia elata (Orchidaceae)	4-Hydroxybenzyl alcohol, 4-hydroxybenzaldehyde, 4,4-Dihydroxydiphenylmethane	**AD** - Delay of paralysis in CL4176 - Improvement of mobility, pharyngeal pumping - Resistance to acute oxidative and heat stress - Delay of aging and reduction of lipofuscin accumulation - Reduction of Aâ aggregation and Aâ toxicity - Down-regulation of the expression of NLP-29 and UCR-11 expression - Upregulation of the expression of SOD-3, CAT, SOD, SKN-1, GST-4, PQN-75, LYS-3; *gst-25, hsp-12.3, hsp-12.6, ugt-37* - Downregulation of *dod-22, fat-7, ins-7, ins-23, rgba-1* - Nuclear localization of DAF-16	Shi et al. 2023; Yu et al. 2024

continued on following page

Table 3. Continued

Plant species Type of extract	Main PSM	Bioactivity in *C. elegans*	References
Ginkgo biloba (Ginkgoaceae)	Ginkgo flavone glycosides, Terpene lactones (ginkgolide, bilobalide), ginkgolic acids	**AD** - Reduction of the number of Aâ aggregates - Delayed Aâ-induced paralysis in CL4176 - Improved chemotaxis **HD** - Reduced the number of polyQ40 aggregates - Reduction of polyQ mediated neurotoxicity	Heiner 2017
Glochidion zeylanicum (Phyllanthaceae)	Gallic acid and catechins	**AD** - Reduced Aâ-induced paralysis on CL4176 and CL2006 - Improved chemotaxis in CL2122 and CL2355	Duangjan et al. 2021
***Glycine max* and other legumes** (Fabaceae)	Isoflavonoids: Genistein	**AD** - Delayed Aâ-induced paralysis in CL4176 and CL2006 - Reduced lipofuscin accumulation - Down-regulation of *vit-3* and *vit-6,* upregulation of *hsp-16.2* - Nuclear translocation of the DAF-16 - Increased survival under heat stress	Li et al. 2022b
Glycyrrhiza glabra; G. uralensis (Fabaceae)	Isoliquiritigenin, liquiritigenin, glycyrrhizic acid, and glycyrrhetinic acid	**AD** - EGCG reduced Aâ-deposits and aggregate formation in CL2006 - Delayed Aâ-induced paralysis in CL4176 - Improved survival under acute oxidative stress in CL2006 - Stimulation of SOD and CAT, reduction of MDA - Nuclear translocation of DAF-16 and SKN-1	Link et al. 2015; Chen et al. 2023b
Hedera helix (Araliaceae)	Triterpene saponins: hederagenin	**AD** - Increase of SOD and ROS tolerance in CL4176 - Reduction of Aâ-induced oxidative damage - Reduction of Aâ deposition - Delayed senescence and paralysis in CL4176 **PD** - Induction of mitophagy - Reduction of á-synuclein aggregation in NL5901 - Improvement of mobility - Reduction of loss of dopaminergic neurons in 6-OHDA-induced BZ555	Li et al. 2024b; Xie et al. 2025
Humulus lupulus (Cannabaceae)	Chlorogenic acids, proanthocyanidines, flavonoids, xanthohumol, lupulone, humulone	**AD** - Reduction of Aâ deposition in CL2006 - Delayed Aâ-induced paralysis in CL2006	Palmioli et al. 2022

continued on following page

Table 3. Continued

Plant species Type of extract	Main PSM	Bioactivity in *C. elegans*	References
Hypericum perforatum (Hypericaceae)	Flavonoids, hyperizin, hyperforin	- Reduces ROS accumulation - Reduces juglone induced hsp-16 expression **AD** - Reduction of the number of Aâ aggregates - Delayed Aâ-induced paralysis in CL4176 - Improved chemotaxis **PD** - Reduction of 6-OHDA induced neurotoxicity in BZ555	Heiner 2017
Ligusticum chuanxiong (Apiaceae)	Polyphenols: phenolic acids, flavonoids, anthocyanins and simple phenols	-Improved resistance under oxidative stress and antioxidant enzyme (GSH-Px, SOD)activities in N2 -Lifespan elongation in N2 -Reduction of lipofuscin, MDA and ROS accumulation in N2 **AD** -Reduction of Aâ-induced paralysis in CL4176s - Improved chemotaxis in CL2355s - Reduction of Aâ accumulation and ROS, depending on DAF-16 and HSF-1 - Activation of SOD in CL4176s - Upregulation of *sod-3, sod-5, hsp-16.1* and *hsp-70* genes	Qin et al. 2002
Lycium barbarum (Solanaceae)	Flavonoids: rutin, chlorogenic acid, and kaempferol; anthocyanins: petunidin-3-*O*-glucoside; polysaccharides	**AD** - Substantial antioxidant potential - Reduction of Aâ accumulation in CL2006 - Delay of Aâ-induced paralysis in CL2006 - Improved mobility - Reduction of ROS via SKN-1 pathway - Upregulation of *dve-1*, *ubl-5*, *xbp-1, skn1-, sod-1* and *sod-2* genes - Inhibition of mitochondrial damage - Induction of FSHR-1-mediated activation of mtUPR	Meng et al. 2022

continued on following page

Table 3. Continued

Plant species Type of extract	Main PSM	Bioactivity in *C. elegans*	References
***Malus* spec.** (Rosaceae)	Chalcones: phloridzin	- Reduction of acute oxidative stress and ROS accumulation - Improved motility - Extension of lifespan - Increase of *hsp-16.2* and *sod-3* expression - Nuclear localization of DAF-16 - Upregulation of the expression of *skn-1, ctl-1, sod-3, gst-4, bec-1* and *lgg-1* genes (regulating autophagy and oxidative activities) **AD** - Delayed Aâ-induced paralysis was dependent on DAF-16 and SKN-1. - Reduction of mortality induced with a high-glucose diet via SKN-1 **PD** - Reduction of loss of dopaminergic neurons in 6-OHDA-induced PD	Park et al. 2022
Morus nigra (Moraceae)	Flavonoids: Rutin, isoquercitrin, chlorogenic acid; anthocyanins: cyanidin-3-O glucoside	**AD** - Delayed Aâ-induced paralysis in CL4176 - Reduction of the number of Aâ aggregates in CL2006 and CL4176 - Reduction of serotonin hypersensitivity - Reduction of ROS and acute oxidative stress in N2 and CL4176 - Nuclear translocation of DAF-16 - Upregulation of *sod-3, gst-4, daf-16* genes - Lifespan elongation in N2 and CL4176	Wang et al. 2022d; Casedas et al. 2024
Nelumbo nucifera (Nymphaceae)	Nuciferine, leonticine, dauriciline, sinomenine, chrysoeriol, and kaempferol	**AD** - Reduction of the number of Aâ aggregates - Delayed Aâ-induced paralysis in CL4176 and CL2006 - Improved mobility and food searching behavior in CL2355 - Improved SOD, GST-4, HSP-4, HSP-6, GSH-Px, and CAT activities in CL4176 - Reduction of acute oxidative stress - Induction of autophagy	Wen et al. 2024

continued on following page

Table 3. Continued

Plant species Type of extract	Main PSM	Bioactivity in *C. elegans*	References
Panax ginseng (Araliaceae)	Ginsenoside RD (GS-Rd)	**AD** - RNA-Sec analysis of GS-Rd-treated CL4176 (94 genes were upregulated and 203 genes were downregulated) - Downregulation of *daf-16* and *skn-1* expression - Importance of MAPK signaling pathway - Life time extension in in Cl2006 - Higher survival under heat stress and CL4176 - Delay of paralysis - Reduction of ROS in CL4176 - Increase of SOD activity - Translocation of DAF-16 to the nucleus - Reduction of Aâ aggregation - Reduction of tauopathy	Mi et al. 2022; Zhang et al. 2022d
Paullinia cupana (Sapindaceae)	Methylxanthines (caffeine, theobromine and theophylline), polyphenols (catechins and epicatechin)	**AD** - Delayed Aâ-induced paralysis in a SKN-1- and DAF-16-dependent manner (independently of caffeine) **HD** - Decreased the number of polyQ40 aggregates; - Reduced polyQ-mediated neuronal death in ASH neurons - Increased proteasomal and lysosomal degradation	Boasquivis et al. 2018; Peixoto et al. 2017
Ocymum sanctum (Lamiaceae)	Eugenol	- Increase of lifespan - Enhanced resistance under oxidative stress **AD** - Improved lifespan and reduction of paralysis in CL4176 -Longevity improvement independent of DAF-16	Parween et al. 2022
Olea europaea (Oleaceae)	Polyphenols: oleuropein	**AD** - Reduction of ROS and lifespan elongation in N2 - Reduction of Aâ deposition in CL4176 - Improved paralysis in CL4176 - Nuclear translocation of DAF-16 - Improvement from tau expression in BR5706 - Involvement of DAF-16, SKN-, HSP-16.2 in oleuropein activity	Romero-Márquez et al. 2022; Chen et al. 2022b

continued on following page

Table 3. Continued

Plant species Type of extract	Main PSM	Bioactivity in *C. elegans*	References
Piper wallichii (Piperaceae)	2-Methoxycinnamic, acid, phenethyl acetate, á-kojibiose, pentose, momor-cerebroside I, and kikemanine	**AD** - Activation of autophagy (LGG-1 foci and decreased GFP-p62 expression) - Lifespan and health span elongation via autophagy induction - Improvement of body bends and pharyngeal pumping rates, - Delayed Aâ-induced paralysis - Decrease of lipofuscin accumulation - Resistance to oxidative, heat, and pathogenic stress - Alleviation of Aâ and Tau pathology	Zhu et al. 2023a
Polygonum multiflorum (Polygonaceae)	2,3,5,4 -Tetrahydroxystilbene-2-*O*-*â*-D-glucoside (TSG)	**AD** - Counteracts proteotoxicity of Aâ-amyloid and tau - Improved motility and chemotaxis	Sun et al. 2024
Rehmannia glutinosa (Orobanchaceae)	Oligosaccharides (stachyose raffinose, melibiose, mannotriose); catalpol (iridoid glucoside)	**AD** - Reduction of ROS in CL4176 - Reduced deposition of Aâ in CL2006 and paralysis in CL4176 - Improved chemotaxis in CL2355 - Alleviation of serotonin hypersensitivity in CL2355 - Upregulation of the expression of *sir-2.1, daf-16, sod-3,* and *hsp-16.2* genes - Down-regulation of *amy-1* gene - Nuclear localization of DAF-16 - Increase of lifespan	Kang et al. 2022
Reineckia carnea (Asparagaceae)	saponins, flavonoids, and polysaccharides	**AD** - Reduction of Aâ and Tau aggregates - Reduction of paralysis and improved motility in CL4176 - Attenuation of neurotoxicity from Tau proteins BR5270 - Reduction of oxidative stress - Induction of autophagy	Fu et al. 2023
Rhodiola rosea (Crassulaceae)	Rosavin, salidroside	- Reduces ROS - Reduces juglone induced hsp-16 expression - DAF-16 translocation to nucleus **AD** - Reduction of the number of Aâ aggregates - Improved chemotaxis **PD** - Reduced alpha-synuclein formation	Heiner 2017

continued on following page

Table 3. Continued

Plant species **Type of extract**	**Main PSM**	**Bioactivity in *C. elegans***	**References**
Rosa setate x R. rugosa (Rosaceae)	Essential oil: Citronellol, Geraniol, and Octadiene	**HD** - Reduction of á-synuclein aggregations - Counteracting DA neuron degeneration induced by 6-OHDA - Improved food-sensing behavior and SOD activity - Increase of lipid deposits - Reduced ROS level - Enhanced proteasome activity in OW13 - Prolongation of lifespan	Muhammad et al. 2023
Salvia castanea, S. miltiorrhiza (Lamiaceae)	Cryptotanshinone	**AD** - Reduction of ROS - Upregulation of *sod-3*, and *hsp-16.2* and downregulation of *ace-2* - DAF-16 translocation to the nucleus - Reduction of Aâ monomers and toxic oligomers - Delay of Aâ-induced paralysis in CL4176 **HD** - Reduction of polyglutamine protein accumulation in AM14	Cui et al. 2002
Salvia leucantha (Lamiaceae)	Lipids: 2,4-Di-tert-butylphenol	- Extension of the longevity in N2 - Delay of CL4176 paralysis - Upregulation of *gst-5* - 927 genes were significantly regulated in longevity regulatory pathways	Zhao et al. 2024b

continued on following page

Table 3. Continued

Plant species Type of extract	Main PSM	Bioactivity in *C. elegans*	References
***Salvia rosmarinus* (syn. *Rosmarinus officinalis*)** (Lamiaceae)	Rosmarinic acid; carnosic acid	- Reduction of ROS and MDA - Upregulation of SOD-3, GSH-Px, CAT **AD** - Delay of CL4176 paralysis; improvement of motility - Reduction of Aâ monomers and toxic oligomers - Down-regulation of *ace-1* and *ace-2* genes, - Upregulation of *phb-1, phb-2, eat-3, drp-1, cha-1* and *unc-17* genes - Reduction of AChE activity - Improvement of mitochondrial function **HD** - Decreased oxidative damage of polyQ40 aggregates AM140, HA759 - Induction of Wnt Signaling and Notch Signaling - Involvement of IIS, MAPK signaling, and HSF-1 signaling pathways - Decreased the number of polyQ40 aggregates - Improvement of mitochondrial dynamic homeostasis **PD** - Decreased oxidative damage of alpha-synuclein formation NL5901 - Induction of Wnt signaling and Notch signaling - Involvement of IIS, MAPK signaling, and HSF-1 signaling pathways - Reduced alpha-synuclein formation - Improvement of mitochondrial dynamic homeostasis	Chen et al. 2022, 2024
Sambucus nigra (Adoxaceae)	Flavonoids: narcissoside	**PD** - Reduction of 6-OHDA-mediated dopaminergic neuron degeneration - Reduction of ROS - Increase of GSH content - Enhanced expression of *Skn-1, Gcs-1*, and *E01A2.1* - Improved lifespan in 6-OHDA-treated nematodes - Reduction of alpha-synuclein accumulation - Stimulation of autophagy	Fu et al. 2022
Sideritis scardica, Sideritis clandestina (Lamiaceae)	Sideridiol, verbascoside, chlorogenic acid, caffeoylquinic acids, acteoside, and flavonoids	**AD** - Reduced the number of Aâ aggregates (influence of peptide conformation) - Delayed Aâ-induced paralysis.	Heiner et al. 2018; Nishioka et al. 2020; Gioran et al. 2024

continued on following page

Table 3. Continued

Plant species Type of extract	Main PSM	Bioactivity in *C. elegans*	References
Styphnolobium japonicum (Fabaceae)	Fruit extract: Phenolic acids, flavonoids, flavan-3-ols, and proanthocyanidins	**AD** - Delayed Aâ-induced paralysis **HD** - Decreased the number of polyQ40 aggregates **PD** - Reduced alpha-synuclein formation	Thabit et al. 2023
Syzygium nervosum (Myrtaceae)	Anthocyanins	**AD** - Extended lifespan of Aâ-expressing worms indicating potential neuroprotective effect.	Prasanth et al. 2019
Vitis vinifera (Vitaceae)	Seeds: procyanidins	**AD** - Delayed Aâ-induced paralysis - Enhanced longevity in Aâ- expressing CL2006 - Improved chemotaxis - Improved autophagy	González-Manzano et al. 2024
Withania somnifera (Solanaceae)	Withaferin A	**PD** - Improved motility, survival and reduced neurotoxicity after N-methyl-4-phenylpyridinium (MPP+) and 6-hydroxydopamine (6-OHDA) treatment	Parrales et al. 2025
Zingiber officinale (Zingiberaceae)	Polyphenols: apigenin, kaempferol, and quercetin derivatives	**AD** - Increased survival under oxidative stress CL4176 - Reduced ROS levels under basal stress - Increased the expression of *jnk-1, daf-16, sod-3, hasp-16.2* and *cat* - Reduction of paralysis induced by Aâ in CL4176 - Reduction of Aâ-aggregates - Improved motility, chemotaxis and longevity	Gao et al. 2025
Ziziphus jujuba (Rhamnaceae)	Triterpenes: Ursonic acid	**AD** - Improved survival under oxidative stress - Increase of the expression of *sod-1*, *sod-3*, *gcs-1*, and *gst-4* in SKN-1 pathway - Higher expression of *hsp-16.2*, *bec-1*, and *lgg-1* - Improved chemotaxis in CL2355 worms expressing Aâ1–42 proteins - Improved lifespan in UM0001with Aâ and pro-aggregation tau - Reduction of lipofuscin accumulation	Wang et al. 2025

When *C. elegans* is treated with many plant extracts (Table 2 and 3), a prominent antioxidative activity was determined, which was often accompanied by a lifespan elongation of 10 to 30%. The following effects were recorded (Figure 3; Table 2 and 3); it was not intended to discuss these biochemical effects and their implications in detail (for more information consult Lee and Johnson 2004; Kampkötter et al. 2007; Chiang et al. 2012; Chen et al. 2013a,b,c; de Freitas Bonomo et al. 2014; Peixoto et al. 2019a,b; Guerrero-Rubio et al. 2020; Kenyon 2011; Conte et al. 2015; Zheng et al. 2018; Sural et al. 2019; Adedara et al. 2025). Many of the PSM and extracts have been studied in cell cultures, other animal models and even in humans; a discussion of the observed effects in these system would be out of scope for this chapter.

- Inhibition of the *daf-2* pathway
- ROS and MDA reduction under normal conditions in N2 wild-type nematodes
- Increased survival of nematodes under acute oxidative and/or heat stress
- Nuclear translocation of the transcription factors DAF-16 and/or SKN-1 and activation of DAF-16 and SKN-1 by SIR-2.1 signaling
- Down-regulation of *daf-2, age-1, fat-5, acs-2, vit-2, (sek-1, pmk-1, nsy-1, lipl-4, ist-1* and *kgb-1* genes
- Upregulation of *sir-2.1, aak-2, daf-16, skn-1, hsf-1, jnk-1, sod-3, mlt-1, ctl-1, hsp16.2, gst-4, sip-1, clpp-1, dve-1, ama-1, gcs-1gab-1, ace-1, dop-1, mod-1, eat-4, hlh-30, lgg-1, par-4 jnk-1, jkk-1, ist-1, pha-4, lipl-4, kgb-2*, and *fat-6*
- Increased activity of CAT, SOD-3, SIR-2, GSH-Px, GST
- Improved pharyngeal pumping, muscle quality, motility and chemotaxis
- Reduced accumulation of aging-related pigment lipofuscin
- Lifespan extension depending on DAF-16 and/or SKN-1 (but not in DAF-16, SKN-1 and HSF-1 mutants) and involvement of IIS, MAPK, HSF, JNK-1, mtUPR, and JNK pathways
- Lifespan elongation by activating autophagy, mitophagy, and UPRmt

In case of models for the neurodegenerative disorders AD, HD, and PD, the following effects were recorded after treatment with above-mentioned extracts or isolated PSM (Table 2 and 3):

AD:

- Inhibition of AChE and MAO-A activity
- Reduction of the number of Aβ aggregates and their oligomerization
- Delay of paralysis depending on DAF-16, SKN-1 and HSF-1
- Improvement of chemotaxis, mobility and pharyngeal pumping
- Delay of senescence, aging and reduction of lipofuscin accumulation
- Nuclear translocation of DAF-16 and SKN-1
- Upregulation of *sir-2.1, daf-16, sod-3, gst-4, rpt-3, acr-16, hsp-16.1, dve-1, ubl-5, xbp-1, skn-1,* p*myo-3, phb-1, phb-2, eat-3, drp-1, cha-1* and *unc-17* genes and proteasome activity,
- Activation of the autophagy genes *lgg-1 & bec-1*
- Enhanced expression of SOD-3, CAT, SOD, SKN-1, GST-4, PQN-75, LYS-3; HSP-4, GSH-Px
- Down-regulation of *amy-1, ace-1* and *ace-2* genes,
- Inhibition of mitochondrial damage and induction of FSHR-1-mediated activation of mtUPR

HD

- Reduction of polyQ40 aggregation in AM141
- Reduction of polyQ40-induced oxidative stress, neurotoxicity via autophagy induction
- Induction of Wnt signaling and Notch signaling
- Involvement of IIS, MAPK, and HSF-1 signaling pathways
- Increased proteasomal and lysosomal degradation
- Improved food-sensing behavior and SOD activity
- Prolongation of lifespan

PD

- Reduction of ROS and amelioration of dyskinesia
- Reduced alpha-synuclein accumulation and of 6-OHDA induced neurotoxicity
- Upregulation of *skn-1, gcs*-1, *gst-4, gcs-1, sod-3,* and *daf-16*; under $MPP^{(+)}$ treatment
- Improving food-sensing behavior and stimulation of ubiquitin-like proteasomes
- Induction of mitophagy and autophagy
- Lifespan extension
- Induction of Wnt Signaling and Notch Signaling
- Involvement of IIS, MAPK, and HSF-1 signaling pathways

Many of the plant extracts investigated Table 2 and 3 contain phenolics and polyphenols. The phenolics represent a major class of PSM, including structurally diverse molecules with one or more phenolic hydroxyl (OH) groups, their typical functional group (Wink 2008, 2015; Wink and Schimmer, 2010; van Wyk and Wink 2017). The class of phenolics consists of phenolic acids, flavonoids, stilbenes, catechin, cyanidins, procyanidins and tannins (van Wyk and Wink 2017). Flavonoids, the largest group of polyphenols, include the subclasses of flavanones, flavones, flavanols, flavonols and anthocyanins, and are predominantly sequestered in plant vacuoles as O-glycosides.

A typical property of isolated phenolics and of polyphenol-rich plant extracts is a prominent *in vitro* antioxidant activity, which can easily be determined in the laboratory. The *C. elegans* studies revealed that many of the phenolics are at least partly bioavailable, although they are polar molecules. Many lipophilic or amphiphilic other PSM in the extracts apparently facilitate their uptake (Wink 2008, 2015). In the *C. elegans* model the phenolics are able to reduce the intracellular levels of ROS and improve resistance of the nematodes to acute oxidative stress caused by H_2O_2, juglone, paraquat or the expression of Aβ-peptides in AD and polyQ in HD models of neurodegeneration (Tables 2 and 3).

As discussed in 1.2 and 1.3, ROS can oxidize cellular macromolecules such as proteins, lipids and nucleic acids. Apparently, antioxidants can counteract such oxidative processes: Several polyphenolic compounds can indeed protect proteins, nucleic acids and lipids from oxidative damage by simply scavenging ROS (Wink 2008, 2015; Fraga et al. 2010). The antioxidant activity of polyphenols is strictly related to their structural properties, namely the number and distribution of phenolic OH groups, the three-dimensional structure and degree of polymerization. The molecular mechanisms of the antioxidative properties of phenolics and polyphenols is apparently mediated by hydrogen atom transfer and single electron transfer (Leopoldini et al. 2011). In hydrogen atom transfer reactions, the dissociation of the phenolic OH bond allows polyphenols to stabilize free radicals by donating a hydrogen atom. Through single electron transfer, phenolics reduce the free radical by transferring an electron. The positively charged polyphenol radical formed in this reaction is later deprotonated by water. Moreover, polyphenols may indirectly reduce the formation of ROS by chelating ionic metals, thus impeding Fenton-like reactions (Perron and Brumaghin 2009).

In addition, another important mode of action of phenolics and other PSM is mediated directly by interaction with proteins (enzymes, receptors) and importantly with transcription factors (Wink 2015) which can explain many activities summarized in Table 2 and 3. Molecular interactions between phenolics and polyphenols with proteins are mostly of non-covalent nature, including hydrophobic, hydrogen and ionic bonding and Vanderwal's interactions; however, covalent bonding may also occur (Wink 2015; Ozdal et al. 2013). Hydrogen bonds are established between the phenolic and non-phenolic OH groups and the carboxyl and amino groups of amino acids. Ionic bonds are facilitated under physiological conditions due to the dissociation of the phenolic OH group into negatively charged phenolate ions, which bind to the positively charged amino groups and amino acid side chains. These transient polyphenol-protein interactions enable polyphenols to modulate the functional activity of enzymes, transcription factors and receptors; they can also target proteins for cellular degradation, which may be important in case of neurodegenerative diseases. Moreover, by binding to proteins, polyphenols may avoid their oxidative modification, which could otherwise lead to conformation changes and irreversible aggregation, a common pathological hallmark of neurodegenerative diseases.

Even as polyphenol-protein interactions are very important, it should be mentioned that phenolics and polyphenols can also interact with nucleic acids mostly via intercalation, groove binding, ionic or hydrophobic interactions (Chanphai and Tajmir-Riahi, 2019). We assume, that phenolics can bind to the potential target sites for free radicals on DNA, thus avoiding oxidative damage to nucleic acids. Furthermore, such an activity could prevent mutations or translational errors potentially compromising the function of proteins. In addition, direct polyphenol-DNA interactions can modulate gene expression, for example through blocking the access of transcription factors to their DNA-binding sites (Choi et al. 2007). As shown in many studies, plant extracts rich in polyphenols can change the gene expression patterns in many systems, suggesting an interaction with DNA/RNA or directly the transcription factors. However, polyphenol-DNA interactions can also cause negative effects, such as causing mutations or inhibition of replication (Wink and Schimmer 2010). Thus, an excessive application of polyphenol-rich plant extracts or nutraceuticals could also be harmful - remember the famous conclusion of Paracelsus- "*Dosis sola facit venenum*".

In addition to proteins and nucleic acids, polyphenols can also interact with lipids via hydrophobic interactions and hydrogen bonding. By binding to the polar head groups of the lipid bilayer, polyphenols form a barrier on the membrane surface, protecting biomembranes from ROS-induced damage (de Granada-Flor et al. 2019; Košinová et al. 2012; Oteiza et al. 2005; Sirk et al. 2009). A planar structure of phenolics apparently favors this type of interactions. Lipophilic polyphenols can even intercalate into the hydrophobic core of the biomembrane, thus being able to inhibit ROS-mediated lipid peroxidation by neutralizing intramembrane lipid radicals or by increasing membrane fluidity (Fadel et al. 2011). Changes in membrane fluidity can disrupt the organization of lipid chains, which may prevent the propagation of lipid and oxygen radicals and facilitate polyphenol-radical interactions.

As seen in Tables 2 and 3, PSM, especially phenolics and polyphenols, but also carotenoids, isothiocyanates and some polysaccharides, saponins and even chlorophyll can influence the ROS levels in *C. elegans*, and modulate stress resistance to pro-oxidants and heat. They can up- or down-regulate a large number of genes, involved in IIS, MAPK, HSF, JNK-1, mtUPR, and JNK pathways, which are involved in ROS homoeostasis, stress response, longevity and aging and also in the modulation of neurodegeneration in AD, HD and PD models (Table 4).

Table 4. Estimated number of plant specialized metabolites (PSM) (Wink and van Wyk 2008; van Wyk & Wink 2015, 2017), their potential antioxidant, antiaging and neuroprotectant activities and occurrence [graded in few species (*), some species (**), many species (***), and very abundant (****)].

Class of PSM	Estimated numbers of secondary metabolites	Antioxidant activities	Antiaging activities	Activity against neurodegeneration
With nitrogen				
Alkaloids	27000	**	*	*
Non-protein amino acids	1000			
Amines	100	*	*	
Cyanogenic glucosides	60	*		
Glucosinolates/isothiocyanates	130	**	**	
Without nitrogen				
Monoterpenes	2500	**	*	*
Iridoids	600	**	**	**
Sesquiterpenes	8000	*	**	*
Diterpenes	10000	*	*	*
Triterpenes, steroids, saponins	20000	*	**	**
Tetraterpenes (carotenoids)	750	***	**	*
Phenylpropanoids, phenolic acids, coumarins, lignans, lignin	4000	****	****	***
Flavonoids, anthocyanins, xanthones, and tannins	5000	****	****	****
Polyacetylenes	2000	**	*	
Polyketides, quinones	10000	***	*	
Oligosaccharides, polysaccharides	1000	*	**	*

3. CONCLUSIONS

The nematode *C. elegans* is an important model organism which has greatly contributed to our understanding of molecular and cell biology, development, physiology and pharmacology (Alberts et al. 2015). It was and is an important tool to study the effect of antioxidant, neuroprotective and lifespan prolongating PSM, medicinal plants, food and beverages. The *C. elegans* model also allows insides into the molecular mechanisms and pathways which regulate oxidative stress, aging and neurodegeneration (Kenyon 2011; Lublin and Link 2013; Leonov et al. 2015; Barardo et al. 2017). Although several mechanisms have been elucidated, we still lack knowledge on transport of PSM within the nematodes and cellular uptake, and on metabolization of PSM in the microbiome of the nematodes and intracellularly.

Many medicinal plants, especially those storing phenolics, polyphenols and carotenoids exhibit apparent antioxidant, longevity promoting and neuroprotective activities in *C. elegans*, in cell culture and other animal modelsThese PSM can directly influence the level of ROS in cells and tissues, but can also affect the activity of proteins (enzymes, receptors and particularly transcription factors), thus regulation important signal pathways involved with antioxidative defense and longevity.

To some degree, these substances are also relevant for humans and there is good evidence that medicinal plants, herbs, spices and nutraceuticals with phenolics, polyphenols, carotenoids, isothiocyanates, allicin and even chlorophyll are useful for the prevention and therapy of ROS-mediated and age-related health conditions as well as for promoting a longer and healthier life (van Wyk and Wink 2017; Wink 2022, 2024). Although substantial evidence exists for the beneficial properties of PSM in *C. elegans* and other model systems, we need more clinical and intervention studies with humans to improve the selection of plants, extracts as well as their dosage, delivery and application form in order to produce safe and efficient therapeutics or nutritional supplements.

ACKNOWLEDGEMENT

I would like to thank my PhD students in the *C. elegans* projects for their continuous support and excellent work, especially Mariana Roxo, Shaoxiong Zhang, Erjia Wang, Hanmei Li, Junxian Zhou, Sara Shody Thabit, Markus Braun, Felix Heiner, Sonja Krstin, Herbenya Peixoto, Mansour Sobeh, Pille Link, Leila Rezaizadehnajafi, Wei Chen, Shan Su, and Sami Abbas.

Our research was funded by grants of German Science Foundation (DFG), German Academic Exchange Service (DAAD), Chinese Scholarship Council (CSC), Cusanuswerk, Coordenação de Aperfeiçoamento de Pessoal de Nível Superior (CAPES), National Council of Science and Technology (CONACYT), Science and Technology Development Fund (STDF).

REFERENCES

Abbas, S., & Wink, M. (2010). 2010 Epigallocatechin gallate inhibits beta-amyloid oligomerization in *Caenorhabditis elegans* and affects the *daf-2*/insulin-like signaling pathway. *Phytomedicine*, *17*(11), 902–909. DOI: 10.1016/j.phymed.2010.03.008 PMID: 20382008

Abbas, S., & Wink, M. (2014). Green tea extract induces the resistance of *Caenorhabditis elegans* against oxidative stress. *Antioxidants*, *3*(1), 129–143. DOI: 10.3390/antiox3010129 PMID: 26784668

Abbas, S. M. W., & Wink, M. (2009). Epigallocatechin gallate (EGCG) from green tea (*Camellia sinensis*) increases lifespan and stress resistance in *Caenorhabditis elegans.Planta Medica*, *75*(3), 216–221. DOI: 10.1055/s-0028-1088378 PMID: 19085685

Abdelfattah, M. A. O., Dmirieh, M., Bakrim, W. B., Mouhtady, O., Ghareeb, M. A., Wink, M., & Sobeh, M. (2022). Antioxidant and anti-aging effects of *Warburgia salutaris* bark aqueous extract: Evidence from in silico, in vitro and in vivo studies. *Journal of Enzyme Inhibition and Medicinal Chemistry*, *37*(1), 2710–2724. DOI: 10.1080/14756366.2022.2127700 PMID: 36168121

Adedara, I. A., Weis, G. C. C., Monteiro, C. S., Soares, F. A. A., Rocha, J. B. T., Schetinger, M. R. C., Emanuelli, T., & Aschner, M. (2025, January 25). Versatility of Caenorhabditis elegans as a Model Organism for Evaluating Foodborne Neurotoxins and Food Bioactive Compounds in Nutritional Neuroscience. *Molecular Neurobiology*, *62*(6), 7205–7229. Advance online publication. DOI: 10.1007/s12035-025-04705-y PMID: 39863742

Alberts, B.. (2015). [Ed.; Garland Science: New York, NY, USA]. *Molecular Biology of the Cell*, •••, 6.

Ayoub, I. M., Eldahshan, O. A., Roxo, M., & Zhang, S. (2024). M Wink A N B. Singab, 2024 Stress resistance, anti-aging, and neuroprotective activities of baicalein 5,6-dimethyl ether and *Alnus rugosa* extract in *Caenorhabditis elegans.Archiv der Pharmazie*, •••. Advance online publication. DOI: 10.1002/ardp.202400464 PMID: 39361247

Azevedo, B., Pereira, A. M. S., Roxo, M., Borges, M. C., Peixoto, H., Bertoni, B. W., Contini, S. H. T., Lopes, A., França, S. C., & Wink, M. (2019). 2019 Antioxidant activity of an aqueous leaf extract from *Uncaria tomentosa* and its major alkaloids mitraphylline and isomitraphylline in *Caenorhabditis elegans.Molecules (Basel, Switzerland)*, *24*, 3299. DOI: 10.3390/molecules24183299 PMID: 31510078

Bai, X., Wang, M., Xu, T., Zhou, S., & Chu, W. (2025, March). Antioxidant and anti-aging activities of Acanthopanax senticosus polysaccharide CQ-1 in nematode Caenorhabditis elegans. *International Journal of Biological Macromolecules*, *297*, 139925. DOI: 10.1016/j.ijbiomac.2025.139925 PMID: 39824422

Bakrim, W. B., Nurcahyanti, A. D. R., Dmirieh, M., Mahdy, I., Elgamal, A. M., El Raey, M. A., Wink, M., & Sobeh, M. (2022). Phytochemical profiling of the leaf extract of *Ximenia americana* var. *caffra* and its antioxidant, antibacterial, and antiaging activities *in vitro* and in *Caenorhabditis elegans*: A cosmeceutical and dermatological approach. *Oxidative Medicine and Cellular Longevity*, *2022*, 1–11. Advance online publication. DOI: 10.1155/2022/3486257 PMID: 35387261

Barardo, D., Thornton, D., Thoppil, H., Walsh, M., Sharifi, S., Ferreira, S., Anžič, A., Fernandes, M., Monteiro, P., Grum, T., Cordeiro, R., De-Souza, E. A., Budovsky, A., Araujo, N., Gruber, J., Petrascheck, M., Fraifeld, V. E., Zhavoronkov, A., Moskalev, A., & de Magalhães, J. P. (2017). The DrugAge database of aging-related drugs. *Aging Cell*, *16*(3), 594–597. DOI: 10.1111/acel.12585 PMID: 28299908

Barsyte, D., Lovejoy, D. A., & Lithgow, G. J. (2001). LITHGOW GJ. Longevity and heavy metal resistance in *daf-2* and *age-1* long-lived mutants of *Caenorhabditis elegans.The FASEB Journal*, *15*(3), 627–634. DOI: 10.1096/fj.99-0966com PMID: 11259381

Bhatt, V., & Tiwari, A. K. (2023, December). *Sirtuins*, a key regulator of ageing and age-related neurodegenerative diseases. *The International Journal of Neuroscience*, *133*(10), 1167–1192. DOI: 10.1080/00207454.2022.2057849 PMID: 35549800

Blackwell, T. K., Steinbaugh, M. J., Hourihan, J. M., Ewald, C. Y., & Isik, M. (2015). SKN-1/Nrf, stress responses, and aging in *Caenorhabditis elegans.Free Radical Biology & Medicine*, *88*, 290–301. DOI: 10.1016/j.freeradbiomed.2015.06.008 PMID: 26232625

Blumenthal, T., & Steward, K. (1997). C. elegans II; Riddle D, Blumenthal T, Meyer B, Priess J, eds.

Boasquívis, P. F., Silva, G. M. M., Paiva, F. A., Cavalcanti, R. M., Nunez, C. V., & de Paula Oliveira, R. (2018). Guarana (Paullinia cupana) extract protects Caenorhabditis elegans models for Alzheimer disease and Huntington disease through activation of antioxidant and protein degradation pathways. *Oxidative Medicine and Cellular Longevity*, *2018*(1), 9241308.

Bogari, H. A., Rashied, R. M. H., Abdelfattah, M. A. O., Malatani, R. T., Khinkar, R. M., Hareeri, R. H., Wink, M., & Sobeh, M. (2022). *Euclea divinorum* Hiern: Chemical Profiling of the Leaf Extract and Its Antioxidant Activity In Silico, In Vitro and in *Caenorhabditis elegans* Model. *Metabolites*, *12*(11), 1031. DOI: 10.3390/metabo12111031 PMID: 36355114

Brignull, H. R., Moore, F. E., Tang, S. J., & Morimoto, R. I. (2006). Polyglutamine proteins at the pathogenic threshold display neuron-specific aggregation in a pan-neuronal *Caenorhabditis elegans* model. *The Journal of Neuroscience : The Official Journal of the Society for Neuroscience*, *26*(29), 7597–7606. DOI: 10.1523/JNEUROSCI.0990-06.2006 PMID: 16855087

Cásedas, G., Moliner, C., Abad-Longas, A., Núñez, S., Gómez-Rincón, C., Maggi, F., & López, V. (2024, August 17). Black Mulberries (*Morus nigra* L.) Modulate Oxidative Stress and Beta-Amyloid-Induced Toxicity, Becoming a Potential Neuroprotective Functional Food. *Foods*, *13*(16), 2577. DOI: 10.3390/foods13162577 PMID: 39200504

Cesari, M., Pahor, M., Bartali, B., Cherubini, A., Penninx, B. W., Williams, G. R., Atkinson, H., Martin, A., Guralnik, J. M., & Ferrucci, L. (2004). Antioxidants and physical performance in elderly persons: The Invecchiare in Chianti (InCHIANTI) study. *The American Journal of Clinical Nutrition*, *79*(2), 289–294. DOI: 10.1093/ajcn/79.2.289 PMID: 14749236

Chanphai, P., & Tajmir-Riahi, H. (2019). Structural dynamics of DNA binding to tea catechins. *International Journal of Biological Macromolecules*, *125*, 238–243. DOI: 10.1016/j.ijbiomac.2018.12.054 PMID: 30528995

Chen, L., Chen, G., Gai, T., Zhou, X., Zhu, J., Wang, R., Wang, X., Guo, Y., Wang, Y., & Xie, Z. (2024, June 6). 2024a. L-Theanine Prolongs the Lifespan by Activating Multiple Molecular Pathways in Ultraviolet C-Exposed *Caenorhabditis elegans.Molecules (Basel, Switzerland)*, *29*(11), 2691. DOI: 10.3390/molecules29112691 PMID: 38893565

Chen, Q., Yang, X., Capanoglu, E., Amrouche, A. T., Wu, L., Luo, J., Zhu, Y., Wang, Y., Jiang, X., Zhang, D., & Lu, B. (2023, January 3). 2023a. *Eucommia ulmoides* male flower as a remarkable edible floral resource exerts lifespan/healthspan-promoting effects on *Caenorhabditis elegans.Food & Function*, *14*(1), 457–470. DOI: 10.1039/D2FO03006C PMID: 36519399

Chen, W., He, L., Pei, H., Li, J., Zhao, Y., Zong, Y., Kan, H., He, Z., & Du, R. (2023, April 4). 2023b. Neuroprotective effect of total flavonoids in stems and leaves of *Glycyrrhiza uralensis* Fisch. on oxidative stress in HT-22 cells and *Caenorhabditis elegans.Aging (Albany NY)*, *15*(12), 5290–5303. DOI: 10.18632/aging.204627 PMID: 37367832

Chen, W., Joubert, E., van Wyk, B. E., & Wink, M. (2013a). Ameliorative effect of aspalathin from rooibos (*Aspalathus linearis*) on acute oxidative stress in *Caenorhabditis elegans.Phytomedicine*, *20*(3-4), 380–386. DOI: 10.1016/j.phymed.2012.10.006 PMID: 23218401

Chen, W., Müller, D., Richling, E., & Wink, M. (2013). 2013c. Anthocyanin-rich purple wheat prolongs the life span of *Caenorhabditis elegans* probably by activating the DAF-16/FOXO transcription factor. *Journal of Agricultural and Food Chemistry*, *61*(12), 3047–3053. DOI: 10.1021/jf3054643 PMID: 23470220

Chen, W., Rezaizadehnajafi, L., & Wink, M. (2013b). Influence of resveratrol on oxidative stress resistance and life span in *Caenorhabditis elegans*. *The Journal of Pharmacy and Pharmacology*, *65*(5), 682–688. DOI: 10.1111/jphp.12023 PMID: 23600385

Chen, X., Bahramimehr, F., Shahhamzehei, N., Fu, H., Lin, S., Wang, H., Li, C., Efferth, T., & Hong, C. (2024, July). Anti-aging effects of medicinal plants and their rapid screening using the nematode Caenorhabditis elegans. *Phytomedicine*, *129*, 155665. DOI: 10.1016/j.phymed.2024.155665 PMID: 38768535

Chen, Y., Hamidu, S., Yang, X., Yan, Y., Wang, Q., Li, L., Oduro, P. K., & Li, Y. (2022, April 28). 2022a. Dietary Supplements and Natural Products: An Update on Their Clinical Effectiveness and Molecular Mechanisms of Action During Accelerated Biological Aging. *Frontiers in Genetics*, *13*, 880421. DOI: 10.3389/fgene.2022.880421 PMID: 35571015

Chen, Y., Wang, Y., Qin, Q., Zhang, Y., Xie, L., Xiao, J., Cao, Y., Su, Z., Chen, Y., Romero-Márquez, J. M., Navarro-Hortal, M. D., Jiménez-Trigo, V., Vera-Ramírez, L., Forbes-Hernández, T. J., Esteban-Muñoz, A., Giampieri, F., Bullón, P., Battino, M., Sánchez-González, C., & Quiles, J. L. (2022, April). 2022b. An oleuropein rich-olive (Olea europaea L.) leaf extract reduces β-amyloid and tau proteotoxicity through regulation of oxidative- and heat shock-stress responses in Caenorhabditis elegans. *Food and Chemical Toxicology*, *162*, 112914. DOI: 10.1016/j.fct.2022.112914 PMID: 35276233

Chen, Y., Xu, R., Liu, Q., Zeng, Y., Chen, W., Liu, Y., Cao, Y., Liu, G., & Chen, Y. (2024, December). Rosmarinic acid ameliorated oxidative stress, neuronal injuries, and mitochondrial dysfunctions mediated by polyglutamine and α-synuclein in Caenorhabditis elegans models. *Molecular Neurobiology*, *61*(12), 10138–10158. DOI: 10.1007/s12035-024-04206-4 PMID: 38703342

Chiang, W.-C., Ching, T.-T., Lee, H. C., Mousigian, C., & Hsu, A.-L. (2012). HSF-1 regulators DDL-1/2 link insulin-like signaling to heat-shock responses and modulation of longevity. *Cell*, *148*(1-2), 322–334. DOI: 10.1016/j.cell.2011.12.019 PMID: 22265419

Cho, M., Kim, Y., You, S., Hwang, D. Y., & Jang, M. (2023, February 3). Chlorogenic Acid of *Cirsium japonicum* Resists Oxidative Stress Caused by Aging and Prolongs Healthspan via SKN-1/Nrf2 and DAF-16/FOXO in *Caenorhabditis elegans.Metabolites*, *13*(2), 224. DOI: 10.3390/metabo13020224 PMID: 36837843

Choi, P. G., Park, S. H., Nirmala, F. S., Kim, H. S., Kim, M. J., Hahm, J. H., Seo, H. D., Ahn, J., Ha, T., & Jung, C. H. (2023, July 8). Geniposide-Rich Gardenia jasminoides Ellis Fruit Extract Increases Healthspan in Caenorhabditis elegans. *The Journals of Gerontology. Series A, Biological Sciences and Medical Sciences*, *78*(7), 1108–1115. DOI: 10.1093/gerona/glad066 PMID: 36821434

Choi, S.-Y., Hwang, J.-H., Ko, H.-C., Park, J.-G., & Kim, S.-J. (2007). Nobiletin from citrus fruit peel inhibits the DNA-binding activity of NF-κB and ROS production in LPS-activated RAW 264.7 cells. *Journal of Ethnopharmacology*, *113*(1), 149–155. DOI: 10.1016/j.jep.2007.05.021 PMID: 17611060

Conte Jr D, MacNeil LT, Walhout AJ, Mello CC. RNA interference in *Caenorhabditis elegans*. Curr Prot Mol Biol 2015; 109: 26.3.1-.3.30.

Corsi, A. K., Wightman, B., & Chalfie, M. (2015). A transparent window into biology: A primer on *Caenorhabditis elegans.Genetics*, *200*(2), 387–407. DOI: 10.1534/genetics.115.176099 PMID: 26088431

Cui, W. B., Zhang, Z. P., Bai, X., Wang, S. S., Chen, X. H., Liu, X., Su, P. J., Zhi, D. J., Fei, D. Q., Zhang, Z. X., & Wang, D. S. (2022, September 2). Cryptotanshinone Alleviates Oxidative Stress and Reduces the Level of Abnormally Aggregated Protein in *Caenorhabditis elegans* AD Models. *International Journal of Molecular Sciences*, *23*(17), 10030. DOI: 10.3390/ijms231710030 PMID: 36077432

de Araújo, L. C. A., Leite, N. R., da Rocha, P. D. S., Baldivia, D. D. S., Agarrayua, D. A., Ávila, D. S., da Silva, D. B., Carollo, C. A., Campos, J. F., Souza, K. P., & Dos Santos, E. L. (2023, November 16). Campomanesia adamantium O Berg. fruit, native to Brazil, can protect against oxidative stress and promote longevity. *PLoS One*, *18*(11), e0294316. DOI: 10.1371/journal.pone.0294316 PMID: 37972127 de Freitas Bonomo, L., Silva, D. N., Boasquivis, P. F., Paiva, F. A., da Costa Guerra, J. F., & Martins, T. A. F.. (2014). Açaí (*Euterpe oleracea* Mart.) modulates oxidative stress resistance in *Caenorhabditis elegans* by direct and indirect mechanisms. *PLoS One*, *9*(3), e89933. DOI: 10.1371/journal.pone.0089933 PMID: 24594796

de Granada-Flor, A., Sousa, C., Filipe, H. A., Santos, M. S. C., & de Almeida, R. F. (2019). Quercetin dual interaction at the membrane level. *Chemical Communications*, *55*(12), 1750–1753. DOI: 10.1039/C8CC09656B PMID: 30664132

Devore, E. E., Kang, J. H., Breteler, M. M., & Grodstein, F. (2012). Dietary intakes of berries and flavonoids in relation to cognitive decline. *Annals of Neurology*, *72*(1), 135–143. DOI: 10.1002/ana.23594 PMID: 22535616

Dong, Q., Cui, Z., Wu, X., Li, L., Lu, F., & Liu, F. (2024, April 22). Natural flavonoid hesperetin blocks amyloid β-protein fibrillogenesis, depolymerizes preformed fibrils and alleviates cytotoxicity caused by amyloids. *Food & Function*, *15*(8), 4233–4245. DOI: 10.1039/D3FO05566C PMID: 38517352

Dosanjh, L. E., Brown, M. K., Rao, G., Link, C. D., & Luo, Y. (2010). Behavioral phenotyping of a transgenic *Caenorhabditis elegans* expressing neuronal amyloid-β. *Journal of Alzheimer's Disease*, *19*(2), 681–690. DOI: 10.3233/JAD-2010-1267 PMID: 20110612

Dostal, V., & Link, C. D. (2010). Assaying β-amyloid toxicity using a transgenic *C. elegans* model. *Journal of Visualized Experiments*, •••(44), e2252. DOI: 10.3791/2252 PMID: 20972410

Duangjan, C., Rangsinth, P., Gu, X., Wink, M., & Tencomnao, T. (2019). Lifespan extending and oxidative stress resistance properties of a leaf extracts from Anacardium occidentale L. in Caenorhabditis elegans. *Oxidative Medicine and Cellular Longevity*, *2019*(1), 9012396.

Duangjan, C., Rangsinth, P., Gu, X., Zhang, S., Wink, M., & Tencomnao, T. (2019b). *Glochidion zeylanicum* leaf extracts exhibit lifespan extending and oxidative stress resistance properties in *Caenorhabditis elegans* via DAF-16/FoxO and SKN-1/Nrf-2 signaling pathways. *Phytomedicine*, *64*, 153061. DOI: 10.1016/j.phymed.2019.153061 PMID: 31401497

Duangjan, C., Rangsinth, P., Gu, X., Zhang, S., Wink, M., & Tencomnao, T. (2021b). *Vitis vinifera* leaf extract protects against glutamate-induced oxidative toxicity in HT22 hippocampal neuronal cells and increases stress resistance in *Caenorhabditis elegans.Frontiers in Nutrition*, *8*, 634100. DOI: 10.3389/fnut.2021.634100 PMID: 34179052

Duangjan, C., Rangsinth, P., Zhang, S., Gu, X., Wink, M., & Tencomnao, T. (2021). 2021a Neuroprotective effects of *Glochidion zeylanicum* leaf extract against H2O2/glutamate-induced toxicity in cultured neuronal cells and Aß-induced toxicity in *Caenorhabditis elegans.Biology (Basel)*, *10*(8), 800. DOI: 10.3390/biology10080800 PMID: 34440032

Elkhedir, A., Iqbal, A., Albahi, A., Tao, M., Rong, L., & Xu, X. (2022, March). Capsaicinoid-Glucosides of Fresh Hot Pepper Promotes Stress Resistance and Longevity in Caenorhabditis elegans. *Plant Foods for Human Nutrition (Dordrecht, Netherlands)*, *77*(1), 30–36. DOI: 10.1007/s11130-021-00939-y PMID: 35119578

Estrada-Valencia, R., Hurtado-Díaz, M. E., Rangel-López, E., Retana-Márquez, S., Túnez, I., Tinkov, A., Karasu, C., Ferrer, B., Pedraza-Chaverri, J., Aschner, M., & Santamaría, A. (2022, April). Alpha-Mangostin Alleviates the Short-term 6-Hydroxydopamine-Induced Neurotoxicity and Oxidative Damage in Rat Cortical Slices and in Caenorhabditis elegans. *Neurotoxicity Research*, *40*(2), 573–584. DOI: 10.1007/s12640-022-00493-8 PMID: 35380367

Fadel, O., El Kirat, K., & Morandat, S. (2011). The natural antioxidant rosmarinic acid spontaneously penetrates membranes to inhibit lipid peroxidation *in situ*. Biochimica et Biophysica Acta (BBA)-. *Biomembranes*, *1808*(12), 2973–2978. DOI: 10.1016/j.bbamem.2011.08.011 PMID: 21864504

Farias-Pereira, R., Camayoc, P., & Raskin, I. (2024, October 10). Isothiocyanate-Rich Moringa Seed Extract Activates SKN-1/Nrf2 Pathway in *Caenorhabditis elegans.International Journal of Molecular Sciences*, *25*(20), 10917. DOI: 10.3390/ijms252010917 PMID: 39456700

Filaferro, M., Codeluppi, A., Brighenti, V., Cimurri, F., González-Paramás, A. M., Santos-Buelga, C., Bertelli, D., Pellati, F., & Vitale, G. (2022, January 22). Disclosing the Antioxidant and Neuroprotective Activity of an Anthocyanin-Rich Extract from Sweet Cherry (*Prunus avium* L.) Using In Vitro and In Vivo Models. *Antioxidants*, *11*(2), 211. DOI: 10.3390/antiox11020211 PMID: 35204092

Fraga, C. G., Galleano, M., Verstraeten, S. V., & Oteiza, P. I. (2010). Basic biochemical mechanisms behind the health benefits of polyphenols. *Molecular Aspects of Medicine*, *31*(6), 435–445. DOI: 10.1016/j.mam.2010.09.006 PMID: 20854840

Franceschi, C., Garagnani, P., Morsiani, C., Conte, M., Santoro, A., Grignolio, A., Monti, D., Capri, M., & Salvioli, S. (2018). The continuum of aging and age-related diseases: Common mechanisms but different rates. *Frontiers in Medicine*, *5*, 61. DOI: 10.3389/fmed.2018.00061 PMID: 29662881

Fu, H. J., Zhou, X. Y., Li, Y. P., Chen, X., He, Y. N., Qin, D. L., Yu, L., Yu, C. L., Wu, J. M., Wu, A. G., & Zhou, X. G. (2023, November 20). The Protective Effects of *Reineckia carnea* Ether Fraction against Alzheimer's Disease Pathology: An Exploration in *Caenorhabditis elegans* Models. *International Journal of Molecular Sciences*, *24*(22), 16536. DOI: 10.3390/ijms242216536 PMID: 38003724

Fu, R. H., Tsai, C. W., Liu, S. P., Chiu, S. C., Chen, Y. C., Chiang, Y. T., Kuo, Y. H., Shyu, W. C., & Lin, S. Z. (2022, October 23). Neuroprotective Capability of Narcissoside in 6-OHDA-Exposed Parkinson's Disease Models through Enhancing the MiR200a/Nrf-2/GSH Axis and Mediating MAPK/Akt Associated Signaling Pathway. *Antioxidants*, *11*(11), 2089. DOI: 10.3390/antiox11112089 PMID: 36358461

Gao, L., Liu, X., Luo, X., Lou, X., Li, P., Li, X., & Liu, X. (2023). Antiaging effects of dietary supplements and natural products. *Frontiers in Pharmacology*, *14*, 1192714. DOI: 10.3389/fphar.2023.1192714 PMID: 37441528

Gao, T., Yan, N., Pu, Y., Zhang, Z., Duan, Z., Tang, Z., Huang, D., Chen, Y., Yuan, S., Yan, X., & Yuan, M. (2025, February 3). Ginger leaf polyphenols mitigate β-amyloid toxicity *via* JNK/FOXO pathway activation in *Caenorhabditis elegans.Food & Function*, *16*(3), 1072–1085. DOI: 10.1039/D4FO03238A PMID: 39829385

Gioran, A., Paikopoulos, Y., Panagiotidou, E., Rizou, A. E. I., Nasi, G. I., Dimaki, V. D., Vraila, K. D., Bezantakou, D. S., Spatharas, P. M., Papandreou, N. C., Magafa, V., Lamari, F. N., Iconomidou, V. A., & Chondrogianni, N. (2024, February 21). Beneficial Effects of *Sideritis clandestina* Extracts and Sideridiol against Amyloid β Toxicity. *Antioxidants, 13*(3), 261. DOI: 10.3390/antiox13030261 PMID: 38539796

Giunti, S., Andersen, N., Rayes, D., & De Rosa, M. J. (2021). Drug discovery: Insights from the invertebrate *Caenorhabditis elegans.Pharmacology Research & Perspectives, 9*(2), e00721. DOI: 10.1002/prp2.721 PMID: 33641258

González-Manzano, S., Ayuda-Durán, B., Martín-Sanz, R., Garzón-García, L., Santos-Buelga, C., & González-Paramás, A. M. (2024, November 29). Exploring the Neuroprotective Effects of Grape Seed Procyanidins on Amyloid-β-Induced Toxicity in *Caenorhabditis elegans.Foods, 13*(23), 3865. DOI: 10.3390/foods13233865 PMID: 39682936

Guerrero-Rubio, M. A., Hernández-García, S., Escribano, J., Jiménez-Atiénzar, M., Cabanes, J., García-Carmona, F., & Gandía-Herrero, F. (2020). Betalain health-promoting effects after ingestion in *Caenorhabditis elegans* are mediated by DAF-16/FOXO and SKN-1/Nrf2 transcription factors. *Food Chemistry, 330*, 127228. DOI: 10.1016/j.foodchem.2020.127228 PMID: 32535316

Han, S., Hu, F., Ji, X., Liu, Y., Zhang, S., Wang, Z., & Qiao, K. (2024, December). Polysaccharides from Ziziphus jujuba prolong lifespan and attenuate oxidative stress in Caenorhabditis elegans via DAF-16 and SKN-1. *International Journal of Biological Macromolecules, 282*(Pt 6), 137482. DOI: 10.1016/j.ijbiomac.2024.137482 PMID: 39528176

Han, X., Chen, X., Zheng, X., & Yan, F. (2025, February 17). Strawberry anthocyanin pelargonidin-3-glucoside attenuated OA-induced neurotoxicity by activating UPR^{mt}. *Food & Function, 16*(4), 1330–1346. DOI: 10.1039/D4FO04639K PMID: 39873116

Hayden, A. N., Leptich, E. J., & Arey, R. N. (2022, May). Invited review: Unearthing the mechanisms of age-related neurodegenerative disease using Caenorhabditis elegans. *Comparative Biochemistry and Physiology. Part A, Molecular & Integrative Physiology, 267*, 111166. DOI: 10.1016/j.cbpa.2022.111166 PMID: 35176489

Heiner, F. (2017) Neuroprotektive Wirkung von *Sideritis scardica* Griseb. In *Caenorhabditis elegans* als Modellorganismus für neurodegenerative Erkrankungen. PhD Thesis, Faculty of Lifesciences, Heidelberg University, Germany

Heiner, F., Feistel, B., & Wink, M. (2018). *Sideritis scardica* extracts inhibit aggregation and toxicity of amyloid-β in *Caenorhabditis elegans* used as a model for Alzheimer's disease. *PeerJ, 6*, e4683. DOI: 10.7717/peerj.4683 PMID: 29736334

Henderson, S. T., & Johnson, T. E. (2001). *daf-16* integrates developmental and environmental inputs to mediate aging in the nematode *Caenorhabditis elegans.Current Biology, 11*(24), 1975–1980. DOI: 10.1016/S0960-9822(01)00594-2 PMID: 11747825

Hertweck, M., Göbel, C., & Baumeister, R. (2004). *C. elegans* SGK-1 is the critical component in the Akt/PKB kinase complex to control stress response and life span. *Developmental Cell, 6*(4), 577–588. DOI: 10.1016/S1534-5807(04)00095-4 PMID: 15068796

Imamura, T., Isozumi, N., Higashimura, Y., Koga, H., Segawa, T., Desaka, N., Takagi, H., Matsumoto, K., Ohki, S., & Mori, M. (2022, March). Red-Beet Betalain Pigments Inhibit Amyloid-β Aggregation and Toxicity in Amyloid-β Expressing Caenorhabditis elegans. *Plant Foods for Human Nutrition (Dordrecht, Netherlands)*, *77*(1), 90–97. DOI: 10.1007/s11130-022-00951-w PMID: 35088214

Kampkötter, A., Nkwonkam, C. G., Zurawski, R. F., Timpel, C., Chovolou, Y., & Wätjen, W.. (2007). Effects of the flavonoids kaempferol and fisetin on thermotolerance, oxidative stress and FoxO transcription factor DAF-16 in the model organism *Caenorhabditis elegans.Archives of Toxicology*, *81*(12), 849–858. DOI: 10.1007/s00204-007-0215-4 PMID: 17551714

Kang, N., Luan, Y., Jiang, Y., Cheng, W., Liu, Y., Su, Z., Liu, Y., & Tan, P. (2022, June 17). Neuroprotective Effects of Oligosaccharides in Rehmanniae Radix on Transgenic *Caenorhabditis elegans* Models for Alzheimer's Disease. *Frontiers in Pharmacology*, *13*, 878631. DOI: 10.3389/fphar.2022.878631 PMID: 35784741

Kenyon, C. (2011). The first long-lived mutants: Discovery of the insulin/IGF-1 pathway for ageing. *Philosophical Transactions of the Royal Society of London. Series B, Biological Sciences*, *366*(1561), 9–16. DOI: 10.1098/rstb.2010.0276 PMID: 21115525

Kim, H. J., Mun, J. S., Oh, S. H., & Kim, J. H. (2024, November 30). Antioxidant and Antiaging Activity of *Houttuynia cordata* Thunb. Ethyl Acetate Fraction in *Caenorhabditis elegans.Nutrients*, *16*(23), 4168. DOI: 10.3390/nu16234168 PMID: 39683560

Kim, W., Underwood, R. S., Greenwald, I., & Shaye, D. D. (2018). OrthoList 2: A new comparative genomic analysis of human and *Caenorhabditis elegans* genes. *Genetics*, *210*(2), 445–461. DOI: 10.1534/genetics.118.301307 PMID: 30120140

Kim, Y., Lee, S. B., Cho, M., Choe, S., & Jang, M. (2023, December 20). Indian Almond (*Terminalia catappa* Linn.) Leaf Extract Extends Lifespan by Improving Lipid Metabolism and Antioxidant Activity Dependent on AMPK Signaling Pathway in *Caenorhabditis elegans* under High-Glucose-Diet Conditions. *Antioxidants*, *13*(1), 14. DOI: 10.3390/antiox13010014 PMID: 38275634

Kirchweger, B., Zwirchmayr, J., Grienke, U., & Rollinger, J. M. (2023, December 13). The role of *Caenorhabditis elegans* in the discovery of natural products for healthy aging. *Natural Product Reports*, *40*(12), 1849–1873. DOI: 10.1039/D3NP00021D PMID: 37585263

Koch, K., Weldle, N., Baier, S., Büchter, C., & Wätjen, W. (2020). *Hibiscus sabdariffa* L. extract prolongs lifespan and protects against amyloid-β toxicity in *Caenorhabditis elegans*: Involvement of the FoxO and Nrf2 orthologues DAF-16 and SKN-1. *European Journal of Nutrition*, *59*(1), 137–150. DOI: 10.1007/s00394-019-01894-w PMID: 30710163

Košinová, P., Berka, K., Wykes, M., Otyepka, M., & Trouillas, P. (2012). Positioning of antioxidant quercetin and its metabolites in lipid bilayer membranes: Implication for their lipid-peroxidation inhibition. *The Journal of Physical Chemistry B*, *116*(4), 1309–1318. DOI: 10.1021/jp208731g PMID: 22201287

Kotecha, R., Takami, A., & Espinoza, J. L. (2016). Dietary phytochemicals and cancer chemoprevention: A review of the clinical evidence. *Oncotarget*, *7*(32), 52517–52529. DOI: 10.18632/oncotarget.9593 PMID: 27232756

Kumar, S., Akhila, P. V., & Suchiang, K. (2023). Hesperidin ameliorates amyloid-β toxicity and enhances oxidative stress resistance and lifespan of Caenorhabditis elegans through acr-16 mediated activation of the autophagy pathway. *Free Radical Biology & Medicine*, *209*, 366–380.

Kutscher, L. M., & Shaham, S. (2014). Forward and reverse mutagenesis in C. elegans. WormBook: the online review of C. elegans biology, 1.

Labuschagne, C. F., & Brenkman, A. B. (2013). Current methods in quantifying ROS and oxidative damage in *Caenorhabditis elegans* and other model organism of aging. *Ageing Research Reviews*, *12*(4), 918–930. DOI: 10.1016/j.arr.2013.09.003 PMID: 24080227

Landis, J. N., & Murphy, C. T. (2010). Integration of diverse inputs in the regulation of *C. elegans* DAF-16/FOXO. *Developmental Dynamics*, *239*(5), 1405–1412. DOI: 10.1002/dvdy.22244 PMID: 20140911

Lee, J.-M., & Johnson, J. A. (2004). An important role of Nrf2-ARE pathway in the cellular defense mechanism. *BMB Reports*, *37*(2), 139–143. DOI: 10.5483/BMBRep.2004.37.2.139 PMID: 15469687

Lee, S. S., Kennedy, S., Tolonen, A. C., & Ruvkun, G. (2003). DAF-16 target genes that control *C. elegans* life-span and metabolism. *Science*, *300*(5619), 644–647. DOI: 10.1126/science.1083614 PMID: 12690206

Leiers, B., Kampkötter, A., Grevelding, C. G., Link, C. D., Johnson, T. E., & Henkle-Dührsen, K. (2003). A stress-responsive glutathione S-transferase confers resistance to oxidative stress in *Caenorhabditis elegans.Free Radical Biology & Medicine*, *34*(11), 1405–1415. DOI: 10.1016/S0891-5849(03)00102-3 PMID: 12757851

Leonov, A., Arlia-Ciommo, A., Piano, A., Svistkova, V., Lutchman, V., Medkour, Y., & Titorenko, V. (2015). Longevity extension by phytochemicals. *Molecules (Basel, Switzerland)*, *20*(4), 6544–6572. DOI: 10.3390/molecules20046544 PMID: 25871373

Leopoldini, M., Russo, N., & Toscano, M. (2011). The molecular basis of working mechanism of natural polyphenolic antioxidants. *Food Chemistry*, *125*(2), 288–306. DOI: 10.1016/j.foodchem.2010.08.012

Li, H., Roxo, M., Cheng, X., Zhang, S., Cheng, H., & Wink, M. (2019). Pro-oxidant and lifespan extension effects of caffeine and Related methylxanthines in *Caenorhabditis elegans.Food Chemistry: X*, *1*, 100005. Advance online publication. DOI: 10.1016/j.fochx.2019.100005 PMID: 31432005

Li, K., Zhang, S., Sun, Y., Chen, Y., Chen, W., Ruan, W., & Liu, Y. (2022b, July). Antiamyloid β toxicity effect of genistein via activation of DAF-16 and HSP-16.2 signal pathways in Caenorhabditis elegans. *Journal of Biochemical and Molecular Toxicology*, *36*(7), e23055. DOI: 10.1002/jbt.23055 PMID: 35373417

Li, R., Tao, M., Xu, T., Huang, Y., Zogona, D., Pan, S., Wu, T., & Xu, X. (2022a, August 30). *Artemisia selengensis* Turcz. leaf extract promotes longevity and stress resistance in Caenorhabditis elegans. *Journal of the Science of Food and Agriculture*, *102*(11), 4532–4541. DOI: 10.1002/jsfa.11808 PMID: 35122267

Li, R., Yi, Q., Wang, J., Miao, Y., Chen, Q., Xu, Y., & Tao, M. (2024a, April). Paeonol promotes longevity and fitness in Caenorhabditis elegans through activating the DAF-16/FOXO and SKN-1/Nrf2 transcription factors. *Biomedicine and Pharmacotherapy*, *173*, 116368. DOI: 10.1016/j.biopha.2024.116368 PMID: 38471269

Li, X., Hu, M., Zhou, X., Yu, L., Qin, D., Wu, J., Deng, L., Huang, L., Ren, F., Liao, B., Wu, A., & Fan, D. (2024b, November 1). Hederagenin inhibits mitochondrial damage in Parkinson's disease via mitophagy induction. *Free Radical Biology & Medicine*, *224*, 740–756. DOI: 10.1016/j.freeradbiomed.2024.09.030 PMID: 39313012

Li, X., Wang, X., Wang, K., Yang, X., Liu, X., Chen, J., Li, J., Wang, J., Guo, Q., & Wang, H. (2023, March). Black rice anthocyanin extract enhances the antioxidant capacity in PC12 cells and improves the lifespan by activating IIS pathway in Caenorhabditis elegans. *Comparative Biochemistry and Physiology. Toxicology & Pharmacology : CBP*, *265*, 109533. DOI: 10.1016/j.cbpc.2022.109533 PMID: 36549628

Liang, L., Yue, Y., Zhong, L., Liang, Y., Shi, R., Luo, R., Zhao, M., Cao, X., Yang, M., Du, J., Shen, X., Wang, Y., & Shu, Z. (2023, December 31). Anti-aging activities of Rehmannia glutinosa Libosch. crude polysaccharide in Caenorhabditis elegans based on gut microbiota and metabonomic analysis. *International Journal of Biological Macromolecules*, *253*(Pt 8), 127647. DOI: 10.1016/j.ijbiomac.2023.127647 PMID: 37884235

Libina, N., Berman, J. R., & Kenyon, C. (2003). Tissue-specific activities of *C. elegans* DAF-16 in the regulation of lifespan. *Cell*, *115*(4), 489–502. DOI: 10.1016/S0092-8674(03)00889-4 PMID: 14622602

Lima, M. E., Colpo, A. C., Salgueiro, W. G., Sardinha, G. E., Ávila, D. S., & Folmer, V. (2014). *Ilex paraguariensis* extract increases lifespan and protects against the toxic effects caused by paraquat in *Caenorhabditis elegans.International Journal of Environmental Research and Public Health*, *11*(10), 10091–10104. DOI: 10.3390/ijerph111010091 PMID: 25264684

Lin, K., Hsin, H., Libina, N., & Kenyon, C. (2001). Regulation of the *Caenorhabditis elegans* longevity protein DAF-16 by insulin/IGF-1 and germline signaling. *Nature Genetics*, *28*(2), 139–145. DOI: 10.1038/88850 PMID: 11381260

Link, C. D. (2006). *C. elegans* models of age-associated neurodegenerative diseases: Lessons from transgenic worm models of Alzheimer's disease. *Experimental Gerontology*, *41*(10), 1007–1013. DOI: 10.1016/j.exger.2006.06.059 PMID: 16930903

Link, C. D., Cypser, J. R., Johnson, C. J., & Johnson, T. E. (1999). Direct observation of stress response in *Caenorhabditis elegans* using a reporter transgene. *Cell Stress & Chaperones*, *4*(4), 235. DOI: 10.1379/1466-1268(1999)004<0235:DOOSRI>2.3.CO;2 PMID: 10590837

Link, C. D., & Johnson, C. J. (2002). *Reporter transgenes for study of oxidant stress in Caenorhabditis elegans. Meth Enzymol 353*. Elsevier.

Link, C. D., Taft, A., Kapulkin, V., Duke, K., Kim, S., & Fei, Q.. (2003). Gene expression analysis in a transgenic *Caenorhabditis elegans* Alzheimer's disease model. *Neurobiology of Aging*, *24*(3), 397–413. DOI: 10.1016/S0197-4580(02)00224-5 PMID: 12600716

Link, P., Fu, Y., Wetterauer, B., & Wink, M. (2015). Extracts of *Glycyrrhiza uralensis* and isoliquiritigenin, one of its compounds, counteract amyloid-beta toxicity in *Caenorhabditis elegans.Planta Medica, 81*(5), 357–362. DOI: 10.1055/s-0035-1545724 PMID: 25782036

Link, P., Roth, K., Sporer, F., & Wink, M. (2016). Carlina acaulis exhibits antioxidant activity and counteracts Aβ toxicity in Caenorhabditis elegans. *Molecules (Basel, Switzerland), 21*(7), 871.

Link, P., & Wink, M. (2019). Isoliquiritigenin exerts antioxidant activity in *Caenorhabditis elegans* via insulin-like signaling pathway and SKN-1. *Phytomedicine, 55*, 119–124. DOI: 10.1016/j.phymed.2018.07.004 PMID: 30668421

Long, T., Tang, Y., He, Y. N., He, C. L., Chen, X., Guo, M. S., Wu, J. M., Yu, L., Yu, C. L., Yuen-Kwan Law, B., Qin, D. L., Wu, A. G., & Zhou, X. G. (2022, November 21). Citri Reticulatae Semen Extract Promotes Healthy Aging and Neuroprotection via Autophagy Induction in Caenorhabditis elegans. *The Journals of Gerontology. Series A, Biological Sciences and Medical Sciences, 77*(11), 2186–2194. DOI: 10.1093/gerona/glac136 PMID: 35788666

Loo, J., Shah Bana, M. A. F., Tan, J. K., & Goon, J. A. (2023, October 15). Effect of dietary restriction on health span in Caenorhabditis elegans: A systematic review. *Experimental Gerontology, 182*, 112294. DOI: 10.1016/j.exger.2023.112294 PMID: 37730186

Lublin, A., & Link, C. (2013). Alzheimer's disease drug discovery: *In vivo* screening using *Caenorhabditis elegans* as a model for β-amyloid peptide-induced toxicity. *Drug Discovery Today. Technologies, 10*(1), e115–e9. DOI: 10.1016/j.ddtec.2012.02.002 PMID: 24050239

Luo, J., Zhang, X., Li, W., Lan, Y., Li, F., Xiao, J., & Chen, Y. (2024). Pentagalloyl glucose enhanced the stress resistance to delay aging process in Caenorhabditis elegans. *Process Biochemistry, 146*, 462–472.

Luo, S., Jiang, X., Jia, L., Tan, C., Li, M., Yang, Q., Du, Y., & Ding, C. (2019). *In vivo* and *in vitro* antioxidant activities of methanol extracts from olive leaves on *Caenorhabditis elegans.Molecules (Basel, Switzerland), 24*(4), 704. DOI: 10.3390/molecules24040704 PMID: 30781358

Markaki, M., & Tavernarakis, N. (2010). Modeling human diseases in *Caenorhabditis elegans.Biotechnology Journal, 5*(12), 1261–1276. DOI: 10.1002/biot.201000183 PMID: 21154667

McIntyre, R. L., Liu, Y. J., Hu, M., Morris, B. J., Willcox, B. J., Donlon, T. A., Houtkooper, R. H., & Janssens, G. E. (2022, June). Pharmaceutical and nutraceutical activation of FOXO3 for healthy longevity. *Ageing Research Reviews, 78*, 101621. DOI: 10.1016/j.arr.2022.101621 PMID: 35421606

Meng, J., Lv, Z., Guo, M., Sun, C., Li, X., Jiang, Z., Zhang, W., & Chen, C. (2022, February). A Lycium barbarum extract inhibits β-amyloid toxicity by activating the antioxidant system and mtUPR in a Caenorhabditis elegans model of Alzheimer's disease. *The FASEB Journal, 36*(2), e22156. DOI: 10.1096/fj.202101116RR PMID: 35044707

Mi, L., Fan, M., Liu, T., Wu, D., Wang, Y., Li, F., Cai, Y., Qiu, Z., Liu, D., & Cao, L. (2022, December 15). Ginsenoside Rd protects transgenic *Caenorhabditis elegans* from β-amyloid toxicity by activating oxidative resistant. *Frontiers in Pharmacology, 13*, 1074397. DOI: 10.3389/fphar.2022.1074397 PMID: 36588689

Mishra, S. K., Balendra, V., Esposto, J., Obaid, A. A., Maccioni, R. B., Jha, N. K., Perry, G., Moustafa, M., Al-Shehri, M., Singh, M. P., Khan, A. A., Vamanu, E., & Singh, S. K. (2022, October 8). Therapeutic Antiaging Strategies. *Biomedicines*, *10*(10), 2515. DOI: 10.3390/biomedicines10102515 PMID: 36289777

Mohanty, S. K., & Suchiang, K. (2023, September 15). Baicalein mitigates oxidative stress and enhances lifespan through modulation of Wnt ligands and GATA factor: ELT-3 in Caenorhabditis elegans. *Life Sciences*, *329*, 121946. DOI: 10.1016/j.lfs.2023.121946 PMID: 37463652

Morley, J. F., Brignull, H. R., Weyers, J. J., & Morimoto, R. I. (2002). The threshold for polyglutamine-expansion protein aggregation and cellular toxicity is dynamic and influenced by aging in *Caenorhabditis elegans.Proceedings of the National Academy of Sciences of the United States of America*, *99*(16), 10417–10422. DOI: 10.1073/pnas.152161099 PMID: 12122205

Morton, E. A., & Lamitina, T. (2013). *Caenorhabditis elegans* HSF-1 is an essential nuclear protein that forms stress granule-like structures following heat shock. *Aging Cell*, *12*(1), 112–120. DOI: 10.1111/acel.12024 PMID: 23107491

Muhammad, F., Liu, Y., Wang, N., Zhao, L., Zhou, Y., Yang, H., & Li, H. (2022, December). Neuroprotective effects of cannabidiol on dopaminergic neurodegeneration and α-synuclein accumulation in C. elegans models of Parkinson's disease. *Neurotoxicology*, *93*, 128–139. DOI: 10.1016/j.neuro.2022.09.001 PMID: 36108815

Muhammad, F., Liu, Y., Wang, N., Zhao, L., Zhou, Y., Yang, H., & Li, H. (2023, July). Rose essential oil diminishes dopaminergic neuron degenerations and reduces α-synuclein aggregation in Caenorhabditis elegans models of Parkinson's disease. *Phytotherapy Research*, *37*(7), 2877–2893. DOI: 10.1002/ptr.7783 PMID: 36920348

Murphy, C. T., & Hu, P. J. (2018). Insulin/insulin-like growth factor signaling in C. elegans. WormBook: The online review of C. elegans biology [Internet].

Murphy, C. T., McCarroll, S. A., Bargmann, C. I., Fraser, A., Kamath, R. S., Ahringer, J., Li, H., & Kenyon, C. (2003). Genes that act downstream of DAF-16 to influence the lifespan of *Caenorhabditis elegans.Nature*, *424*(6946), 277–283. DOI: 10.1038/nature01789 PMID: 12845331

Mursu, J., Virtanen, J. K., Tuomainen, T.-P., Nurmi, T., & Voutilainen, S. (2014). Intake of fruit, berries, and vegetables and risk of type 2 diabetes in Finnish men: The Kuopio Ischaemic Heart Disease Risk Factor Study. *The American Journal of Clinical Nutrition*, *99*(2), 328–333. DOI: 10.3945/ajcn.113.069641 PMID: 24257723

N'Soukpoe-Kossi, C., Bourassa, P., Mandeville, J., Bekale, L., & Tajmir-Riahi, H. (2015). Structural modeling for DNA binding to antioxidants resveratrol, genistein and curcumin. *Journal of Photochemistry and Photobiology. B, Biology*, *151*, 69–75. DOI: 10.1016/j.jphotobiol.2015.07.007 PMID: 26188387

Naskar, R., Ghosh, A., Bhattacharya, R., & Chakraborty, S. (2024, November). A critical appraisal of geroprotective activities of flavonoids in terms of their bio-accessibility and polypharmacology. *Neurochemistry International*, *180*, 105859. DOI: 10.1016/j.neuint.2024.105859 PMID: 39265701

Nishioka, Y., Nishikawa, S., & Shibata, T. (2020). *A hot water extract of Sideritis scardica prolongs life span and enhances heat shock resistance in Caenorhabditis elegans*. Nat Prod Comm. DOI: 10.1177/1934578X20917283

Niu, Y., Liao, J., Zhou, H., Wang, C. C., Wang, L., & Fan, Y. (2022, August 3). Flavonoids from *Lycium barbarum* Leaves Exhibit Anti-Aging Effects through the Redox-Modulation. *Molecules (Basel, Switzerland)*, *27*(15), 4952. DOI: 10.3390/molecules27154952 PMID: 35956901

Ösz, A., Takács-Vellai, K., & Farkas, Z. (2025). Mutations of the Electron Transport Chain Affect Lifespan and ROS Levels in *C. elegans.Antioxidants*, *14*(1), 76. DOI: 10.3390/antiox14010076 PMID: 39857410

Oteiza, P. I., Erlejman, A. G., Verstraeten, S. V., Keen, C. L., & Fraga, C. G. (2005). Flavonoid-membrane interactions: A protective role of flavonoids at the membrane surface? *Clinical & Developmental Immunology*, *12*, 19–25. PMID: 15712595

Ozdal, T., Capanoglu, E., & Altay, F. (2013). A review on protein–phenolic interactions and associated changes. *Food Research International*, *51*(2), 954–970. DOI: 10.1016/j.foodres.2013.02.009

Palmioli, A., Mazzoni, V., De Luigi, A., Bruzzone, C., Sala, G., Colombo, L., Bazzini, C., Zoia, C. P., Inserra, M., Salmona, M., De Noni, I., Ferrarese, C., Diomede, L., & Airoldi, C. (2022, November 16). Alzheimer's Disease Prevention through Natural Compounds: Cell-Free, In Vitro, and In Vivo Dissection of Hop (*Humulus lupulus* L.) Multitarget Activity. *ACS Chemical Neuroscience*, *13*(22), 3152–3167. DOI: 10.1021/acschemneuro.2c00444 PMID: 36283035

Park, S., & Park, S. K. (2022, October 8). Anti-Oxidant and Anti-Aging Effects of Phlorizin Are Mediated by DAF-16-Induced Stress Response and Autophagy in *Caenorhabditis elegans.Antioxidants*, *11*(10), 1996. DOI: 10.3390/antiox11101996 PMID: 36290719

Park, S.-H. (2024). Role of Phytochemicals in Treatment of Aging and Cancer: Focus on Mechanism of FOXO3 Activation. *Antioxidants*, *13*(9), 1099. DOI: 10.3390/antiox13091099 PMID: 39334758

Parrales, V., Arcile, G., Laserre, L., Normant, S., Le Goff, G., Da Costa Noble, C., Ouazzani, J., Callizot, N., Haïk, S., Rabhi, C., & Bizat, N. (2025). Guillaume Arcile, Louise Laserre, Sébastien Normant, Géraldine Le Goff, Christian Da Costa Noble, Jamal Ouazzani, Noelle Callizot, Stéphane Haïk, Chérif Rabhi, and Nicolas Bizat Neuroprotective Effect of Withaferin Derivatives toward MPP^+ and 6-OHDA Toxicity to Dopaminergic Neurons. *ACS Chemical Neuroscience*, *16*(5), 802–817. DOI: 10.1021/acschemneuro.4c00655 PMID: 39946298

Parween, N., Jabeen, A., & Prasad, B. (2022). Eugenol Elicits Prolongevity by Increasing Resistance to Oxidative Stress in C. elegans. *CNS & Neurological Disorders - Drug Targets*, *21*(9), 841–853. DOI: 10.2174/1871527320666211008150347 PMID: 34629046

Peixoto, H., Roxo, M., Koolen, H., da Silva, F., Silva, E., Braun, M., Wang, X., & Wink, M. (2018). M Wink 2018 *Calycophyllum spruceanum* (Benth.), the Amazonian "tree of youth" prolongs longevity and enhances stress resistance in *Caenorhabditis elegans.Molecules (Basel, Switzerland)*, *23*(3), 534. DOI: 10.3390/molecules23030534 PMID: 29495517

Peixoto, H., Roxo, M., Krstin, S., Röhrig, T., Richling, E., & Wink, M. (2016a). An anthocyanin-rich extract of acai (*Euterpe precatoria* Mart.) increases stress resistance and retards aging-related markers in *Caenorhabditis elegans.Journal of Agricultural and Food Chemistry*, *64*(6), 1283–1290. DOI: 10.1021/acs.jafc.5b05812 PMID: 26809379

Peixoto, H., Roxo, M., Krstin, S., Wang, X., & Wink, M. (2016b). Anthocyanin-rich extract of Acai (*Euterpe precatoria* Mart.) mediates neuroprotective activities in *Caenorhabditis elegans.Journal of Functional Foods*, *26*, 385–393. DOI: 10.1016/j.jff.2016.08.012

Peixoto, H., Roxo, M., Röhrig, T., Richling, E., Wang, X., & Wink, M. (2017). Anti-aging and antioxidant potential of *Paullinia cupana* var. *sorbilis*: Findings in *Caenorhabditis elegans* indicate a new utilization for roasted seeds of guarana. *Medicines (Basel, Switzerland)*, *4*(3), 61. DOI: 10.3390/medicines4030061 PMID: 28930275

Peixoto, H., Roxo, M., Silva, E., Valente, K., Braun, M., Wang, X., & Wink, M. (2019). Bark extract of the amazonian tree *Endopleura uchi* (Humiriaceae) extends lifespan and enhances stress resistance in *Caenorhabditis elegans.Molecules (Basel, Switzerland)*, *24*(5), 915. DOI: 10.3390/molecules24050915 PMID: 30845642

Perron, N. R., & Brumaghim, J. L. (2009). A review of the antioxidant mechanisms of polyphenol compounds related to iron binding. *Cell Biochemistry and Biophysics*, *53*(2), 75–100. DOI: 10.1007/s12013-009-9043-x PMID: 19184542

Phoraksa, O., Chimkerd, C., Thiyajai, P., Judprasong, K., Tuntipopipat, S., Tencomnao, T., Charoenkiatkul, S., Muangnoi, C., & Sukprasansap, M. (2023, July 10). Neuroprotective Effects of *Albizia lebbeck* (L.) Benth. Leaf Extract against Glutamate-Induced Endoplasmic Reticulum Stress and Apoptosis in Human Microglial Cells. *Pharmaceuticals (Basel, Switzerland)*, *16*(7), 989. DOI: 10.3390/ph16070989 PMID: 37513900

Phoraksa, O., Vongthip, W., Juntranggoor, P., Maiuthed, A., Tuntipopipat, S., Charoenkiatkul, S., & Sukprasansap, M. (2025). Bioavailable fraction from edible leaf of Albizia lebbeck (L.) Benth. Inhibits neurotoxicity in human microglial HMC3 cells, and promotes lifespan in Caenorhabditis elegans. *International Journal of Food Science & Technology*, •••, vvae067.

Prasanth, M. I., Brimson, J. M., Chuchawankul, S., Sukprasansap, M., & Tencomnao, T. (2019). Antiaging, stress resistance, and neuroprotective efficacies of Cleistocalyx nervosum var. paniala fruit extracts using Caenorhabditis elegans model. *Oxidative Medicine and Cellular Longevity*, *2019*(1), 7024785.

Proshkina, E., Koval, L., Platonova, E., Golubev, D., Ulyasheva, N., Babak, T., Shaposhnikov, M., & Moskalev, A. (2024, March). Polyphenols as Potential Geroprotectors. *Antioxidants & Redox Signaling*, *40*(7-9), 564–593. DOI: 10.1089/ars.2023.0247 PMID: 38251662

Qi, Z., Ji, H., Le, M., Li, H., Wieland, A., Bauer, S., Liu, L., Wink, M., & Herr, I. (2021). Sulforaphane promotes *C. elegans* longevity and health span by DAF-16/DAF-2 insulin/IGF-1 signaling. *Aging (Albany NY)*, *13*(2), 2021. DOI: 10.18632/aging.202512

Qin, Y., Chen, F., Tang, Z., Ren, H., Wang, Q., Shen, N., Lin, W., Xiao, Y., Yuan, M., Chen, H., Bu, T., Li, Q., & Huang, L. (2022, October 26). *Ligusticum chuanxiong* Hort as a medicinal and edible plant foods: Antioxidant, anti-aging and neuroprotective properties in *Caenorhabditis elegans.Frontiers in Pharmacology, 13*, 1049890. DOI: 10.3389/fphar.2022.1049890 PMID: 36386171

Ramatchandirane, M., Rajendran, P., Athira, M. P., & Suchiang, K. (2024, December 14). Coniferaldehyde activates autophagy and enhances oxidative stress resistance and lifespan of Caenorhabditis elegans via par-4/aak-2/skn-1 pathway. *Biogerontology, 26*(1), 25. DOI: 10.1007/s10522-024-10163-1 PMID: 39674829

Rangsinth, P., Prasansuklab, A., Duangjan, C., Gu, X., Meemon, K., Wink, M., & Tencomnao, T. (2019). Leaf extract of *Caesalpinia mimosoides* enhances oxidative stress resistance and prolongs lifespan in *Caenorhabditis elegans.BMC Complementary and Alternative Medicine, 19*(1), 1–13. DOI: 10.1186/s12906-019-2578-5 PMID: 31286949

Regitz, C., Fitzenberger, E., Mahn, F. L., Dußling, L. M., & Wenzel, U. (2016). Resveratrol reduces amyloid-beta (Aβ 1–42)-induced paralysis through targeting proteostasis in an Alzheimer model of *Caenorhabditis elegans.European Journal of Nutrition, 55*(2), 741–747. DOI: 10.1007/s00394-015-0894-1 PMID: 25851110

Rezaizadehnajafi, L., & Wink, M. (2014). EPs7630® from *Pelargonium sidoides* increases stress resistance in *Caenorhabditis elegans* and enhances life span probably via the DAF-16/FOXO pathway. *Phytomedicine, 21*, 547–550. DOI: 10.1016/j.phymed.2013.10.027 PMID: 24252337

Robida-Stubbs, S., Glover-Cutter, K., Lamming, D. W., Mizunuma, M., Narasimhan, S. D., Neumann-Haefelin, E., Sabatini, D. M., & Blackwell, T. K. (2012). TOR signaling and rapamycin influence longevity by regulating SKN-1/Nrf and DAF-16/FoxO. *Cell Metabolism, 15*(5), 713–724. DOI: 10.1016/j.cmet.2012.04.007 PMID: 22560223

Romero-Márquez, J. M., Navarro-Hortal, M. D., Jiménez-Trigo, V., Vera-Ramírez, L., Forbes-Hernández, T. J., Esteban-Muñoz, A., Giampieri, F., Bullón, P., Battino, M., Sánchez-González, C., & Quiles, J. L. (2022, April). An oleuropein rich-olive (Olea europaea L.) leaf extract reduces β-amyloid and tau proteotoxicity through regulation of oxidative- and heat shock-stress responses in Caenorhabditis elegans. *Food and Chemical Toxicology, 162*, 112914. DOI: 10.1016/j.fct.2022.112914 PMID: 35276233

Roxo, M., Peixoto, H., Wetterauer, P., Lima, E., & Wink, M. (2020). Piquiá shells (Caryocar villosum): A fruit by-product with antioxidant and antiaging properties in Caenorhabditis elegans. *Oxidative Medicine and Cellular Longevity, 2020*(1), 7590707.

Roxo, M., & Wink, M. (2022). The use of the nematode Caenorhabditis elegans to study antioxidant and longevity-promoting plant secondary metabolites. *New Find Nat Subs, 6*, 133–163.

Saier, C., Gommlich, I., Hiemann, V., Baier, S., Koch, K., Horn, G., Kowalewsky, T., Bartelt, J., Seemann, M., & Wätjen, W. (2018). *Agrimonia procera* Wallr. Extract Increases stress resistance and prolongs life span in *Caenorhabditis elegans* via transcription factor DAF-16 (FoxO Orthologue). *Antioxidants, 7*(12), 192. DOI: 10.3390/antiox7120192 PMID: 30558122

Savova, M. S., Todorova, M. N., Binev, B. K., Georgiev, M. I., & Mihaylova, L. V. (2025, January 24). Curcumin enhances the anti-obesogenic activity of orlistat through SKN-1/NRF2-dependent regulation of nutrient metabolism in Caenorhabditis elegans. *International Journal of Obesity*, *49*(3), 516–526. Advance online publication. DOI: 10.1038/s41366-025-01724-6 PMID: 39856245

Scalbert, A., Manach, C., Morand, C., Rémésy, C., & Jiménez, L. (2005). Dietary polyphenols and the prevention of diseases. *Critical Reviews in Food Science and Nutrition*, *45*(4), 287–306. DOI: 10.1080/1040869059096 PMID: 16047496

Scerbak, C., Vayndorf, E., Hernandez, A., McGill, C., & Taylor, B. (2018). Lowbush cranberry acts through DAF-16/FOXO signaling to promote increased lifespan and axon branching in aging posterior touch receptor neurons. *GeroScience*, *40*(2), 151–162. DOI: 10.1007/s11357-018-0016-0 PMID: 29717416

Selkoe, D. J., & Hardy, J. (2016). The amyloid hypothesis of Alzheimer's disease at 25 years. *EMBO Molecular Medicine*, *8*(6), 595–608. DOI: 10.15252/emmm.201606210 PMID: 27025652

Sen, I., Zhou, X., Chernobrovkin, A., Puerta-Cavanzo, N., Kanno, T., Salignon, J., Stoehr, A., Lin, X.-X., Baskaner, B., Brandenburg, S., Björkegren, C., Zubarev, R. A., & Riedel, C. G. (2020). DAF-16/FOXO requires Protein Phosphatase 4 to initiate transcription of stress resistance and longevity promoting genes. *Nature Communications*, *11*(1), 1–17. DOI: 10.1038/s41467-019-13931-7 PMID: 31919361

Senchuk, M. M., Dues, D. J., & Van Raamsdonk, J. M. (2017). Measuring oxidative stress in *Caenorhabditis elegans*: Paraquat and juglone sensitivity assays. *Bio-Protocol*, *7*(1), e2086. DOI: 10.21769/BioProtoc.2086 PMID: 29276721

Seo, K., Choi, E., Lee, D., Jeong, D. E., Jang, S. K., & Lee, S. J. (2013). Heat shock factor 1 mediates the longevity conferred by inhibition of TOR and insulin/IGF-1 signaling pathways in *C. elegans.Aging Cell*, *12*(6), 1073–1081. DOI: 10.1111/acel.12140 PMID: 23879233

Shi, X., Yu, X., Yang, L., & Duan, X. (2023, July 7). Ethyl acetate extract of *Gastrodia elata* protects *Caenorhabditis elegans* from oxidative stress and amyloid β peptide toxicity. *Experimental and Therapeutic Medicine*, *26*(2), 405. DOI: 10.3892/etm.2023.12104 PMID: 37522064

Sies, H., & Jones, D. P. (2020). Reactive oxygen species (ROS) as pleiotropic physiological signalling agents. *Nature Reviews. Molecular Cell Biology*, *21*(7), 363–383. DOI: 10.1038/s41580-020-0230-3 PMID: 32231263

Sirk, T. W., Brown, E. F., Friedman, M., & Sum, A. K. (2009). Molecular binding of catechins to biomembranes: Relationship to biological activity. *Journal of Agricultural and Food Chemistry*, *57*(15), 6720–6728. DOI: 10.1021/jf900951w PMID: 19572638

Siswanto, F. M., Sakuma, R., Oguro, A., & Imaoka, S. (2022, August 12). Chlorogenic Acid Activates Nrf2/SKN-1 and Prolongs the Lifespan of Caenorhabditis elegans via the Akt-FOXO3/DAF16a-DDB1 Pathway and Activation of DAF16f. *The Journals of Gerontology. Series A, Biological Sciences and Medical Sciences*, *77*(8), 1503–1516. DOI: 10.1093/gerona/glac062 PMID: 35279029

Sobeh, M., ElHawary, E., Peixoto, H., Labib, R. M., Handoussa, H., Swilam, N., El-Khatib, A. H., Sharapov, F., Mohamed, T., Krstin, S., Linscheid, M. W., Singab, A. N., Wink, M., & Ayoub, N. (2016). Identification of phenolic secondary metabolites from *Schotia brachypetala* Sond. (Fabaceae) and demonstration of their antioxidant activities in *Caenorhabditis elegans.PeerJ*, *4*, e2404. DOI: 10.7717/peerj.2404 PMID: 27896020

Sobeh, M., Mahmoud, M. F., Abdelfattah, M. A., Cheng, H., El-Shazly, A. M., & Wink, M. (2018). A proanthocyanidin-rich extract from *Cassia abbreviata* exhibits antioxidant and hepatoprotective activities *in vivo.Journal of Ethnopharmacology*, *213*, 38–47. DOI: 10.1016/j.jep.2017.11.007 PMID: 29126990

Song, L., & Zhang, S. (2023, October 31). Anti-Aging Activity and Modes of Action of Compounds from Natural Food Sources. *Biomolecules*, *13*(11), 1600. DOI: 10.3390/biom13111600 PMID: 38002283

Spotorno, V. G., Roxo, M., Lópeza, M., Zabalc, O. A., & Wink, M. (2025). Effects on neuroprotection and alpha-synuclein expression of a *Canna coccinea* rhizome extract. *Fitoterapia*, *181*, 106380. Advance online publication. DOI: 10.1016/j.fitote.2025.106380 PMID: 39765315

Strange, K. (2006). *An overview of C. elegans biology. C elegans*. Springer.

Sun, M., Wei, C., Gao, Y., Chen, X., Zhong, K., Li, Y., Yang, Z., Gao, Y., & Wang, H. (2024, September 4). TSG Extends the Longevity of *Caenorhabditis elegans* by Targeting the DAF-16/SKN-1/SIR-2.1-Mediated Mitochondrial Quality Control Process. *Antioxidants*, *13*(9), 1086. DOI: 10.3390/antiox13091086 PMID: 39334745

Sural, S., Lu, T.-C., Jung, S. A., & Hsu, A.-L. (2019). HSB-1 inhibition and HSF-1 overexpression trigger overlapping transcriptional changes to promote longevity in *Caenorhabditis elegans.G3 (Bethesda, Md.)*, *9*(5), 1679–1692. DOI: 10.1534/g3.119.400044 PMID: 30894454

Tambara, A. L., de Los Santos Moraes, L., Dal Forno, A. H., Boldori, J. R., Gonçalves Soares, A. T., de Freitas Rodrigues, C., Mariutti, L. R. B., Mercadante, A. Z., de Ávila, D. S., & Denardin, C. C. (2018). Purple pitanga fruit (*Eugenia uniflora* L.) protects against oxidative stress and increase the lifespan in *Caenorhabditis elegans* via the DAF-16/FOXO pathway. *Food and Chemical Toxicology*, *120*, 639–650. DOI: 10.1016/j.fct.2018.07.057 PMID: 30077708

Tao, M., Li, R., Xu, T., Zhang, Z., Zheng, D., Xia, Z., Wu, T., Pan, S., & Xu, X. (2023, September). Vitexin and isovitexin delayed ageing and enhanced stress-resistance through the activation of the SKN-1/Nrf2 signaling pathway. *International Journal of Food Sciences and Nutrition*, *74*(6), 685–694. DOI: 10.1080/09637486.2023.2243055 PMID: 37604809

Thabit, S., Handoussa, H., El Sayed, N. S., Breitinger, H., Breitinger, U., & Wink, M. (2023). A fruit extract of *Styphnolobium japonicum* (L.) counteracts oxidative stress and mediates neuroprotection in *Caenorhabditis elegans* possibly through the SKN-1/Nrf-2 pathway. *BMC Complementary Medicine and Therapies*, *23*(1), 333. DOI: 10.1186/s12906-023-04149-8

Thabit, S., Handoussa, H., Roxo, M., El Sayed, N. S., de Azevedo, B. C., & Wink, M. (2018). Evaluation of antioxidant and neuroprotective activities of *Cassia fistula* (L.) using the *Caenorhabditis elegans* model. *PeerJ*, *6*, e5159. DOI: 10.7717/peerj.5159 PMID: 30023139

Thew, H. Y., Boon Keat, K., Tan, Y. C., Ong, Y. S., Parat, M. O., Murugaiyah, V., Goh, B. H., & Khaw, K. Y. (2024, May 1). Probing the anti-Aβ42 aggregation and protective effects of prenylated xanthone against Aβ42-induced toxicity in transgenic Caenorhabditis elegans model. *Chemico-Biological Interactions, 394*, 110978. DOI: 10.1016/j.cbi.2024.110978 PMID: 38552766

Thomas, C., Erni, R., Wu, J. Y., Fischer, F., Lamers, G., Grigolon, G., Mitchell, S. J., Zarse, K., Carreira, E. M., & Ristow, M. (2023, December 8). A naturally occurring polyacetylene isolated from carrots promotes health and delays signatures of aging. *Nature Communications, 14*(1), 8142. DOI: 10.1038/s41467-023-43672-7 PMID: 38065964

Todorova, M. N., Savova, M. S., Mihaylova, L. V., & Georgiev, M. I. (2023, December 26). Icariin Improves Stress Resistance and Extends Lifespan in *Caenorhabditis elegans* through *hsf-1* and *daf-2*-Driven Hormesis. *International Journal of Molecular Sciences, 25*(1), 352. DOI: 10.3390/ijms25010352 PMID: 38203522

Tullet, J. M., Hertweck, M., An, J. H., Baker, J., Hwang, J. Y., Liu, S., Oliveira, R. P., Baumeister, R., & Blackwell, T. K. (2008). Direct inhibition of the longevity-promoting factor SKN-1 by insulin-like signaling in *C. elegans.Cell, 132*(6), 1025–1038. DOI: 10.1016/j.cell.2008.01.030 PMID: 18358814

Upadhayay, S., Jamwal, S., & Kumar, P. (2023, May). Animal models of Huntington's disease and their applicability to novel drug discovery and development. *Expert Opinion on Drug Discovery, 18*(5), 527–538. DOI: 10.1080/17460441.2023.2201493 PMID: 37042034

van Wyk, B.-E., & Wink, M. (2017). *Medicinal plants of the World* (2nd ed.). Briza.

Wang, E., Wang, N., Zou, Y., Fahim, M., Zhou, Y., Yang, H., Liu, Y., & Li, H. (2022d). Black mulberry (*Morus nigra*) fruit extract alleviated AD-Like symptoms induced by toxic Aβ protein in transgenic Caenorhabditis elegans via insulin DAF-16 signaling pathway. *Food Research International, 160*, 111696. DOI: 10.1016/j.foodres.2022.111696 PMID: 36076399

Wang, E., & Wink, M. (2016). Chlorophyll enhances oxidative stress tolerance in *Caenorhabditis elegans* and extends its lifespan. *PeerJ, 4*, e1879. DOI: 10.7717/peerj.1879 PMID: 27077003

Wang, J., Yang, J., Lu, J., Lu, J., Ling, B., Song, Y., & Chen, G. (2025, January 23). Ursonic Acid Ameliorates H_2O_2-Induced Oxidative Damage in PC12 Cells and Prolonged the Lifespan in C. elegans by Activating MAPKs/Nrf2/HO-1 Signaling Pathway. *Molecular Neurobiology, 62*(5), 6598–6611. Advance online publication. DOI: 10.1007/s12035-025-04701-2 PMID: 39849276

Wang, J., Zhu, D., Cui, H., Xu, Y., Shang, S., Miao, Y., Xu, Z., & Li, R. (2024a, December 24). Molecular mechanism of culinary herb *Artemisia argyi* in promoting lifespan and stress tolerance. *NPJ Science of Food, 8*(1), 111. DOI: 10.1038/s41538-024-00358-8 PMID: 39719452

Wang, K., Zhang, X., Zhang, M., Li, X., Xie, J., Liu, S., Huang, Q., Wang, J., Guo, Q., & Wang, H. (2023a, December). Hyperoside Prevents Aβ42-Induced Neurotoxicity in PC12 Cells and *Caenorhabditis elegans.Molecular Neurobiology, 60*(12), 7136–7150. DOI: 10.1007/s12035-023-03521-6 PMID: 37535309

Wang, R., Ding, A., Wang, J., Wang, J., Zhou, Y., Chen, M., Ju, S., Tan, M., & Xiang, Z. (2024c). Astragalin from *Thesium chinense*: A Novel Anti-Aging and Antioxidant Agent Targeting IGFR/CD38/ *Sirtuins.Antioxidants*, *13*(7), 859. DOI: 10.3390/antiox13070859 PMID: 39061927

Wang, R. J., Ni, Y. J., & Liu, Y. Q. (2024b, December 6). Hesperetin Increases Lifespan and Antioxidant Ability Correlating with IIS, HSP, mtUPR, and JNK Pathways of Chronic Oxidative Stress in *Caenorhabditis elegans.International Journal of Molecular Sciences*, *25*(23), 13148. DOI: 10.3390/ijms252313148 PMID: 39684858

Wang, S., Melnyk, J. P., Tsao, R., & Marcone, M. F. (2011). How natural dietary antioxidants in fruits, vegetables and legumes promote vascular health. *Food Research International*, *44*(1), 14–22. DOI: 10.1016/j.foodres.2010.09.028

Wang, X., Kang, N., Liu, Y., & Xu, G. (2024, November 14). Formononetin Exerts Neuroprotection in Parkinson's Disease via the Activation of the Nrf2 Signaling Pathway. *Molecules (Basel, Switzerland)*, *29*(22), 5364. DOI: 10.3390/molecules29225364 PMID: 39598753

Wang, X., Li, X., Li, L., Yang, X., Wang, J., Liu, X., Chen, J., Liu, S., Zhang, N., Li, J., & Wang, H. (2022a). Hawthorn fruit extract ameliorates H2O2-induced oxidative damage in neuronal PC12 cells and prolongs the lifespan of Caenorhabditis elegans via the IIS signaling pathway. *Food & Function*, *13*(20), 10680–10694. Advance online publication. DOI: 10.1039/D2FO01657E PMID: 36172739

Wang, Y., Cao, X., Ma, J., Liu, S., Jin, X., & Liu, B. (2024, November 13). Unveiling the Longevity Potential of Natural Phytochemicals: A Comprehensive Review of Active Ingredients in Dietary Plants and Herbs. *Journal of Agricultural and Food Chemistry*, *72*(45), 24908–24927. DOI: 10.1021/acs.jafc.4c07756 PMID: 39480905

Wang, Y., Cheng, Q., Su, Q., Yu, X., Shen, T., Yang, X., & Jia, W. (2022c, February 15). Aesculin offers increased resistance against oxidative stress and protective effects against Aβ-induced neurotoxicity in Caenorhabditis elegans. *European Journal of Pharmacology*, *917*, 174755. DOI: 10.1016/j.ejphar.2022.174755 PMID: 35016885

Wang, Z., Wang, W., Zhu, C., Gao, X., & Chu, W. (2022b, June 21). Evaluation of Antioxidative and Neuroprotective Activities of Total Flavonoids From Sea Buckthorn (*Hippophae rhamnoides* L.). *Frontiers in Nutrition*, *9*, 861097. DOI: 10.3389/fnut.2022.861097 PMID: 35799585

Wen, Y. P., Fu, H. J., Chen, Q., Lan, C., Qin, D. L., Wu, J. M., Wu, A. G., & Zhou, X. G. (2024, June 24). Exploring the therapeutic potential of *Nelumbo nucifera* leaf extract against amyloid-beta-induced toxicity in the *Caenorhabditis elegans* model of Alzheimer's disease. *Frontiers in Pharmacology*, *15*, 1408031. DOI: 10.3389/fphar.2024.1408031 PMID: 38983916

Whitley, A. C., Stoner, G. D., Darby, M. V., & Walle, T. (2003). Intestinal epithelial cell accumulation of the cancer preventive polyphenol ellagic acid—Extensive binding to protein and DNA. *Biochemical Pharmacology*, *66*(6), 907–915. DOI: 10.1016/S0006-2952(03)00413-1 PMID: 12963477

WHO. (2015). *World report on ageing and health*. World Health Organization.

Wink, M. (2003). Evolution of secondary metabolites from an ecological and molecular phylogenetic perspective. *Phytochemistry*, *64*(1), 3–19. DOI: 10.1016/S0031-9422(03)00300-5 PMID: 12946402

Wink, M. (2008). Evolutionary advantage and molecular modes of action of multi-component mixtures used in phytomedicine. *Current Drug Metabolism, 9*(10), 996–1009. DOI: 10.2174/138920008786927794 PMID: 19075616

Wink, M. (2010). Introduction. In Wink, M. (Ed.), *Functions and Biotechnology of plant secondary metabolites, Wiley-Blackwell, Annual Plant Reviews 39, 1-20.* DOI: 10.1002/9781444318876.ch1

Wink, M. (2015). Modes of action of herbal medicines and plant secondary metabolites. *Medicines (Basel, Switzerland), 2*(3), 251–286. DOI: 10.3390/medicines2030251 PMID: 28930211

Wink, M. (2022). 2022 Current understanding of modes of action of multicomponent bioactive phytochemicals: Potential for nutraceuticals and antimicrobials. *Annual Review of Food Science and Technology, 13*(1), 337–359. DOI: 10.1146/annurev-food-052720-100326 PMID: 35333591

Wink, M. (2024). Antioxidant properties of food plants, spices, beverages and nutraceuticals - Potential health and anti-ageing totentials. In Upadhyay, S. K., & Singh, S. P. (Eds.), *Herbal Nutraceuticals: Products and Processes*. Wiley., DOI: 10.1002/9781394241576.ch5

Wink, M., & Schimmer, O. (2010). Molecular modes of action of defensive secondary metabolites. *Ann Plant Rev, 39*, 21–161. DOI: 10.1002/9781444318876.ch2

Wolff, S., Ma, H., Burch, D., Maciel, G. A., Hunter, T., & Dillin, A. (2006). SMK-1, an essential regulator of DAF-16-mediated longevity. *Cell, 124*(5), 1039–1053. DOI: 10.1016/j.cell.2005.12.042 PMID: 16530049

Wu, Y., Wu, Z., Butko, P., Christen, Y., Lambert, M. P., Klein, W. L., Link, C. D., & Luo, Y. (2006). Amyloid-β-induced pathological behaviors are suppressed by *Ginkgo biloba* extract EGb 761 and ginkgolides in transgenic *Caenorhabditis elegans.The Journal of Neuroscience : The Official Journal of the Society for Neuroscience, 26*(50), 13102–13113. DOI: 10.1523/JNEUROSCI.3448-06.2006 PMID: 17167099

Xiao, M., Chen, B., Niu, K., Long, Z., Yang, F., & Xie, Y. (2022, November 24). *Alpiniae oxyphylla* fructus extract promotes longevity and stress resistance of *C. elegans via* DAF-16 and SKN-1. *Frontiers in Pharmacology, 13*, 1034515. DOI: 10.3389/fphar.2022.1034515 PMID: 36506568

Xiao, X., Wu, F., Wang, B., Cai, Z., Wang, L., Zhang, Y., Yu, X., & Luo, Y. (2024, September 6). *Clerodendranthus spicatus* (Thunb.) Water Extracts Reduce Lipid Accumulation and Oxidative Stress in the Caenorhabditis elegans. *International Journal of Molecular Sciences, 25*(17), 9655. DOI: 10.3390/ijms25179655 PMID: 39273603

Xiao, Y., Zhang, L., Zhou, H., Cui, Y., Chen, K., Zhang, H., Wu, Q., & Liu, F. (2025, January). Berberine extends healthspan and delays neurodegenerative diseases in Caenorhabditis elegans through ROS-dependent PMK-1/SKN-1 activation. *Archives of Gerontology and Geriatrics, 128*, 105644. DOI: 10.1016/j.archger.2024.105644 PMID: 39357500

Xie, K., Wang, H., Yao, X., Lv, J., Wang, Q., Zhao, Y., Yang, S., Xu, L., Shi, Y., Hu, J., & Shan, Y. (2025, February 13). Hederagenin reduces Aβ-induced oxidative damage, decreases Aβ deposition, and promotes cell survival by the P13K/Akt signaling pathway. *Journal of Leukocyte Biology, 117*(2), qiae124. Advance online publication. DOI: 10.1093/jleuko/qiae124 PMID: 38814954

Xu, J., Du, P., Liu, X., Xu, X., Ge, Y., & Zhang, C. (2023, June 6). Curcumin supplementation increases longevity and antioxidant capacity in *Caenorhabditis elegans.Frontiers in Pharmacology*, *14*, 1195490. DOI: 10.3389/fphar.2023.1195490 PMID: 37346299

Xu, Q., Zheng, B., Li, T., & Liu, R. H. (2025, March 15). Black goji berry anthocyanins extend lifespan and enhance the antioxidant defenses in Caenorhabditis elegans via the JNK-1 and DAF-16/FOXO pathways. *Journal of the Science of Food and Agriculture*, *105*(4), 2282–2293. DOI: 10.1002/jsfa.13998 PMID: 39483065

Xu, R., Li, A. P., Tan, X., Tang, X., He, X. P., Wang, L. X., Kang, J. J., Li, S. H., & Liu, Y. (2025, January 1). Patchouli essential oil extends the lifespan and healthspan of Caenorhabditis elegans through JNK-1/DAF-16. *Life Sciences*, *360*, 123270. DOI: 10.1016/j.lfs.2024.123270 PMID: 39581459

Yasuda, K., Miyazawa, M., Ishii, T., & Ishii, N. (2023, November). The role of nutrition and oxidative stress as aging factors in *Caenorhabditis elegans.Journal of Clinical Biochemistry and Nutrition*, *73*(3), 173–177. DOI: 10.3164/jcbn.23-44 PMID: 37970544

Yen, P.-L., Lin, T.-A., Chuah, W. L., Chang, C.-Y., Tseng, Y.-H., Huang, C.-Y., Yang, J.-C., Hsu, F.-L., & Liao, V. H.-C. (2023). Methanol Extracts from *Cirsium japonicum* DC. var. *australe* Kitam. and Their Active Components Reduce Intracellular Oxidative Stress in *Caenorhabditis elegans.Molecules (Basel, Switzerland)*, *28*(19), 6923. DOI: 10.3390/molecules28196923 PMID: 37836767

Youssef, F. S., Sobeh, M., Dmirieh, M., Bogari, H. A., Koshak, A. E., Wink, M., Ashour, M. L., & El-hady, S. S. (2022). 2022 Metabolomics based profiling of *Clerodendrum speciosum* (Lamiaceae) leaves using LC/ESI/MS-MS and in vivo evaluation of its antioxidant activity using *Caenorhabditis elegans* model. *Antioxidants*, *11*(2), 330. DOI: 10.3390/antiox11020330 PMID: 35204212

Yu, X., Tao, J., Xiao, T., & Duan, X. (2024, May 22). *P*-hydroxybenzaldehyde protects *Caenorhabditis elegans* from oxidative stress and β-amyloid toxicity. *Frontiers in Aging Neuroscience*, *16*, 1414956. DOI: 10.3389/fnagi.2024.1414956 PMID: 38841104

Yuan, X., Ni, H., Shi, F., Huang, Y., Hou, Y., & Hu, S. Q. (2025). 2025 The anti-aging and anti-Alzheimer's disease potential of kinsenoside prepared from *Anoectochilus roxburghii*. *Fitoterapia*, *182*, 106441. DOI: 10.1016/j.fitote.2025.106441 PMID: 39938659

Zamberlan, D. C., Amaral, G. P., Arantes, L. P., Machado, M. L., Mizdal, C. R., Campos, M. M. A., & Soares, F. A. A. (2016). Rosmarinus officinalis L. increases Caenorhabditis elegans stress resistance and longevity in a DAF-16, HSF-1 and SKN-1-dependent manner. *Brazilian Journal of Medical and Biological Research = Revista Brasileira de Pesquisas Médicas e Biológicas*, *49*(9), e5235.

Zhang, H., Zhu, Z., Wei, W., Liu, Z., Zhou, H., Gong, Y., Yan, X., Du, J., Li, H., Chen, L., & Sheng, L. (2024a, November 11). *Aronia melanocarpa* extract extends the lifespan and health-span of *Caenorhabditis elegans via* mitogen-activated protein kinase 1. *Food & Function*, *15*(22), 11020–11035. DOI: 10.1039/D4FO02479F PMID: 39450574

Zhang, J., He, L., Wang, A., Wu, B., Zhang, P., Zhu, Y., Jiang, Y., Bai, J., & Xiao, X. (2022b, December). Responses of bitter melon saponins to oxidative stress and aging via the IIS pathway linked with sir-2.1 and hlh-30. *Journal of Food Biochemistry*, *46*(12), e14456. DOI: 10.1111/jfbc.14456 PMID: 36226991

Zhang, K., Zhu, J., Liu, P., Guo, R., Yan, Y., Mi, J., & Zeng, X. (2024b). Petunidin-3-O-[rhamnopyranosyl-(trans-p-coumaroyl)]-5-O-(β-D-glucopyranoside), the main anthocyanin from the fruits of Lycium ruthenicum murray, enhances the lifespan of Caenorhabditis elegans by activating DAF-16 and improving the gut microbiota. *Food Bioscience*, *61*, 104642.

Zhang, S., Duangjan, C., Tencomnao, T., Liu, J., Wink, M., & Lin, J. (2020a). 2020 Neuroprotective effects of oolong tea extracts against glutamate-induced toxicity in cultured neuronal cells and Aβ-induced toxicity in *Caenorhabditis elegans.Food & Function*, *11*(9), 8179–8192. DOI: 10.1039/D0FO01072C PMID: 32966472

Zhang, S., Duangjan, C., Tencomnao, T., Wu, L., Wink, M., & Lin, J. (2022). Oolonghomobisflavans exert neuroprotective activities in cultured neuronal cells and anti-aging effects in *Caenorhabditis elegans.Frontiers in Aging Neuroscience*, *14*, 967316. DOI: 10.3389/fnagi.2022.967316 PMID: 36158534

Zhang, S., Wang, H., Wang, J., Jin, W., Yan, X., Chen, X., Wang, D., Zhao, D., Wang, Y., Cong, D., & Sun, L. (2022d, May 5). Ginsenoside Rf inhibits human tau proteotoxicity and causes specific LncRNA, miRNA and mRNA expression changes in Caenorhabditis elegans model of tauopathy. *European Journal of Pharmacology*, *922*, 174887. DOI: 10.1016/j.ejphar.2022.174887 PMID: 35306001

Zhang, X. Y., Wang, D. S., Li, X., Miao, Y. C., Gao, J. M., & Zhang, Q. (2023). A new utilization of total flavonoids from Acer truncatum samara and leaves: Anti-aging and metabolic regulation. *Industrial Crops and Products*, *203*, 117207.

Zhang, Y., Li, H., Jin, S., Lu, Y., Peng, Y., Zhao, L., & Wang, X. (2022c, March 15). Cannabidiol protects against Alzheimer's disease in C. elegans via ROS scavenging activity of its phenolic hydroxyl groups. *European Journal of Pharmacology*, *919*, 174829. DOI: 10.1016/j.ejphar.2022.174829 PMID: 35181336

Zhang, Z., Li, J., Li, F., Wang, T., Luo, X., Li, B., You, Y., Wu, C., & Liu, X. (2024b, June 14). Jujubae Fructus extract prolongs lifespan and improves stress tolerance in *Caenorhabditis elegans* dependent on DAF-16/SOD-3. *Scientific Reports*, *14*(1), 13713. DOI: 10.1038/s41598-024-64045-0 PMID: 38877105

Zhang, Z. P., Bai, X., Cui, W. B., Chen, X. H., Liu, X., Zhi, D. J., Zhang, Z. X., Fei, D. Q., & Wang, D. S. (2022b, June 20). Diterpenoid Caesalmin C Delays Aβ-Induced Paralysis Symptoms via the DAF-16 Pathway in *Caenorhabditis elegans.International Journal of Molecular Sciences*, *23*(12), 6871. DOI: 10.3390/ijms23126871 PMID: 35743309

Zhao, J., Jiang, Y., Bi, Y., & Wei, J. (2024a, June 25). Antioxidant and Stress Resistance Properties of Flavonoids from Chinese Sea Buckthorn Leaves from the Qinghai-Tibet Plateau. *Antioxidants*, *13*(7), 763. DOI: 10.3390/antiox13070763 PMID: 39061832

Zhao, P., Wang, Z., Liao, S., Liao, Y., Hu, S., Qin, J., Zhang, D., & Yan, X. (2024b, September 23). Components in SLPE Alleviate AD Model Nematodes by Up-Regulating Gene *gst-5.International Journal of Molecular Sciences*, *25*(18), 10188. DOI: 10.3390/ijms251810188 PMID: 39337674

Zheng, S., Chiu, H., Boudreau, J., Papanicolaou, T., Bendena, W., & Chin-Sang, I. (2018). A functional study of all 40 *Caenorhabditis elegans* insulin-like peptides. *The Journal of Biological Chemistry*, *293*(43), 16912–16922. DOI: 10.1074/jbc.RA118.004542 PMID: 30206121

Zhu, A., Zheng, F., Zhang, W., Li, L., Li, Y., Hu, H., Wu, Y., Bao, W., Li, G., Wang, Q., & Li, H. (2022, April 2). Oxidation and Antioxidation of Natural Products in the Model Organism *Caenorhabditis elegans.Antioxidants*, *11*(4), 705. DOI: 10.3390/antiox11040705 PMID: 35453390

Zhu, F. D., Chen, X., Yu, L., Hu, M. L., Pan, Y. R., Qin, D. L., Wu, J. M., Li, L., Law, B. Y., Wong, V. K., Zhou, X. G., Wu, A. G., & Fan, D. S. (2023, August). Targeting autophagy to discover the Piper wallichii petroleum ether fraction exhibiting antiaging and anti-Alzheimer's disease effects in *Caenorhabditis elegans.Phytomedicine*, *117*, 154916. DOI: 10.1016/j.phymed.2023.154916 PMID: 37327643

Zhu, J., Jia, Y., Wang, C., Zhou, W., Shu, Y., Zhang, K., Zeng, X., & Guo, R. (2023b, February 28). Lonicera japonica polysaccharides improve longevity and fitness of *Caenorhabditis elegans* by activating DAF-16. *International Journal of Biological Macromolecules*, *229*, 81–91. DOI: 10.1016/j.ijbiomac.2022.12.289 PMID: 36586650

Chapter 2
Biology, Genetics and Molecular Aspects of Aging:
An Update

Elakkiya Maruthamuthu Rathinam
https://orcid.org/0009-0004-8001-3203
PSGR Krishnammal College for Women, India

Krishnasreya Mohandas
https://orcid.org/0009-0001-3311-6638
PSGR Krishnammal College for Women, India

Tharani Sureshkumar
https://orcid.org/0009-0000-9898-3225
PSGR Krishnammal College for Women, India

Chithra Devi Balasundaram Saraswathy
https://orcid.org/0000-0002-6205-9556
PSGR Krishnammal College for Women, India

ABSTRACT

Aging is a complicated process influenced by various factors that disturb cellular function and alter organism equilibrium over time. This chapter provides an updated overview, focusing on mechanisms like genomic instability, telomere attrition, mitochondrial failure, and DNA damage buildup. Cellular senescence is addressed in age-related illnesses, highlighting irreversible cell cycle arrest and pro-inflammatory aspects. Epigenetic processes, specifically DNA methylation and inherited histone modifications, contribute to age-related phenotypes. Longevity research covers factors like FOXO, SIRT, and autophagy. Nutrient-sensing pathways and the microbiome's role in aging are explored, along with therapeutic interventions targeting these pathways. This synthesis of recent discoveries in genetics, molecular biology, and translational research provides a comprehensive perspective on aging biology and future clinical applications. By integrating insights from various fields, this chapter aims to develop innovative strategies to promote healthy aging and longevity.

DOI: 10.4018/979-8-3693-9730-5.ch002

INTRODUCTION

Aging constitutes a multifaceted biological phenomenon that is affected by diverse elements such as environmental, genetic, and molecular factors. These components work in concert to undermine cellular operations and disrupt the organism's overall stability over time (Gonzalo, 2010). It involves the progressive buildup of molecular, cellular, and tissue damage that occurs throughout the lifetime. This continuous deterioration generally hinders the capacity of a species to uphold homeostasis when subjected to stress, leading to greater susceptibility to a range of diseases, including cardiovascular, cancer, and neurodegenerative ailments along with increased chance of mortality (Gladyshev et al., 2021; Rodríguez-Rodero et al., 2011). The process of aging, or senescence, represents a systematic reduction of physiological functions, which results in decreased survival and reproductive rates as with progression of age, eventually leading to death (Flatt & Schmidt, 2009).

Essential mechanisms including the shortening of telomere, genomic instability, mitochondrial impairment, and the buildup of DNA damage significantly influence the aging process at both the cellular and organismal levels. Genomic instability emerges from the ongoing damage to DNA inflicted by environmental influences and metabolic byproducts, which leads to mutations and chromosomal anomalies (Gerasymchuk, 2021; Langie et al., 2015). The phenomenon of telomere attrition, marked by the progressive shortening of chromosomal ends during cellular division, ultimately causes cellular aging or programmed cell death, thereby restricting the ability of the tissues to regenerate (Aubert & Lansdorp, 2008). Additionally, mitochondrial dysfunction, which arises from a decrease in the efficiency of the electron transport chain and an increase in the production of reactive oxygen species, further intensifies cellular injury and energy shortages. Over time, the accumulation of DNA damage compromises the integrity of genetic information, thereby contributing to a decline in cellular functionality (Facecchia et al., 2011; Vijg, 2021).

Epigenetic modifications, including histone modifications, and DNA methylation, represent a dynamic level of regulation that generates age-related phenotypes. The process of DNA methylation, which involves adding methyl groups to cytosine residues within the DNA, can effectively silence gene expression and is pivotal in the developmental and metabolic pathway regulation (Ciccarone et al., 2018). Histone modifications, like methylation, phosphorylation, and acetylation, modify the structure of chromatin and influences the accessibility of genes. Recent advancements in the field of gene expression and phase hysteresis have offered important perspectives on how temporal alterations in these epigenetic marks contribute to the process of aging (Bheda, 2020; Quina et al., 2006).

Longevity-related pathways, involving key regulators such as FOXO transcription factors, sirtuins (SIRT), and autophagy, remain central to understanding the genetic regulation of lifespan (Y. Zhao & Liu, 2021). FOXO transcription factors are activated due to nutrient deprivation, and oxidative stress, promoting the expression of gene involved in metabolism, cell cycle regulation, and stress resistance (Klotz et al., 2015). Sirtuins, a group of NAD+ dependent deacetylases, regulates various cellular processes, including DNA repair, inflammation, and mitochondrial function. Autophagy, the process of cellular self-digestion and recycling, maintains cellular equilibrium by eliminating the damaged proteins and cells. These pathways offer potential targets for research aimed at fostering healthy aging and extending lifespan (Hurley & Schulman, 2014; Santos et al., 2023). The interaction between cellular communication and nutrient-detection pathways provides crucial knowledge on how metabolic and signalling networks influence aging independently. Key nutrient-sensing pathways, including the mTOR and insulin/ IGF-1 signalling pathways, detect the availability of nutrients and modulate growth, metabolism, and aging.

Caloric restriction, a proven strategy for promoting longevity, exerts its effects by modulating these nutrient-sensing pathways (Bettedi & Foukas, 2017; Templeman & Murphy, 2017).

The growing significance of the microbiome in modulating age-associated processes emphasizes the complexity and interconnectedness of biological systems. Composed of trillions of microorganisms, the gut microbiome, has a crucial role in regulating numerous aspects of host physiology, including immune function, metabolism, and inflammation (Pathak & Banerjee, 2024). Dysbiosis, or the imbalance in the gut flora, is linked to the development of age-associated illnesses and a decline in overall health. Recent research indicates that therapeutic approaches targeting the microbiome present in the gut, such as pro- and prebiotics, and faecal microbiota transplantation, can positively influence health and potentially extend lifespan in various animal models (Ahmadi et al., 2024; Haran & McCormick, 2021; Vaiserman et al., 2017). The development of molecular and clinical therapeutic strategies focuses on targeting pathways that may help to postpone senescence and reduce the incidence of age-associated diseases. Notable approaches include senolytics, that are designed to particularly remove aging cells, as well as the use of genetic modifications or small molecules to modulate epigenetic markers (Burdusel et al., 2024; Z. Li et al., 2021). Such strategies exhibit encouraging results in the *in vitro*, and *in vivo* studies aiming to determine the efficacy and safety in humans.

Figure 1. Factors contributing to aging

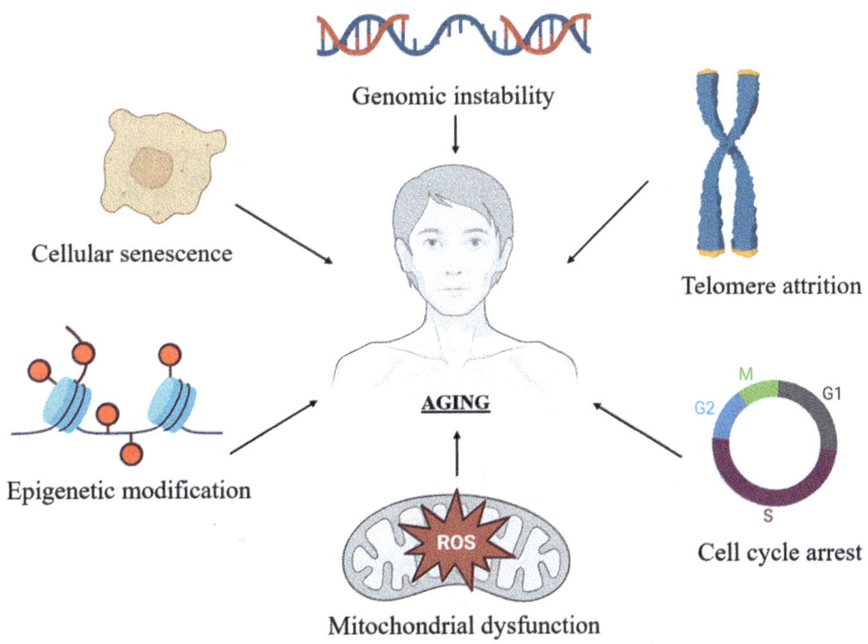

Genetic and Molecular Mechanisms of Aging

Genomic Instability

Aging is accompanied by an increased susceptibility to genomic instability. This phenomenon results from continuous DNA damage instigated by various external and internal factors, including ultraviolet (UV) radiation, environmental toxins, and metabolic by-products. The resultant damage can lead to chromosomal aberrations, mutations, and inefficiencies in DNA repair processes (Iakovou & Kourti, 2022). The progressive buildup of genetic modifications in due course compromises the genomic stability of cells, leading to diminished cellular function and an elevated vulnerability to diseases that are associated with aging, such as cancer. (Adams et al., 2015; Guo et al., 2022). Mechanisms responsible for maintaining genomic stability include DNA repair mechanisms like mismatch repair, base excision repair, and nucleotide excision repair. Nonetheless, the efficiency of these pathways weakens over time. (Gorbunova et al., 2007). The absence of telomerase in non-reproductive cells also leads to genomic instability, as it facilitates the shortening of telomeres and the occurrence of terminal fusions between chromosomes. Elucidating the relationship between accelerated aging and genomic instability is essential for the establishment of therapeutic interventions focused on preserving genomic integrity and promoting longevity (Muraki et al., 2012; Z. Wu et al., 2024).

Telomere Attrition

Telomeres, which consist of repetitive nucleotides at the chromosome ends, are crucial for the preventing the chromosomal ends from fusion and degradation. During cellular proliferation, telomeres progressively decrease in length because of the end-replication, eventually leading to a minimum length that can induce either apoptosis or cellular aging. This progressive telomere attrition acts as a biological clock, thereby restricting the proliferative capacity of the cells and contributing to the aging process (O'Sullivan & Karlseder, 2010). Research has shown that the enzyme telomerase can elongate telomeres and extend cellular lifespan. Nevertheless, in majority of the somatic cells, the activity telomerase enzyme is insufficient to counteract telomere shortening (Aubert & Lansdorp, 2008). Telomere attrition is associated with various age-related illnesses, including cardio - and neurodegenerative diseases (Iskandar et al., 2025). Approaches that focus on increasing the of activity the telomerase or protecting the telomeres from attrition may hold promise in delaying aging.

Mitochondrial Dysfunction

As the energy-producing organelles of the cell, mitochondria are essential for the production of energy through oxidative phosphorylation. As organisms age, the efficiency of these organelles diminishes, primarily as a result of the combined impact of reactive oxygen species that arise from mitochondrial respiration (Venditti & Di Meo, 2020). This mitochondrial dysfunction leads to impaired cellular function, increased levels of the ROS, and decreased production of ATP. Mitochondrial DNA is especially prone to injury because of its close association with the electron transport chain and the absence of protective histones (Nilsson & Tarnopolsky, 2019; Sena & Chandel, 2012). Accumulation of mtDNA mutations aggravates mitochondrial dysfunction and contributes to the process of aging (Cui et al., 2012; Haas, 2019; Pinto & Moraes, 2015). Interventions aimed at improving the functions of mitochondria, such as promoting mitophagy, enhancing the biogenesis, and reducing oxidative stress, are potential strategies for mitigating age-related decline.

Accumulation of DNA Damage

The aggregation of damage to DNA is recognized as a fundamental aspect of aging, arising from both endogenous sources, such as metabolic byproducts, and exogenous sources, like UV radiation. As time progresses, the efficacy of DNA repair processes declines, resulting in the persistence of DNA lesions. These lesions can interfere with transcription, replication, and cellular function, thereby contributing to the aging phenotype. The DNA damage response (DDR) comprises a series of interconnected signalling pathways that identify and rectify DNA damage (Ma & Zhou, 2025; Panich et al., 2016). Prominent components of the DDR include the p53, tumour suppressor protein and the ATM/ATR kinases, which play critical roles in mediating the arrest of the cell cycle and facilitating the repair of DNA. The persistent activation of DDR can lead to cellular aging or programmed cell death, which thereby contributes to the tissue dysfunction and aging. A thorough knowledge of the factors that drive the accumulation of DNA damage and its subsequent effects on cellular operations is important for the development of approaches intended to improve genomic stability and promoting DNA repair (Kelly & Bischof, 2025; X. Zhao et al., 2025). Potential strategies include the use of small molecules or gene therapy to enhance the function of enzymes involved in DNA repair, ultimately reducing the adverse effects of degradation in DNA associated with aging (Dong et al., 2025).

Cellular Senescence and Age-Associated Diseases

Mechanisms of Cellular Senescence

Cellular aging or senescence constitutes a vital physiological process that are marked by the perpetual loss of proliferative capacity in cells when exposed to various stressors. This irreversible growth arrest serves as a protective function to inhibit the proliferation of damaged or non-functional cells (Chen et al., 2024; Tufail et al., 2024). The onset of aging is influenced by several factors, including shortening of telomere, DNA damage, oxidative stress, oncogene activation, and mitochondrial dysfunction, many of which are intricately connected to the aging (Iskandar et al., 2025).

At the molecular level, senescence is orchestrated by key regulatory pathways involving tumour suppressor proteins such as p53, $p16^{INK4a}$, and $p21^{CIP1/WAF1}$. These proteins respond to cellular stress by activating cell cycle inhibitors that halt progression through the cell cycle. The p53 activation leads to p21 transcription, that prevents the cyclin-dependent kinases (CDKs), while $p16^{INK4a}$ directly inhibits CDK4/6 (Asciolla et al., 2025; Feroz et al., 2024). This coordinated inhibition prevents the retinoblastoma protein phosphorylation, maintaining it in an active state that suppresses E2F target genes necessary for cell cycle progression (Longworth & Damania, 2025; Pellarin et al., 2025).

Senescent cells undergo major changes in the gene expression, morphology, and function. They exhibit enlarged cell size, altered chromatin organization characterized by senescence-associated heterochromatin foci (SAHF), and increased metabolic activity. Despite their non-proliferative state, senescent cells continue to be metabolically active and can affect their microenvironment through the release of various factors (Della Vedova et al., 2025; Ramponi et al., 2025).

Irreversible Cell Cycle Arrest

Cellular senescence is characterized by a permanent cessation of the cell cycle, primarily at the G1 phase. Unlike quiescent cells, which possess the ability to re-engage in the cell cycle when conditions are favourable, senescent cells are irreversibly removed from the cell cycle. This arrest is enforced by sustained expression of CDK inhibitors and is resistant to mitogenic stimuli (Berardi, 2005; Liao et al., 2021; Roger et al., 2021). The irreversibility of the state of senescence is critical for its role in suppression of tumour, as it prohibits the damaged cells from proliferating and potentially acquiring oncogenic mutations (Ohtani et al., 2009). However, the aggregation of senescent cells over time can have degenerating effects on the functions of cells and tissues. Their inability to divide impairs tissue regeneration and repair, contributing to age-associated reduction in tissue function (Ogrodnik et al., 2019; Schmitt et al., 2022; Shvedova et al., 2022).

Pro-inflammatory Prospects

Senescent cells are not merely inert bystanders; they actively release a variety of pro-inflammatory growth factors, proteases, cytokines, and chemokines which is a collective phenomenon called Senescence-Associated Secretory Phenotype (SASP). The SASP has the potential to yield both beneficial outcomes and detrimental consequences. In simple terms, the SASP aids the immune system in eliminating senescent cells and enhances the process of tissue regeneration (Chambers et al., 2021; Docherty et al., 2020). The continuous presence of senescent cells is associated with prolonged SASP activity, resulting in persistent low-grade inflammation, or "inflammaging." This persistent inflammatory state can disrupt normal structure and functionality of the tissues, promote fibrosis, and create a microenvironment conducive to the development of age-associated illness (X. Li et al., 2023; Xiao et al., 2023). The paracrine senescence in neighbouring cells can also be induced by the SASP factors, amplifying the senescence response and further exacerbating tissue dysfunction. Additionally, they can influence stem cell function, impairing the regenerative capacity of tissues (Khalil et al., 2023).

Link to Age-Associated Illnesses

The presence of senescent cells and the ongoing activation of the SASP are intimately linked to the onset of multiple diseases that are prevalent in older populations. In the cardiovascular network, senescent endothelial cells play a significant role in the development of atherosclerosis through their promotion of inflammatory responses and the deterioration of endothelial function. (Luan et al., 2024). In the musculo-skeletal system, senescent cells in cartilage and the tissues in bones are associated with osteoarthritis and osteoporosis, respectively (Hamerman, 1997; Xie et al., 2021). Senescent glial cells are recognized as key contributors to the processes of neuroinflammation and neuronal dysfunction in neurodegenerative diseases, such as Alzheimer's disease and Parkinson's disease (Kritsilis et al., 2018; Martínez-Cué & Rueda, 2020). The SASP factors can disrupt neuronal communication and promote the deposition of pathological proteins. Moreover, while cellular senescence plays a critical role in tumour suppression by preventing the growth of damaged cells, the SASP can, in contrast, facilitate the progression of tumour. Pro-inflammatory and pro-angiogenic factors released by the senescent cells have the potential to promote the tumour growth, invasion, and metastasis (Chambers et al., 2021; Giroud et al., 2023; Xiong et al., 2024).

Epigenetic Processes in Aging

DNA Methylation

DNA methylation is primarily characterized by the addition of a methyl group to the C5 position of a cytosine base. Nonetheless, it is essential to recognize that other forms of nucleic acid modifications, such as DNA adenine methylation, have been shown to have significant biological implications (Musheev et al., 2020). In mammalian cells, the majority of DNA methylation occurs at CPG dinucleotides, and this process undergoes substantial changes during cell differentiation (Smallwood & Kelsey, 2012; Rotriguez et al., 2020). Furthermore, non-CPG methylation is predominantly found in oocytes and embryonic stem cells (Ramsahoye et al., 2000; Yu et al., 2017).

Studies comparing subjects of various ages have established that DNA methylation is modified as a result of aging. Initial findings pointed to a reduction in global methylation levels over time. However, more recent research has shown that different genomic regions may experience either hypermethylation or hypomethylation. It has been observed that about 2% of the CPG sites in the genome are subject to age-related changes across different tissues in humans and mice (Unnikrishnan et al., 2019).

DNA methylation is pivotal in the modulation of gene expression, the safeguarding of genomic stability, and the differentiation of cellular identities. Aging is a complex biological process that entails a gradual decline in physiological functions and an augmented susceptibility to numerous diseases. This process is fundamentally driven by the accumulation of molecular and cellular damage over time. Furthermore, epigenetic modifications, particularly those related to DNA methylation, are recognized as significant contributors to the aging process (Salameh et al., 2020).

Epigenetic clocks are sophisticated models utilized for the accurate prediction of chronological age, developed through the analysis of the methylation patterns of a select group of age-associated CPG sites. The most widely referenced clock for humans comprises 353 CPG sites and was created using data derived from 8,000 samples across 51 healthy tissues and cell types (Horvath, 2013). Should a relationship exist between DNA damage and age-related epigenetic modifications, it would be reasonable to expect that increased DNA damage could accelerate the advancement of the epigenetic clock. Prominent examples of epigenetic clocks include Horvath's clock and Hannum's clock.

- **Horvath's Clock**: In 2013, Steve Horvath introduced this clock, which employs DNA methylation measurements at 353 CPG sites to assess biological age across different tissues and cell types. It is regarded as a strong biomarker of aging and has connections to various age-associated illnesses.
- **Hannum's Clock**: Jeffrey Hannum's clock, also developed in 2013, focuses on 71 CPG sites and has shown accuracy in estimating biological age from blood samples.

Mechanisms and Implications

DNA methylation affects aging through several mechanisms:

1. **Gene Expression Regulation**: The modification of methylation patterns may contribute to the dysregulation of genes that are significant in the context of aging, including those related to the control of the cell cycle, the repair of DNA, and the processes of inflammation. Generally, hypo-

methylation in the promoter regions is correlated with the upregulation of gene expression, while hyper-methylation is known to suppress gene function.

2. **Genomic Instability**: Age-related hypo-methylation of repetitive DNA elements can result in the instability in the genome, contributing to cellular senescence and age-associated diseases (Salameh et al., 2020 & Seale et al., 2024).
3. **Epigenetic Drift**: Over time, stochastic changes in the methylation of DNA accumulate, which is known as epigenetic drift. This drift contributes to individual variations in aging processes and susceptibility to diseases.
4. **Epigenetic Reprogramming**: Interventions like diet, exercise, and pharmacological treatments can influence DNA methylation patterns, potentially slowing aging or mitigating age- associated pathologies (Xiao et al., 2019).

Understanding how patterns of methylation change can lead to early diagnosis of age- associated ailments, development of anti-aging therapies, and strategies to promote healthy aging.

- **Cancer**: Aberrant DNA methylation is a defining trait of cancer. Age-related methylation changes can predispose cells to malignant transformation. Epigenetic clocks can potentially predict cancer risk based on methylation patterns.
- **Cardiovascular Diseases**: Methylation changes in genes related to cardiovascular function can lead to heart disease and other cardiovascular conditions.

5. **Neurodegenerative Disorders**: Altered methylation patterns in the brain are linked to conditions like Alzheimer's and Parkinson's. Identifying these modifications can aid in early diagnosis and intervention (Salameh et al., 2020 & Seale et al., 2024).

Post Translational Histone Modification

Epigenetic modifications of histones, alongside DNA methylation, significantly contribute to the DNA damage response, DNA repair, and the aging process. Modifications like acetylation, methylation, and phosphorylation alter the chromatin architecture, facilitating both transcription and DNA repair mechanism (Polo & Jackson, 2011 & Sanchez et al., 2021).

Histone Acetylation

Acetylation of histones occurs on the lysine residues of histones H2A, H2B, H3, and H4. This modification disrupts the binding of histones to DNA, leading to a more relaxed chromatin structure that promotes the transcription of nearby genes. The enzymatic processes involved in histone acetylation and deacetylation are mediated by histone acetyltransferases and histone deacetylases, respectively. Moreover, histone acetylation is essential for the DNA damage response. The nature and extent of DNA damage can trigger either hyperacetylation or hypoacetylation of lysine residues on histones in specific regions. This modification aids in the recruitment of repair proteins to the sites of DNA damage. Once the repair mechanisms are completed, histones revert to their original post-translational modification state (Gong et al., 2016).

The HAT TIP-60 is responsible for the acetylation of H4K-16, which promotes homologous recombination repair. Meanwhile, HDAC-1 and HDAC-2 are crucial in the repair of double-strand breaks as they deacetylate H3K-56ac and H4K16-ac (Miller *et al.,* 2010). A study comparing brain samples from young and elderly individuals, and patients with Alzheimer's condition, identified significant variations in H4K16-ac levels. In aged brain samples, levels of H4K16-ac are elevated; conversely, Alzheimer's patients exhibit a widespread reduction in H4K16-ac. Notably, there is a significant reduction of H4K16-ac in the regulatory regions in the genes that are predominantly exhibited in neurons, along with a consistent transcriptional alteration pattern observed across various Alzheimer's patients. These alterations in transcription are associated with processes like cell death, myeloid differentiation, and signalling pathways, indicating the presence of a transcriptional program unique to Alzheimer's disease (Nativio et al., 2018). The transcriptional corepressor expression REST rises with age in human brain neuronal populations but declines in Alzheimer's, indicating a potential protective function. REST is responsible for the deacetylation of H3K9ac. Consequently, H3K9-ac levels are generally reduced in neurons of normal aging, while they are elevated in Alzheimer's patients, where the evidence of gene derepression that contributes to the disease pathology. Overall, these findings underscore the significant role of histone acetylation and deacetylation in maintaining genomic stability and epigenetic balance during aging and in age-associated ailments (Lu et al., 2014).

Histone Methylation

Histone methylation is a crucial post-translational modification where methyl groups are added to histone proteins in the lysine or arginine residues. This change plays a significant role in regulating expression of genes by altering chromatin structure and influencing cellular processes. Histone methylation patterns are dynamically regulated throughout an organism's lifespan. During aging, the balance between different histone methylation marks is often disrupted (Qin et al., 2024 & Singh & Paramanik, 2025).

Transcriptional Regulation

In young and healthy cells, precise histone methylation maintains genes in an optimal state for either activation or repression. Aging cells, however, often exhibit an imbalance, leading to aberrant gene expression patterns associated with reduced cellular function, senescence, and age-associated illnesses.

Stem Cell Function and Regeneration

Histone methylation plays a major role in conserving the function of stem cells and regenerative potential. Altered histone methylation patterns in aging stem cells can impair their ability to regenerate and differentiate, contributing to tissue degeneration and impaired repair mechanisms prevalent in aging.

Neurodegenerative Diseases

Aberrant histone methylation is linked to neurodegenerative conditions like Alzheimer's and Parkinson's disease. These modifications can cause dysregulation of genes involved in memory formation, synaptic plasticity, and neuronal function.

Inflammation and Immune Response

Age-related changes in histone methylation can also affect the inflammatory gene expression. Increased inflammatory gene expression, driven by altered histone methylation, is a sign of aging and contributes to chronic inflammation and immune system deterioration (Singh & Paramanik, 2025 & Cauley et al., 2014)

Therapeutic Implications

Targeting Histone Methyltransferases and Demethylases

Modulating the activity of enzymes responsible for adding or removing methyl groups from histones has shown promise in preclinical models. Small molecule inhibitors targeting specific HMTs and HDMs can potentially restore youthful methylation patterns, thereby delaying or reversing aging-related changes

Epigenetic Drugs

Compounds that can modulate histone methylation are being explored as potential therapeutics. For example, drugs targeting H3K27me3 or H3K9me3 marks are used to treat certain cancers and could potentially be repurposed for age-related diseases.

Lifestyle and Dietary Interventions

Emerging research suggests that lifestyle factors like exercise, diet, and exposure to environmental stress can influence the patterns of histone methylation. Interventions aimed at promoting healthy methylation patterns through lifestyle modifications hold promise for enhancing the health and longevity (Singh & Paramanik, 2025 & Cauley et al., 2014).

Longevity-Related Criteria

FoxO Transcription factors in Aging

The FoxO transcription factor family is classified within the Forkhead box transcription factors, which includes DAF-16 in *Caenorhabditis elegans*, dFOXO in *Drosophila melanogaster*, and four mammalian variants: FoxO1, FoxO3, FoxO4, and FoxO6. These proteins are integral to the process of receiving and integrating multiple upstream signals. They govern a variety of downstream targets across both peripheral tissues and the central nervous system (CNS) through post-translational modifications and their translocation from the cytoplasm to the nucleus. The dysfunction of this pathway significantly contributes to the onset of type 2 diabetes, a metabolic disorder linked to aging. Additionally, emerging studies indicate a correlation between type 2 diabetes and an elevated risk of developing Alzheimer's disease (AD), the most common type of dementia in older populations (Du & Zheng, 2021)

Molecular Characteristics of FoxO Transaction Factors

The FoxO proteins, identified by their forkhead box DNA-binding domain, are key transcription factors that contribute significantly to various cellular functions. These proteins respond to multiple upstream signals, including oxidative stress, nutrient availability, and growth factors. Once they are activated, FoxO proteins relocate from the cytoplasm to the nucleus, where they play a pivotal role in regulating the expression of target genes that are important for cell cycle management, apoptosis, DNA repair, and the cellular response to stress (Santos et al., 2023 & Guan et al., 2025)

The regulation of FoxO proteins is significantly influenced by post-translational modifications. Phosphorylation, typically carried out by kinases like Akt, causes FoxO proteins to be retained in the cytoplasm, which subsequently diminishes their transcriptional capabilities (Calissi et al., 2021). In contrast, dephosphorylation enables the movement and activation of these proteins within the nuclear compartment. Moreover, the modifications of acetylation and ubiquitination are essential for determining the stability and operational effectiveness of FoxO, thereby fine-tuning their involvement in cellular homeostasis (Gao et al., 2024).

FoxO transcription factors are recognized as essential regulators of aging and lifespan. Investigations utilizing model organisms such as *Caenorhabditis elegans* and *Drosophila melanogaster* have demonstrated that FoxO proteins significantly influence lifespan determination. For instance, the overexpression of DAF-16, the FoxO counterpart in *C. elegans*, leads to increased resistance to stress and an extended lifespan. These findings highlight the evolutionary conservation of FoxO's function in longevity regulation (Du & Zheng, 2021). In mammals, particular emphasis has been placed on FoxO3 due to its links to human longevity (Colman et al., 2024). Genetic analyses have revealed specific polymorphisms within the FOXO3 gene that are associated with longer lifespans and a lower incidence of age-related diseases (Zhao & Liu, 2021). At a mechanistic level, FoxO3 modulates a diverse range of genes that are pivotal in oxidative stress responses, apoptosis, and autophagy, all of which are vital for cellular upkeep and longevity (Bernardo et al., 2023).

Cellular Functions

FoxOs are involved in many cellular processes that are crucial for aging. They regulate apoptosis (programmed cell death) and autophagy (cellular degradation), which help remove damaged cells and maintain tissue health (Cao et al., 2023). Dysregulation of these pathways can lead to age-related ailments. FoxOs can induce the of pro-apoptotic gene expression such as Bim and Fas ligand, promoting the elimination of damaged cells (Park, 2024). Similarly, FoxOs activate genes engaged in autophagy, such as Atg genes, to facilitate the removal of damaged organelles and proteins (Virgilio et al., 2022).

Role of Sirtuins on Aging

Sirtuins are a group of proteins that significantly influence the regulation of various cellular functions associated with aging and longevity. In mammals, there are seven identified sirtuins, referred to as SIRT1 through SIRT7, each possessing unique functions and specific cellular locations (Watroba et al., 2017). SIRT1 and SIRT6, in particular, are key players in the mechanisms of DNA repair and maintenance. They help uphold genomic stability by deacetylating histones and other proteins involved in DNA repair processes. SIRT6, for example, is crucial for the base excision repair pathway, which addresses single-strand breaks in DNA. This activity is vital for preventing the accumulation of DNA damage, a significant factor contributing to the aging process (Presegué & Vaquero, 2015).

Located in the mitochondria, SIRT3, SIRT4, and SIRT5 are pivotal in the regulation of mitochondrial function and energy metabolism. SIRT3 specifically deacetylates and activates key enzymes that play a role in oxidative phosphorylation, the process through which ATP is synthesized in cells. This activity is essential for sustaining mitochondrial integrity and functionality, which are vital for cellular health and longevity. In addition, SIRT4 and SIRT5 also participate in the regulation of metabolic pathways within the mitochondria, further supporting energy homeostasis (Parihar et al., 2015).

Sirtuins are integral to the cellular mechanisms that respond to stress, aiding cells in managing oxidative stress and various environmental adversities. They influence the expression of genes that are pivotal for antioxidant protection and stress resistance (Saha et al., 2024). Specifically, SIRT1 is known to activate the transcription factor FOXO3a, which subsequently promotes the expression of antioxidant enzymes such as superoxide dismutase and catalase. This action is crucial for defending cells against oxidative injury and prolonging cellular lifespan (Alanazi et al., 2024).

Sirtuins play a major role in regulating the metabolic pathways, including lipid and glucose metabolism. SIRT1 activates and deacetylates PGC-1α, which is a primary regulator in the biogenesis of mitochondria and energy metabolism. This enhances the cell's ability to adapt to changes in nutrient availability and maintain metabolic homeostasis (Kim et al., 2024). Additionally, SIRT1 influences insulin sensitivity, glucose homeostasis, and lipid metabolism, which are critical for preventing metabolic disorders associated with aging (Wang et al., 2024). They are engaged in regulating immune responses and inflammation. SIRT1 inhibits the activity of a transcription factor, NF-κB that promotes the expression of pro-inflammatory cytokines. By modulating NF-κB activity, SIRT1 helps reduce serious inflammation, which is a sign of aging. Sirtuins also regulate the differentiation and function of immune cells, contributing to a balanced immune response (Sun et al., 2024).

Role of Autophagy in Aging

Autophagy is a fundamental cellular mechanism responsible for the degradation and recycling of damaged cellular constituents. This process plays a critical role in sustaining cellular homeostasis and facilitating adaptation to various stressors. With advancing age, the significance of autophagy escalates, as it helps to alleviate age-associated cellular damage and dysfunction (Sedaghatmehr & Balazadeh, 2024). Autophagy can be categorized into three primary forms: macroautophagy, microautophagy, and chaperone-mediated autophagy (CMA). Macroautophagy is characterized by the formation of autophagosomes, which are double-membraned vesicles that encapsulate cellular materials and transport them to lysosomes for degradation. In contrast, microautophagy entails the direct uptake of cytoplasmic substances by lysosomes, while CMA is a selective process that targets specific proteins for degradation within lysosomes (Manastireanu et al., 2024).

Autophagy plays a major role in aging by conserving the cellular quality control. It helps eliminate damaged organelles, and proteins, inhibiting their buildup and the subsequent cellular dysfunction. Dysregulation of autophagy has been linked to various age-associated illnesses, including cardiovascular, neurodegenerative disorders, and metabolic syndromes (Wu et al., 2024). Research has shown that enhancing autophagy can extend longevity in wide range of model organisms. Dietary interventions such as the inhibition of nutrient-sensing pathways and caloric restriction like, IIS, and TOR have been shown to activate autophagy and promote longevity. These findings suggest that autophagy is vital process in the aging and a potential objective for anti-aging therapies (Hardin, 2024).

Autophagy dysfunction is a contributing factor in numerous diseases associated with aging. For example, when autophagy is disrupted, it can result in the accumulation of protein aggregates, which are commonly observed in neurodegenerative diseases such as Alzheimer's and Parkinson's. Additionally, dysfunctional autophagy may lead to mitochondrial impairment and cellular senescence, both of which are key features of aging and age-related illnesses (Palmer et al., 2025). The process of autophagy is essential for cellular health and is closely linked to the aging process and its associated diseases. Interventions aimed at boosting autophagy through dietary and pharmacological means present a promising avenue for extending lifespan (Raza, 2024).

Recent Advances in Therapeutic Interventions

Aging research has seen numerous breakthroughs in recent years, aiming to extend longevity and alleviate age-associated ailments. The recent advances include:

Gene Therapy

Gene therapy for aging focuses on modifying genes that play critical roles in the process of aging and age-associated illnesses (Yu et al., 2023).

- **Delivery Systems:** Researchers have improved viral vectors and nanoparticle systems for efficient delivery of therapeutic genes. Adeno-associated viruses (AAVs) and lentiviruses are frequently used vectors that target specific tissues (Yu et al., 2023).
- **CRISPR/Cas9 Technique:** This revolutionary gene-editing technology allows specific editing of gene sequences. It has been used to remove senescent cells and correct genetic mutations associated with aging (Jia et al., 2024).
- **Gene Targets:** Key genes targeted include telomerase reverse transcriptase (TERT) to extend telomeres, SIRT6 for DNA repair and metabolic regulation, and FOXO3 for stress resistance and longevity (Vitiello et al., 2017, Khor & Wong, 2024)

Stem Cell Therapy

Stem cell therapy aims to replenish and repair damaged cells, thereby combating the effects of senescence.

- **Mesenchymal stem cells:** These are widely studied because of their ability to differentiate into various types of cells and their immunomodulatory properties. They show promise in treating cardiovascular ailments, osteoarthritis, and skin aging (Wei et al., 2024).
- **Induced Pluripotent Stem Cells:** These are reprogrammed from adult cells and have the ability to differentiate into any type of cells. This technology offers a renewable source of cells for regenerative therapies. Recent advances include creating iPSC-derived organoids for disease modelling and personalized medicine (Mohite et al., 2024).
- **Hematopoietic Stem Cells (HSCs):** HSC transplantation is being explored to rejuvenate the aging immune system and improve overall health (Zhang et al., 2024).

Nanomedicine

Nanomedicine uses nanoscale materials to deliver therapeutic agents with high precision.

- **Drug Delivery Systems:** The utilization of nanoparticles for drug encapsulation serves to protect these substances from degradation and enables their directed delivery to specific cellular or tissue targets. This strategy effectively minimizes side effects and enhances the therapeutic impact (Elumalai et al., 2024).
- **Nanoparticle Types:** Lipid nanoparticles (LNPs), polymeric nanoparticles, and gold nanoparticles are among the types used in aging research. LNPs has been notably effective in delivering the mRNA for gene therapy (Soroudi et al., 2024).
- **Combination Therapies:** Researchers are exploring nanoparticles that can simultaneously deliver multiple therapeutic agents, such as antioxidants and anti-inflammatory drugs, to address various aspects of aging (Singh et al., 2024).

Monoclonal Antibodies

Monoclonal antibodies (mAbs) are specifically designed to interact with specific molecules involved in age-related diseases.

- **Alzheimer's Disease:** Monoclonal antibodies, such as aducanumab, targets amyloid-beta plaques in the brain, seeking to decrease the progression of Alzheimer's disease. Other mAbs target tau proteins, another defining feature of Alzheimer's (Shenhav, 2024).
- **Cancer:** A category of monoclonal antibodies, immune checkpoint inhibitors improve the immune system's proficiency in detecting and eradicating cancer cells. Prominent examples of such inhibitors are pembrolizumab, an anti-PD-1 agent, and ipilimumab, an anti-CTLA-4 agent (Rotriguez et al., 2024)

Digital Health Technologies

Digital health technologies enhance monitoring, early detection, and management of age-related conditions.

- **Smart watches:** Smartwatches and fitness tracking devices monitor physical activity, sleep patterns, vital signs, and other health metrics. These devices help detect early signs of disease and track the effectiveness of interventions (Jafleh et al., 2024).
- **Telemedicine:** Remote consultations enable continuous care and monitoring, especially for individuals with mobility issues or those living in remote areas. By incorporating wearable technology, telemedicine platforms facilitate the provision of immediate health data to healthcare providers (Nwankwo et al., 2024).
- **Artificial Intelligence:** AI algorithms analyse large datasets from wearables and electronic health records to uncover patterns and predict health outcomes. AI-powered tools provide personalized health recommendations and support clinical decision-making (Elhaddad & Hamam, 2024).

These therapeutic advances hold great promise in improving health span and addressing the challenges of aging.

Translational Science and Future Directions

Translational science bridges the gap between laboratory research and clinical applications, aiming to convert scientific discoveries into practical therapies and interventions. Recent advancements have shown promise in several areas, including targeting cellular senescence to reduce age-related damage, utilizing stem cell therapy for tissue regeneration, and progressing in the field of gene editing through technologies like CRISPR-Cas9 aimed to rectify genetic abnormalities (Abusalah et al., 2024). Epigenetic modulation, pharmacological interventions such as rapamycin, and microbiome modulation are also studied for their capability to elevate lifespan and mitigate age-associated illnesses (Yu et al., 2024).

Looking to the future, personalized medicine and digital health technologies are expected to play crucial roles in aging research. Advances in genomics, big data, and artificial intelligence will enable tailored interventions based on individual genetic profiles. As research continues, these innovative approaches will contribute to longevity, enhancing standard of living, and addressing the complex challenges of aging (Jafleh et al., 2024, Elhaddad & Hamam, 2024).

CONCLUSION

Aging is a complex multifaceted shaped by a wide array of molecular, genetic, and environmental influences. This chapter has delved into the biology and genetics of aging, illuminating the molecular processes that contribute to this intricate issue. We have explored the collection of genetic mutations, epigenetic modifications, mitochondrial dysfunction, and cellular senescence, enhancing our comprehension of the processes that influence aging and age-associated illnesses. Recent breakthroughs in therapeutic strategies, such as nanomedicine, stem cell, and gene therapy, present promising opportunities to alleviate the impacts of aging and improve health. Translational science is vital in connecting research with clinical applications, ensuring that these innovative findings can be effectively utilized to enhance human health. Looking ahead, personalized medicine, regenerative medicine, and cutting-edge digital health technologies are set to revolutionize aging research, providing new possibilities for extending health span and enhancing quality of life. The exploration of understanding and tackling the complexities of aging is a vibrant and promising field, poised for ongoing advancements and innovative therapeutic solutions in the future.

REFERENCES

Abusalah, M. A. H., Abd Rahman, E. N. S. E., & Choudhary, O. P. (2024). Evolving trends in stem cell therapy: An emerging and promising approach against various diseases. *International Journal of Surgery*, *110*(11), 6862–6868. DOI: 10.1097/JS9.0000000000001948 PMID: 39699861

Adams, P. D., Jasper, H., & Rudolph, K. L. (2015). Aging-Induced Stem Cell Mutations as Drivers for Disease and Cancer. *Cell Stem Cell*, *16*(6), 601–612. DOI: 10.1016/j.stem.2015.05.002 PMID: 26046760

Ahmadi, S., Hasani, A., Khabbaz, A., Poortahmasbe, V., Hosseini, S., Yasdchi, M., Mehdizadehfar, E., Mousavi, Z., Hasani, R., Nabizadeh, E., & Nezhadi, J. (2024). Dysbiosis and fecal microbiota transplant: Contemplating progress in health, neurodegeneration and longevity. *Biogerontology*, *25*(6), 957–983. DOI: 10.1007/s10522-024-10136-4 PMID: 39317918

Alanazi, S. T., Salama, S. A., Althobaiti, M. M., Alotaibi, R. A., AlAbdullatif, A. A., Musa, A., & Harisa, G. I. (2024). Alleviation of Copper-Induced Hepatotoxicity by Bergenin: Diminution of Oxidative Stress, Inflammation, and Apoptosis via Targeting SIRT1/FOXO3a/NF-κB Axes and p38 MAPK Signaling. *Biological Trace Element Research*, •••, 1–13. DOI: 10.1007/s12011-024-04401-3 PMID: 39347884

Asciolla, J. J., Wu, X., Adamopoulos, C., Gavathiotis, E., & Poulikakos, P. I. (2025). Resistance mechanisms and therapeutic strategies of CDK4 and CDK6 kinase targeting in cancer. *Nature Cancer*, *6*(1), 24–40. DOI: 10.1038/s43018-024-00893-z PMID: 39885369

Aubert, G., & Lansdorp, P. M. (2008). Telomeres and Aging. *Physiological Reviews*, *88*(2), 557–579. DOI: 10.1152/physrev.00026.2007 PMID: 18391173

Berardi, P. (2005). *Genetic and epigenetic events regulating cellular senescence and aging*. http://hdl.handle.net/1880/44818

Bernardo, V. S., Torres, F. F., & Da Silva, D. G. H. (2023). FoxO3 and oxidative stress: A multifaceted role in cellular adaptation. *Journal of Molecular Medicine*, *101*(1), 83–99. DOI: 10.1007/s00109-022-02281-5 PMID: 36598531

Bettedi, L., & Foukas, L. C. (2017). Growth factor, energy and nutrient sensing signalling pathways in metabolic ageing. *Biogerontology*, *18*(6), 913–929. DOI: 10.1007/s10522-017-9724-6 PMID: 28795262

Bheda, P. (2020). Metabolic transcriptional memory. *Molecular Metabolism*, *38*, 100955. DOI: 10.1016/j.molmet.2020.01.019 PMID: 32240621

Bosch-Presegué, L., & Vaquero, A. (2015). Sirtuin-dependent epigenetic regulation in the maintenance of genome integrity. *The FEBS Journal*, *282*(9), 1745–1767. DOI: 10.1111/febs.13053 PMID: 25223884

Burdusel, D., Doeppner, T. R., Surugiu, R., Hermann, D. M., Olaru, D. G., & Popa-Wagner, A. (2024). The Intersection of Epigenetics and Senolytics in Mechanisms of Aging and Therapeutic Approaches. *Biomolecules*, *15*(1), 18. DOI: 10.3390/biom15010018 PMID: 39858413

Cao, G., Lin, M., Gu, W., Su, Z., Duan, Y., Song, W., Liu, H., & Zhang, F. (2023). The rules and regulatory mechanisms of FOXO3 on inflammation, metabolism, cell death and aging in hosts. *Life Sciences*, *328*, 121877. DOI: 10.1016/j.lfs.2023.121877 PMID: 37352918

Chambers, C. R., Ritchie, S., Pereira, B. A., & Timpson, P. (2021). Overcoming the senescence-associated secretory phenotype (SASP): A complex mechanism of resistance in the treatment of cancer. *Molecular Oncology*, *15*(12), 3242–3255. DOI: 10.1002/1878-0261.13042 PMID: 34137158

Chen, J., Li, H., Liang, R., Huang, Y., & Tang, Q. (2024). Aging through the lens of mitochondrial DNA mutations and inheritance paradoxes. *Biogerontology*, *26*(1), 33. DOI: 10.1007/s10522-024-10175-x PMID: 39729246

Ciccarone, F., Tagliatesta, S., Caiafa, P., & Zampieri, M. (2018). DNA methylation dynamics in aging: How far are we from understanding the mechanisms? *Mechanisms of Ageing and Development*, *174*, 3–17. DOI: 10.1016/j.mad.2017.12.002 PMID: 29268958

Cui, H., Kong, Y., & Zhang, H. (2012). Oxidative Stress, Mitochondrial Dysfunction, and Aging. *Journal of Signal Transduction*, *2012*(1), 646354. DOI: 10.1155/2012/646354 PMID: 21977319

Della Vedova, L., Baron, G., Morazzoni, P., Aldini, G., & Gado, F. (2025). The Potential of Polyphenols in Modulating the Cellular Senescence Process: Implications and Mechanism of Action. *Pharmaceuticals (Basel, Switzerland)*, *18*(2), 2. Advance online publication. DOI: 10.3390/ph18020138 PMID: 40005954

Docherty, M. H., Baird, D. P., Hughes, J., & Ferenbach, D. A. (2020). Cellular Senescence and Senotherapies in the Kidney: Current Evidence and Future Directions. *Frontiers in Pharmacology*, *11*, 755. Advance online publication. DOI: 10.3389/fphar.2020.00755 PMID: 32528288

Dong, X.-M., Chen, L., Xu, Y.-X., Wu, P., Xie, T., & Liu, Z.-Q. (2025). Exploring metabolic reprogramming in esophageal cancer: The role of key enzymes in glucose, amino acid, and nucleotide pathways and targeted therapies. *Cancer Gene Therapy*, *32*(2), 1–19. DOI: 10.1038/s41417-024-00858-5 PMID: 39794467

Du, S., & Zheng, H. (2021). Role of FoxO transcription factors in aging and age-related metabolic and neurodegenerative diseases. *Cell & Bioscience*, *11*(1), 188. DOI: 10.1186/s13578-021-00700-7 PMID: 34727995

Elhaddad, M., & Hamam, S. (2024). AI-Driven clinical decision support systems: An ongoing pursuit of potential. *Cureus*, *16*(4). Advance online publication. DOI: 10.7759/cureus.57728 PMID: 38711724

Elumalai, K., Srinivasan, S., & Shanmugam, A. (2024). Review of the efficacy of nanoparticle-based drug delivery systems for cancer treatment. *Biomedical Technology*, *5*, 109–122. DOI: 10.1016/j.bmt.2023.09.001

Facecchia, K., Fochesato, L.-A., Ray, S. D., Stohs, S. J., & Pandey, S. (2011). Oxidative Toxicity in Neurodegenerative Diseases: Role of Mitochondrial Dysfunction and Therapeutic Strategies. *Journal of Toxicology*, *2011*(1), 683728. DOI: 10.1155/2011/683728 PMID: 21785590

Feroz, M., Jan, A., Yasin, J., & Mir, M. A. (2024). Control of Cell Cycle Dynamics in Breast Cancer: Maintaining a Balance between Arrest and Proliferation. In *Breast Cancer* (p. 53). CRC Press.

Flatt, T., & Schmidt, P. S. (2009). Integrating Evolutionary and Molecular Genetics of Aging. *Biochimica et Biophysica Acta*, *1790*(10), 951–962. DOI: 10.1016/j.bbagen.2009.07.010 PMID: 19619612

Gao, M., Shi, J., Xiao, X., Yao, Y., Chen, X., Wang, B., & Zhang, J. (2024). PD-1 regulation in immune homeostasis and immunotherapy. *Cancer Letters, 216726*, 216726. Advance online publication. DOI: 10.1016/j.canlet.2024.216726 PMID: 38401888

Gerasymchuk, M. (2021). Genomic instability and aging: Causes and consequences. In Kovalchuk, I., & Kovalchuk, O. (Eds.), *Genome Stability* (2nd ed., Vol. 26, pp. 533–553). Academic Press., DOI: 10.1016/B978-0-323-85679-9.00028-3

Gladyshev, V. N., Kritchevsky, S. B., Clarke, S. G., Cuervo, A. M., Fiehn, O., de Magalhães, J. P., Mau, T., Maes, M., Moritz, R. L., Niedernhofer, L. J., Van Schaftingen, E., Tranah, G. J., Walsh, K., Yura, Y., Zhang, B., & Cummings, S. R. (2021). Molecular damage in aging. *Nature Aging*, *1*(12), 1096–1106. DOI: 10.1038/s43587-021-00150-3 PMID: 36846190

Gómez-Virgilio, L., Silva-Lucero, M. D. C., Flores-Morelos, D. S., Gallardo-Nieto, J., Lopez-Toledo, G., Abarca-Fernandez, A. M., Zacapala-Gómez, A.-E., Luna-Muñoz, J., Montiel-Sosa, F., Soto-Rojas, L. O., Pacheco-Herrero, M., & Cardenas-Aguayo, M. D. C. (2022). Autophagy: a key regulator of homeostasis and disease: an overview of molecular mechanisms and modulators. *Cells*, *11*(15), 2262. DOI: 10.3390/cells11152262 PMID: 35892559

Gong, F., Chiu, L. Y., & Miller, K. M. (2016). Acetylation reader proteins: Linking acetylation signaling to genome maintenance and cancer. *PLOS Genetics*, *12*(9), e1006272. DOI: 10.1371/journal.pgen.1006272 PMID: 27631103

Gonzalo, S. (2010). Epigenetic alterations in aging. *Journal of Applied Physiology*, *109*(2), 586–597. DOI: 10.1152/japplphysiol.00238.2010 PMID: 20448029

Gorbunova, V., Seluanov, A., Mao, Z., & Hine, C. (2007). Changes in DNA repair during aging. *Nucleic Acids Research*, *35*(22), 7466–7474. DOI: 10.1093/nar/gkm756 PMID: 17913742

Guan, G., Chen, Y., & Dong, Y. (2025). Unraveling the AMPK-SIRT1-FOXO Pathway: The In-Depth Analysis and Breakthrough Prospects of Oxidative Stress-Induced Diseases. *Antioxidants*, *14*(1), 70. DOI: 10.3390/antiox14010070 PMID: 39857404

Guo, J., Huang, X., Dou, L., Yan, M., Shen, T., Tang, W., & Li, J. (2022). Aging and aging-related diseases: From molecular mechanisms to interventions and treatments. *Signal Transduction and Targeted Therapy*, *7*(1), 1–40. DOI: 10.1038/s41392-022-01251-0 PMID: 36522308

Haas, R. H. (2019). Mitochondrial Dysfunction in Aging and Diseases of Aging. *Biology (Basel)*, *8*(2), 2. Advance online publication. DOI: 10.3390/biology8020048 PMID: 31213034

Hamerman, D. (1997). Aging and the musculoskeletal system. *Annals of the Rheumatic Diseases*, *56*(10), 578–585. DOI: 10.1136/ard.56.10.578 PMID: 9389217

Haran, J. P., & McCormick, B. A. (2021). Aging, Frailty, and the Microbiome—How Dysbiosis Influences Human Aging and Disease. *Gastroenterology*, *160*(2), 507–523. DOI: 10.1053/j.gastro.2020.09.060 PMID: 33307030

Hardin, R. (2024). The Effect Of Intermittent Fasting, Caloric Restriction And Exercise On Aging And Longevity. *Systematic Reviews*.

Horvath, S. (2013). DNA methylation age of human tissues and cell types. *Genome Biology*, *14*(10), 3156. DOI: 10.1186/gb-2013-14-10-r115 PMID: 24138928

Hurley, J. H., & Schulman, B. A. (2014). Atomistic Autophagy: The Structures of Cellular Self-Digestion. *Cell*, *157*(2), 300–311. DOI: 10.1016/j.cell.2014.01.070 PMID: 24725401

Iakovou, E., & Kourti, M. (2022). A Comprehensive Overview of the Complex Role of Oxidative Stress in Aging, The Contributing Environmental Stressors and Emerging Antioxidant Therapeutic Interventions. *Frontiers in Aging Neuroscience*, *14*, 827900. DOI: 10.3389/fnagi.2022.827900 PMID: 35769600

Iskandar, M., Xiao Barbero, M., Jaber, M., Chen, R., Gomez-Guevara, R., Cruz, E., & Westerheide, S. (2025). A Review of Telomere Attrition in Cancer and Aging: Current Molecular Insights and Future Therapeutic Approaches. *Cancers (Basel)*, *17*(2), 257. DOI: 10.3390/cancers17020257 PMID: 39858038

Jafleh, E. A., Alnaqbi, F. A., Almaeeni, H. A., Faqeeh, S., Alzaabi, M. A., & Al Zaman, K. (2024). The role of wearable devices in chronic disease monitoring and patient care: A comprehensive review. *Cureus*, *16*(9), e68921. DOI: 10.7759/cureus.68921 PMID: 39381470

Jia, S., Liang, R., Chen, J., Liao, S., Lin, J., & Li, W. (2024). Emerging technology has a brilliant future: The CRISPR-Cas system for senescence, inflammation, and cartilage repair in osteoarthritis. *Cellular & Molecular Biology Letters*, *29*(1), 64. DOI: 10.1186/s11658-024-00581-x PMID: 38698311

Kelly, L., & Bischof, E. (2025). Unraveling the threads of time: Longevity and DNA repair mechanisms. In Kelly, L., & Stanford, W. P. (Eds.), *Implementation of Personalized Precision Medicine* (pp. 377–395). Academic Press., DOI: 10.1016/B978-0-323-98808-7.00016-3

Khalil, R., Diab-Assaf, M., & Lemaitre, J.-M. (2023). Emerging Therapeutic Approaches to Target the Dark Side of Senescent Cells: New Hopes to Treat Aging as a Disease and to Delay Age-Related Pathologies. *Cells*, *12*(6), 6. Advance online publication. DOI: 10.3390/cells12060915 PMID: 36980256

Khor, Y. S., & Wong, P. F. (2024). MicroRNAs-associated with FOXO3 in cellular senescence and other stress responses. *Biogerontology*, *25*(1), 23–51. DOI: 10.1007/s10522-023-10059-6 PMID: 37646881

Kim, J. T., Jeon, D. H., & Lee, H. J. (2024). Molecular mechanism of skeletal muscle loss and its prevention by natural resources. *Food Science and Biotechnology*, *33*(15), 3387–3400. DOI: 10.1007/s10068-024-01678-x PMID: 39493391

Klotz, L.-O., Sánchez-Ramos, C., Prieto-Arroyo, I., Urbánek, P., Steinbrenner, H., & Monsalve, M. (2015). Redox regulation of FoxO transcription factors. *Redox Biology*, *6*, 51–72. DOI: 10.1016/j.redox.2015.06.019 PMID: 26184557

Langie, S. A. S., Koppen, G., Desaulniers, D., Al-Mulla, F., Al-Temaimi, R., Amedei, A., Azqueta, A., Bisson, W. H., Brown, D., Brunborg, G., Charles, A. K., Chen, T., Colacci, A., Darroudi, F., Forte, S., Gonzalez, L., Hamid, R. A., Knudsen, L. E., Leyns, L., & Collins, A. R. (2015). Causes of genome instability: The effect of low dose chemical exposures in modern society. *Carcinogenesis*, *36*(Suppl_1), S61–S88. DOI: 10.1093/carcin/bgv031 PMID: 26106144

Lei, K., Wu, R., Wang, J., Lei, X., Zhou, E., Fan, R., & Gong, L. (2024). Sirtuins as potential targets for neuroprotection: Mechanisms of early brain injury induced by subarachnoid hemorrhage. *Translational Stroke Research*, *15*(6), 1017–1034. DOI: 10.1007/s12975-023-01191-z PMID: 37779164

Li, X., Li, C., Zhang, W., Wang, Y., Qian, P., & Huang, H. (2023). Inflammation and aging: Signaling pathways and intervention therapies. *Signal Transduction and Targeted Therapy*, *8*(1), 1–29. DOI: 10.1038/s41392-023-01502-8 PMID: 37291105

Li, Z., Zhang, Z., Ren, Y., Wang, Y., Fang, J., Yue, H., Ma, S., & Guan, F. (2021). Aging and age-related diseases: From mechanisms to therapeutic strategies. *Biogerontology*, *22*(2), 165–187. DOI: 10.1007/s10522-021-09910-5 PMID: 33502634

Liao, Z., Yeo, H. L., Wong, S. W., & Zhao, Y. (2021). Cellular Senescence: Mechanisms and Therapeutic Potential. *Biomedicines*, *9*(12), 12. Advance online publication. DOI: 10.3390/biomedicines9121769 PMID: 34944585

Longworth, S., & Damania, B. (2025). Modulation of Cell Cycle Kinases by Kaposi's Sarcoma-Associated Herpesvirus. *Journal of Medical Virology*, *97*(1), e70157. DOI: 10.1002/jmv.70157 PMID: 39804127

Lu, T., Aron, L., Zullo, J., Pan, Y., Kim, H., Chen, Y., Yang, T.-H., Kim, H.-M., Drake, D., Liu, X. S., Bennett, D. A., Colaiácovo, M. P., & Yankner, B. A. (2014). REST and stress resistance in ageing and Alzheimer's disease. *Nature*, *507*(7493), 448–454. DOI: 10.1038/nature13163 PMID: 24670762

Luan, Y., Zhu, X., Jiao, Y., Liu, H., Huang, Z., Pei, J., Xu, Y., Yang, Y., & Ren, K. (2024). Cardiac cell senescence: Molecular mechanisms, key proteins and therapeutic targets. *Cell Death Discovery*, *10*(1), 1–15. DOI: 10.1038/s41420-023-01792-5 PMID: 38355681

Lv, J., Zhang, C., Liu, X., Gu, C., Liu, Y., Gao, Y., Huang, Z., Jiang, Q., Chen, B., He, D., Wang, T., Xu, Z., & Su, W. (2024). An aging-related immune landscape in the hematopoietic immune system. *Immunity & Ageing*, *21*(1), 3. DOI: 10.1186/s12979-023-00403-2 PMID: 38169405

Ma, W., & Zhou, S. (2025). Metabolic Rewiring in the Face of Genomic Assault: Integrating DNA Damage Response and Cellular Metabolism. *Biomolecules*, *15*(2), 2. Advance online publication. DOI: 10.3390/biom15020168 PMID: 40001471

Manastireanu, D. M., Salazar, N. A., Bejarano, E., & Nieto-Torres, J. L. (2024). Selective autophagy: A therapeutic target for healthy aging? *Aging Advances*, *1*(1), 2–22. DOI: 10.4103/AGINGADV.AGINGADV-D-24-00002

Martínez-Cué, C., & Rueda, N. (2020). Cellular Senescence in Neurodegenerative Diseases. *Frontiers in Cellular Neuroscience*, *14*, 16. Advance online publication. DOI: 10.3389/fncel.2020.00016 PMID: 32116562

McCauley, B. S., & Dang, W. (2014). Histone methylation and aging: Lessons learned from model systems. *Biochimica et Biophysica Acta*, *1839*(12), 1454–1462. DOI: 10.1016/j.bbagrm.2014.05.008 PMID: 24859460

Miller, K. M., Tjeertes, J. V., Coates, J., Legube, G., Polo, S. E., Britton, S., & Jackson, S. P. (2010). Human HDAC1 and HDAC2 function in the DNA-damage response to promote DNA nonhomologous end-joining. *Nature Structural & Molecular Biology*, *17*(9), 1144–1151. DOI: 10.1038/nsmb.1899 PMID: 20802485

Mohite, P., Puri, A., Dave, R., Budar, A., Munde, S., Ghosh, S. B., Alqahtani, T., Shmrany, H. A., Kumer, A., & Dhara, B. (2024). Unlocking the therapeutic potential: Odyssey of induced pluripotent stem cells in precision cell therapies. *International Journal of Surgery*, *110*(10), 6432–6455. DOI: 10.1097/JS9.0000000000001892 PMID: 38963728

Muraki, K., Nyhan, K., Han, L., & Murnane, J. P. (2012). Mechanisms of telomere loss and their consequences for chromosome instability. *Frontiers in Oncology*, *2*, 135. DOI: 10.3389/fonc.2012.00135 PMID: 23061048

Musheev, M. U., Baumgärtner, A., Krebs, L., & Niehrs, C. (2020). The origin of genomic N 6-methyl-deoxyadenosine in mammalian cells. *Nature Chemical Biology*, *16*(6), 630–634. DOI: 10.1038/s41589-020-0504-2 PMID: 32203414

Nativio, R., Donahue, G., Berson, A., Lan, Y., Amlie-Wolf, A., Tuzer, F., Toledo, J. B., Gosai, S. J., Gregory, B. D., Torres, C., Trojanowski, J. Q., Wang, L.-S., Johnson, F. B., Bonini, N. M., & Berger, S. L. (2018). Dysregulation of the epigenetic landscape of normal aging in Alzheimer's disease. *Nature Neuroscience*, *21*(4), 497–505. DOI: 10.1038/s41593-018-0101-9 PMID: 29507413

Niedernhofer, L. J., Bohr, V. A., Sander, M., & Kraemer, K. H. (2011). Xeroderma pigmentosum and other diseases of human premature aging and DNA repair: Molecules to patients. *Mechanisms of Ageing and Development*, *132*(6-7), 340–347. DOI: 10.1016/j.mad.2011.06.004 PMID: 21708183

Nilsson, M. I., & Tarnopolsky, M. A. (2019). Mitochondria and Aging—The Role of Exercise as a Countermeasure. *Biology (Basel)*, *8*(2), 2. Advance online publication. DOI: 10.3390/biology8020040 PMID: 31083586

Nwankwo, E. I., Emeihe, E. V., Ajegbile, M. D., Olaboye, J. A., & Maha, C. C. (2024). Integrating telemedicine and AI to improve healthcare access in rural settings. International Journal of Life science Research Archives, 7(1), 59-77. DOI: DOI: 10.53771/ijlsra.2024.7.1.0061

O'Sullivan, R. J., & Karlseder, J. (2010). Telomeres: Protecting chromosomes against genome instability. *Nature Reviews. Molecular Cell Biology*, *11*(3), 171–181. DOI: 10.1038/nrm2848 PMID: 20125188

Ogrodnik, M., Salmonowicz, H., & Gladyshev, V. N. (2019). Integrating cellular senescence with the concept of damage accumulation in aging: Relevance for clearance of senescent cells. *Aging Cell*, *18*(1), e12841. DOI: 10.1111/acel.12841 PMID: 30346102

Ohtani, N., Mann, D. J., & Hara, E. (2009). Cellular senescence: Its role in tumor suppression and aging. *Cancer Science*, *100*(5), 792–797. DOI: 10.1111/j.1349-7006.2009.01123.x PMID: 19302284

Palmer, J. E., Wilson, N., Son, S. M., Obrocki, P., Wrobel, L., Rob, M., Takla, M., Korolchuk, V. I., & Rubinsztein, D. C. (2025). Autophagy, aging, and age-related neurodegeneration. *Neuron*, *113*(1), 29–48. DOI: 10.1016/j.neuron.2024.09.015 PMID: 39406236

Panich, U., Sittithumcharee, G., Rathviboon, N., & Jirawatnotai, S. (2016). Ultraviolet Radiation-Induced Skin Aging: The Role of DNA Damage and Oxidative Stress in Epidermal Stem Cell Damage Mediated Skin Aging. *Stem Cells International*, *2016*(1), 7370642. DOI: 10.1155/2016/7370642 PMID: 27148370

Parihar, P., Solanki, I., Mansuri, M. L., & Parihar, M. S. (2015). Mitochondrial sirtuins: Emerging roles in metabolic regulations, energy homeostasis and diseases. *Experimental Gerontology*, *61*, 130–141. DOI: 10.1016/j.exger.2014.12.004 PMID: 25482473

Park, S. H. (2024). Role of Phytochemicals in Treatment of Aging and Cancer: Focus on Mechanism of FOXO3 Activation. *Antioxidants*, *13*(9), 1099. DOI: 10.3390/antiox13091099 PMID: 39334758

Pathak, S., & Banerjee, A. (2024). *Gut Microbiome and Brain Ageing: Brain Aging*. Springer Nature. DOI: 10.1007/978-981-99-8803-7

Pellarin, I., Dall'Acqua, A., Favero, A., Segatto, I., Rossi, V., Crestan, N., Karimbayli, J., Belletti, B., & Baldassarre, G. (2025). Cyclin-dependent protein kinases and cell cycle regulation in biology and disease. *Signal Transduction and Targeted Therapy*, *10*(1), 1–62. DOI: 10.1038/s41392-024-02080-z PMID: 39800748

Pinto, M., & Moraes, C. T. (2015). Mechanisms linking mtDNA damage and aging. *Free Radical Biology & Medicine*, *85*, 250–258. DOI: 10.1016/j.freeradbiomed.2015.05.005 PMID: 25979659

Polo, S. E., & Jackson, S. P. (2011). Dynamics of DNA damage response proteins at DNA breaks: a focus on protein modifications. *Genes & development*, 25(5), 409-433. DOI: http://www.genesdev.org/cgi/doi/10.1101/gad.2021311

Qin, Y., Yang, P., He, W., Li, D., Zeng, L., Li, J., Zhou, T., Peng, J., Cao, L., & Huang, W. (2024). Novel histone post-translational modifications in Alzheimer's disease: Current advances and implications. *Clinical Epigenetics*, *16*(1), 39. DOI: 10.1186/s13148-024-01650-w PMID: 38461320

Quina, A. S., Buschbeck, M., & Di Croce, L. (2006). Chromatin structure and epigenetics. *Biochemical Pharmacology*, *72*(11), 1563–1569. DOI: 10.1016/j.bcp.2006.06.016 PMID: 16836980

Ramponi, V., Richart, L., Kovatcheva, M., Stephan-Otto Attolini, C., Capellades, J., Lord, A. E., Yanes, O., Ficz, G., & Serrano, M. (2025). H4K20me3-Mediated Repression of Inflammatory Genes Is a Characteristic and Targetable Vulnerability of Persister Cancer Cells. *Cancer Research*, *85*(1), 32–51. DOI: 10.1158/0008-5472.CAN-24-0529 PMID: 39476057

Ramsahoye, B. H., Biniszkiewicz, D., Lyko, F., Clark, V., Bird, A. P., & Jaenisch, R. (2000). Non-CpG methylation is prevalent in embryonic stem cells and may be mediated by DNA methyltransferase 3a. *Proceedings of the National Academy of Sciences of the United States of America*, *97*(10), 5237–5242. DOI: 10.1073/pnas.97.10.5237 PMID: 10805783

Raza, S. (2024). Autophagy and metabolic aging: Current understanding and future applications. Biochimica et Biophysica Acta (BBA)-. *Biochimica et Biophysica Acta. Molecular Cell Research*, *119753*(6), 119753. Advance online publication. DOI: 10.1016/j.bbamcr.2024.119753 PMID: 38763302

Rodriguez, M. A., Bucktrout, R., Orlando, A., Serganova, I., & Zappasodi, R. (2024). Mechanism of Action and Pharmacologic Features of Drugs Targeting PD-1/PDL-1 and CTLA-4. Precision Cancer Therapies vol 2-Immunologic Approaches for the Treatment of Lymphoid Malignancies-From Concept to Practice, 139-155. DOI: https://doi.org/DOI: 10.1002/9781119824572.ch11

Rodríguez-Aguilera, J. R., Ecsedi, S., Goldsmith, C., Cros, M. P., Domínguez-López, M., Guerrero-Celis, N., Pérez-Cabeza de Vaca, R., Chemin, I., Recillas-Targa, F., Chagoya de Sánchez, V., & Hernández-Vargas, H. (2020). Genome-wide 5-hydroxymethylcytosine (5hmC) emerges at early stage of in vitro differentiation of a putative hepatocyte progenitor. *Scientific Reports*, *10*(1), 7822. DOI: 10.1038/s41598-020-64700-2 PMID: 32385352

Rodriguez-Colman, M. J., Dansen, T. B., & Burgering, B. M. (2024). FOXO transcription factors as mediators of stress adaptation. *Nature Reviews. Molecular Cell Biology*, *25*(1), 46–64. DOI: 10.1038/s41580-023-00649-0 PMID: 37710009

Rodríguez-Rodero, S., Fernández-Morera, J. L., Menéndez-Torre, E., Calvanese, V., Fernández, A. F., & Fraga, M. F. (2011). Aging Genetics and Aging. *Aging and Disease*, *2*(3), 186–195. PMID: 22396873

Saha, A., Sanyal, T., Mukherjee, P., Sen, K., & Madhu, N. R. (2024). Response of Cellular Stress Toward the Hormetic Phytochemicals in Brain Aging. In *Neuroprotective Effects of Phytochemicals in Brain Ageing* (pp. 57–95). Springer Nature Singapore., DOI: 10.1007/978-981-99-7269-2_4

Salameh, Y., Bejaoui, Y., & El Hajj, N. (2020). DNA methylation biomarkers in aging and age-related diseases. *Frontiers in Genetics*, *11*, 480672. DOI: 10.3389/fgene.2020.00171 PMID: 32211026

Sanchez, A., Lee, D., Kim, D. I., & Miller, K. M. (2021). Making connections: Integrative signaling mechanisms coordinate DNA break repair in chromatin. *Frontiers in Genetics*, *12*, 747734. DOI: 10.3389/fgene.2021.747734 PMID: 34659365

Santos, B. F., Grenho, I., Martel, P. J., Ferreira, B. I., & Link, W. (2023). FOXO family isoforms. *Cell Death & Disease*, *14*(10), 702. DOI: 10.1038/s41419-023-06177-1 PMID: 37891184

Santos, L., Benitez-Rosendo, A., Bresque, M., Camacho-Pereira, J., Calliari, A., & Escande, C. (2023). Sirtuins: The NAD+-Dependent Multifaceted Modulators of Inflammation. *Antioxidants & Redox Signaling*, *39*(16–18), 1185–1208. DOI: 10.1089/ars.2023.0295 PMID: 37767625

Schmitt, C. A., Wang, B., & Demaria, M. (2022). Senescence and cancer—Role and therapeutic opportunities. *Nature Reviews. Clinical Oncology*, *19*(10), 619–636. DOI: 10.1038/s41571-022-00668-4 PMID: 36045302

Seale, K., Teschendorff, A., Reiner, A. P., Voisin, S., & Eynon, N. (2024). A comprehensive map of the aging blood methylome in humans. *Genome Biology*, 25(1), 240. DOI: Sedaghatmehr, M., & Balazadeh, S. (2024). Autophagy: a key player in the recovery of plants from heat stress. *Journal of Experimental Botany*, *75*(8), 2246–2255. DOI: 10.1093/jxb/erae018 PMID: 38236036

Sena, L. A., & Chandel, N. S. (2012). Physiological Roles of Mitochondrial Reactive Oxygen Species. *Molecular Cell*, *48*(2), 158–167. DOI: 10.1016/j.molcel.2012.09.025 PMID: 23102266

Shenhav, O. (2024). Next generation in Alzheimer's therapeutic strategies (Doctoral dissertation, University of Zagreb. School of Medicine. Department of Neurology).

Shvedova, M., Samdavid Thanapaul, R. J. R., Thompson, E. L., Niedernhofer, L. J., & Roh, D. S. (2022). Cellular Senescence in Aging, Tissue Repair, and Regeneration. *Plastic and Reconstructive Surgery*, *150*, 4S–11S. DOI: 10.1097/PRS.0000000000009667 PMID: 36170430

Singh, P., & Paramanik, V. (2025). DNA methylation, histone acetylation in the regulation of memory and its modulation during aging. *Frontiers in Aging*, *5*, 1480932. DOI: 10.3389/fragi.2024.1480932 PMID: 39835300

Singh, S. K., Parihar, S., Jain, S., Ho, J. A. A., & Vankayala, R. (2024). Light-responsive functional nanomaterials as pioneering therapeutics: A paradigm shift to combat age-related disorders. *Journal of Materials Chemistry. B*, *12*(34), 8212–8234. DOI: 10.1039/D4TB00578C PMID: 39058026

Smallwood, S. A., & Kelsey, G. (2012). De novo DNA methylation: A germ cell perspective. *Trends in Genetics*, *28*(1), 33–42. DOI: 10.1016/j.tig.2011.09.004 PMID: 22019337

Soroudi, S., Jaafari, M. R., & Arabi, L. (2024). Lipid nanoparticle (LNP) mediated mRNA delivery in cardiovascular diseases: Advances in genome editing and CAR T cell therapy. *Journal of Controlled Release*, *372*, 113–140. DOI: 10.1016/j.jconrel.2024.06.023 PMID: 38876358

Sun, H., Li, D., Wei, C., Liu, L., Xin, Z., Gao, H., & Gao, R. (2024). The relationship between SIRT1 and inflammation: A systematic review and meta-analysis. *Frontiers in Immunology*, *15*, 1465849. DOI: 10.3389/fimmu.2024.1465849 PMID: 39676853

Templeman, N. M., & Murphy, C. T. (2017). Regulation of reproduction and longevity by nutrient-sensing pathways. *The Journal of Cell Biology*, *217*(1), 93–106. DOI: 10.1083/jcb.201707168 PMID: 29074705

Tufail, M., Huang, Y.-Q., Hu, J.-J., Liang, J., He, C.-Y., Wan, W.-D., Jiang, C.-H., Wu, H., & Li, N. (2024). Cellular Aging and Senescence in Cancer: A Holistic Review of Cellular Fate Determinants. *Aging and Disease*, 0. Advance online publication. DOI: 10.14336/AD.2024.0421 PMID: 38913050

Unnikrishnan, A., Freeman, W. M., Jackson, J., Wren, J. D., Porter, H., & Richardson, A. (2019). The role of DNA methylation in epigenetics of aging. *Pharmacology & Therapeutics*, *195*, 172–185. DOI: 10.1016/j.pharmthera.2018.11.001 PMID: 30419258

Vaiserman, A. M., Koliada, A. K., & Marotta, F. (2017). Gut microbiota: A player in aging and a target for anti-aging intervention. *Ageing Research Reviews*, *35*, 36–45. DOI: 10.1016/j.arr.2017.01.001 PMID: 28109835

Van Der Heide, L. P., Hoekman, M. F., & Smidt, M. P. (2004). The ins and outs of FoxO shuttling: Mechanisms of FoxO translocation and transcriptional regulation. *The Biochemical Journal*, *380*(2), 297–309. DOI: 10.1042/bj20040167 PMID: 15005655

Venditti, P., & Di Meo, S. (2020). The Role of Reactive Oxygen Species in the Life Cycle of the Mitochondrion. *International Journal of Molecular Sciences*, *21*(6), 6. Advance online publication. DOI: 10.3390/ijms21062173 PMID: 32245255

Vijg, J. (2021). From DNA damage to mutations: All roads lead to aging. *Ageing Research Reviews, 68*, 101316. DOI: 10.1016/j.arr.2021.101316 PMID: 33711511

Vitiello, M., Zullo, A., Servillo, L., Mancini, F. P., Borriello, A., Giovane, A., Della Ragione, F., D'Onofrio, N., & Balestrieri, M. L. (2017). Multiple pathways of SIRT6 at the crossroads in the control of longevity, cancer, and cardiovascular diseases. *Ageing Research Reviews, 35*, 301–311. DOI: 10.1016/j.arr.2016.10.008 PMID: 27829173

Wang, Y., Liu, S., Ying, L., Zhang, K., Li, H., Liang, N., Xiao, L., & Luo, G. (2024). Nicotinamide Mononucleotide (NMN) Ameliorates Free Fatty Acid-Induced Pancreatic β-Cell Dysfunction via the NAD+/AMPK/SIRT1/HIF-1α Pathway. *International Journal of Molecular Sciences, 25*(19), 10534. DOI: 10.3390/ijms251910534 PMID: 39408861

Wątroba, M., Dudek, I., Skoda, M., Stangret, A., Rzodkiewicz, P., & Szukiewicz, D. (2017). Sirtuins, epigenetics and longevity. *Ageing Research Reviews, 40*, 11–19. DOI: 10.1016/j.arr.2017.08.001 PMID: 28789901

Wei, B., Wei, M., Huang, H., Fan, T., Zhang, Z., & Song, X. (2024). Mesenchymal Stem Cell-Derived Exosomes: A Promising Therapeutic Strategy for Age-Related Diseases. *Cell Proliferation, 13795*, e13795. Advance online publication. DOI: 10.1111/cpr.13795 PMID: 39704104

Wu, N., Zheng, W., Zhou, Y., Tian, Y., Tang, M., Feng, X., Ashrafizadeh, M., Wang, Y., Niu, X., Tambuwala, M., Wang, L., Tergaonkar, V., Sethi, G., Klionsky, D., Huang, L., & Gu, M. (2024). Autophagy in aging-related diseases and cancer: Principles, regulatory mechanisms and therapeutic potential. *Ageing Research Reviews, 102428*, 102428. Advance online publication. DOI: 10.1016/j.arr.2024.102428 PMID: 39038742

Wu, Z., Qu, J., & Liu, G.-H. (2024). Roles of chromatin and genome instability in cellular senescence and their relevance to ageing and related diseases. *Nature Reviews. Molecular Cell Biology, 25*(12), 979–1000. DOI: 10.1038/s41580-024-00775-3 PMID: 39363000

Xiao, F. H., Wang, H. T., & Kong, Q. P. (2019). Dynamic DNA methylation during aging: A "prophet" of age-related outcomes. *Frontiers in Genetics, 10*, 107. DOI: 10.3389/fgene.2019.00107 PMID: 30833961

Xiao, P., Zhang, Y., Zeng, Y., Yang, D., Mo, J., Zheng, Z., Wang, J., Zhang, Y., Zhou, Z., Zhong, X., & Yan, W. (2023). Impaired angiogenesis in ageing: The central role of the extracellular matrix. *Journal of Translational Medicine, 21*(1), 457. DOI: 10.1186/s12967-023-04315-z PMID: 37434156

Xie, J., Wang, Y., Lu, L., Liu, L., Yu, X., & Pei, F. (2021). Cellular senescence in knee osteoarthritis: Molecular mechanisms and therapeutic implications. *Ageing Research Reviews, 70*, 101413. DOI: 10.1016/j.arr.2021.101413 PMID: 34298194

Xiong, J., Dong, L., Lv, Q., Yin, Y., Zhao, J., Ke, Y., Wang, S., Zhang, W., & Wu, M. (2024). Targeting senescence-associated secretory phenotypes to remodel the tumour microenvironment and modulate tumour outcomes. *Clinical and Translational Medicine, 14*(9), e1772. DOI: 10.1002/ctm2.1772 PMID: 39270064

Yu, B., Dong, X., Gravina, S., Kartal, Ö., Schimmel, T., Cohen, J., Tortoriello, D., Zody, R., Hawkins, R. D., & Vijg, J. (2017). Genome-wide, single-cell DNA methylomics reveals increased non-CpG methylation during human oocyte maturation. *Stem Cell Reports*, *9*(1), 397–407. DOI: 10.1016/j.stemcr.2017.05.026 PMID: 28648898

Yu, J., Li, T., & Zhu, J. (2023). Gene therapy strategies targeting aging-related diseases. *Aging and Disease*, *14*(2), 398. DOI: 10.14336/AD.2022.00725 PMID: 37008065

Yu, W., Yu, Y., Sun, S., Lu, C., Zhai, J., Lei, Y., Bai, F., Wang, R., & Chen, J. (2024). Immune Alterations with Aging: Mechanisms and Intervention *Strategies.Nutrients*, *16*(22), 3830. DOI: 10.3390/nu16223830 PMID: 39599617

Zhao, X., Wei, T., Hou, Y., Wu, Y., Zhou, H., Meng, J., Wang, Q., & Liu, Y. (2025). ATM/ATR-Mediated DNA Damage Response Facilitates SARS-CoV-2 Spike Protein-Induced Syncytium Formation. *Journal of Medical Virology*, *97*(1), e70137. DOI: 10.1002/jmv.70137 PMID: 39740081

Zhao, Y., & Liu, Y. S. (2021). Longevity factor FOXO3: A key regulator in aging-related vascular diseases. *Frontiers in Cardiovascular Medicine*, *8*, 778674. DOI: 10.3389/fcvm.2021.778674 PMID: 35004893

Zhao, Y., & Liu, Y.-S. (2021). Longevity Factor FOXO3: A Key Regulator in Aging-Related Vascular Diseases. *Frontiers in Cardiovascular Medicine*, *8*, 778674. Advance online publication. DOI: 10.3389/fcvm.2021.778674 PMID: 35004893

Chapter 3
Exploring the Role of Telomere Dynamics and Homocysteine Levels in Aging and Potential Intervention Strategies

Tanushree Kar
https://orcid.org/0009-0005-2840-6584
VIT Bhopal University, India

D. Lakshmi
https://orcid.org/0000-0003-4018-1208
VIT Bhopal University, India

Mahendran Botlagunta
VIT Bhopal University, India

ABSTRACT

Aging is an inevitable biological process that affects every living organism. It is influenced by a complex interplay of factors like genetics, environment, and lifestyle. These factors gradually lead to changes in an individual's body's physiological functions over a period of time. With modern society's increased workload and bustling lifestyles, many individuals are gradually neglecting their health, which accelerates the aging process and contributes to the development of critical health conditions. This chapter will explore two of the key biological mechanisms associated with aging—telomere shortening and elevated homocysteine levels—and examine potential interventions to mitigate their effects.

1. INTRODUCTION TO AGING

The process of aging is an influential and complex multitude of factors, including genetics, environment, lifestyle, telomere shortening, levels of homocysteines, mitochondrial genome damage, and cumulative "wear and tear" on the body. Genetic factors, such as inherited mutations and epigenetic changes play a crucial role in determining the rate of aging and susceptibility to age-related diseases. Environmental

DOI: 10.4018/979-8-3693-9730-5.ch003

factors, including exposure to UV radiation, pollution, and oxidative stress, also contribute significantly to the aging process by causing cellular damage. Lifestyle choices, such as diet, exercise, smoking, alcohol consumption, and sleep patterns, also play a significant role in determining an individual's aging trajectory (Pandey, 2018; Accardi & Aiello, 2021).

After extensive years of research on the aging process, scientists categorized the major factors responsible into ten major domains: genetic factors, cellular factors, biochemical factors, metabolic factors, environmental factors, lifestyle factors, social and psychological factors, immunological factors, microbiome, and extracellular matrix and tissue factors (Pandey, 2018; Accardi & Aiello, 2021).

These factors blend and interact with each other to form a network kind of process that cumulatively influences aging. Factors like lifestyle and diet are modifiable and can be regulated and monitored, while genetics are not. But understanding all these factors and their mechanisms can lead us to develop anti-aging interventions that target multiple pathways.

1.1 Genetic Factors

Genetics is one of the multiple factors that affect and influence aging. These factors have a grand total of 27estimated influences on aging, as shown in Figure 1. These factors are subdivided into 4 factors: DNA damage and mutation, telomere shortening, epigenetic changes, and genetic predisposition.

Figure 1. The domains of factors that determine the aging process in an individual with their estimated influence on this process.

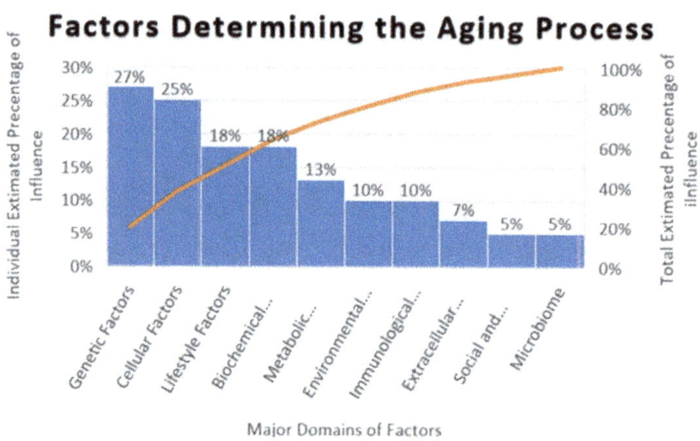

With the passing time, it is observed that the DNA in cells gradually starts to accumulate damages that they receive from internal processes like replication errors and external factors like UV radiation and other toxins. These types of mutations in the body can impair the cellular functions, leading to aging. Telomeres are the protective caps of the chromosomes that are present at the end but gradually shorten with each passing cell division. Cellular senscence or apoptosis, is the result of shortened telomeres. We will learn more about telomeres in the later parts of this chapter. Epigenetic changes suggest the chemical modifications of DNA and the role of histones in changing the gene expression pattern without altering the DNA sequence. Studies observe that with time, these little modifications can result in the disruption of cellular functions, leading to aging. Research shows that genes like FOXO3A are associated with longevity or increased lifespan (Pandey, 2018; Accardi & Aiello, 2021).

1.2 Cellular Factors

Cellular is one of the multiple factors that affect and influence aging. These factors have a grand total of 25estimated influences on aging as shown in Figure 1. These factors are subdivided into 4 factors: cellular senescence, mitochondrial dysfunction, proteostasis decline, and stem cell exhaustion.

During cellular senescence, the cells that have stopped dividing due to conditions like stress or damage can accumulate in the tissues, then start secreting inflammatory factors that harm the neighboring cells and tissues, which add on to the aging process. Mitochondria is well-known as the powerhouse of the cell. But, with passing time, it accumulates damages that result in the production of less efficient energies, which results in increased production of reactive oxygen species (ROS) that damages the cells. With age, studies evidently show that the mechanical processes responsible for proteostasis (i.e., protein folding and degradation) decline, resulting in the accumulation of misfolded or damaged proteins that have the potential to disrupt cellular functions. Stem cells are known for their ability to repair damaged tissue, but they can gradually lose function and potential, leading to an age-related decline in tissue repair and function (Pandey, 2018; Accardi & Aiello, 2021).

1.3 Biochemical Factors

Biochemicals are one of the multiple factors that affect and influence aging. These factors have a grand total of 18estimated influences on aging (Figure 1). These factors are subdivided into 4 factors: oxidative stress, inflammation, advanced glycation end-products (AGEs), and homocysteine.

Oxidative stress occurs due to the accumulation of ROS that can cause changes to DNA, proteins, and lipid profiles, contributing to aging. While over time these systems can become less effective due to the presence of the body's antioxidant defenses. Chronic low-grade inflammation is also a significant sign of aging. Research suggests that inflammatory markers gradually increase with age, resulting in damage to tissues and other age-related diseases. When proteins or fats combine with sugars in the bloodstream, ACEs form. With time, AEGs accumulate and impair the cellular functioning of the body, resulting in aging and diseases like diabetes and Alzheimer's. Studies show that the elevated levels of homocysteine in the blood are associated with the increased risk of cardiovascular diseases, neurodegenerative disorders, and osteoporosis. Basically, homocysteine is a byproduct of methionine metabolism; it can accumulate in the body when not properly metabolized due to the deficiencies in vitamin B (B6, B12, and folate), which leads to the development of oxidative stress, endothelial damage, and accelerated aging (Pandey, 2018; Accardi & Aiello, 2021). We will learn more about homocysteine in the later parts of this chapter.

1.4 Metabolic Factors

Metabolism is one of the multiple factors that affect and influence aging. These factors have a grand total of 13estimated influences on aging (Figure 1). These factors are subdivided into 4 factors: caloric intake, hormonal changes, nutrient-sensing pathways, and homocysteine metabolism.

Intakes of high-calorie food items can lead to accelerated aging, as through this there is an increase in metabolic stress. Studies conducted on animal models depicted an extended lifespan and delay in the onset of age-related diseases just by restricting caloric intake (without malnutrition). Hormones like insulin, growth hormones, and sex hormones (e.g., estrogen, testosterone) show a significantly positive decline with age. Slight changes in the levels of these hormones can affect the metabolism, immune function, and cellular repair mechanisms. In the regulation of growth, metabolism, and lifespan pathways, like mTOR (mechanistic target of rapamycin), AMPK (AMP-activated protein kinase), and IGF-1 (insulin-like growth factor) play an important role. The aging process is linked to the dysregulation of these pathways. Elevated homocysteine levels also cause disruption in metabolic balance, especially in pathways that depend on methylation and one-carbon metabolism. Adequate levels of folate, vitamin B12, and vitamin B6 are crucial for the proper metabolism of homocysteine. If a deficiency of these nutrients is seen, then it is evident that to observe a risen level of homocysteine leading to cellular and vascular aging (Pandey, 2018; Accardi & Aiello, 2021). We will learn more about homocysteine in the later parts of this chapter.

1.5 Environmental Factors

The environment also acts as one of the multiple factors that affect and influence aging. These factors have a grand total of 10estimated influences on aging (Figure 1). These factors are subdivided into 3 factors: UV radiation, pollution, and toxins and chemicals.

Studies suggest that ultraviolet (UV) light exposure from the sun damages skin cells, which accelerates skin aging, like wrinkles and loss of elasticity, etc., and also increases the chances of skin cancer. Exposure to environmental pollutants like air pollution, heavy metals, and pesticides can cause skin irritation, oxidative stress, and even inflammation that leads to accelerated aging. Damaging cells and tissues can be evident due to smoking, consumption of alcohol, and exposure to harmful chemicals, which can lead to accelerated aging (Pandey, 2018; Accardi & Aiello, 2021).

1.6 Lifestyle Factors

Lifestyle also acts as one of the multiple factors that affect and influence aging. These factors have a grand total of 18estimated influences on aging (Figure 1). These factors are subdivided into 4 factors: diet, physical activity, sleep, and stress.

Diets that contain high sugar, unhealthy fats, and processed foods accelerate aging, while diets rich in antioxidants like fruits and vegetables can act as a counteract for oxidative stress and inflammation, leading to the deacceleration of aging. It is advisable to maintain an optimal level of vitamin B in the body, as it is crucial for regulating homocysteine levels and supporting overall health. We will learn more about homocysteine in the later parts of this chapter. Years of extensive research have shown that regular exercise has the potential to improve one's mitochondrial function, enhance autophagy (cellular cleaning), and also promote a longer lifespan by decreasing inflammation and maintaining cardiovascular health in an individual. Oxidative stress and impaired cognitive function can also be the result of poor sleep quality and quantity, which increases the risk of age-related diseases. Many studies link increased inflammation, shortened telomeres, and accelerated aging to chronic psychological stress. In order to maintain and manage the stress levels, mindfulness, yoga, or meditation are advised; these practices can also slow down the aging process (Pandey, 2018; Accardi & Aiello, 2021).

1.7 Social and Psychological Factors

Society and psychology also act as one of the multiple factors that affect and influence aging. These factors have a grand total of 5estimated influences on aging (Figure 1). These factors are subdivided into 3 factors: social engagement, cognitive stimulation, and mental health.

Studies say that positive interactions and a strong support network are linked to a longer life expectancy and a better quality of mental health. Learning new skills or solving a complex problem, like mental activities that usually challenge the brain, can help in maintaining cognitive function as one ages. Poorer physical health, increased inflammation, and accelerated aging are considered contributing factors of depression, anxiety, and other mental health-related conditions (Pandey, 2018; Accardi & Aiello, 2021).

1.8 Immunological Factors

Immunity also acts as one of the multiple factors that affect and influence aging. These factors have a grand total of 10estimated influences on aging (Figure 1). These factors are subdivided into 2 factors: immunosenescence and autoimmunity.

Research suggests that with declining age, the immune system loses its effectiveness, which results in an increased risk of susceptibility to infections, cancers, and other chronic diseases. Due to the immune system's lessened responsiveness, the body also gets susceptible to chronic inflammations. As an individual ages, his immune system gradually declines, which may lead to misjudging the body's own tissues and attacking them. This misinterpretation leads to many autoimmune diseases that exacerbate the rate of the aging process (Pandey, 2018; Accardi & Aiello, 2021).

1.9 Microbiome

Immunity also acts as one of the multiple factors that affect and influence aging. These factors have a grand total of 5estimated influences on aging (Figure 1). This factor is subdivided into 1 factor: gut microbiota changes.

Studies suggest that with age, the composition of the gut microbiota shifts. This shift can affect metabolism, inflammation, and immune function. This imbalance in the gut microbiota is responsible for many age-related changes and diseases and the overall health decline of an individual (Pandey, 2018; Accardi & Aiello, 2021).

1.10 Extracellular Matrix and Tissue Factors

The extracellular matrix and tissue also act as one of the multiple factors that affect and influence aging. These factors have a grand total of 7estimated influences on aging (Figure 1). These factors are subdivided into 2 factors: extracellular matrix degradation and tissue-specific aging.

The ECM (extracellular matrix) provides structural support to tissues. ECM is composed of components like collagen and elastin. But as we age, the components of the ECM degrade, which leads to tissue stiffness, wrinkles, and decreased organ function. All of the body's tissues and organs have a specific age of their own. Their aging primarily depends on their exposure to environmental stress, metabolic demands, and regenerative capacity (Pandey, 2018; Accardi & Aiello, 2021).

2. INTRODUCTION TO HOMOCYSTEINE

It is a metabolite of the essential amino acid methionine. Homocysteine (Hcy) acts as a stepping stone in a metabolic pathway where methionine is converted into cysteine, termed transsulfuration (Bruce, 2012). Typically, it is a sulfur-containing amino acid that plays a vital role in the functioning of one's body's metabolism. Basically, it is obtained from dietary sources. Understanding and recognizing its function, metabolism, and implications for health are very crucial to identify the homocysteine's role in different physiological processes and to know about its potential impacts on a disease.

2.1 Transsulfuration and Homocysteine Role

This process can be dangerous in homocysteine due to its chances of disturbing cellular sulfur catabolism, contributing to various health-related issues. When homocysteine deviates towards transsulfuration, it undergoes several biochemical transformations to produce cysteine. But for some reason, if this pathway gets dysfunctional or overloaded, then it can cause the accumulation of homocysteine or its toxic derivatives. A rise in the levels of homocysteine in the body will lead to an increase in oxidative stress, endothelial dysfunction, and inflammation, all of which will result in various diseases like cardiovascular disorders, neurodegenerative disorders, pregnancy complications like preeclampsia, and several types of cancer. Cysteine synthesis during the transsulfuration process is essential for the body, but imbalance can cause severe diseases and, in some cases, death (Kumar et al., 2017).

2.2 The Discovery of Homocysteine

It was first used by Du Vigneaud and his coworkers in 1932 in an investigation that required the study of all the individual amino acids towards the Folin-Marenzi reagent. During that, when methionine was heated with strong sulfuric acid, it produced a reaction that yielded a positive result, which was then tested with the Folin-Marenzi reagent. In this experiment, the researchers noticed that when they tested a certain protein, they only got a small reaction with methionine under normal conditions. However, when they added more sulfuric acid to the test, the positive result increased. At first, they thought that it was dimethyl disulfide that was causing this reaction, as its odor was mostly noticeable, but very soon it became clear that only a relatively small amount of this compound was present in the result, and the material that was causing this reaction was non-volatile. Hence, a detailed study, isolation, and identification of this non-volatile cystine-reacting substance revealed the conditions responsible for this mind-blowing decomposition. This is how, during an investigation, they discovered the compound homocysteine. (Lewis & Vincent, 1932)

As the research on elevated levels of homocysteine progresses, the major health conditions related to cardiovascular diseases, dementia, and bone-related issues come into play. which are commonly seen in aging populations. Studies see the role of homocysteine in aging as a part of a complex interplay between oxidative stress, inflammation, and mitochondrial dysfunction whose contribution leads to senescence and cellular damages (Ostrakhovitch & Tabibzadeh, 2019).

Many efforts have been taken to maintain the levels of homocysteine through lifestyle interventions like supplementation with folate, vitamin B6, and vitamin B12. These interventions have shown positive and promising outcomes in terms of lowering homocysteine and mitigating some of the age-associated risks. By studying the homocysteine's broader role in aging, there is a significant chance that we can come up with some concrete strategies and solutions to improve longevity and start targeting healthy aging approaches (Ostrakhovitch & Tabibzadeh, 2019).

2.3 Homocysteine Cycle

The homocysteine cycle includes both the biosynthesis and metabolism of homocysteine. All the reactions that are regulated by SAM are either positive or negative, as mentioned in Figure 2. The homocysteine cycle is regulated by four enzymes.

A. Methyltetrahydrofolate-homocysteine methyltransferase or methionine synthase,
B. Betaine-homocysteine methyltransferase,
C. Cystathionine beta-synthase,
D. MTHFR (a cofactor of vitamin B2) (Miller, 2013).

At first, methionine is activated by the addition of an adenosyl group (i.e., derived from ATP energy currency for many cellular activities) to form SAM (i.e., S-adenosylmethionine, which is a metabolite that plays a crucial role in many biochemical processes in the body). It plays an important role as a universal methyl donor that is crucial for the survival of all living beings. It takes part in many essential reactions, like the synthesis of DNA, RNA, proteins, polyamines, and phospholipids. Additionally, it is a co-substrate in transsulfuration (i.e., a metabolic pathway that is involved in the transfer of sulfur from homocysteine to cysteine), aminopropylation (i.e., a pathway that follows the conversion of SAM into its decarboxylated metabolite), and transmethylation reactions (i.e., organic reactions that transfer the methyl groups from one form of compound to another). Now a product of SAM called SAH (S-adenosylhomocysteine) comes into play, which forms adenosine and homocysteine when it is metabolized. This led homocysteine to a metabolic crossroad, meaning now it can either be remethylated to form methionine or catabolized through cystathionine synthesis (Miller, 2013).

Figure 2. The complex homocysteine cycle

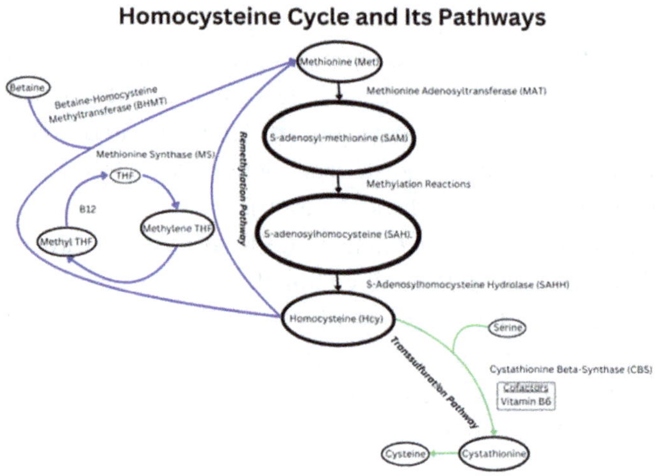

2.3.1 Causes of Homocysteine

We all need to agree on the fact that homocysteine is an essential amino acid of the human body and plays an important role in cellular homeostasis (i.e., it is the ability of the cell to sense internal and external cues and adjust its metabolism accordingly). In normal conditions, the levels of homocysteine are low. But again, extremely low levels can cause cellular dysfunction and damage, which leads to the accumulation of toxins in the body. Studies show that hyperhomocysteinemia (a condition of elevated levels of homocysteine) acts as a critical factor and is linked to many age-related diseases like cardiovascular disorders, cognitive decline, and neurodegeneration. Factors affecting the elevation of levels are deficiency of vitamins, genetic factors, oxidative stress, renal function degradation, diet and lifestyle factors, hormonal changes, chronic inflammation, and medication usage (Wu et al., 2024).

Vitamin B, like B6, B12, and folate, has played a major role in regulating the metabolism of homocysteine. Generally, as we age, a common problem of malabsorption of nutrients is frequently reported. These create deficiencies in some of the crucial vitamins that convert homocysteine back into methionine or cysteine. A reduction in the intake or absorption rate of vitamin B leads to the accumulation of homocysteine in the body. If there is a decline in the direct intake or absorption of folate, then that directly elevates the levels of homocysteine by converting it through the remethylation pathway (Simonenko et al., (2024)..

The variants of the MTHFR gene that are responsible for folate metabolism can impair the homocysteine to methionine conversion, which ultimately leads to a rise in levels of homocysteine. Generally, aging amplifies genetic predisposition that leads to further homocysteine accumulation (Gołębiowska et al., 2023; Ostrakhovitch & Tabibzadeh, 2019).

Elevated levels of oxidative stress are often associated with aging by affecting enzymes responsible for the metabolism of homocysteine. Primarily, oxidative stress damages and impairs the activities of CBS (cystathionine beta-synthase) and other important enzymes that manage and regulate the conversion of homocysteine that ultimately leads to accumulations (Gołębiowska et al., 2023; Ostrakhovitch & Tabibzadeh, 2019).

Declined kidney function is a commonly reported problem in elderly populations. As we know, the kidney acts as a body's natural filter to clean and filter out essential nutrients and minerals from the bloodstream; this condition is equally true for homocysteine. But in elderly populations, due to the declined renal clearance, elevated levels of plasma homocysteine are evident (Gołębiowska et al., 2023; Ostrakhovitch & Tabibzadeh, 2019).

In the elderly population, intake of diets that are low in essential nutrients, mainly vitamin B, folates, and antioxidants, is commonly observed. Studies suggest that the main reason for this type of dietary choice is due to changes in appetite, digestive pattern, and lifestyle habits. Lifestyle habits like smoking, alcohol consumption, and physical inactivity also act as important components that contribute to the elevated levels of homocysteine by breaking the metabolism pattern and increasing the oxidative stress level (Gołębiowska et al., 2023; Ostrakhovitch & Tabibzadeh, 2019).

Estrogen in women is considered to boost the metabolism of homocysteine. It is observed in women with postmenopause that they experience an elevated homocysteine level due to the declined levels of estrogen, which leads to aging in women that is contributed by increased plasma homocysteine (Gołębiowska et al., 2023; Ostrakhovitch & Tabibzadeh, 2019).

Studies often link aging with a state of low-grade chronic inflammation. This inflammation contributes to the promotion of oxidative stress, leading to oxidative damage that interferes with the homocysteine's metabolism and clearance, resulting in its elevated levels (Gołębiowska et al., 2023; Ostrakhovitch & Tabibzadeh, 2019).

Medications like methotrexate, metformin, and anti-epileptic drugs are commonly used by elderly individuals. This medication interferes with the metabolism of folate and homocysteine clearance, which results in elevated homocysteiene levels with time (Gołębiowska et al., 2023; Ostrakhovitch & Tabibzadeh, 2019).

2.3.2 Technology Intervention in Measuring Homocysteine

The technological intervention in measuring homocysteine plays a crucial role in its early detection, which helps in curing and treating patients easily. There are several technologies on the market. Some technologies are lab-based and some patients themselves can detect potential health hazards. Some such lab-based technologies are automated immunoassay systems, high-performance liquid chromatography (HPLC) and mass spectrometry (MS). In automated immunoassay systems, advanced laboratory setups are used, which give precise and effective results by employing various methods like sample handling, dispensing, incubation, and detection. An example of such a technique is ELISA (enzyme-linked immunosorbent assay). Features it includes for the effective detection of homocysteine are high throughput, precision and accuracy, workflow efficiency, quality control, and data management. High-Performance Liquid Chromatography (HPLC) uses physiochemical properties (i.e., size, polarity, and affinity in the case of the stationary phase) to segregate homocysteine from other compounds that are present in the sample matrix. It is widely used in clinical and research laboratory applications because it offers high resolution, sensitivity, and reproducibility in homocysteine analysis. Fluorescence or UV-Vis spectroscopy, is used to enhance resolution and sensitivity. Mass spectrometry (MS) helps to get a precise and sensitive quantification of homocysteine molecules present in biological samples based on their mass-to-charge ratio and detecting the resulting ions. Techniques used in this process include electrospray ionization (ESI) or matrix-assisted laser desorption/ionization (MALDI), a mass analyzer, and a detector. This technology is associated with health conditions like cardiovascular diseases, neural tube defects, and certain genetic disorders. The advantages of using this technology to do homocysteine analysis are its high sensitivity, specificity, and ability to simultaneously measure multiple analytes (McCaddon & Miller, 2023).

Technologies that enable patients themselves to detect potential health hazards are point-of-care testing (POCT), lab-on-a-chip (LOC) technologies, biosensors, and digital health solutions. Point-of-care testing (POCT) offers a way to rapidly and conveniently test for homocysteine levels outside of the laboratory setup. For the quantitative measurement of homocysteine concentrations in biological samples, technologies like immunoassays or enzymatic assays are used. The advantages this technology offers are rapid results, accessibility, point-of-care management, patient convenience, and reduced sample volume. Lab-on-a-chip (LOC) technologies are microfluidic devices that offer innovative solutions that help with the rapid and sensitive detection of this biomarker in the biological sample. These devices typically consist of channels, chambers, and detection elements (i.e., fabricated on a small chip). The advantages of these in the measurement of homocysteine are miniaturization, automation, rapid analysis, portability, and multiplexing. Biosensors use recognition elements (these bind to homocysteine molecules, and upon binding, they convert into a quantifiable output like color change or electrical signals) that selectively interact with the homocysteine molecules. Its applications are widely seen in clinical diagnostics, POCT, and environmental monitoring. It's advantages are rapid, sensitive, and specific detection of homocysteine, and it can be used in many other applications. Digital Health Solutions aims to provide real-time access to homocysteine data, personalized health insights, and tools for proactive management that help empower individuals, healthcare professionals, and researchers. This technology may also include mobile applications, wearable technology, digital platforms, data analytics, AI remote monitoring and telemedicine, and integration with electronic health records (Tseng & Huang, 2021).

2.3.3 Nutrients and Solutions

The main source of homocysteine is dietary methionine, which is found in food items like meats, fish, eggs, nuts, beef, lamb, cheese, turkey, pork, soya, coffee, etc. The deficiencies in one or all of the below-mentioned vitamin B's may affect both remethylation and transsulfuration processes and this will deplete abnormalities in the levels of homocysteine. The major nutrients involved in the metabolism include folate, vitamin B12, vitamin B6, riboflavin, and choline. Although it has been observed that supplementation with folate, vitamin B6, and vitamin B12 successfully reduces concentrations of homocysteine in the blood, most importantly, there is no significant effect on cardiovascular disease risk (Mary Hanna et al., 2022; Olaso-Gonzalez et al., 2021).

Vitamin B6 is also known as pyridoxine. The main functions are that it helps in the conversion of food into energy, helps in the making of red blood cells, and helps normalize the levels of homocysteine in the blood by converting it into cysteine through the transsulfuration pathway. With age, a gradual decline in the efficiency of enzymatic reactions may be observed, which leads to a reduction in the effective homocysteine metabolism. The daily recommended intake for adults (19-50), men (+51 years), and women (+51 years) are 1.3mg/day, 1.7mg/day, and 1.5mg/day, respectively. Hence, the daily recommended intake for all adults is 2mg. Vitamin B6 is added to the refined grains in the US. Excessive supplementation intake can lead to nerve damage and skin lesions. Good sources of it are fish (salmon, tuna, and halibut), poultry (turkey, chicken, and duck), and nuts (hazelnuts and walnuts), as mentioned in Figure 3 (Mary Hanna et al., 2022; Olaso-Gonzalez et al., 2021).

Vitamin B12 is also known as cobalamin. It plays the role of a crucial cofactor in the remethylation of homocysteine into methionine. There is a reduction in the absorption of it if it encounters antacids. Age plays an important role in the ability to absorb it, as with age the gastric acid production and intrinsic factors levels reduce in the body. Deficiency symptoms include tingling (an abnormal feeling that may occur when a nerve is irritated and sends some extra signals), numbness in the extremities (loss of sensation either partially or fully in the affected area of the body), nerve damage, and memory loss. Fortified foods or supplements are recommended for older adults and dietary vegans. Good sources of it are seafood (shellfish and fish), poultry (turkey, chicken, and duck), and red meat (beef, pork, and lamb), as mentioned in Figure 3. The daily recommended intake for adults (19-50 years) and adults (51+ years) are 2.4µg and 100-400µg, respectively. The main functions are to help in the making of red blood cells, which are necessary for the proper functioning of the nerve, and to help normalize the levels of homocysteine in the blood. Supplements of vitamin B12 in its bioavailable form have shown positive results in optimally maintaining levels of homocysteine (Mary Hanna et al., 2022; Olaso-Gonzalez et al., 2021).

Folate is also called vitamin B9. It directly plays a vital role in remythylating homocysteine to methionine via the MTHFR enzyme. Adequate intakes of folate are required to maintain the levels of homocysteine. In the elderly population, a decline in folate absorption or low dietary intake is commonly seen. It is used to reduce the risk of neural tube defects. Supplement intake could be beneficial, especially the active form of folate supplements. It is advised that pregnant women consume folic acid daily to obtain folate from varied diets. Good sources of it are legumes (beans, peas, and lentils), green leafy vegetables (kale, spinach), fortified foods, and supplements, as mentioned in Figure 3. The daily recommended intakes for adults and pregnant women are 400µg DFE (dietary folate equivalents) and 600µg DFE, respectively. The main functions are requirements for DNA synthesis, supporting cell growth and repair, and helping in the prevention of neural tube defects. Direct intake (i.e., from food) or indirect intake (i.e., folic acid from supplements) results in a reduction of homocysteine concentration (Mary Hanna et al., 2022; Olaso-Gonzalez et al., 2021).

Riboflavin is also known as vitamin B2. It easily gets destroyed upon light exposure. In individuals with a genetic mutation in MTHFR (an enzyme involved in folate metabolism), a low dose of its supplementation may result in lowering blood pressure. Riboflavin, by assisting the enzyme MTHFR, aids in the conversion of folate to a form that is required for the transformation of homocysteine to methionine. The main functions are to promote the conversion of food into usable energy and aid several antioxidant enzymes. The deficiency of riboflavin is also not uncommon in elderly populations; this results in an exacerbation of the effects of elevated homocysteine levels. It is important to intake adequate riboflavin intakes in order to optimize the levels of homocysteine. The good sources of it are dairy products (milk, yogurt, cheese), meat (chicken, beef, fish), and eggs, as mentioned in Figure 3. The daily recommended intake for men and women is 1.3mg and 1.1mg, respectively (Mary Hanna et al., 2022; Olaso-Gonzalez et al., 2021).

Choline is also known as vitamin B4. It can be synthesized in the human body but the amount is pretty small. That is not enough for the functions to support good health. It may play a role in lowering plasma homocysteine concentrations. It is involved in the methylation of homocysteine to methionine through a betaine (the successor of choline)-dependent pathway. This provides an alternative channel for the clearance of homocysteine, primarily when the folate or vitamin B12 levels are insufficient for the process. Its main functions are as the structural component of all the cell membranes, fat and cholesterol transport, metabolism, helping in the building of some important neurotransmitters and helping normalize homocysteine levels in the blood. In the elderly population, it is evident that they may experience a reduced efficiency in the homocysteine-methionine cycle, which makes betaine supplementation an important alternative way to lower the levels of homocysteine. So, we need to consume eggs, meat (beef and poultry), and seafood (fish and shellfish) to compensate, as mentioned in Figure 4. The daily recommended intakes for men and women are 550mg and 425mg, respectively. While beets are advised as supplements for betaine due to their high betaine concentrations, as mentioned in Figure 4 (Mary Hanna et al., 2022; Olaso-Gonzalez et al., 2021).

Omega-3 fatty acids, mainly EPA (eicosapentanenoic acid) and DHA (docosahexaenoic acid), have shown potential results in reducing homocysteine levels and decreasing cardiovascular risks by providing supports to the requisite supporting endothelial function and reducing the inflammation rate. Studies have shown intakes of Omega-3 to be often reduced in the elderly population. This results in increased chances of homocysteine and inflammation. This situation can be handled and managed with the increased dietary intake of omega-3 or supplementation. Good dietary sources of omega-3 are fatty fish like salmon, mackerel, and sardines; flaxseeds; chia seeds; and omega-3 supplements like fisk oil or algae oil, which have shown promising results, as mentioned in Figure 4 (Sohouli et al.,2022; Rizzo & Laganà, 2020).

Studies prove the involvement of magnesium in numerous enzymatic reactions. These include the enzymatic reactions that are linked to homocysteine metabolism. It plays a crucial role as a supporting factor for all the functions of enzymes that require vitamin B for the conversion of homocysteine into cysteine or methionine. In the elderly population, the deficiency of magnesium is also commonly seen. This deficiency is majorly associated with elevated levels of homocysteines. Intakes of magnesium supplements can prove beneficial in regulating the levels of homocysteine. Nuts, seeds, leafy greens, and whole grains have been certified as magnesium-rich sources, as mentioned in Figure 4 (Dhillon et al., 2023; Zhao et al., 2022; Luzzi et al., 2022).

Antioxidants have proven to reduce oxidative stress levels, resulting in the repair of homocysteine metabolism that is hampered by damaging enzymes involved in its clearance. Vitamin C and E, the two vitamins containing antioxidant properties. They protect the body against this oxidative damage and support vascular health by reducing the risk of homocysteine-induced endothelialdysfunction. Studies have shown that oxidative stress increases with age. Causing the necessary requirement of supplementation with antioxidants in order to regulate and maintain homocysteine metabolism and ultimately protect the body against age-related damage. Sources like citrus fruits, berries, nuts, seeds, and vegetable oils are some of the antioxidant-rich sources, as mentioned in Figure 4 (Fusco et al., 2007).

Figure 3. Food sources of vitamin B6 (pyridoxine), vitamin B12 (cobalamin), vitamin B9 (folate), and vitamin B2 (riboflavin)

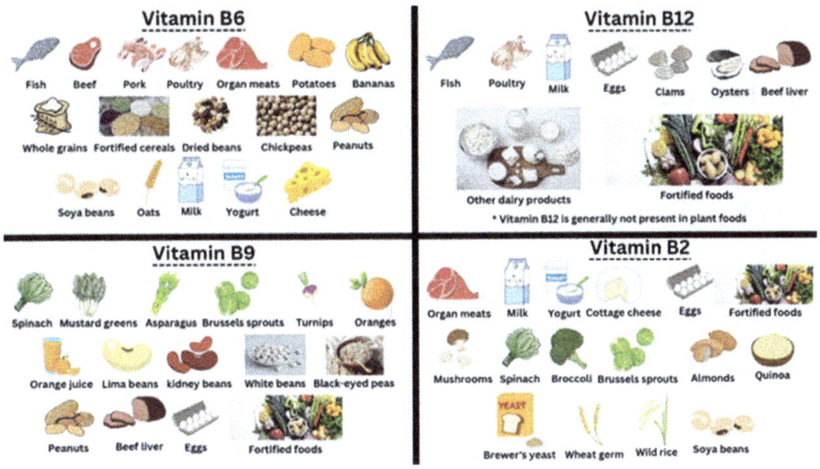

Figure 4. Food sources of vitamin B4 (choline), omega-3 fatty acids, magnesium, and antioxidants (vitamins C and E)

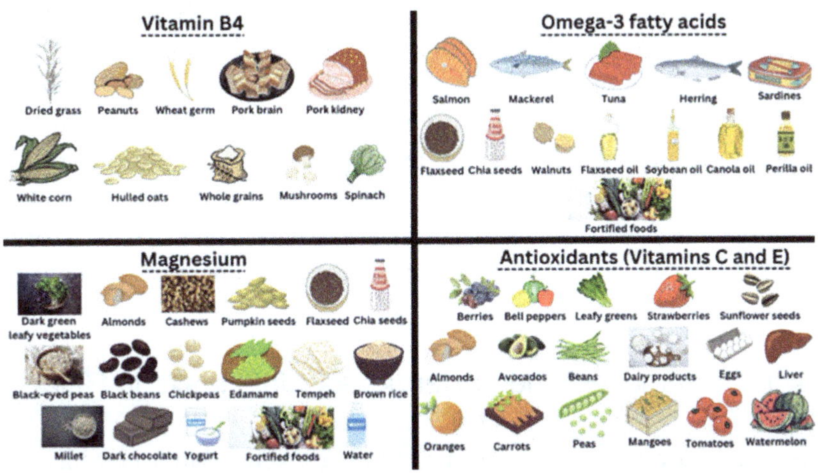

Studies prove that physical activity has the potential to reduce elevated levels of homocysteine by enhancing metabolism and improving cardiovascular health. Exercise also has the potential to lower inflammation and oxidative stress that significantly contribute to elevated levels of homocysteine. Changing our unhealthy dietary plans to diets rich in fruits, vegetables, whole grains, and lean proteins supplies the body with necessary nutrients like vitamin B, omega-3s, and magnesium for the regulation of homocysteine. Processed food and refined sugar are also the reasons for impaired homocysteine metabolism. Hence, limiting their consumption could help in reducing oxidative stress and inflammation. Smoking is a most common practice that is observed mainly from teenagers to the elderly population. Smoking acts as a booster to promote oxidative stress and reduce the bioavailability of vitamin B, which leads to an increase in homocysteine levels. Reducing or most appropriately quitting smoking could prove to be one of the most effective ways to reduce the smoking population's homocysteine levels (de Oliveira et al., 2021; Deminice et al., 2016).

2.4 Association Between Homocysteine and Cardiovascular Diseases in Relation to Aging

Elevated homocysteine, an amino acid involved in methionine metabolism, is a well-documented risk factor for cardiovascular diseases (CVD), especially as individuals age. Aging contributes to various metabolic changes, including decreased nutrient absorption and renal function, which often result in elevated homocysteine levels. These elevated levels are closely linked to several age-related cardiovascular conditions such as stroke, heart attack, thrombosis, coronary artery disease (CAD), peripheral arterial disease, carotid artery disease, systemic atherosclerosis, heart failure, thoracic aortic atherosclerosis, atrial fibrillation, hypertension, myocardial infarction (MI), ischemic heart disease, deep vein thrombosis, and pulmonary embolism.

In recent decades, CVD has become a major public health concern worldwide, particularly in aging populations (Sapha et al., 2024). Homocysteine contributes to vascular damage by causing endothelial dysfunction and promoting clot formation, which increases the risk of heart attacks and strokes. It induces a pro-thrombotic and pro-oxidant environment, leading to platelet hyperreactivity and further endothelial injury, both of which are critical factors in CVD. Hyperhomocysteinemia (plasma levels of homocysteine above 10 μmol/L) is therefore recognized as a significant marker and risk factor for cardiovascular diseases in elderly individuals (Yun-Ah et al., 2024).

Routine monitoring of homocysteine levels in older adults can aid in assessing cardiovascular risk and guiding preventative and therapeutic measures. Elevated homocysteine levels correlate with increased risks of heart attack, stroke, and clot formation, making homocysteine testing an important tool for cardiologists and healthcare providers. This connection was first identified by Kilmer McCully, who highlighted the role of homocysteine in vascular pathology (Miller, 2013), underscoring its importance in cardiovascular health, particularly as part of a comprehensive approach to managing aging-related CVD risk.

2.4.1 Mechanisms of Homocysteine in Cardiovascular Health in Relation to Aging

Elevated homocysteine levels are strongly linked to endothelial damage, which results in vascular dysfunction and is a key contributor to cardiovascular disease (CVD). With aging, the risk of hyperhomocysteinemia increases, often exacerbating the effects of aging-related vascular changes. Elevated homocysteine promotes oxidative stress, leading to increased production of reactive oxygen species (ROS) and lipid peroxidation. This oxidative damage contributes to endothelial dysfunction by degrading cell membranes and increasing inflammation. Lipid peroxidation products, such as malondialdehyde (MDA) and 4-hydroxynonenal (4-HNE), serve as biomarkers of oxidative stress and are linked to age-related vascular inflammation. Homocysteine disrupts endothelial cell function by decreasing nitric oxide (NO) bioavailability, which is essential for vascular relaxation. Reduced NO levels lead to impaired vasodilation, which contributes to hypertension and vascular stiffness, both prevalent in aging populations. Homocysteine induces apoptosis in endothelial cells, further weakening the integrity of blood vessels. This loss of endothelial cells exacerbates vascular dysfunction and accelerates atherosclerotic processes associated with aging. Elevated homocysteine enhances inflammatory responses by activating cytokine production. Chronic inflammation is common in aging, and hyperhomocysteinemia amplifies this by promoting pro-inflammatory states that contribute to vascular damage and plaque formation, key factors in CVD. Homocysteine increases the risk of thrombotic events by promoting platelet activation and coagulation factor activation, which facilitates thrombin formation. This hypercoagulable state impairs thrombolysis, where increased plasminogen activator inhibitor-1 (PAI-1) levels slow down the natural breakdown of clots. Hypercoagulability, paired with impaired thrombolysis, is a significant risk factor for heart attacks and strokes in aging individuals. Homocysteine-induced oxidative stress accelerates lipid peroxidation, a process that damages lipid membranes in cells, contributing to atherosclerosis. Lipid peroxidation products not only damage cells directly but also induce further inflammation and endothelial dysfunction, driving CVD progression. Elevated homocysteine increases platelet aggregation, making clot formation more likely. Aging itself is associated with higher platelet reactivity, and hyperhomocysteinemia further enhances this condition, contributing to the formation of blood clots within vessels. Fibrinolysis is the body's mechanism for dissolving blood clots to maintain blood flow and prevent clot buildup. Elevated homocysteine impairs fibrinolysis by inhibiting plasmin activity, reducing the breakdown of fibrin clots, and leading to persistent thrombotic risk (Paul & Shreyoshi, 2015).

2.4.2 Impact of Homocysteine on the Cardiovascular System

Elevated levels of homocysteine are strongly linked to adverse effects on cardiovascular health, particularly in aging individuals. Hyperhomocysteinemia affects blood pressure regulation and interacts with other cardiovascular risk factors and is influenced by age, lifestyle choices, and certain medical conditions.

Studies have shown that individuals with hypertension tend to have higher concentrations of homocysteine compared to those with normal blood pressure. However, the direct association between elevated homocysteine and other cardiovascular disease risk factors, like dyslipidemia, may be less consistent (Dinavahi & Falkner, 2004). The relationship becomes more complex when genetic factors, such as the MTHFR C677T mutation, are considered. This genetic mutation is associated with higher blood pressure values and increases the risk of hypertension, especially in aging populations (Elias & Brown, 2022).

Hyperhomocysteinemia exacerbates the negative effects of several established risk factors, such as hypertension, smoking, and lipid metabolism disorders. These interactions can result in endothelial damage, decreased vascular elasticity, and disruptions in hemostasis, all of which contribute to an elevated risk of cardiovascular events like heart attacks and strokes (Ganguly & Alam, 2015). This is particularly concerning for older adults, who are more vulnerable to vascular complications.

Elevated homocysteine damages the endothelium, the inner lining of blood vessels, reducing their flexibility and compromising their ability to regulate blood flow. Age-related stiffening of blood vessels, when combined with hyperhomocysteinemia, further accelerates vascular dysfunction and increases the likelihood of cardiovascular disease.

Lifestyle factors, such as smoking and high coffee consumption, have been shown to increase homocysteine levels. High coffee intake, in particular, adds to the complexity of homocysteine's role in cardiovascular health. Moreover, aging individuals often experience compounded effects from these lifestyle factors, heightening their cardiovascular risk.

Conditions like chronic kidney disease (CKD) and metabolic disorders such as diabetes further complicate the relationship between homocysteine and cardiovascular health. As kidney function declines with age, homocysteine clearance decreases, resulting in higher blood levels and increased cardiovascular risk (Marcus et al., 2007; Ganguly & Alam, 2015). Diabetes, which is also prevalent in aging populations, aggravates the pro-inflammatory and pro-thrombotic environment created by elevated homocysteine, worsening cardiovascular outcomes.

The risk of elevated homocysteine is influenced by age, gender, dietary habits, and other lifestyle choices. Aging itself is a risk factor for higher homocysteine levels, partly due to changes in metabolism and reduced nutrient absorption. Gender differences, with men typically having higher levels than women, also contribute to variations in cardiovascular risk. Furthermore, inadequate dietary intake of B-vitamins, which are crucial for homocysteine metabolism, is common among older adults and exacerbates cardiovascular risks.

2.4.3 Physiological Effects of Elevated Homocysteine

Elevated homocysteine levels in the blood, known as hyperhomocysteinemia (HHCys), have numerous physiological effects on cardiovascular health that become increasingly significant with aging. As people age, metabolic efficiency and nutrient absorption decline, often leading to higher homocysteine levels. HHCys impacts cardiovascular health through mechanisms including atherosclerosis, endothelial dysfunction, thrombosis, inflammation, oxidative stress, and disrupted methylation pathways. These factors collectively increase cardiovascular risk in aging populations (Yuan et al., 2023).

With age, the risk of arterial plaque formation increases. Elevated homocysteine damages the arterial endothelium, accelerating atherosclerosis by promoting plaque buildup. This narrowing of arteries restricts blood flow and raises the likelihood of heart attacks and strokes, both of which are particularly prevalent in older adults (Yuan et al., 2023).

Homocysteine impairs endothelial cells, which line blood vessels and regulate vascular health. Aging itself compromises endothelial function, and elevated homocysteine intensifies this effect, contributing to conditions like hypertension, atherosclerosis, and thrombosis. This decline in endothelial health is often the first step toward cardiovascular diseases common in aging populations (Yuan et al., 2023).

Aging is associated with increased coagulability and a greater risk of clot formation, a process further promoted by high homocysteine levels. Hyperhomocysteinemia encourages thrombus (clot) formation, raising the risk of heart attacks and strokes by obstructing blood flow. This risk is particularly concerning in older adults, who are already prone to vascular complications.

Homocysteine promotes inflammation in blood vessels, a factor that accelerates atherosclerosis and contributes to cardiovascular disease progression. Aging is often accompanied by a state of chronic low-grade inflammation (termed "inflammaging"), and elevated homocysteine levels further exacerbate this, compounding cardiovascular risk in older adults (Yuan et al., 2023).

High homocysteine levels increase oxidative stress, leading to cellular and tissue damage. With age, the body's antioxidant defenses decline, making cells more vulnerable to oxidative damage. This stress contributes to hypertension, atherosclerosis, and heart failure, common age-related cardiovascular disorders (Yuan et al., 2023).

Homocysteine is essential in the methylation process, which supports numerous biochemical reactions. However, high homocysteine levels disrupt these pathways, affecting DNA methylation and gene expression related to cardiovascular health. Aging can impair methylation efficiency, and elevated homocysteine exacerbates this disruption, which may contribute to age-related cardiovascular conditions (Yuan et al., 2023).

2.5 Association Between Homocysteine and Cancer in Relation to Aging

The relationship between homocysteine and cancer has been a topic of considerable research and debate within the medical community. Homocysteine, an amino acid produced from the breakdown of methionine, is essential for various metabolic processes. Hyperhomocysteinemia conditions have been associated with several health risks; the list also includes cancer. Aging is a critical factor that influences homocysteine metabolism and cancer risk. As individuals age, metabolic processes often become less efficient, and the accumulation of homocysteine is more likely due to a decline in the function of enzymes and vitamins that regulate its breakdown.

Homocysteine metabolism is intricately linked to the methylation cycle, which plays a crucial role in DNA synthesis and repair. Disruptions in methylation, which are more prevalent with aging, can lead to DNA damage and genomic instability, creating a permissive environment for cancer development. This is particularly relevant in rapidly dividing tissues, such as those of the breast and digestive tract (Lin et al., 2010; Xu et al., 2018).

Elevated homocysteine levels promote oxidative stress and chronic inflammation, both of which are hallmarks of aging and cancer. Oxidative damage to DNA, proteins, and lipids increases the likelihood of mutations and malignant transformations. Chronic inflammation, often exacerbated by hyperhomocysteinemia, contributes to a tumor-promoting environment, especially in older adults whose inflammatory regulation is already compromised (Lin et al., 2010; Xu et al., 2018).

Studies have shown a correlation between high homocysteine levels and certain cancer types, such as breast cancer and digestive tract cancer (Lin et al., 2010; Xu et al., 2018). Aging-related changes in the immune system, combined with the pro-inflammatory and pro-oxidant effects of homocysteine, may facilitate tumor growth and metastasis. Additionally, homocysteine may influence angiogenesis, the formation of new blood vessels, which tumors use to support their growth.

2.5.1 Mechanisms of Homocysteine in Cancer in Relation to Aging

Elevated homocysteine levels have been increasingly linked to the development and progression of cancer, and aging serves as a critical factor that amplifies these effects. Numerous scientific studies have demonstrated how homocysteine contributes to carcinogenesis through mechanisms such as DNA methylation alterations, proinflammatory gene activation, endothelial injury, enhanced cellular proliferation, and disruptions in methionine metabolism.

Aging is associated with natural changes in DNA methylation patterns, often leading to genomic instability. Elevated homocysteine exacerbates these age-related changes by disrupting DNA methylation machinery, which regulates gene expression. This disruption may cause hypomethylation in specific regions of the genome, leading to the activation of oncogenes and proinflammatory pathways (Koklesova et al., 2021). This age-accelerated methylation dysfunction can increase cancer susceptibility, especially in older adults whose methylation processes are already compromised.

Homocysteine can enhance the expression of proinflammatory genes, creating a chronic inflammatory state that is characteristic of aging and associated with increased cancer risk. By targeting hypomethylated regions, homocysteine promotes the upregulation of these genes, accelerating cancer development. The impact of inflammation becomes more significant in aging as the body's ability to control inflammatory responses diminishes over time (Ferroni et al., 2009).

Aging naturally reduces endothelial function, a situation worsened by elevated homocysteine. Homocysteine contributes to endothelial damage by inhibiting the enzyme that degrades asymmetric dimethylarginine (ADMA), an endogenous inhibitor of nitric oxide (NO) synthesis. The resulting decrease in NO bioavailability impairs vascular health, promoting an environment conducive to tumor growth and metastasis (Yuan et al., 2023). This mechanism is particularly concerning for older individuals, who are more prone to vascular dysfunction.

Aging tissues are more susceptible to unregulated cell growth, a risk factor for cancer. Elevated homocysteine levels have been linked to increased cellular proliferation, a key process in cancer development. For example, studies have shown that homocysteine promotes proliferation in cancer cell lines, such as Caco-2 cells, by creating a microenvironment favorable to tumor expansion (Hasan et al., 2019). In the context of aging, where cellular repair mechanisms are already weakened, this proliferative effect becomes even more pronounced.

Alterations in methionine metabolism, often seen in cancer cells, are further affected by elevated homocysteine. Research indicates that tumor cells may alter methionine metabolism, leading to an accumulation of homocysteine. This metabolic disruption is more prevalent in older individuals, as age-related metabolic inefficiencies amplify these effects. Interestingly, while high homocysteine levels can support tumor growth, extremely elevated concentrations may be cytotoxic to cancer cells, suggesting a complex, dose-dependent relationship (Yuan et al., 2023; Hasan et al., 2019).

2.5.2 Impact of Homocysteine on Cancer in Relation to Cancer

Elevated levels of homocysteine have been associated with an increased risk of various cancers, including colorectal cancer, breast cancer, and digestive tract cancer. Aging plays a crucial role in modulating these effects, as age-related physiological changes can influence homocysteine metabolism and cancer susceptibility.

Studies indicate that hyperhomocysteinemia, a condition characterized by elevated homocysteine levels, may contribute to the development of colorectal cancer (Keshteli et al., 2015). The impact of aging on homocysteine metabolism, coupled with a natural decline in DNA repair mechanisms, enhances the potential for DNA damage and genomic instability, thereby increasing cancer risk in older adults.

Research has shown that elevated homocysteine levels may raise the risk of breast cancer, particularly in women with low folate status. This risk is even more pronounced in aging populations, where nutrient absorption and metabolism often decline. The combination of high homocysteine and low folate disrupts DNA methylation processes, promoting carcinogenesis (Lin et al., 2010).

A dose-response analysis suggests that for every 5 μmol/L increase in homocysteine levels, the risk of developing digestive tract cancer rises by 7% (Xu et al., 2018). Aging exacerbates this risk due to cumulative oxidative stress, inflammation, and weakened metabolic pathways that are less effective at regulating homocysteine.

As people age, there is often a dysregulation of enzymes involved in critical biochemical pathways, such as those producing hydrogen sulfide, which is involved in cancer progression. The altered expression or activity of these enzymes in aging bodies may further facilitate cancer development and progression (Majumder, 2023).

2.5.3 Physiological Effects of Elevated Homocysteine in Relation to Aging and Cancer

Hyperhomocysteinemia, a condition characterized by elevated levels of homocysteine in the blood, has wide-ranging and complex physiological effects that can significantly impact cancer development and progression, especially as one ages. The interconnected mechanisms include oxidative stress, disrupted DNA methylation, enhanced angiogenesis, chronic inflammation, impaired DNA repair, cell cycle alterations, metabolic reprogramming, endothelial dysfunction, and compromised immune responses (Anugerawati et al., 2024).

Aging naturally increases oxidative stress, and high homocysteine levels exacerbate this effect by boosting reactive oxygen species (ROS) production. This leads to DNA damage and a weakened antioxidant defense, primarily through the depletion of glutathione. Older individuals are particularly vulnerable, as the cumulative oxidative damage over the years may accelerate the risk of cancer.

Homocysteine disrupts the methylation cycle, resulting in abnormal DNA methylation patterns. This involves hypomethylation of oncogenes and hypermethylation of tumor suppressor genes, which can initiate cancer. With aging, the body's ability to maintain proper DNA methylation declines, making these epigenetic disruptions more detrimental (Mikkelsen & Apostolopoulos, 2024).

Elevated homocysteine promotes angiogenesis, the formation of new blood vessels that feed tumors, supporting their growth and metastatic potential. This is critical in aging populations, as angiogenesis-related changes become more pronounced with age, potentially hastening cancer progression.

Aging is associated with a low-grade chronic inflammatory state, which is exacerbated by high homocysteine levels. Homocysteine activates inflammatory pathways, leading to the release of pro-inflammatory cytokines that support tumor growth and survival. This aging-associated inflammation creates a fertile ground for cancers to thrive.

The ability to repair DNA diminishes with age. Hyperhomocysteinemia further impairs DNA repair mechanisms, causing the accumulation of genetic damage, which heightens the risk of malignant transformations. This is particularly concerning in older individuals whose genomic integrity is already compromised.

Elevated homocysteine disrupts cell cycle regulation, leading to uncontrolled cell division and resistance to apoptosis (programmed cell death). As cellular turnover and repair processes become less efficient with age, this dysregulation significantly contributes to cancer development and reduced treatment efficacy.

Cancer cells often undergo metabolic reprogramming to fuel rapid proliferation. Homocysteine aids this process by altering one-carbon metabolism, crucial for synthesizing biomolecules needed for cell division. Aging slows down metabolism, making this reprogramming even more impactful in sustaining cancer cell growth.

Homocysteine induces endothelial dysfunction, promoting a pro-thrombotic state and disrupting normal blood flow within tumors. Aging exacerbates vascular dysfunction, facilitating tumor metastasis and complicating treatment outcomes.

The immune system's efficacy declines with age, and high homocysteine levels further suppress immune surveillance, allowing cancer cells to evade detection and spread. This diminished immune response is a key factor in the increased cancer risk observed in aging populations (Badawy, 2024).

Understanding these physiological effects is critical for developing strategies to manage homocysteine levels, especially in older individuals, to reduce cancer risk and slow disease progression (Amado-Garzan et al., 2024).

3. INTRODUCTION TO TELOMERE

Telomeres play a crucial role in aging. Telomeres are repetitive sequences at the ends of chromosomes that protect the length of the DNA and control cell division. In humans, the telomere sequence is TTAGGG. Thus, one section of telomere is made of six "base pairs." This sequence is usually repeated about 3,000 times and can reach up to 15,000 base pairs in length. Each time it divides, an approximation of 30 to 200 cells lose their base pairs from the ends of their telomeres. Cells under normal conditions continue to divide only 50 to 70 times with the telomeres getting progressively larger; this process continues until the cells reach senescence. This telomerase shortening is not applicable to tissues like heart muscles, whose cells do not continually divide. In order to inhibit or reduce the shortening process, lifestyle changes like regular exercise, a balanced diet rich in antioxidants, stress reduction, and the avoidance of smoking are considered beneficial. In addition to this, telomerase is an enzyme that prevents telomere shortening by helping in maintaining the length by adding DNA sequences to the ends of the chromosomes, although its activities are limited to some specific cells like stem cells and germ cells. There is ongoing research on increasing the activity of telomerases, but the likelihood of getting cancer is a potential risk that may come into play with this invention (Shay., 2018).

3.1 Discovery of Telomere

The discovery of telomeres has been a stepping stone in the understanding of cellular aging, replication, and chromosome stability. Scientific journals have unfolded over several decades, shaped by major research and remarkable discoveries. In the 1930s, when *Hermann Muller* and *Barbara McClintock* were independently conducting research on fruit flies and maize, respectively, they discovered protective structures at the ends of chromosomes. Muller termed these structures as "telomeres" (Greek word—telos meaning "end" and *meros* meaning "part"). Both the researchers have similar observations that these endings prevent abnormal chromosomal fusions and degradation, functioning as they act as a "cap" to safeguard genetic materials. Later they were awarded with Nobel Prizes for their pioneering work (Chuaire., 2006).

In the 1970s researchers began to uncover the molecular nature of telomeres. *Elizabeth Blackburn* was working on *Tetrahymena thermophila* when she identified telomeres that consisted of repetitive nucleotide sequences (TTGGGG in *Tetrahymena*). This groundbreaking discovery of Blackburn's was published in 1978, highlighting the sequence-specific nature of telomeres and sparking interest in their biological function (Blackburn and Gall., 1978).

Carol Greider and *Elizabeth Blackburn,* in the year 1984, discovered an enzyme that adds telomeric repeats to chromosome ends and solves the "end-replication problem" found in eukaryotic cells. termed as telomerase. Basically, telomerase is a ribonucleoprotein that consists of an RNA component that serves as a template strand and a protein component that acts as a reverse transcriptase (Greider and Blackburn., 1985).

Leonard Hayflick's earlier work in 1961 demonstrated the finite capacity of cells to replicate (i.e., the Hayflick limit), as a lead to the later research on telomere shortening (Hayflick and Moorhead., 1961). Researchers during the 1990s linked telomeres and telomerase to cellular senescence, aging, and cancer. Further research on telomerase found that the enzyme is active in germ cells and cancer cells while largely inactive in most of the somatic cells. This characteristic of telomerase suggests its role in immortality and uncontrolled cell proliferation.

Elizabeth Blackburn, Carol Greider, and Jack Szostak received the 2009 Nobel Prize in Physiology or Medicine for their milestone discovery of how chromosomes are protected by telomeres and telomerase.

3.2 Telomerase

Telomerase is an enzyme that adds the TTAGGG (in humans) telomere sequence to the ends of chromosomes. There are 300 to 8000 times repeated telomere sequences in humans. Telomerase is found in high concentrations in germline cells (like sperm and egg), stem cells, and cancer cells. The maintenance of telomere length after DNA replication, leading to the cells not showing signs of aging, is the main reason for the high concentration. But, in somatic cells (like muscle cells, bone cells, etc.), there are low concentrations of telomerase. Because these cells do not regularly use telomerase (as they do not often undergo replication), this leads to a reduction in the age and normal function of the cell. The result of aging cells is an aging body (Smith et al., 2020). Telomerase is also found in high concentrations in cancer cells. This concentration enables the cancer cells to be immortal and continue replicating themselves. If by any means the telomerase activity was turned off in cancer cells, then their telomeres would shorten until they attain a "critical length." This would prevent the cancer cells from dividing uncontrollably to form tumors (Jafri et al., 2016).

Telomerase is composed of telomerase reverse transcriptase (TERT), telomerase RNA component, and accessory proteins. TERT is the catalytic protein component that adds nucleotide repeats. TERC provides the RNA template for the addition of telomeric repeats. Accessory proteins (like Gar1, Nhp2, and dyskerin) aid in the assembly, localization, and activity of telomerase. In order to compensate for the loss of DNA at the ends of chromosomes that occurs during DNA replication, telomerase extends the 3' primer overhang of telomeres by adding specific nucleotide sequences (Lee & Pellegrini, 2022). Telomerase has a lot of biological importance, like it helps in preventing telomere shortening, chromosomal stability, maintaining cellular aging, tumor immortality, therapeutic targets, regenerative medicine, and roles in aging-related diseases. It claims huge potential for cancer therapy, anti-aging interventions, and stem cell research.

3.2.1 Causes of Telomere Shortening

Telomeres are the repetitive nucleotide sequences at the ends of chromosomes that protect the genetic material during cell division by acting like aglets. With each passing cell cycle, telomeres naturally shorten during replication (S phase) due to the inability of DNA polymerase to fully replicate the chromosomal ends, which is also known as the end-replication problem. With time, this contributes to cellular aging, leading to reduced cellular function and eventually senescence or apoptosis. Factors like biological aging, oxidative stress, chronic inflammation, psychological stress, lifestyle factors, environmental toxins, genetic factors, telomerase deficiency, replicative stress and high cell turnover, diseases and genetic disorders, and viral infections accelerate this process, ultimately speeding up the aging process. Understanding these processes is vital for exploring the interventions that may slow down telomere shortening and promote healthier aging.

Natural aging is caused by telomere shortening. Each passing cell cycle gradually causes shortening of telomeres, which eventually triggers the Hayflick limit, which causes the cessation of cell division. This acts as a biological clock that regulates and indicates one's lifespan and tissue renewal (Victorelli & Passos, 2017).

Reactive oxygen species (ROS) are generated during metabolism and can damage telomeres. These are very harmful because telomeres lack the ability of efficient repair mechanisms, and oxidative stress accelerates this shortening beyond what occurs normally. Conditions like obesity, autoimmune disorders, and chronic infections contribute to worsening of chronic inflammation. In chronic inflammation, the inflammatory processes like the release of cytokines and ROS cause sustained stress on telomeric DNA, which accelerates the aging process (Mangaonkar & Patnaik, 2019).

Chronic psychological stress leads to the activation of pathways that increase cortisol levels by promoting inflammation and oxidative stress. Studies often establish connections between high stress and reduced telomerase activity. The enzyme responsible for telomere maintenance accelerates the decline of telomere length, which significantly impacts cellular aging and health. Lifestyle factors like poor diet, smoking, sedentary lifestyle, and excessive alcohol play a significant role in the declination of telomeres. Intake of a diet with low antioxidants and high processing can increase oxidative damage to telomeres. Chemicals contained in tobacco directly damage DNA and increase oxidative stress. Lack of physical activity results in higher oxidative stress and shorter telomeres. Consumption of alcohol leads to the generation of free radicals, which contributes to oxidative telomere damage. Exposure to toxins like pollutants, UV radiation, and heavy metals accelerates oxidative damage to telomeres. These factors increase ROS production, which leads to acceleration of declined telomere length (Verma et al., 2022).

Studies have shown a chance that our genetics influence the rate at which our telomere shortens. Mutations in the genes regulating telomerase enzymes or the DNA repair mechanisms can speed up the shortening of telomere length. Telomerase is the enzyme that is responsible for extending telomeres. But in most of the somatic cells, it is not active, leading to insufficient telomere repair and maintenance, contributing to shortening. Tissues that experience rapid cell division, like the tissues of the skin, bone marrow, and gut lining, experience a faster telomere shortening than the rest of the tissues. The telomere shortening rate also gets massively accelerated due to injury, disease, or hyperplasia (Nag, 2019).

Dyskeratosis congenita is a rare disorder that is caused by mutations in genes related to telomerase, leading to extremely short telomeres and premature aging. Hutchinson-Gilford progeria syndrome is a rare genetic condition due to defective nuclear envelope protein that causes children to age rapidly, which leads to rapid telomere shortening. Certain viral infections can also contribute to the telomere attrition in affected cells by increasing cellular turnover or triggering immune responses (Rossiello et al, 2022).

3.2.2 Technology Intervention in Measuring Homocysteine

Precise measurement and analysis of telomeres have been enabled by advances in technology that offer critical insights into aging, cellular health, and disease progression. These techniques provide quantitative and qualitative data on telomere length, structure, and dynamics, which is crucial for research in aging, cancer, and regenerative medicine. Techniques like quantitative polymerase chain reaction (qPCR), terminal restriction fragment (TRF) analysis, single telomere length analysis (STELA), telomere fluorescence in situ hybridization (Flow-FISH), telomere shortest length assay (TeSLA), quantitative fluorescence in situ hybridization (Q-FISH), long-read sequencing, whole-genome sequencing (WGS) and computational approaches, and super-resolution microscopy.

qPCR works on the principle of measuring the average telomere length relative to a reference gene. This technique is advantageous in context to high throughput and cost-effectiveness and requires minimal DNA and is disadvantageous in context to providing relative, not absolute, telomere length and susceptibility to technical variability (Cawthon, 2002). TRF is a

Southern blot-based method that measures the average telomere length by digesting genomic DNA with restriction enzymes that do not cut within telomeric repeats, which is followed by gel electrophoresis. This technique is advantageous in the context of the gold standard for absolute telomere length measurements and to provide detailed information about telomere length distribution and disadvantageous in the context of labor-intensive and low-throughput and the requirement of a large amount of high-quality DNA (Kimura et al., 2010). STELA is a PCR-based method that helps in measuring telomere length at specific chromosomal ends. This technique is highly sensitive and can detect very short telomeres. This technique is advantageous in the context of high resolution and specificity and is useful for studying telomere shortening in individual chromosome ends and disadvantageous in context to limitation to single telomeres; it is not suitable for global telomere length measurement (Britt-Compton et al., 2006). U-STELA is an advanced and powerful version of STELA that is designed to analyze individual telomeres without requiring sequence-specific primers. It can effectively measure telomeres across all chromosomes. This technique is advantageous in the context of being more universal than traditional STELA and effective for measuring critically short telomeres across the genome and disadvantageous in context to being complex and labor-intensive (Yu et al., 2024). The Flow-FISH technique is a combination of flow cytometry and fluorescence in situ hybridization to measure telomere length in specific cell populations using telomere-specific fluorescent probes. This technique is advantageous in the context of quantifying telomere length in individual cells and useful for studying heterogeneity in telomere length and disadvantageous in context to the requirement of specialized equipment and expertise and limited sensitivity for very short telomeres (Baerlocher et al., 2006). Q-FISH technique uses fluorescent probes to measure telomere length in metaphase chromosomes or interphase nuclei. This technique is advantageous in the context of providing chromosome-specific telomere analysis and disadvantageous in context to limited sensitivity for very short telomeres (Slijepcevic, 2001). Long-read sequencing includes platforms like Oxford Nanopore and PacBio that enable a direct measurement of telomeric repeats at the ends of chromosomes. This technique is advantageous in the context that it can measure length genome-wide and detect structural variations and repetitive sequences and disadvantageous in context to high cost and computational demands (Sanchez et al., 2024). WGS and computational approaches include algorithms that estimate telomere length from reads mapping to telomeric repeat regions. This technique is advantageous in the context of providing genome-wide telomere information and disadvantageous in context to the requirement of high-coverage sequencing data (Lee et al., 2017). Super-resolution microscopy enables nanoscale visualization and quantification of telomeres. This technique is advantageous in the context of providing structural details about telomeres and disadvantageous in context to the requirement of specialized equipment (Phipps et al., 2016).

3.2.3 Nutrients and Solutions

Studies suggest that a diet consisting of nutrients like folate, vitamin B, vitamin C, vitamin D, vitamin E, zinc, magnesium, polyphenols (plant-based compounds), and omega-3 fatty acids may support telomerase activity and potentially help maintain telomere length. While a diet that comprises alcohol, saturated fats, sugary drinks, and high consumption of processed meat will very likely result in a greater shortening of telomeres (Galiè et al., 2020). In addition to diet, positive changes in life, like meditation and mindfulness, regular exercise, and sleep hygiene, could be helpful in maintaining and managing telomere length (Boccardi et al., 2016).

Folate is also called vitamin B9. Folate or folic acid, is greatly related to the immune system and the integrity of DNA and its methylation, which has a significant impact on telomeres. Vitamin B9 is mainly found in green leafy vegetables like broccoli, spinach, and arugula, and legumes including beans and chickpeas. Intake of vitamin B9 supports cellular replication and telomere preservation. Vitamin B complex includes vitamins like vitamin B6 and vitamin B12 that aid in DNA synthesis and repair while reducing oxidative stress. These vitamins collaborate with folate to regulate the homocysteine levels, ultimately preventing telomere shortening. Good sources of these vitamins are whole grains, eggs, dairy, and lean meats. Vitamin C is known for its antioxidant properties. It also combats oxidative stress, a major driver of telomere attrition and enhances collagen production that supports tissue health at the cellular level. This vitamin is majorly found in citrus fruits, bell peppers, and berries. Vitamin D acts on reducing inflammation and oxidative stress, which are the key elements in telomere degeneration. This vitamin is also crucial for genomic stability and immune function that indirectly results in protecting telomeres. Mainly obtained from sunlight, fortified foods, and fatty fish (Galiè et al., 2020). Vitamin E is also well known for its antioxidant (i.e., fat-soluble antioxidant) properties. This vitamin preserves telomere integrity by preventing lipid peroxidation and protecting cellular membranes. It also supports other antioxidants in reducing cellular aging. Mainly found in nuts, seeds, and vegetable oils. Zinc acts as a cofactor for numerous enzymatic reactions, including those that are involved in antioxidant defenses. By weakening the oxidative damage, zinc provides support to telomere health. Major sources are shellfish, seeds, and whole grains. Magnesium is an essential mineral for DNA synthesis and repair, which characteristic makes it critical for the maintenance of telomeres. It promotes cellular resilience. It also helps in the reduction of oxidative stress and inflammation. Found in nuts, seeds, spinach, and whole grains. Polyphenols are plant-based compounds like resveratrol, curcumin, and epigallocatechin gallate (EGCG) that activate protective pathways like SIRT1 and AMPK. It reduces inflammations and enhances telomerase activity. Majorly found in green tea, berries, and dark chocolate (Crous-Bou et al., 2019). Omega-3 fatty acids play a major role in reducing inflammation and oxidative stress. Especially in contexts of cardiovascular and metabolic health, these essential fats protect cellular membranes and promote telomere preservation. Abundantly found in fish oil, flaxseed, and walnuts.

Figure 5. Food sources of vitamin B9, vitamin B6, vitamin B12, and vitamin C

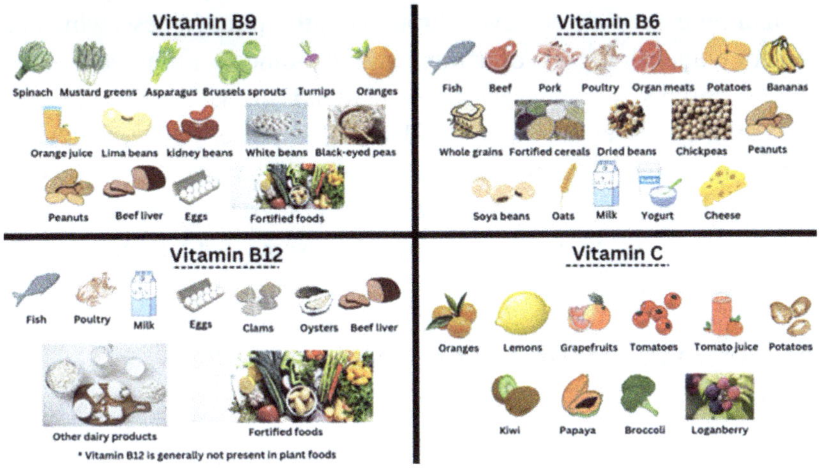

Figure 6. Food sources of vitamin D, vitamin E, zinc, and magnesium

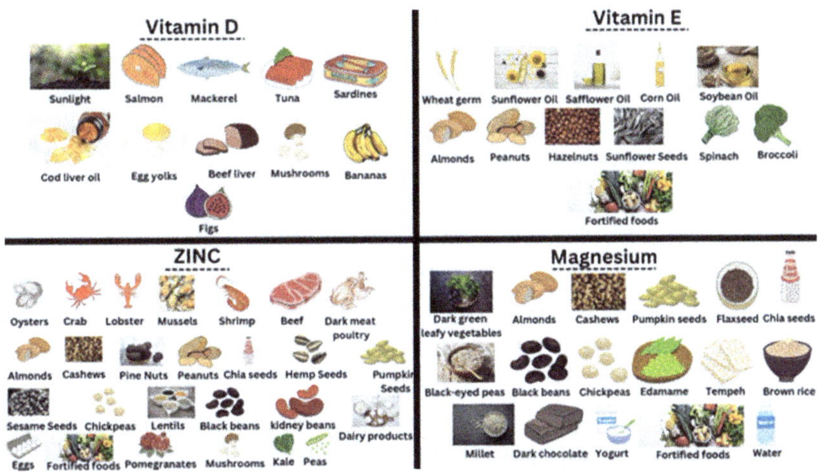

Figure 7. Food sources of polyphenols and omega-3 fatty acids

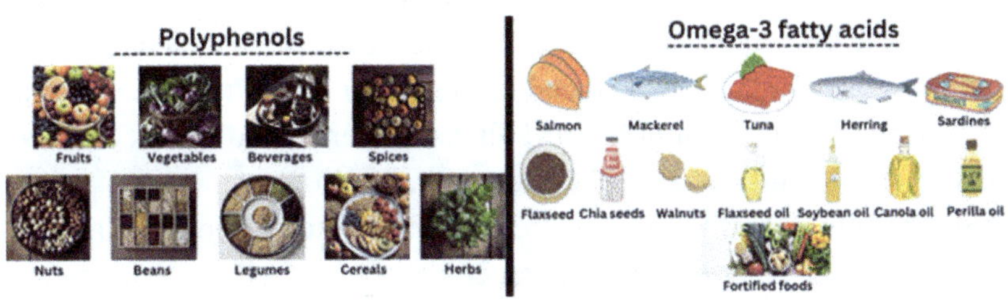

Polyphenols
Fruits Vegetables Beverages Spices
Nuts Beans Legumes Cereals Herbs
Omega-3 fatty acids
Salmon Mackerel Tuna Herring Sardines
Flaxseed Chia seeds Walnuts Flaxseed oil Soybean oil Canola oil Perilla oil
Fortified foods

Studies blame chronic stress for being the reason for accelerated telomere shortening. But mindfulness practices have proven an enhancement to telomerase activity, especially meditation. Reduction in cortisol levels and promotion of relaxation are achieved through regular mindfulness, which ultimately protects cellular health. Moderate-intensity levels of aerobic and resistance training help in the maintenance of telomeres by improving antioxidant defenses and reducing inflammation. Production of growth factors that support cellular repair and renewal is also stimulated by exercise. Hence, regular exercise is advised to maintain telomeres that ultimately contribute to reduced aging. Quality of sleep is a key determining factor for DNA repair and reduction of oxidative stress.A consistent sleep pattern helps in promoting hormonal balance and cellular recovery, which ultimately ensures that telomeres are not shortened prematurely (Boccardi et al., 2016).

3.3 Association Between Telomere and Cardiovascular Diseases in Relation to Aging

Telomeres are protective, cap-like structures present at the ends of the chromosomes that play a crucial role in cellular aging and are also associated with the development of cardiovascular diseases, especially with reference to aging. Gradually, with each cell division, the telomeres shorten progressively, which results in cellular senescence and reduced regenerative capacity. This telomere shortening is often linked to many key cardiovascular conditions like atherosclerosis, hypertension, and heart failure (De Meyer et al., 2018). For instance, consider the atherosclerosis condition where the shortening of telomeres in endothelial and smooth muscle cells impairs their ability to repair vascular damage by promoting chronic inflammation and plaque formation. In a similar fashion, telomere dysfunction in cardiomyocytes occurs by contributing to heart failure by restricting the heart's ability to repair damage while telomere shortening in vascular cells exacerbates hypertension and arterial stiffness (Gruber et al., 2021).

Moreover, aging is a process that is further compounded by chronic inflammation and oxidative stress; both of these result in an accelerated shortening of telomeres and also lead to the progression of cardiovascular diseases. The length of telomere has hence emerged as a potential biomarker for cardiovascular aging and determination of disease risk. The shorter the telomere, the higher the incidences of coronary artery disease, myocardial infarction, and stroke. Studies have come up with various therapeutic strategies that aim to protect telomeres by reducing oxidative stress through lifestyle modification and exploration of telomerase activators that promise to offer directions to mitigate cardiovascular decline and improve healthspan in aging populations (Yeh et al., 2019).

3.3.1 Mechanisms of Telomere in Cardiovascular Health in Relation to Aging

In context to aging, telomeres play a vital role in cardiovascular health. It acts like a "molecular clock" that progressively shortens with each cell division, which leads to cellular senescence and potential; it also contributes to the development of cardiovascular diseases. Primary mechanisms that are involved in this are impaired endothelial function, reduced tissue repair capacity when telomeres become critically short in size, and increased inflammation. This is further fueled by accelerated risk factors like hypertension, oxidative stress, and smoking (Gruber et al., 2021).

Mechanisms that are often linked with telomere dysfunction to cardiovascular diseases include cellular senescence, DNA damage response, and epigenetic changes. Cellular senescence is a condition in which telomeres become critically short in size, which results in cells entering senescence (i.e., a state where cells stop dividing) and releasing inflammatory factors, which contributes to the formation of plaque in arteries. Studies have shown that short telomeres have the potential to trigger DNA's damage response pathways, resulting in additional cellular dysfunction and increased oxidative stress. Telomere shortening can also be associated with changes in epigenetic marks, which impact gene expression and contribute to cardiovascular disease development (Yeh et al., 2019).

3.3.2 Impact of Telomere on the Cardiovascular System

Telomeres play a key role in cardiovascular health by influencing functions and aging. Shortened telomeres in vascular endothelial and smooth muscles result in cellular senescence, impair blood vessel integrity and additionally promote conditions like atherosclerosis and hypertension. This situation is furthermore compounded by oxidative stress and chronic inflammation that led to accelerated telomere erosion, which creates a chain reaction of endothelial dysfunction and plaque formation. Due to telomere shortening, cardiac tissues limit the regenerative capacity of progenitor cells and this leads to mitochondrial dysfunction in myocytes, exacerbating into heart failure and other cardiovascular diseases (Yeh et al., 2019).

Studies have shown that telomere length is recently increasingly recognized as a biomarker of cardiovascular aging and disease risk. Telomerase activation, antioxidants, and lifestyle modifications like stress management and regular exercise are the suggested interventions. These interventions have shown potential in mitigating telomere shortening and even improving the cardiovascular outcome. Understanding telomere dynamics leads us to a pathway that provides novel strategies for preventing and even managing cardiovascular diseases while enhancing overall longevity (Deng et al., 2022).

3.3.3 Physiological Effects of Elevated Telomere in Relation to Cardiovascular Disease

In the context of cardiovascular diseases, the elevated telomerase activity (i.e., the counterpart of telomere shortening) has both protective and potentially adverse effects. Although prolonged telomere length can preserve endothelial cell function, which improves vascular repair and also mitigates age-related vascular stiffness, excessive telomerase activation might lead to consequences like promoting cellular proliferation, wrestling with vascular hyperplasia, or tumorigenesis, which is a rare case. In elderly populations it is crucial to maintain balanced telomere dynamics to prevent both cellular senescence and uncontrolled growth (Arsenis et al., 2017).

From an aging perspective, elevated telomerase-activating can act like a counterbalance of oxidative stress and inflammation, which leads to telomere shortening in cardiovascular cells. This protective effect of elevated telomerase activity helps in maintaining vascular elasticity and reduces the risk of heart failure and atherosclerosis. However, the therapeutic strategies targeting telomerase finely balance the requirement to avoid the potential adverse effects by ensuring elongation of telomeres to support healthy aging and to get cardiovascular resilience without even triggering the pathological proliferation (Shammas, 2011).

3.4 Association Between Telomere and Cancer in Relation to Aging

Telomeres and cancer relationships are intricately linked to aging, which points out a delicate balance between cellular protection and risk. Telomeres can be precisely called a biological clock, resulting in limiting the cellular divisions to prevent uncontrolled growth. Telomere shortening in aging cells leads to genomic instability that triggers cellular senescence (i.e., a mechanism that has the capacity to suppress tumor formation). However, studies suggest that in some cases even critically short telomeres can promote chromosomal rearrangements leading to an increasing likelihood of mutations and the development of age-related cancers (Lansdorp, 2022).

But, often cancer cells bypass this limitation by reactivating telomerase, leading to enabling limitless replications. This telomerase activation characteristic is a hallmark of most cancers and represents a major divergence from the normal aging procedure. While maintenance of telomeres supports healthy tissue renewal, its dysregulation in aging creates a dual-edged sword (i.e., where insufficient telomere repair accelerates aging and tissue degeneration, and excessive repairs foster oncogenesis). Hence, balancing telomere dynamics is important for minimizing the risk of cancer while promoting healthy aging (Son et al., 2022).

3.4.1 Mechanisms of Telomere in Cancer in Relation to Aging

The mechanisms revolve around the dual role of telomere dynamics in maintaining genomic stability and also enabling the unchecked cell proliferation. Aging cells face progressive telomere shortening that limits a number of cell divisions that a cell can undergo, triggering cellular senescence, which is a protective mechanism against tumorigenesis. But critically shortened telomeres can result in end-to-end chromosome fusions and genomic instability, fostering the mutations that are initiated by cancer (Jafri et al., 2016).

Cancer cells often overpower these safeguards by reactivating telomerase or by utilizing alternative lengthening of telomeres (ALT) pathways. These mechanisms help cancer cells to maintain telomere integrity while supporting uncontrolled proliferation despite their inherently high rates of DNA damage. Aging boosts this process by increasing oxidative stress and chronic inflammation that results in accelerated shortening of telomeres and mutilation accumulation (Bordeira et al., 2018).

3.4.2 Impact of Telomere on Cancer in Relation to Cancer

Telomeres serve both as barriers and facilitators of oncogenesis with an unmatched impact on cancer development and progression. In the case of normal cells, telomere shortening is considered a tumor-suppressive mechanism by limiting cell division numbers and inducing senescence in critically short telomeres. But this same shortening could backfire as the reason for increasing the likelihood of mutations and the emergence of cancerous cells by leading to genomic instability as unprotected chromosome ends undergo fusion and rearrangements (Jafri et al., 2016).

In cancerous cells the telomere maintenance mechanisms are often hijacked in order to enable unlimited proliferation. Mostly, it reactivates telomerase, preventing critical shortening and allowing for continuous division. Some cancers utilize an alternative method to maintain telomere length called the alternative lengthening of telomeres pathway (ALT pathway). These adaptations help cancer cells to achieve the replicative immortality required. Hence, although telomeres play a protective role in preventing tumor formation, their dysregulation ends up in the initiation of cancer and progression (Zhu et al., 2016).

3.4.3 Physiological Effects of Elevated Telomere in Relation to Aging and Cancer

The elevated telomerase activity and longer telomeres can have a mixed physiological effect when it comes to aging and cancer. On one hand, by maintaining telomere length, delaying cellular aging, preserving tissue regeneration, and protecting against age-related degenerative diseases. In stem and progenitor cells, longer telomeres enhance their ability to repair and replace the old and damaged tissues, promoting overall health and longevity (Lansdorp, 2022).

But when it comes to cancer, the elevated telomerase activity acts as a double-edged sword. It undoubtedly helps in preventing genomic instability caused by critically shortening telomeres but it also blesses cancer cells with replicative immortality, which allows them to escape normally the limitations of cell division and fuels tumor growth and progression. Thus this highlights the importance of a delicate balance between telomere maintenance to optimize health while minimizing cancer risk (Boccardi & Marano, 2024).

4. CONCLUSION

Aging is a complicated process that is influenced by an intricate interplay of cellular, biochemical, environmental, and genetic factors. Among all the above-mentioned factors, telomere dynamics and homocysteine levels have emerged as critical determinants of aging and age-associated diseases. Telomere shortening is considered a hallmark of cellular aging because it underscores the importance of genomic stability in maintaining cellular function and longevity. On the other hand, elevated homocysteine levels highlight the biochemical and metabolic pathways that accelerate aging and also contribute to a wide range of pathologies (like cardiovascular diseases and neurodegeneration).

Intervention strategies targeting these two factors hold major importance for delaying aging and extending lifespan. Telomerase activation, telomere elongation, and gene editing are some of the telomere-based therapies that are at the leading edge of anti-aging research. Meanwhile, lifestyle modification (like balanced nutrition rich in folate, Vitamin B6, and B12), along with emerging pharmacological approaches, has shown great promise in reducing homocysteine levels and mitigating its harmful effects.

However, while these strategies are promising, their implementation requires a meaningful understanding of the broader implications. For example, the telomerase activation needs to be carefully controlled in order to prevent any unplanned consequences like oncogenesis. Likewise, the interventions that are targeting homocysteine levels should consider individual variability, genetic predispositions, and potential interactions with other metabolic processes.

As the research advances, centralized approaches are needed that combine genetic, biochemical, and lifestyle interventions that may offer the most effective path towards a healthier aging. The scientific community has the opportunity to unlock the full potential of telomere- and homocysteine-targeted therapies by bridging the gap between basic research and clinical application. This approach will ultimately pave the way for life-changing advancements in human longevity and quality of life.

REFERENCES

Accardi, G., & Aiello, A. (2021). Ways to become old: Role of lifestyle in modulation of the hallmarks of aging. In *Human Aging* (pp. 273–293). Academic Press. DOI: 10.1016/B978-0-12-822569-1.00009-3

Amado-Garzon, S. B., Molina-Pimienta, L., Vejarano-Pombo, A., Vélez-Bonilla, M., Moreno-Chaparro, J., & Buitrago-Lopez, A. (2024). Elevated Vitamin B12, Risk of Cancer, and Mortality: A Systematic Review. *Cancer Investigation*, *42*(6), 515–526. DOI: 10.1080/07357907.2024.2366907 PMID: 38953509

Anugerawati, M. T., Samsuria, I. K., Kurnia Setiawan Limijadi, I. E., Retnoningrum, D., & Rachmawati, B. (2024). Differences in Ca 15-3 and Homocysteine Levels in Patients with Benign Tumor and Breast Cancer. *Médico Moderno : MM : Revista Sócio-Econômica e Cultural de Medicina*, *31*(1).

Arsenis, N. C., You, T., Ogawa, E. F., Tinsley, G. M., & Zuo, L. (2017). Physical activity and telomere length: Impact of aging and potential mechanisms of action. *Oncotarget*, *8*(27), 45008–45019. DOI: 10.18632/oncotarget.16726 PMID: 28410238

Badawy, A. A. B. (2024). The role of nonesterified fatty acids in cancer biology: Focus on tryptophan and related metabolism. *Biochimica et Biophysica Acta (BBA)-. Biochimica et Biophysica Acta. Molecular and Cell Biology of Lipids*, *1869*(7), 159531. DOI: 10.1016/j.bbalip.2024.159531 PMID: 38986804

Baerlocher, G. M., Vulto, I., De Jong, G., & Lansdorp, P. M. (2006). Flow cytometry and FISH to measure the average length of telomeres (flow FISH). *Nature Protocols*, *1*(5), 2365–2376. DOI: 10.1038/nprot.2006.263 PMID: 17406480

Barshop, B. A. (2012). Homocystinuria and Hyperhomocysteinemia. In Goldman's Cecil Medicine (pp. 1361-1363). WB Saunders. DOI: 10.1016/B978-1-4377-1604-7.00216-5

Blackburn, E. H., & Gall, J. G. (1978). A tandemly repeated sequence at the termini of the extrachromosomal ribosomal RNA genes in Tetrahymena. *Journal of Molecular Biology*, *120*(1), 33–53. DOI: 10.1016/0022-2836(78)90294-2 PMID: 642006

Boccardi, V., & Marano, L. (2024). Aging, cancer, and inflammation: The telomerase connection. *International Journal of Molecular Sciences*, *25*(15), 8542. DOI: 10.3390/ijms25158542 PMID: 39126110

Boccardi, V., Paolisso, G., & Mecocci, P. (2016). Nutrition and lifestyle in healthy aging: The telomerase challenge. *Aging (Albany NY)*, *8*(1), 12–15. DOI: 10.18632/aging.100886 PMID: 26826704

Bordeira Gaspar, T., Sá, A., Lopes, J. M., Sobrinho-Simões, M., Soares, P., & Vinagre, J. (2018). Telomere maintenance mechanisms in cancer. *Genes*, *9*(5), 241. DOI: 10.3390/genes9050241 PMID: 29751586

Britt-Compton, B., Rowson, J., Locke, M., Mackenzie, I., Kipling, D., & Baird, D. M. (2006). Structural stability and chromosome-specific telomere length is governed by cis-acting determinants in humans. *Human Molecular Genetics*, *15*(5), 725–733. DOI: 10.1093/hmg/ddi486 PMID: 16421168

Butz, L. W., & du Vigneaud, V. (1932). The formation of a homologue of cystine by the decomposition of methionine with sulfuric acid. *The Journal of Biological Chemistry*, *99*(1), 135–142. DOI: 10.1016/S0021-9258(18)76074-2

Cawthon, R. M. (2002). Telomere measurement by quantitative PCR. *Nucleic Acids Research, 30*(10), e47–e47. DOI: 10.1093/nar/30.10.e47 PMID: 12000852

Chuaire, L. (2006). Telomere and Telomerase: Brief review of a history initiated by Hermann Müller and Barbara McClintock. *Colombia Médica : CM, 37*(4), 332–335. DOI: 10.25100/cm.v37i4.466

Crous-Bou, M., Molinuevo, J. L., & Sala-Vila, A. (2019). Plant-rich dietary patterns, plant foods and nutrients, and telomere length. *Advances in Nutrition, 10*, S296–S303. DOI: 10.1093/advances/nmz026 PMID: 31728493

De Meyer, T., Nawrot, T., Bekaert, S., De Buyzere, M. L., Rietzschel, E. R., & Andrés, V. (2018). Telomere length as cardiovascular aging biomarker: JACC review topic of the week. *Journal of the American College of Cardiology, 72*(7), 805–813. DOI: 10.1016/j.jacc.2018.06.014 PMID: 30092957

de Oliveira, J. J., Silva, A. D. S., Ribeiro, A. G. S. V., Barbosa, C. G. R., de Oliveira Silva, J. A., Pontes, A. G., & Pertille, A. (2021). The effect of physical activity on total homocysteine concentrations and cardiovascular risk in older Brazilian adults with type 2 diabetes. *Journal of Diabetes and Metabolic Disorders, 20*(1), 407–416. DOI: 10.1007/s40200-021-00759-6 PMID: 34178848

Deminice, R., Ribeiro, D. F., & Frajacomo, F. T. T. (2016). The effects of acute exercise and exercise training on plasma homocysteine: A meta-analysis. *PLoS One, 11*(3), e0151653. DOI: 10.1371/journal.pone.0151653 PMID: 26986570

Deng, Y., Li, Q., Zhou, F., Li, G., Liu, J., Lv, J., Li, L., & Chang, D. (2022). Telomere length and the risk of cardiovascular diseases: A Mendelian randomization study. *Frontiers in Cardiovascular Medicine, 9*, 1012615. DOI: 10.3389/fcvm.2022.1012615 PMID: 36352846

Dhillon, V. S., Deo, P., Thomas, P., & Fenech, M. (2023). Low Magnesium in conjunction with high homocysteine and less sleep accelerates telomere attrition in healthy elderly Australian. *International Journal of Molecular Sciences, 24*(2), 982. DOI: 10.3390/ijms24020982 PMID: 36674498

Dinavahi, R., & Falkner, B. (2004). Relationship of homocysteine with cardiovascular disease and blood pressure. *Journal of Clinical Hypertension, 6*(9), 494–500. DOI: 10.1111/j.1524-6175.2004.03643.x PMID: 15365276

Elias, M. F., & Brown, C. J. (2022). New evidence for homocysteine lowering for management of treatment-resistant hypertension. *American Journal of Hypertension, 35*(4), 303–305. DOI: 10.1093/ajh/hpab194 PMID: 34935029

Ferroni, P., Palmirotta, R., Martini, F., Riondino, S., Savonarola, A., Spila, A., & Guadagni, F. (2009). Determinants of homocysteine levels in colorectal and breast cancer patients. *Anticancer Research, 29*(10), 4131–4138. PMID: 19846961

Fusco, D., Colloca, G., Monaco, M. R. L., & Cesari, M. (2007). Effects of antioxidant supplementation on the aging process. *Clinical Interventions in Aging, 2*(3), 377–387. PMID: 18044188

Galiè, S., Canudas, S., Muralidharan, J., García-Gavilán, J., Bulló, M., & Salas-Salvadó, J. (2020). Impact of nutrition on telomere health: Systematic review of observational cohort studies and randomized clinical trials. *Advances in Nutrition, 11*(3), 576–601. DOI: 10.1093/advances/nmz107 PMID: 31688893

Ganguly, P., & Alam, S. F. (2015). Role of homocysteine in the development of cardiovascular disease. *Nutrition Journal*, *14*(1), 1–10. DOI: 10.1186/1475-2891-14-6 PMID: 25577237

Gołębiowska, J., Szymala-Pędzik, M., Żórawska, J., Sobieszczańska, M., & Agrawal, S. (2023). Identification of Factors Affecting the Increased Percentage of CGA Recommendations among Patients on Geriatric Ward. *International Journal of Environmental Research and Public Health*, *20*(3), 2065. DOI: 10.3390/ijerph20032065 PMID: 36767432

Greider, C. W., & Blackburn, E. H. (1985). Identification of a specific telomere terminal transferase activity in Tetrahymena extracts. *cell*, *43*(2), 405-413.

Gruber, H. J., Semeraro, M. D., Renner, W., & Herrmann, M. (2021). Telomeres and age-related diseases. *Biomedicines*, *9*(10), 1335. DOI: 10.3390/biomedicines9101335 PMID: 34680452

Hasan, T., Arora, R., Bansal, A. K., Bhattacharya, R., Sharma, G. S., & Singh, L. R. (2019). Disturbed homocysteine metabolism is associated with cancer. *Experimental & Molecular Medicine*, *51*(2), 1–13. DOI: 10.1038/s12276-019-0216-4 PMID: 30804341

Hayflick, L., & Moorhead, P. S. (1961). The serial cultivation of human diploid cell strains. *Experimental Cell Research*, *25*(3), 585–621. DOI: 10.1016/0014-4827(61)90192-6 PMID: 13905658

Jafri, M. A., Ansari, S. A., Alqahtani, M. H., & Shay, J. W. (2016). Roles of telomeres and telomerase in cancer, and advances in telomerase-targeted therapies. *Genome Medicine*, *8*(1), 1–18. DOI: 10.1186/s13073-016-0324-x PMID: 27323951

Jafri, M. A., Ansari, S. A., Alqahtani, M. H., & Shay, J. W. (2016). Roles of telomeres and telomerase in cancer, and advances in telomerase-targeted therapies. *Genome Medicine*, *8*(1), 1–18. DOI: 10.1186/s13073-016-0324-x PMID: 27323951

Keshteli, A. H., Baracos, V. E., & Madsen, K. L. (2015). Hyperhomocysteinemia as a potential contributor of colorectal cancer development in inflammatory bowel diseases: A review. *World Journal of Gastroenterology*, *21*(4), 1081. DOI: 10.3748/wjg.v21.i4.1081 PMID: 25632180

Kimura, M., Stone, R. C., Hunt, S. C., Skurnick, J., Lu, X., Cao, X., Harley, C. B., & Aviv, A. (2010). Measurement of telomere length by the Southern blot analysis of terminal restriction fragment lengths. *Nature Protocols*, *5*(9), 1596–1607. DOI: 10.1038/nprot.2010.124 PMID: 21085125

Koklesova, L., Mazurakova, A., Samec, M., Biringer, K., Samuel, S. M., Büsselberg, D., Kubatka, P., & Golubnitschaja, O. (2021). Homocysteine metabolism as the target for predictive medical approach, disease prevention, prognosis, and treatments tailored to the person. *The EPMA Journal*, *12*(4), 477–505. DOI: 10.1007/s13167-021-00263-0 PMID: 34786033

Kumar, A., Palfrey, H. A., Pathak, R., Kadowitz, P. J., Gettys, T. W., & Murthy, S. N. (2017). The metabolism and significance of homocysteine in nutrition and health. *Nutrition & Metabolism*, *14*(1), 1–12. DOI: 10.1186/s12986-017-0233-z PMID: 29299040

Lansdorp, P. M. (2022). Telomeres, aging, and cancer: The big picture. *Blood*, *139*(6), 813–821. DOI: 10.1182/blood.2021014299 PMID: 35142846

Lansdorp, P. M. (2022). Telomeres, aging, and cancer: The big picture. *Blood*, *139*(6), 813–821. DOI: 10.1182/blood.2021014299 PMID: 35142846

Lee, J., & Pellegrini, M. V. (2022). Biochemistry, Telomere and Telomerase. In *StatPearls* [Internet]. StatPearls Publishing.

Lee, M., Napier, C. E., Yang, S. F., Arthur, J. W., Reddel, R. R., & Pickett, H. A. (2017). Comparative analysis of whole genome sequencing-based telomere length measurement techniques. *Methods (San Diego, Calif.)*, *114*, 4–15. DOI: 10.1016/j.ymeth.2016.08.008 PMID: 27565742

Lee, Y. A., Kang, S. G., Song, S. W., & Kim, S. H. (2024). Association between Homocysteine and Vitamin D Levels in Asymptomatic Korean Adults. *Nutrients*, *16*(8), 1155. DOI: 10.3390/nu16081155 PMID: 38674846

Lin, J., Lee, I. M., Song, Y., Cook, N. R., Selhub, J., Manson, J. E., Buring, J. E., & Zhang, S. M. (2010). Plasma homocysteine and cysteine and risk of breast cancer in women. *Cancer Research*, *70*(6), 2397–2405. DOI: 10.1158/0008-5472.CAN-09-3648 PMID: 20197471

Luzzi, S., Cherubini, V., Falsetti, L., Viticchi, G., Silvestrini, M., & Toraldo, A. (2022). Homocysteine, cognitive functions, and degenerative dementias: State of the art. *Biomedicines*, *10*(11), 2741. DOI: 10.3390/biomedicines10112741 PMID: 36359260

Majumder, A. (2023). Targeting homocysteine and hydrogen sulfide balance as future therapeutics in cancer treatment. *Antioxidants*, *12*(8), 1520. DOI: 10.3390/antiox12081520 PMID: 37627515

Mangaonkar, A. A., & Patnaik, M. M. (2018, July). Short telomere syndromes in clinical practice: Bridging bench and bedside. [). Elsevier.]. *Mayo Clinic Proceedings*, *93*(7), 904–916. DOI: 10.1016/j.mayocp.2018.03.020 PMID: 29804726

Marcus, J., Sarnak, M. J., Menon, V., & Verma, S. (2007). Homocysteine lowering and cardiovascular disease risk: Lost in translation. *The Canadian Journal of Cardiology*, *23*(9), 707–710. DOI: 10.1016/S0828-282X(07)70814-0 PMID: 17622392

McCaddon, A., & Miller, J. W. (2023). Homocysteine—A retrospective and prospective appraisal. *Frontiers in Nutrition*, *10*, 1179807. DOI: 10.3389/fnut.2023.1179807 PMID: 37384104

Mikkelsen, K., & Apostolopoulos, V. (2024). Mechanistic Effects of Vitamin B6 and B12 on Inflammation and Cancer. In *Hydrophilic Vitamins in Health and Disease* (pp. 279–308). Springer International Publishing. DOI: 10.1007/978-3-031-55474-2_13

Miller, J. W. (2013). Encyclopedia of Human Nutrition || Homocysteine., (), 424–430. DOI: 10.1016/B978-0-12-375083-9.00144-6

Nag, S. (2019). Syndromes associated with telomere shortening. In *Telomerase and non-Telomerase Mechanisms of Telomere Maintenance*. IntechOpen.

Olaso-Gonzalez, G., Inzitari, M., Bellelli, G., Morandi, A., Barcons, N., & Viña, J. (2022). Impact of supplementation with vitamins B6, B12, and/or folic acid on the reduction of homocysteine levels in patients with mild cognitive impairment: A systematic review. *IUBMB Life*, *74*(1), 74–84. DOI: 10.1002/iub.2507 PMID: 34058062

Ostrakhovitch, E. A., & Tabibzadeh, S. (2019). Homocysteine and age-associated disorders. *Ageing Research Reviews*, *49*, 144–164. DOI: 10.1016/j.arr.2018.10.010 PMID: 30391754

Pandey, S. (2018). Factors contributing of ageing: Factors in ageing. In *Handbook of research on geriatric health, treatment, and care* (pp. 393–408). IGI Global. DOI: 10.4018/978-1-5225-3480-8.ch022

Phipps, M. L., Goodwin, P. M., Martinez, J. S., & Goodwin, E. H. (2016). Super-resolution optical microscopy study of telomere structure. *Journal of Biomedical Optics*, *21*(9), 094003–094003. DOI: 10.1117/1.JBO.21.9.094003 PMID: 27685813

Rizzo, G., & Laganà, A. S. (2020). The link between homocysteine and omega-3 polyunsaturated fatty acid: Critical appraisal and future directions. *Biomolecules*, *10*(2), 219. DOI: 10.3390/biom10020219 PMID: 32024302

Rossiello, F., Jurk, D., Passos, J. F., & d'Adda di Fagagna, F. (2022). Telomere dysfunction in ageing and age-related diseases. *Nature Cell Biology*, *24*(2), 135–147. DOI: 10.1038/s41556-022-00842-x PMID: 35165420

Sanchez, S. E., Gu, Y., Wang, Y., Golla, A., Martin, A., Shomali, W., Hockemeyer, D., Savage, S. A., & Artandi, S. E. (2024). Digital telomere measurement by long-read sequencing distinguishes healthy aging from disease. *Nature Communications*, *15*(1), 5148. DOI: 10.1038/s41467-024-49007-4 PMID: 38890274

Shammas, M. A. (2011). Telomeres, lifestyle, cancer, and aging. *Current Opinion in Clinical Nutrition and Metabolic Care*, *14*(1), 28–34. DOI: 10.1097/MCO.0b013e32834121b1 PMID: 21102320

Shay, J. W. (2018). Telomeres and aging. *Current Opinion in Cell Biology*, *52*, 1–7. DOI: 10.1016/j.ceb.2017.12.001 PMID: 29253739

Shibeeb, S., Abdallah, A., & Shi, Z. (2024). Blood homocysteine levels mediate the association between blood lead levels and cardiovascular mortality. *Cardiovascular Toxicology*, *24*(1), 62–70. DOI: 10.1007/s12012-023-09819-0 PMID: 38231351

Simonenko, S. Y., Bogdanova, D. A., & Kuldyushev, N. A. (2024). Emerging Roles of Vitamin B12 in Aging and Inflammation. *International Journal of Molecular Sciences*, *25*(9), 5044. DOI: 10.3390/ijms25095044 PMID: 38732262

Slijepcevic, P. (2001). Telomere length measurement by Q-FISH. *Chromosome Painting: Principles, Strategies and Scope*, 17-22.

Smith, E. M., Pendlebury, D. F., & Nandakumar, J. (2020). Structural biology of telomeres and telomerase. *Cellular and Molecular Life Sciences : CMLS*, *77*(1), 61–79. DOI: 10.1007/s00018-019-03369-x PMID: 31728577

Sohouli, M. H., Roshan, M. M., Olusola, O. F., Fatahi, S., Omidi, H. R., Sharifi, P., Hekmatdoost, A., Kutbi, E., & Abu-Zaid, A. (2022). Impact of Omega-3 supplementation on homocysteine levels in humans: A systematic review and meta-regression analysis of randomized controlled trials. *Nutrition, Metabolism, and Cardiovascular Diseases*, *32*(9), 2013–2025. DOI: 10.1016/j.numecd.2022.05.008 PMID: 35843792

Son, N., Cui, Y., & Xi, W. (2022). Association between telomere length and skin cancer and aging: A mendelian randomization analysis. *Frontiers in Genetics*, *13*, 931785. DOI: 10.3389/fgene.2022.931785 PMID: 35903361

Tseng, F. C., & Huang, T. C. (2021). Using data mining technology to explore homocysteine at low levels. *Medicine*, *100*(33), e26893. DOI: 10.1097/MD.0000000000026893 PMID: 34414944

Verma, A. K., Singh, P., Al-Saeed, F. A., Ahmed, A. E., Kumar, S., Kumar, A., Dev, K., & Dohare, R. (2022). Unravelling the role of telomere shortening with ageing and their potential association with diabetes, cancer, and related lifestyle factors. *Tissue & Cell*, *79*, 101925. DOI: 10.1016/j.tice.2022.101925 PMID: 36137363

Victorelli, S., & Passos, J. F. (2017). Telomeres and cell senescence-size matters not. *EBioMedicine*, *21*, 14–20. DOI: 10.1016/j.ebiom.2017.03.027 PMID: 28347656

Vitamin, B. B. (2022). Vitamins: Functions and Uses in Medicine. *The Permanente Journal*, *26*(2). PMID: 35933667

Wu, D. F., Yin, R. X., & Deng, J. L. (2024). Homocysteine, hyperhomocysteinemia, and H-type hypertension. *European Journal of Preventive Cardiology*, •••, zwae022. PMID: 38236144

Xu, J., Zhao, X., Sun, S., Ni, P., Li, C., Ren, A., Wang, W., & Zhu, L. (2018). Homocysteine and Digestive Tract Cancer Risk: A Dose-Response Meta-Analysis. *Journal of Oncology*, *2018*(1), 3720684. DOI: 10.1155/2018/3720684 PMID: 30662463

Yeh, J. K., Lin, M. H., & Wang, C. Y. (2019). Telomeres as therapeutic targets in heart disease. *JACC. Basic to Translational Science*, *4*(7), 855–865. DOI: 10.1016/j.jacbts.2019.05.009 PMID: 31998853

Yu, H. J., Byun, Y. H., & Park, C. K. (2024). Techniques for assessing telomere length: A methodological review. *Computational and Structural Biotechnology Journal*, *23*, 1489–1498. DOI: 10.1016/j.csbj.2024.04.011 PMID: 38633384

Yuan, D., Chu, J., Lin, H., Zhu, G., Qian, J., Yu, Y., Yao, T., Ping, F., Chen, F., & Liu, X. (2023). Mechanism of homocysteine-mediated endothelial injury and its consequences for atherosclerosis. *Frontiers in Cardiovascular Medicine*, *9*, 1109445. DOI: 10.3389/fcvm.2022.1109445 PMID: 36727029

Zhao, G., Guo, D., Li, L., Yang, C., & Dong, J. (2022). The association between dietary magnesium intake and telomere length in adults with hypertension. *The Journal of Nutrition, Health & Aging*, *26*(11), 1010–1015. DOI: 10.1007/s12603-022-1856-y PMID: 36437769

Zhu, X., Han, W., Xue, W., Zou, Y., Xie, C., Du, J., & Jin, G. (2016). The association between telomere length and cancer risk in population studies. *Scientific Reports*, *6*(1), 22243. DOI: 10.1038/srep22243 PMID: 26915412

Chapter 4
Anti-Aging Pharmacology: Advances and Prospects

Rajasekhar Komarla Kumarachari
https://orcid.org/0000-0001-5611-1410
Meenakshi Faculty of Pharmacy, MAHER University, Chennai, India

Sarad Pawar Naik Bukke
Kampala International University, Uganda

Lokesh Kammara
https://orcid.org/0009-0006-5079-3805
Aston University, Birmingham, UK

Chandrakala Aruga
S.V.U. College of Pharmaceutical Sciences, S.V. University, Tirupati, India

M. Himasaila
https://orcid.org/0000-0001-7432-0494
Sri Padmavathi School of Pharmacy, Tiruchanur, India

Mounika Kamati
MB School of Pharmaceutical Sciences, MB University, Rangampeta, India

ABSTRACT

The field of anti-aging pharmacology has seen remarkable advancements over recent years, driven by the growing understanding of the molecular and genetic mechanisms underlying aging. This chapter explores the latest developments in anti-aging pharmacological interventions, including senolytics, caloric restriction mimetics, and autophagy enhancers. We delve into the role of molecular pathways such as mTOR, sirtuins, and AMPK in aging, and discuss how drugs targeting these pathways hold promise for extending lifespan and improving healthspan. The chapter also examines the challenges of translating these interventions from preclinical models to human applications, considering both efficacy and safety. Ethical considerations and regulatory frameworks will be discussed, along with prospects for future research and clinical implementation in the quest to combat aging and age-related diseases.

1. INTRODUCTION

Aging is a complex biological process marked by the gradual decline in cellular function, ultimately leading to a host of age-related diseases such as cardiovascular disorders, neurodegenerative conditions, cancer, and metabolic dysfunctions. For centuries, aging was regarded as an inevitable consequence of time; however, significant scientific advancements in recent decades have dramatically reshaped this perspective. It is now widely recognized that aging can be modulated and potentially slowed through

DOI: 10.4018/979-8-3693-9730-5.ch004

targeted pharmacological interventions. Anti-aging pharmacology has emerged as a promising field, aiming not only to extend lifespan but, more importantly, to enhance healthspan—the period of life free from significant disease and disability (López-Otín et al., 2023).

Advances in molecular biology and genetics have unveiled critical mechanisms that drive aging at the cellular and organismal levels. Several key molecular pathways—such as mechanistic target of rapamycin / mammalian target of rapamycin (mTOR), sirtuins, and AMP-activated protein kinase (AMPK)—have been identified as central regulators of aging. These pathways are involved in cellular processes like metabolism, stress responses, and autophagy, which are integral to the onset of age-related dysfunction. Pharmacological agents targeting these pathways are now at the forefront of research, holding the potential to decelerate or even reverse certain aspects of the aging process (Guo et al., 2022).

This chapter provides a comprehensive overview of recent developments in anti-aging pharmacology. It highlights some of the most promising strategies, including senolytics, which selectively eliminate senescent cells; caloric restriction mimetics (CRMs), which mimic the beneficial effects of caloric restriction (CR) without the need for dietary changes; and autophagy enhancers, which promote the body's natural cellular repair mechanisms. By intervening at the molecular level, these pharmacological approaches aim to reduce age-related damage and promote healthy aging.

However, the transition from preclinical research to clinical application poses significant challenges. While many of these anti-aging interventions have shown promising results in animal models, translating these findings into human therapies has proven difficult. Issues such as efficacy, safety, and long-term impact remain areas of concern. Additionally, the regulatory frameworks surrounding anti-aging drugs are still evolving, and the ethical implications of such treatments raise important questions regarding access, equity, and societal impact (Ineichen et al., 2024).

As research progresses, there is increasing interest in the development of personalized anti-aging therapies that take into account an individual's unique genetic, environmental, and lifestyle factors. Personalized approaches could optimize the effectiveness of these treatments while minimizing risks. Moreover, the ethical and societal considerations surrounding lifespan extension continue to shape the future of anti-aging pharmacology (Martens et al., 2023).

This chapter is structured to provide a comprehensive understanding of anti-aging pharmacology's scientific foundations, including molecular pathways and therapeutic innovations. We critically assess the prospects for future research and clinical application, addressing the ethical, safety, and regulatory challenges that come with this rapidly evolving field. By illuminating the potential of pharmacology in combating aging and age-related diseases, this chapter offers a glimpse into the transformative impact on human health and longevity in the coming decades.

2. MOLECULAR MECHANISMS OF AGING

Aging is a complex, multifactorial process influenced by a combination of genetic, molecular, and environmental factors. Over the past few decades, significant advancements in anti-aging pharmacology have emerged from a deeper understanding of the molecular pathways that govern the aging process. These discoveries have opened the door to pharmacological interventions aimed at modulating aging, extending lifespan, and promoting a healthier aging experience (da Costa et al., 2016). This section delves into the key molecular mechanisms underlying aging, focusing on the most promising pathways that have been identified for therapeutic targeting.

2.1 The Role of Genetics and Molecular Pathways in Aging

Aging is characterized by several hallmark processes, each contributing to the gradual decline in cellular function and overall organismal health. One key hallmark is genomic instability, characterized by the accumulation of DNA damage over time that impairs cell function and can lead to cell death or mutations that contribute to age-related diseases. Another critical factor is telomere shortening, in which the progressive loss of telomere length triggers cellular senescence and tissue dysfunction, as cells lose their capacity to divide. Epigenetic alterations also play a significant role in aging, with age-associated changes in gene expression regulation, such as DNA methylation and histone modifications, affecting cellular function and leading to dysregulation of various metabolic and signaling pathways.

Mitochondrial dysfunction, another hallmark of aging, involves a decline in mitochondrial efficiency coupled with increased oxidative stress, both of which contribute to cellular damage and the loss of energy production needed for cellular health. Cellular senescence further exacerbates aging, as senescent cells cease to divide but remain metabolically active, secreting inflammatory factors that disrupt tissue structure and function. Together, these interconnected hallmarks of aging drive the physiological deterioration associated with age, impacting overall health and susceptibility to age-related diseases (López-Gil et al., 2023).

Central to these processes are molecular pathways that govern cellular responses to stress, energy availability, and damage. Researchers have identified several critical pathways that play a fundamental role in aging, such as the mTOR, sirtuins, and AMPK. These pathways regulate key aspects of cellular health, including metabolism, growth, and autophagy, making them attractive targets for pharmacological interventions aimed at delaying or mitigating the effects of aging (Pan & Finkel, 2017).

Figure 1. Pharmacological and lifestyle strategies that target aging-related pathways.

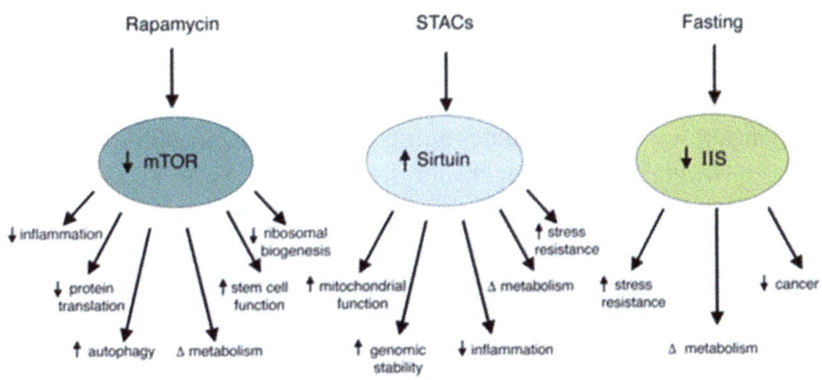

Drugs like rapamycin, along with lifestyle interventions such as fasting and caloric restriction, act on key molecular pathways—namely the mammalian target of rapamycin (mTOR), sirtuin, and insulin/insulin-like growth factor signalling (IIS) pathways. By modulating these pathways, interventions trigger a cascade of biological changes. These changes, whether occurring independently or in synergy, may help decelerate the aging process by promoting cellular resilience, reducing metabolic stress, and enhancing repair mechanisms.

2.2 Key Aging Pathways: mTOR, Sirtuins, and AMPK

The mTOR, sirtuins, and AMPK pathways are three of the most extensively studied in the context of aging and longevity. Pharmacological manipulation of these pathways has shown promise in preclinical models and holds potential for therapeutic application in humans.

2.2.1. mTOR Pathway

The mTOR, also known as FK506-binding protein 12-rapamycin-associated protein 1 (FRAP1), is a protein kinase that plays a central role in regulating cell growth, metabolism, and aging. mTOR integrates signals from nutrients, growth factors, and energy status to control processes such as protein synthesis, autophagy, and lipid metabolism. Importantly, inhibition of the mTOR pathway has been associated with increased lifespan in multiple model organisms, including yeast, worms, flies, and mice (Panwar et al., 2023).

Rapamycin, a well-known mTOR inhibitor, has become one of the most studied pharmacological agents in anti-aging research. By inhibiting mTOR, rapamycin mimics CR—a well-established intervention known to extend lifespan across species. Studies in animal models have shown that rapamycin can delay the onset of age-related diseases, including cancer, cardiovascular disease, and neurodegeneration. However, the translation of mTOR inhibitors to human anti-aging therapies presents challenges, particularly in balancing efficacy with potential side effects such as immunosuppression (Aliper et al., 2017).

2.2.2. Sirtuins

Sirtuins are a family of nicotine adenine dinucleotide+ (NAD+)-dependent histone deacetylases that regulate several cellular processes critical for longevity, including DNA repair, metabolic homeostasis, and stress resistance. Sirtuins are activated in response to environmental stressors, such as CR and exercise, which have been shown to extend lifespan in various species (Wu et al., 2022).

Among the seven known sirtuins, SIRT1 has garnered the most attention due to its role in promoting healthspan and delaying aging. SIRT1 regulates autophagy, mitochondrial function, and inflammation, all of which are key to maintaining cellular health during aging. Sirtuin-activating compounds, such as resveratrol—a polyphenol found in grapes and red wine—have shown potential in mimicking the beneficial effects of CR. Resveratrol has been shown to increase SIRT1 activity and improve lifespan and healthspan in animal models, though its efficacy in humans remains under investigation (Chang et al., 2024).

2.2.3. AMPK Pathway

AMPK is a cellular energy sensor that becomes activated in response to low energy levels, such as during exercise or CR. AMPK activation promotes catabolic processes that generate energy, such as fatty acid oxidation and autophagy, while inhibiting anabolic processes like protein synthesis, which consume energy. By maintaining cellular energy balance, AMPK plays a key role in promoting longevity and metabolic health (Sharma, A. et al., 2023).

Metformin, a widely-used drug for type 2 diabetes, is one of the most prominent pharmacological activators of AMPK. Beyond its glucose-lowering effects, metformin has been shown to activate AMPK, reduce inflammation, and improve mitochondrial function. Epidemiological studies suggest that metformin use is associated with reduced incidence of age-related diseases, such as cancer and cardiovascular disease, as well as potential lifespan extension in diabetic patients (Lv & Guo, 2020). These findings have sparked interest in metformin as a candidate for anti-aging interventions, though large-scale clinical trials are needed to confirm its efficacy in non-diabetic populations.

2.3 Cross-Talk and Synergistic Effects

It is important to note that these pathways do not function in isolation. Cross-talk between mTOR, sirtuins, and AMPK occurs at multiple levels, allowing cells to coordinate responses to various stressors and energy availability. For instance, AMPK activation can inhibit mTOR, while sirtuins are influenced by the cellular energy status regulated by AMPK. Understanding these interactions is crucial for developing combination therapies that may offer synergistic effects, potentially enhancing the efficacy of anti-aging pharmacological interventions (Sadria and Layton, 2021).

In conclusion, targeting the mTOR, sirtuin, and AMPK pathways offers promising avenues for the development of anti-aging therapeutics. Continued research into these molecular mechanisms is essential for understanding how these pathways influence aging and for translating this knowledge into safe, effective therapies that can promote healthy aging and extend both lifespan and healthspan in humans.

3. PHARMACOLOGICAL INTERVENTIONS IN ANTI-AGING

The pharmacological landscape of anti-aging therapies has grown significantly over the past decade, with increasing attention focused on developing drugs that modulate key molecular pathways involved in aging. These interventions aim to delay the onset of age-related diseases, improve healthspan, and potentially extend lifespan (Tenchov et al., 2024). This section explores some of the most promising pharmacological strategies, including senolytics, CR mimetics, and autophagy enhancers, all of which target the underlying mechanisms of aging.

Figure 2. The connection between diverse anti-aging strategies and the specific hallmarks of aging they address.

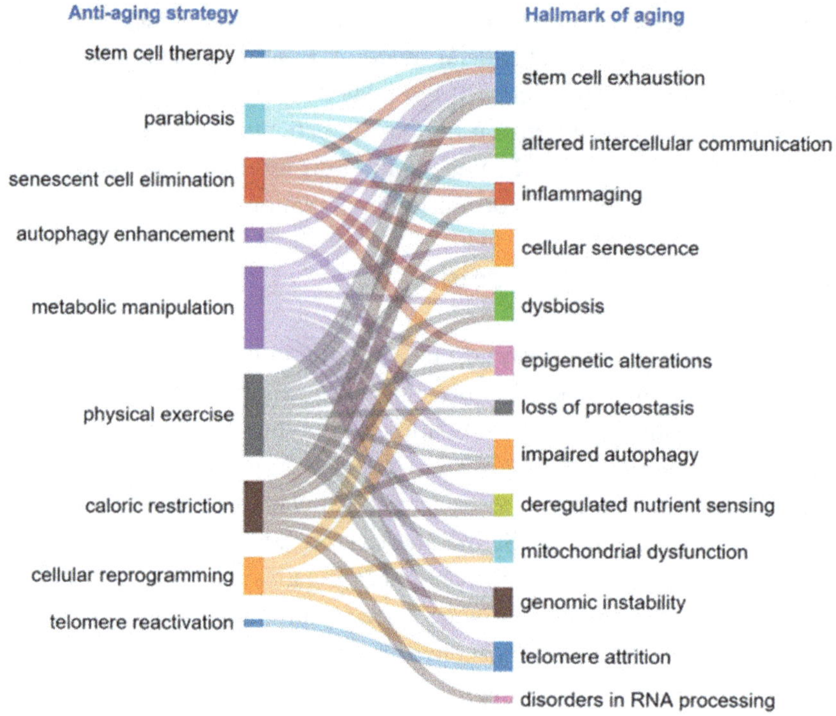

Various approaches, such as parabiosis (blood exchange), metabolic manipulation, senescent cell elimination, and cellular reprogramming, have been investigated for their potential to counteract aging processes. Each of these interventions targets multiple aging hallmarks, suggesting a multifaceted approach to slowing or reversing aging by addressing underlying cellular and molecular dysfunctions that contribute to the aging process.

3.1 Senolytics: Eliminating Senescent Cells

Senolytics represent a groundbreaking area of anti-aging pharmacology, aiming to selectively eliminate senescent cells that accumulate with age and secrete pro-inflammatory factors collectively known as the senescence-associated secretory phenotype (SASP). SASP contributes to inflammation, tissue degradation, and a range of age-related pathologies, including osteoarthritis, cardiovascular disease, and neurodegenerative disorders (Kirkland et al., 2020). Senolytic drugs like dasatinib, quercetin, navitoclax, fisetin, and piperlongumine have shown promise in targeting these senescent cells, reducing their numbers and alleviating SASP-related effects.

Dasatinib, initially developed as a tyrosine kinase inhibitor for cancer treatment, has shown senolytic potential by selectively inducing apoptosis in senescent cells, particularly human preadipocytes and endothelial cells. Orally bioavailable, it reaches peak plasma concentrations within 0.5 to 6 hours and is metabolized by CYP3A4, with a half-life of around 5-6 hours. Though effective, dasatinib's use requires careful monitoring due to side effects such as myelosuppression and QT interval prolongation (Islam et al., 2023).

Quercetin, a natural flavonoid found in various fruits and vegetables, targets senescent endothelial cells and provides antioxidant and anti-inflammatory benefits. Despite its poor bioavailability, it is generally well-tolerated, although high doses can occasionally cause mild side effects. Combined with dasatinib, quercetin has demonstrated efficacy in early human trials, such as in patients with idiopathic pulmonary fibrosis (IPF), where it reduced markers of senescence and improved physical function (Nambiar et al., 2023).

Navitoclax, originally developed as an anticancer agent, acts by inhibiting Bcl-2 family proteins and promoting apoptosis in senescent cells. However, side effects like thrombocytopenia and gastrointestinal symptoms limit its long-term use, despite its promise as a senolytic (Anuar et al., 2020). Fisetin, another naturally occurring flavonoid, targets various types of senescent cells, though its low bioavailability may impact clinical efficacy without pharmacokinetic enhancements. It is generally well tolerated, with high doses only occasionally leading to mild gastrointestinal discomfort (Krishnakumar et al., 2022).

Piperlongumine, an experimental compound obtained from *Piper longum*, works by increasing reactive oxygen species (ROS) in senescent cells, triggering apoptosis selectively within these cells. While promising, it has limited bioavailability, and high doses can be cytotoxic, necessitating further research to ensure safe application (Zhang & Zhou, 2024).

Figure 3. Structures

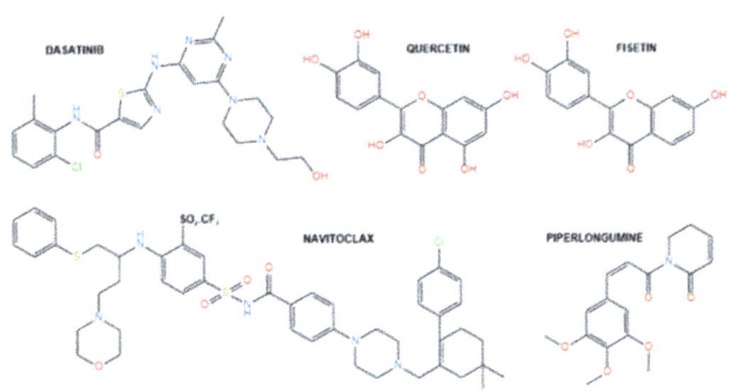

The chemical structures of these senolytics illustrate their diverse mechanisms. Dasatinib's heterocylic core enables kinase inhibition, allowing it to target pathways critical for senescent cell survival. Quercetin and fisetin are polyphenolic compounds with antioxidant properties, while navitoclax's N-sulfonylcarboxamide structure promotes Bcl-2 binding, inducing apoptosis. Piperlongumine's lactone ring is key to its ROS-promoting effects, providing selective action against senescent cells.

Interactions with other drugs and foods highlight the need for careful administration. Dasatinib, as a CYP3A4 substrate, can interact with inhibitors and inducers, such as ketoconazole and rifampin. Navitoclax's side effects necessitate caution with CYP3A4 inhibitors and blood-thinning agents, while quercetin and fisetin have minimal drug interactions. However, dasatinib levels may be increased by grapefruit juice, and high-fat foods can enhance the bioavailability of quercetin and fisetin.

In summary, senolytics hold substantial promise for alleviating age-related diseases by clearing senescent cells, thereby reducing inflammation and promoting healthier aging. Although initial findings are encouraging, ongoing research is needed to optimize the safety and clinical effectiveness of these compounds for broader application in age-related health conditions.

3.2 Caloric Restriction Mimetics

CR, reducing calorie intake without malnutrition, is well-known for extending lifespan and healthspan across various organisms. However, CR's long-term feasibility is limited due to potential physical and mental side effects, prompting the exploration of CRMs. CRMs are compounds that replicate the benefits of CR without requiring dietary changes, targeting cellular pathways linked to aging, stress resistance, and metabolism (Dorling et al., 2020; Martel et al., 2021).

Resveratrol, a polyphenol found in red wine, activates sirtuins, proteins involved in DNA repair and metabolic regulation. This compound's structure, featuring phenolic rings connected by an ethylene bridge, enhances its antioxidant properties and facilitates SIRT1 activation. While promising in animal studies for metabolic and anti-inflammatory benefits, resveratrol has shown mixed results in human trials and can interact with anticoagulants and drugs metabolized by CYP3A4 (Ram W S, 2019; Sarubbo et al., 2018).

Rapamycin inhibits the mechanistic target of rapamycin (mTOR) pathway, promoting autophagy and reducing cellular stress. As a macrolide with a large lactone ring, rapamycin's structure enables it to bind effectively to mTOR. Its metabolism via CYP3A4 creates potential interactions with inhibitors and inducers of this enzyme, and grapefruit juice may significantly increase rapamycin's immunosuppressive effects (Almendáriz-Palacios et al., 2020).

Nicotinamide Mononucleotide (NMN) and Nicotinamide Riboside (NR) are NAD+ precursors, supporting mitochondrial function and DNA repair. With an essential nicotinamide structure, NMN and NR help replenish declining NAD+ levels in aging cells. While they have minimal drug interactions, higher doses could affect vitamin B3-related pathways (Alegre & Pastore, 2023).

Figure 4. Structures

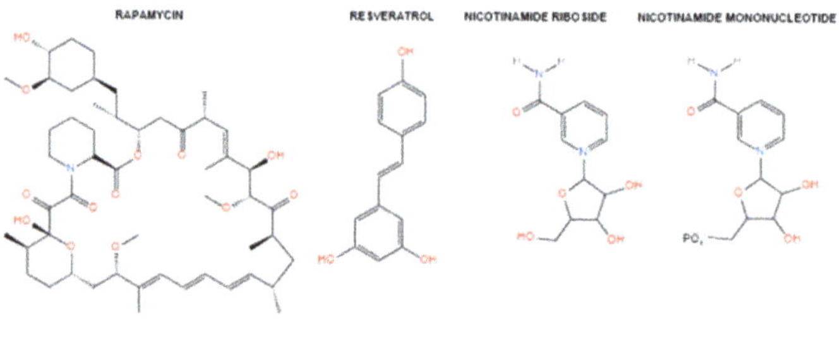

Fisetin, a flavonoid with antioxidant and anti-inflammatory properties, reduces pro-inflammatory cytokines in senescent cells. Its structure, a polyphenolic backbone with hydroxyl groups, enhances cellular uptake and anti-inflammatory effects. Generally well-tolerated, fisetin may amplify anticoagulant effects if combined with blood-thinning medications (Domaszewska-Szostek et al., 2021).

Metformin, a widely used diabetes medication, activates AMP-activated protein kinase (AMPK), promoting energy metabolism and mimicking CR effects. Metformin's structure, with guanidine groups linked by a methylene bridge, is critical to its function. It is primarily cleared by the kidneys, so caution is advised when combined with drugs that affect renal function. Metformin can also interact with other glucose-lowering agents, and taking it with food may reduce gastrointestinal side effects (Goel et al., 2022; Hsu et al., 2021).

Figure 5. Dual mechanisms by which metformin promotes anti-aging effects. In the left panel, metformin influences protein homeostasis, extending longevity by suppressing protein synthesis and enhancing autophagy. Through activation of AMPK, metformin inhibits mTOR, reducing the translation of aging-related proteins like progerin by decreasing phosphorylation of ribosomal protein S6 (rsP6), S6 kinase (S6K), and eIF4E-binding protein 1 (eIF4E-BP1). This inhibition also triggers autophagy, initiated by ULK1 dephosphorylation and subsequent phosphorylation of Beclin-1.

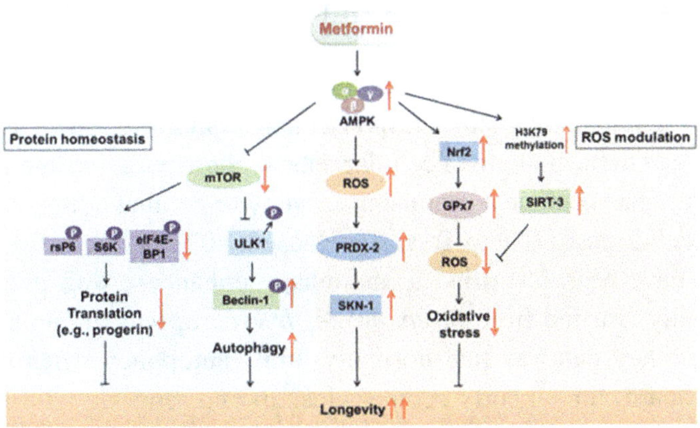

In the right panel, metformin modulates reactive oxygen species (ROS) levels, impacting the aging process through AMPK. ROS act as both promoters and regulators of aging; metformin's AMPK activation enhances ROS-related longevity via the PRDX-2/SKN-1 pathway. Concurrently, AMPK reduces ROS accumulation, extending lifespan by activating the Nrf2/GPx7 axis through SIRT-3. Together, these pathways underscore metformin's potential as an anti-aging agent by maintaining protein balance and regulating oxidative stress.

Spermidine, a polyamine, induces autophagy by inhibiting EP300, aiding cellular maintenance through protein and organelle recycling. Its polyamine structure allows effective cellular uptake, with modifications impacting autophagy. While spermidine has few drug interactions, caution is needed alongside polyamine metabolism inhibitors (Ni & Liu, 2021).

Berberine, an isoquinoline alkaloid, activates AMPK, improving glucose metabolism and insulin sensitivity. Its isoquinoline structure is critical for AMPK activation, though modifications can affect potency. Berberine may interact with drugs metabolized by CYP2D6 and CYP3A4 and is often taken with food to enhance bioavailability (Tian et al., 2023).

Figure 6. Structures

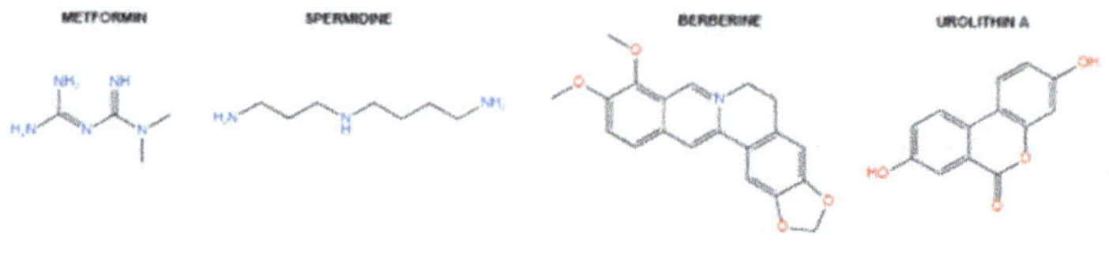

In summary, CRMs offer an innovative approach to extend healthspan by targeting key cellular pathways involved in aging. However, each CRM's unique chemistry, pharmacology, and structure-activity relationships highlight potential interactions with other drugs and foods. Continued research is essential to understand their safety and efficacy in promoting healthy aging and metabolic health.

3.3 Autophagy Enhancers: Promoting Cellular Rejuvenation

Autophagy is an essential cellular process that degrades and recycles damaged proteins and organelles, preserving cellular health, aiding stress response, and supporting longevity. Declining autophagy efficiency with age can lead to the buildup of cellular debris, contributing to age-related diseases. Therefore, enhancing autophagy has become a promising strategy to combat aging, improve healthspan, and protect against age-related diseases (Nieto-Torres & Hansen, 2021).

Several compounds have been identified as autophagy enhancers with potential anti-aging benefits. Rapamycin, originally isolated from *Streptomyces hygroscopicus*, inhibits the mechanistic target of rapamycin (mTOR), a key pathway that normally limits autophagy when nutrients are abundant. By inhibiting mTOR, rapamycin supports cellular cleanup and renewal, with promising applications in anti-aging, neuroprotection, and cancer treatment. Metformin, a synthetic biguanide derived from *Galega officinalis*, activates AMP-activated protein kinase (AMPK), which indirectly inhibits mTOR and enhances autophagy, contributing to improved mitochondrial function and longevity (Wolff et al., 2020; Lamming, 2016; Bang et al., 2024).

Resveratrol, a polyphenol known for its antioxidant properties, also activates AMPK and SIRT1, supporting autophagy and cellular repair. Spermidine, a naturally occurring polyamine found in foods like aged cheese, soybeans, and whole grains, promotes autophagy by inhibiting EP300, a protein that suppresses this process, with potential cardiovascular and cognitive health benefits. Trehalose, a disaccharide present in mushrooms and certain invertebrates, enhances cellular protection by preventing protein aggregation and oxidative stress, independently of mTOR. Lastly, berberine, an isoquinoline alkaloid from Berberis species, activates AMPK and supports autophagy, with benefits in metabolic regulation and neuroprotection (Madeo et al., 2019).

Similarly, urolithin A, a metabolite produced by gut bacteria during the digestion of pomegranates, has been shown to stimulate mitophagy (the selective autophagy of damaged mitochondria). By promoting the removal of dysfunctional mitochondria, urolithin A has demonstrated potential to improve muscle function and delay the onset of age-related decline (Zhao et al., 2023).

Autophagy enhancers are particularly promising because they address one of the fundamental drivers of aging: the accumulation of cellular damage. By promoting cellular cleanup and renewal, these compounds have the potential to improve healthspan, reduce the risk of age-related diseases, and potentially extend lifespan (Park and Lee, 2022). Further studies are needed to fully understand their long-term impacts and efficacy in human populations.

3.4. Sirtuins and Key Activators

Sirtuins are a family of NAD+-dependent enzymes that play a pivotal role in cellular processes tied to aging, metabolism, and stress resilience. In humans, seven sirtuins (SIRT1 to SIRT7) are dispersed across various cellular compartments, exerting effects through deacetylation and ADP-ribosylation of target proteins. This impacts gene expression, DNA repair, mitochondrial function, and cellular metabolism, positioning sirtuins as valuable targets for research in anti-aging and metabolic health. Certain compounds, known as sirtuin activators, promote sirtuin activity, with resveratrol, NMN, NR, quercetin, pterostilbene, and fisetin being particularly notable (Podyacheva and Toropova, 2023).

Resveratrol, a compound found naturally in red wine, grapes, and berries, activates SIRT1, enhancing mitochondrial biogenesis and metabolic health. It is a stilbenoid with anti-inflammatory effects, and interactions with CYP3A4 can affect the metabolism of other drugs, especially in combination with grapefruit (Koushki et al., 2018). NMN and NR are NAD+ precursors found in foods like milk and edamame, which bolster sirtuin activity by replenishing cellular NAD+, aiding in DNA repair and energy metabolism. Quercetin, present in apples and onions, indirectly supports sirtuins by promoting NAD+ biosynthesis and reducing cellular senescence (Kane & Sinclair, 2018). Pterostilbene, a compound obtained from *Pterocarpus marsupium*, shares structural similarity with resveratrol, activating SIRT1 with greater bioavailability and supporting cognitive and metabolic health (Nagarajan et al., 2022). Lastly, fisetin, which is abundant in strawberries, functions as a senolytic agent, reducing the effects of cellular aging and improving cellular resilience (Huard et al., 2023).

3.5 mTOR Inhibitors

The mTOR pathway, essential for cellular growth and metabolism, is a prime target in cancer and immunosuppressive therapies. Inhibitors of mTOR fall into two primary categories: rapalogs, which are analogs of sirolimus (Rapamycin), and ATP-competitive inhibitors that target the mTOR kinase domain directly. Rapalogs such as sirolimus, everolimus (40-O-(2-hydroxyethyl)-rapamycin), and temsirolimus (42-(3-Hydroxy-2-(hydroxymethyl)-2-methylpropanoate)rapamycin) selectively inhibit the mTORC1 complex, while newer, investigational inhibitors like sapanisertib (INK128) and AZD8055 inhibit both mTORC1 and mTORC2, aiming for broader efficacy in cancer treatment (Xie et al., 2016).

Sirolimus, the earliest mTOR inhibitor, binds to FKBP-12 to inhibit mTORC1, suppressing T-cell activation and immune responses. Administered orally, it has variable bioavailability (approximately 14%) and is metabolized by CYP3A4, with a half-life of about 60 hours. Clinically, sirolimus is used as an immunosuppressant in organ transplantation, particularly in kidney transplants. Common side effects include hyperlipidemia, hypertension, and increased infection risk.

Everolimus is second-generation mTORC1 inhibitor that binds FKBP-12 similarly to sirolimus but offers better bioavailability (~30%) and a shorter half-life of 30 hours. It is approved for various cancers, including renal cell carcinoma, hormone receptor-positive breast cancer, and certain neuroendocrine tumors. Adverse effects often include stomatitis, pneumonitis, hyperglycemia, and anemia.

Administered intravenously, temsirolimus has enhanced antiproliferative effects, undergoing CYP3A4-mediated hepatic metabolism. Primarily used in advanced renal cell carcinoma, it has a half-life of 9–15 hours. Side effects include rash, mucositis, thrombocytopenia, and heightened infection risk (Palavra et al., 2017).

3.5.1. Experimental or Off-Label mTOR Inhibitors

Ridaforolimus (Rapamycin 42-(Dimethylphosphinate)): This mTORC1 inhibitor has shown promise in sarcoma and endometrial cancer studies, though it is not fully approved. With a shorter half-life than other rapalogs, it allows for flexible dosing regimens. Fatigue, diarrhea, and increased infection risk are common adverse effects (Wang, L. et al., 2024).

Sapanisertib (INK128): A dual inhibitor of mTORC1 and mTORC2, sapanisertib disrupts cell proliferation more comprehensively and is under investigation for cancers like breast, lung, and pancreatic. Preliminary studies report side effects such as nausea, fatigue, and rash (Subbiah et al., 2024).

AZD8055: This ATP-competitive inhibitor targets both mTORC1 and mTORC2 by occupying the ATP-binding site, a mechanism that inhibits all mTOR signaling pathways. It is being studied in early-phase trials for solid tumors, with initial reports noting gastrointestinal symptoms, fatigue, and elevated liver enzymes (Mao et al., 2022).

XL388: An ATP-competitive inhibitor in preclinical trials for solid tumors, XL388 inhibits both mTOR complexes, potentially enhancing anticancer effects. Side effects observed include gastrointestinal distress and hematological changes (Xiong et al., 2017).

Figure 7. Structures

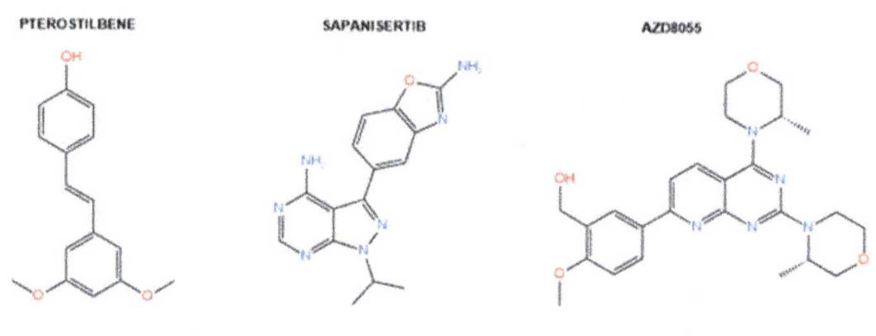

3.5.2. Mechanisms and Structure-Activity Relationships

Rapalogs: Structurally, rapalogs are based on a macrocyclic lactone derived from sirolimus, containing functional groups that interact with FKBP-12. Key structural elements include the macrolide ring, essential for binding, and specific modifications, such as the 2-hydroxyethyl group in everolimus, which improves bioavailability. For instance, temsirolimus includes a dihydroxylpropyl ester for better solubility, facilitating intravenous administration (Waldner et al., 2016).

ATP-Competitive Inhibitors: Compounds like sapanisertib and AZD8055 feature ATP-mimetic cores that enable direct binding to the ATP site in mTOR. This configuration allows dual inhibition of mTORC1 and mTORC2, with unique side chains improving specificity and potency. For example, AZD8055's pyrimidine core enhances selectivity for mTOR over other kinases, and sapanisertib includes substitutions that optimize dual mTOR inhibition (Ali et al., 2022).

3.5.3. Drug Interactions and Dietary Precautions

Most mTOR inhibitors undergo CYP3A4 metabolism, making them susceptible to interactions with CYP3A4-modulating agents. CYP3A4 inhibitors (e.g., ketoconazole, grapefruit juice) can increase toxicity risk, while inducers (e.g., rifampin) may reduce efficacy. Immunosuppressants like cyclosporine, often co-administered in transplants, increase immunosuppressive effects, necessitating close monitoring. Grapefruit should be avoided due to its impact on drug levels, as should high-fat meals with drugs like sirolimus, which can alter bioavailability. Alcohol and St. John's Wort also pose risks of compounded toxicity or reduced efficacy (Veerman et al., 2020).

In summary, while rapalogs offer selective inhibition of mTORC1, newer ATP-competitive inhibitors broaden mTOR pathway inhibition, offering potential advancements in cancer treatment. However, comprehensive dual inhibition may lead to increased toxicity, requiring cautious monitoring of drug interactions and side effects in clinical settings.

The field of anti-aging pharmacology has made significant strides in developing drugs that target key molecular mechanisms of aging. Senolytics offer the potential to clear out senescent cells and reduce inflammation, while CRMs mimic the effects of dietary interventions without the need for drastic lifestyle changes. Autophagy enhancers help rejuvenate cells by promoting the degradation and recycling of damaged components (Liu, 2022). Together, these pharmacological strategies represent exciting avenues for future research and clinical application in the quest to extend both lifespan and healthspan.

4. CLINICAL TRANSLATION AND CURRENT THERAPIES

While significant progress has been made in identifying potential anti-aging pharmacological interventions, translating these findings from preclinical models to humans remains one of the most challenging aspects of anti-aging research. Many compounds that exhibit promising effects in animal models of aging fail to replicate these outcomes in human trials, due to the complexity and variability of human biology (Folch et al., 2018). This section explores the key challenges in clinical translation and the current landscape of drugs and clinical trials aimed at combating aging and age-related diseases.

Figure 8. Illustrates the impact of resveratrol on lifespan extension across various vertebrate and invertebrate preclinical models.

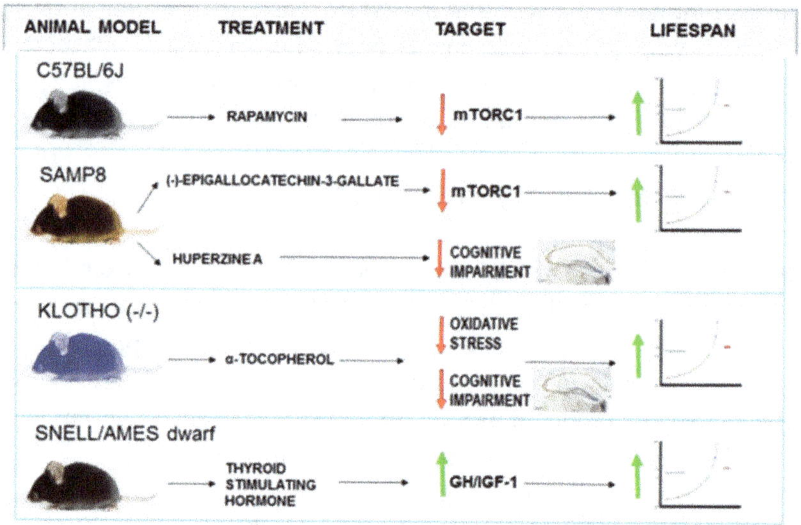

Resveratrol primarily exerts its anti-aging effects by activating SIRT1, a key regulator in cellular health and longevity. Through SIRT1 activation, resveratrol influences numerous cellular processes, such as DNA repair, metabolic regulation, and oxidative stress response, which collectively contribute to enhanced longevity. These findings support resveratrol's potential as an anti-aging compound and its broad applicability across different biological models.

4.1 Challenges in Translating Preclinical Success to Human Applications

One of the primary challenges in translating preclinical success to human applications lies in the complexity of the aging process. Aging is a multifactorial phenomenon that is influenced by genetic, molecular, environmental, and lifestyle factors. While animal models, such as mice and rats, have been instrumental in identifying potential anti-aging drugs, these models do not fully capture the intricacies of human aging (Tenchov et al., 2024). For example, humans experience a longer lifespan, a more complex immune system, and greater environmental variability compared to animal models. This makes it difficult to predict whether drugs that extend lifespan in animals will have the same effect in humans (Cohen, 2018).

Additionally, the genetic diversity among humans poses a challenge in developing anti-aging drugs that work effectively across different populations. Factors such as age, sex, ethnicity, and genetic predispositions can all influence the response to a given therapy, necessitating a more personalized approach to anti-aging pharmacology (Du et al., 2024).

Another major challenge in the clinical translation of anti-aging drugs is the lack of a clear regulatory framework for aging interventions. Aging itself is not classified as a disease, which complicates the regulatory approval process for drugs designed to target aging (Ameya et al., 2022). Without a disease classification, there are no clear endpoints or clinical metrics to evaluate the efficacy of anti-aging therapies in trials. As a result, researchers have turned to using age-related diseases, such as Alzheimer's disease, cardiovascular disease, and osteoarthritis, as surrogate markers for aging. This approach allows for the indirect targeting of aging by treating specific age-related conditions that share common underlying mechanisms with the aging process (Yu et al., 2023).

To address these challenges, regulatory bodies such as the U.S. Food and Drug Administration (FDA) are exploring new pathways to evaluate the safety and efficacy of anti-aging drugs. There is growing interest in redefining aging as a modifiable risk factor for chronic diseases, which would allow for more streamlined approval processes for interventions aimed at promoting healthy aging (Son et al., 2019; Snell et al., 2016).

4.2 Current Drugs and Clinical Trials

Despite the difficulties in translating anti-aging interventions to human applications, several drugs are currently being investigated in clinical trials for their potential to delay aging and improve healthspan. Some of these compounds target the hallmarks of aging, while others aim to mitigate age-related diseases as a proxy for extending lifespan (Zhang, Z. et al., 2024).

One of the most prominent drugs under investigation is metformin, a widely used medication for type 2 diabetes. Metformin has gained attention for its potential anti-aging effects, particularly its ability to activate the AMPK pathway, improve metabolic function, and reduce inflammation. Preclinical studies have shown that metformin can extend lifespan in model organisms such as mice and nematodes, and epidemiological studies suggest that diabetic patients taking metformin experience a reduced incidence of age-related diseases (Novelle et al., 2016; Kulkarni et al., 2020). The TAME (Targeting Aging with Metformin) trial, currently underway, is designed to assess whether metformin can extend healthspan and delay the onset of age-related diseases such as cancer, cardiovascular disease, and cognitive decline in non-diabetic adults. If successful, TAME could provide critical data supporting the use of metformin as an anti-aging therapy (Mohammed et al., 2021).

Another class of drugs that is showing promise in clinical trials are senolytics, which target and eliminate senescent cells. As mentioned in earlier sections, senescent cells accumulate with age and contribute to chronic inflammation, tissue dysfunction, and the progression of age-related diseases. Early-phase clinical trials of senolytic drugs such as dasatinib and quercetin are investigating their efficacy in treating chronic conditions linked to cellular senescence (Robbins et al., 2021). For instance, a combination of dasatinib and quercetin has been tested in patients with IPF, a progressive lung disease associated with aging and senescence. Results from these trials have shown reductions in senescent cell markers and improvements in physical function, suggesting that senolytic therapies may have broad applications in treating diseases associated with aging (Raffaele and Vinciguerra, 2022).

Other senolytic drugs are also being investigated for their potential to treat age-related conditions such as osteoarthritis and Alzheimer's disease, both of which are linked to the accumulation of senescent cells in tissues. As these trials progress, researchers hope to demonstrate that clearing senescent cells can not only alleviate specific disease symptoms but also promote overall healthspan and delay the onset of multiple age-related diseases (Lelarge et al., 2024).

In addition to metformin and senolytics, other drugs are being tested for their potential anti-aging effects. Rapamycin, an inhibitor of the mTOR pathway, has been shown to extend lifespan in animal models and is currently being evaluated for its ability to improve immune function in older adults. Rapamycin is particularly being studied for its potential to reduce immunosenescence (the gradual deterioration of the immune system with age), which could lower the risk of infections and age-related diseases (Barros et al., 2024).

Spermidine, a natural polyamine that induces autophagy, is another compound under investigation. It is currently being studied for its ability to improve cognitive function in older adults by enhancing cellular cleanup processes and reducing oxidative stress (Xu et al., 2020; Rivera et al., 2024).

As these trials advance, they represent crucial steps toward validating the potential of anti-aging drugs in humans. The results of these studies could pave the way for the development of new therapies aimed at not only extending lifespan but also improving the quality of life in older adults. However, the path to widespread clinical use will require continued research into safety, long-term efficacy, and the identification of appropriate biomarkers for aging (Guarente et al., 2024).

In summary, while there are substantial challenges in translating preclinical anti-aging findings to human therapies, significant progress is being made. Trials involving drugs like metformin, senolytics, and rapamycin are advancing our understanding of how to modulate the aging process and treat age-related diseases (Benhamú et al., 2022). These efforts could lead to the development of effective anti-aging therapies that promote healthy aging and extend healthspan in the future.

5. ETHICAL, REGULATORY, AND SAFETY CONSIDERATIONS

The development of anti-aging pharmacology is not without its ethical, regulatory, and safety challenges. As researchers and pharmaceutical companies push forward with promising interventions aimed at extending human lifespan and improving healthspan, it is critical to consider the broader societal, legal, and safety implications of these advances (Pereira et al., 2024). This section explores the key ethical dilemmas, regulatory hurdles, and safety concerns that must be addressed in the pursuit of anti-aging therapies.

Figure 9. Visually summarizes the primary ethical concerns associated with anti-aging research and highlights essential steps needed to responsibly advance the field.

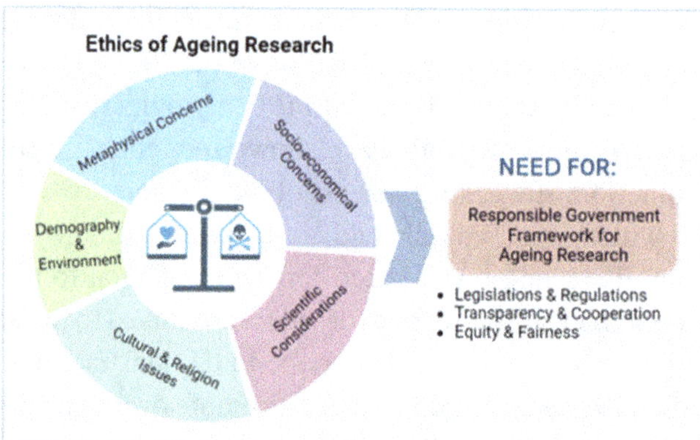

Key ethical issues include equitable access to longevity treatments, potential societal impacts of extended lifespans, and the moral implications of altering human aging processes. To address these concerns and support the responsible growth of longevity science, suggested actions include promoting transparent research practices, implementing regulatory frameworks, and fostering public dialogue around anti-aging interventions. These measures aim to balance scientific progress with societal and ethical considerations in the pursuit of extending healthy lifespans.

5.1 Ethical Dilemmas in Anti-aging Interventions

The potential to extend human lifespan through pharmacological means raises profound ethical questions that society must grapple with. One of the most prominent concerns is the potential exacerbation of existing social inequalities. Access to cutting-edge anti-aging treatments may be limited to individuals or populations with the financial means to afford them, creating a scenario where wealthy individuals could prolong their lives and maintain better health, while disadvantaged populations are left behind. This raises questions about fairness and equity in healthcare, as life-extending treatments could widen the gap between different socioeconomic groups (Pijnenburg & Leget, 2007; Barnett and Helphrey, 2021).

Moreover, the societal implications of significantly extending human lifespan extend beyond issues of access. Prolonging life for decades or more could lead to overpopulation, straining already limited natural resources, social services, and healthcare systems. If anti-aging interventions are successful, society will need to address the impact on global demographics, such as increased pressure on employment, retirement, and healthcare infrastructures. Without careful planning, an extended lifespan could lead to unintended consequences for resource allocation and environmental sustainability (Brown, 2015; Shayan et al., 2022).

Another key ethical dilemma revolves around the fundamental nature of aging. Should aging be viewed as a disease that requires medical intervention, or is it a natural, inevitable part of the human condition that should be accepted? The concept of treating aging as a medical condition challenges long-held societal norms about life and death. If aging becomes a treatable condition, how will this reshape attitudes toward mortality, the life cycle, and intergenerational relationships? These philosophical questions add complexity to the scientific pursuit of anti-aging pharmacology, as society must decide whether it is ethical to intervene in a process that has, until now, been viewed as a natural part of life (Rattan, 2014; Rattan, 2018; Gebremariam and Sadana, 2019).

5.2 Regulatory Landscape and Drug Approval Challenges

The regulatory environment for anti-aging therapies presents another significant barrier to their development and approval. Currently, regulatory agencies such as the FDA do not classify aging as a disease. As a result, anti-aging drugs cannot be approved directly for the treatment of aging. Instead, these therapies must target specific age-related diseases or conditions, such as cardiovascular disease, Alzheimer's disease, or osteoporosis. This regulatory stance complicates the drug development process, as researchers must focus on disease-specific endpoints rather than more generalized markers of aging (Reisman, 2004; Zhavoronkov et al., 2019).

However, there is growing recognition within the scientific and regulatory communities that aging-related biomarkers could serve as viable targets for drug development. For example, researchers are increasingly identifying biomarkers, such as epigenetic clocks and telomere length, which may indicate biological aging. If validated, these biomarkers could serve as surrogate endpoints for clinical trials, enabling the approval of therapies that target the aging process itself. The FDA and other regulatory bodies are beginning to explore ways to accommodate these developments, but significant changes in the regulatory framework will be needed to facilitate the approval of true anti-aging interventions (Moqri et al., 2024).

Another major regulatory challenge is determining the appropriate patient population for clinical trials. Should anti-aging drugs be tested in healthy older adults, or only in individuals with specific age-related diseases? This question has implications for trial design, safety monitoring, and ethical considerations, as testing drugs in healthy individuals presents different risks and benefits than testing them in people who are already ill (Shenoy & Harugeri, 2015; Rolland et al., 2023).

5.3 Safety Concerns in Long-Term Use

Safety is one of the most critical concerns when it comes to anti-aging drugs, especially given that these therapies may need to be administered for long periods—potentially decades. Unlike drugs used to treat acute conditions, anti-aging interventions may require chronic administration to maintain their effects on lifespan and healthspan. As a result, the long-term safety profiles of these drugs must be rigorously evaluated to ensure that they do not cause harm over time (Nadeeshani et al., 2022).

One of the primary safety concerns is the potential for anti-aging drugs to increase the risk of cancer. Many anti-aging pathways, such as those involved in cellular growth and metabolism (e.g., the mTOR pathway), are also implicated in cancer development. Inhibiting mTOR, for instance, has been shown to extend lifespan in animal models, but chronic inhibition of this pathway could have unintended consequences, such as impairing normal cellular growth or promoting tumorigenesis. Balancing the benefits of lifespan extension with the risks of increasing cancer susceptibility will be a key challenge in the development of anti-aging therapies (Marafie et al., 2024; Lee et al., 2024; Mannick and Lamming, 2023).

Another concern is the potential for off-target effects or interactions with other medications. As many older adults take multiple medications for various chronic conditions, introducing anti-aging drugs into this mix could lead to drug-drug interactions that negatively impact health. This is particularly concerning in the case of polypharmacy, where older adults are at higher risk for adverse effects due to the concurrent use of multiple drugs (Zhou et al., 2023; Kurczewska-Michalak et al., 2021; Fialová et al., 2018).

In addition, the potential for immune system dysregulation must be considered. Drugs that modulate cellular pathways involved in aging, such as senolytics or mTOR inhibitors, could inadvertently suppress or overstimulate the immune system. This could lead to increased susceptibility to infections or other immune-related disorders. Careful monitoring of immune function will be essential during clinical trials and long-term use of these therapies (Du et al., 2023; Aiello et al., 2019).

Finally, the ethical dilemma of safety in otherwise healthy individuals must be addressed. If anti-aging drugs are administered to healthy older adults to prevent aging-related decline, there is a high ethical obligation to ensure that these drugs do not cause harm. Since these individuals may not be suffering from a disease at the time of treatment, the risk-benefit analysis becomes more complex, with safety concerns taking on even greater importance (Woo et al., 2019).

In summary, while the pursuit of anti-aging pharmacology holds great promise for extending human lifespan and improving healthspan, it also raises significant ethical, regulatory, and safety considerations. From the ethical challenges of ensuring equitable access and addressing the societal implications of longer lifespans, to the regulatory hurdles of developing drugs that target aging itself, and the safety concerns associated with long-term drug use, these issues must be carefully navigated as the field progresses. Addressing these challenges will be essential to ensuring that anti-aging therapies are developed responsibly, safely, and ethically, with the potential to benefit society as a whole (Penella, 2024).

6. FUTURE DIRECTIONS IN ANTI-AGING PHARMACOLOGY

The future of anti-aging pharmacology is filled with promising innovations and cutting-edge research that may significantly reshape how aging is understood and managed. With advances in biotechnology, molecular biology, and pharmacology, new therapies are emerging that aim to extend both lifespan and healthspan (Li,Y et al., 2024). This section explores two key areas of development: emerging therapies that target the biological underpinnings of aging and the potential for personalized anti-aging medicine, which could revolutionize how treatments are tailored to individuals.

6.1 Emerging Therapies and Innovations

The rapid advancement of gene-editing technologies, particularly CRISPR-Cas9, holds transformative potential in anti-aging pharmacology. CRISPR enables precise modifications of specific genes involved in aging, offering the ability to directly intervene in genetic processes that regulate longevity (Zhu, 2022). For instance, genes related to DNA repair mechanisms, telomere maintenance, and mitochondrial function are critical targets for anti-aging interventions. By editing these genes, researchers may be able to slow or even reverse age-related cellular damage, promoting healthier aging at the molecular level (Schumacher et al., 2021).

In addition to gene editing, epigenetic reprogramming is another exciting area of innovation. Epigenetic changes, which alter gene expression without modifying the DNA sequence, are closely linked to aging. By reversing age-related epigenetic marks, scientists could potentially rejuvenate cells and tissues. Experimental work in this field, such as the partial reprogramming of cells to a more youthful state, has already shown promise in preclinical models (Ji et al., 2023).

The field of stem cell therapies also offers significant potential for addressing the physiological decline associated with aging. Stem cells possess the unique ability to differentiate into various cell types, allowing them to regenerate damaged or aged tissues (Zakrzewski et al., 2019). Researchers are investigating the use of stem cells to replace lost or dysfunctional cells in organs like the heart, brain, and muscles, which are particularly susceptible to age-related deterioration. In theory, stem cell-based treatments could restore tissue function, enhance organ performance, and improve overall vitality in aging individuals. While still in the early stages of clinical development, advances in stem cell therapy could pave the way for regenerative treatments that effectively combat the symptoms of aging (Hoang et al., 2022).

Another emerging area of interest is the development of mitochondrial-targeted therapies. Since mitochondrial dysfunction is a hallmark of aging, enhancing mitochondrial health and function is a key strategy for delaying aging-related decline. Compounds such as mitochondrial-derived peptides and mitochondrial-targeting antioxidants are being explored for their potential to protect against age-related oxidative stress and metabolic dysfunction. These therapies aim to improve energy production and reduce the cellular damage that accumulates with age (Madreiter-Sokolowski et al., 2024).

Extracellular vesicles (EVs), which are small particles released by cells that carry proteins, lipids, and genetic material, are also gaining attention in the field of anti-aging. EVs can influence tissue regeneration and immune responses, making them a potential tool for promoting tissue repair and modulating age-related inflammatory processes. Research on EVs is still in its infancy, but their ability to deliver bioactive molecules to specific tissues may open new doors for anti-aging interventions (Wang, J. et al., 2024; Mas-Bargues & Alique, 2023; Rao et al., 2024).

6.2 Prospects for Personalized Anti-aging Medicine

As the understanding of aging biology grows more sophisticated, the concept of personalized anti-aging medicine is becoming increasingly feasible. Aging is influenced by a complex interplay of genetic, epigenetic, and environmental factors, and it is likely that individuals age at different rates due to their unique biological makeup. Personalized anti-aging medicine seeks to tailor interventions to each person's specific genetic and molecular profile, optimizing the efficacy of treatments while minimizing the risks (Asejeje and Ogunro, 2024).

The field of genomics plays a central role in personalized medicine. By sequencing an individual's genome, researchers can identify genetic variants that influence the aging process. These variants could determine how well a person responds to certain anti-aging therapies, such as senolytics, CRMs, or autophagy enhancers (Brittain et al., 2017). For example, individuals with particular genetic mutations may benefit more from interventions that target specific molecular pathways, such as mTOR inhibition or sirtuin activation (Lambona et al., 2024).

Biomarker-based diagnostics will be critical to enabling personalized anti-aging strategies. Biomarkers such as epigenetic clocks, telomere length, and levels of inflammatory cytokines can provide insights into an individual's biological age—how their body is aging compared to their chronological age. These biomarkers can serve as early indicators of aging-related decline, allowing for the timely initiation of preventative or therapeutic interventions. Moreover, biomarker monitoring can guide the adjustment of treatment regimens to ensure optimal outcomes over time (Tao et al., 2024; Polidori, 2024).

The integration of multi-omics approaches, including genomics, proteomics, metabolomics, and transcriptomics, further enhances the potential for personalized medicine. By analyzing the molecular profiles generated by these technologies, clinicians can obtain a comprehensive picture of an individual's biological state (Babu & Snyder, 2023). This information can be used to design targeted interventions that address the specific mechanisms driving that person's aging process. For instance, an individual with evidence of mitochondrial dysfunction may benefit from therapies that enhance mitochondrial health, while someone with epigenetic alterations may respond better to epigenetic reprogramming techniques (Zhang, C. et al., 2024).

6.3 Artificial Intelligence and Machine Learning

Artificial intelligence (AI) and machine learning (ML) are poised to play transformative roles in personalized anti-aging medicine by analyzing vast clinical, genomic, and patient data to guide treatment decisions. Through pattern recognition, AI-driven tools enable clinicians to tailor anti-aging therapies to individual patients, enhancing precision in care (Barreto et al., 2023; Li, Y.H. et al., 2024).

AI, particularly ML, deep learning, and natural language processing, is advancing drug discovery for aging-related treatments, including autophagy enhancers, sirtuin activators, CRMs, and senolytics. By processing extensive genomic, proteomic, and metabolomic datasets, AI algorithms reveal aging-related drug targets and pathways, such as those involving sirtuins and autophagy modulators, thereby aiding in the identification of potential therapies (Serrano et al., 2024).

AI techniques, such as molecular modeling, quantitative structure-activity relationship (QSAR) modeling, and generative AI (e.g., generative adversarial networks and variational autoencoders), facilitate the design of novel drug compounds with optimized efficacy and safety profiles. Generative models, for example, propose new molecules that mimic known autophagy or sirtuin activators with enhanced bioavailability, while QSAR models design CRMs that emulate the effects of calorie restriction (Samvedna Singh et al., 2024). Additionally, high-throughput virtual screening, powered by convolutional and recurrent neural networks, allows for the rapid identification of compounds that interact with aging-associated proteins, expediting drug discovery (Qureshi et al., 2023).

AI-driven drug repurposing also accelerates the identification of existing drugs with potential anti-aging benefits. For instance, AI has revealed metformin and rapamycin as autophagy enhancers with applications in anti-aging. AI algorithms further predict pharmacokinetic properties and potential toxicity, supporting the development of safe, bioavailable compounds with fewer off-target effects (Cortial et al., 2024).

In clinical applications, AI facilitates patient stratification by identifying biomarkers that predict treatment responses, thereby enhancing the specificity of senolytic therapies, which target senescent cells without affecting healthy ones. Additionally, AI optimizes clinical trial design through predictive modeling, real-time monitoring, and adaptive trial structures, increasing trial efficiency, reducing costs, and enabling more inclusive studies across diverse populations (Xiaoran et al., 2024).

In summary, AI accelerates the development and testing of anti-aging therapies, including autophagy enhancers, sirtuin activators, CRMs, and senolytics, from target discovery through clinical trials. This technological integration offers promising avenues to support healthy aging, metabolic health, and lifespan extension (Dönertaş et al., 2019).

The future of anti-aging pharmacology is not just about extending lifespan but improving the quality of life in later years. Personalized medicine holds the promise of delivering more targeted, individualized care, potentially allowing people to age healthily and maintain higher levels of physical and cognitive function. As research continues to unravel the molecular mechanisms behind aging and as diagnostic tools improve, personalized anti-aging interventions could become a key component of future healthcare, helping individuals live longer, healthier lives tailored to their unique biological makeup (Falshaw et al., 2024).

In conclusion, the future of anti-aging pharmacology is marked by exciting innovations in gene editing, stem cell therapies, mitochondrial-targeted treatments, and personalized medicine. As these areas advance, they hold the potential to not only extend lifespan but to improve healthspan—ensuring that individuals can enjoy better health and quality of life as they age. With ongoing research and clinical trials, the dream of meaningful anti-aging interventions may soon become a reality.

7. CONCLUSION

The field of anti-aging pharmacology has experienced remarkable growth over the past several years, fueled by groundbreaking discoveries in the molecular mechanisms that govern aging and the development of innovative pharmacological interventions. As our understanding of the biological underpinnings of aging has deepened, it has become increasingly clear that the aging process is not an inevitable, uncontrollable decline, but rather one that can be influenced—perhaps even reversed—by targeting specific molecular pathways. With advances in senolytics, CRMs, autophagy enhancers, and other emerging therapies, the potential to significantly extend human healthspan—the period of life free from disease and disability—is rapidly becoming a tangible reality.

This chapter has explored the key molecular pathways involved in aging, including mTOR, sirtuins, and AMPK, and discussed the pharmacological interventions aimed at modulating these pathways. Each of these interventions offers unique opportunities for delaying the onset of age-related diseases and promoting longevity. Senolytics have shown promise in eliminating harmful senescent cells, CRMs offer a feasible alternative to the impracticality of long-term CR, and autophagy enhancers are emerging as a powerful means to maintain cellular homeostasis and promote cellular rejuvenation.

However, despite these advances, translating preclinical success into human therapies remains a formidable challenge. The complexity of human aging, combined with the genetic diversity and environmental influences that vary between individuals, makes it difficult to develop universally effective treatments. The fact that aging itself is not classified as a disease further complicates the regulatory landscape, posing significant hurdles for drug approval. This chapter has also highlighted the ethical dilemmas surrounding anti-aging interventions, particularly in terms of equitable access, the potential societal consequences of extended lifespans, and how we define aging and longevity as a medical condition.

In addition to these obstacles, long-term safety is a major concern, as anti-aging drugs may need to be administered over extended periods. Thorough and ongoing safety evaluations are essential to ensure that these therapies do not introduce unintended consequences, such as increased cancer risk or other serious side effects. As researchers push forward, they must balance the desire to extend lifespan with the need to ensure the interventions are both safe and effective for widespread use.

Looking to the future, the promise of emerging therapies such as gene editing, stem cell treatments, and mitochondrial-targeted interventions suggests that the boundaries of anti-aging pharmacology will continue to expand. The integration of personalized medicine offers the potential for even greater precision, allowing for tailored interventions based on individual genetic, epigenetic, and molecular profiles. This approach could maximize the efficacy of anti-aging treatments, enabling clinicians to offer more effective and personalized solutions for age-related decline.

Ultimately, the future of anti-aging pharmacology is bright. As new technologies emerge and our understanding of the molecular and genetic basis of aging deepens, the field will continue to evolve, offering new avenues for extending both lifespan and healthspan. With sustained research efforts, ethical and regulatory considerations, and a commitment to ensuring safety, anti-aging pharmacology holds the potential to revolutionize how we approach aging, enabling people to live longer, healthier lives.

In conclusion, anti-aging pharmacology stands at the cusp of a transformative era, where the extension of human healthspan is within sight. As we continue to uncover the intricate details of aging and develop therapies to combat its effects, the possibility of a future where age-related diseases are delayed or prevented, and individuals enjoy extended periods of vitality, becomes ever more realistic. While challenges remain, the continued exploration and innovation in this field promise to reshape our understanding of aging and longevity, making healthy aging a primary goal for future healthcare interventions.

REFERENCES

Aiello, A., Farzaneh, F., Candore, G., Caruso, C., Davinelli, S., Gambino, C. M., Ligotti, M. E., Zareian, N., & Accardi, G. (2019). Immunosenescence and its hallmarks: How to oppose aging strategically? A review of potential options for therapeutic intervention. *Frontiers in Immunology, 10*, 2247. DOI: 10.3389/fimmu.2019.02247 PMID: 31608061

Alegre, G. F. S., & Pastore, G. M. (2023). NAD+ precursors nicotinamide mononucleotide (NMN) and nicotinamide riboside (NR): Potential dietary contribution to health. *Current Nutrition Reports, 12*(3), 445–464. DOI: 10.1007/s13668-023-00475-y PMID: 37273100

Ali, E. S., Mitra, K., Akter, S., Ramproshad, S., Mondal, B., Khan, I. N., Islam, M. T., Sharifi-Rad, J., Calina, D., & Cho, W. C. (2022). Recent advances and limitations of mTOR inhibitors in the treatment of cancer. *Cancer Cell International, 22*(1), 284. DOI: 10.1186/s12935-022-02706-8 PMID: 36109789

Aliper, A., Jellen, L., Cortese, F., Artemov, A., Karpinsky-Semper, D., Moskalev, A., Swick, A. G., & Zhavoronkov, A. (2017). Towards natural mimetics of metformin and rapamycin. *Aging (Albany NY), 9*(11), 2245–2268. DOI: 10.18632/aging.101319 PMID: 29165314

Almendáriz-Palacios, C., Mousseau, D. D., Eskiw, C. H., & Gillespie, Z. E. (2020). Still living better through chemistry: An update on caloric restriction and caloric restriction mimetics as tools to promote health and lifespan. *International Journal of Molecular Sciences, 21*(23), 9220. DOI: 10.3390/ijms21239220 PMID: 33287232

Ameya, S. K., Aleksic, S., Berger, D. M., Sierra, F., Kuchel, G. A., & Barzilai, N. (2022). Geroscience-guided repurposing of FDA-approved drugs to target aging: A proposed process and prioritization. *Aging Cell, 21*(4), e13596. DOI: 10.1111/acel.13596 PMID: 35343051

Anuar, N. N. M., Nor Hisam, N. S., Liew, S. L., & Ugusman, A. (2020). Clinical review: Navitoclax as a pro-apoptotic and anti-fibrotic agent. *Frontiers in Pharmacology, 11*, 564108. DOI: 10.3389/fphar.2020.564108 PMID: 33381025

Asejeje, F. O., & Ogunro, O. B. (2024). Deciphering the mechanisms, biochemistry, physiology, and social habits in the process of aging. *Archives of Gerontology and Geriatrics Plus, 1*(1), 100003. DOI: 10.1016/j.aggp.2023.100003

Babu, M., & Snyder, M. (2023). Multi-Omics profiling for health. *Molecular & Cellular Proteomics, 22*(6), 100561. DOI: 10.1016/j.mcpro.2023.100561 PMID: 37119971

Bang, S., Kim, D.-E., Kang, H.-T., & Lee, J. H. (2024). Metformin restores autophagic flux and mitochondrial function in late passage myoblast to impede age-related muscle loss. *Biomedicine and Pharmacotherapy, 164*, 116981. DOI: 10.1016/j.biopha.2024.116981 PMID: 39533541

Barnett, M. D., & Helphrey, J. H. (2021). Who wants to live forever? Age cohort differences in attitudes toward life extension. *Journal of Aging Studies, 57*, 100931. DOI: 10.1016/j.jaging.2021.100931 PMID: 34083000

Barreto, V. S., Quintanilla, A., Elliott, R., Dawson, J. C., Sun, J., Campa, V. M., & Lorente-Macias, A. (2023, June 10). UncitiBroceta, A., Carragher, N. O., Acosta, J. C., & Oyarzún, D. A. (2023). Discovery of senolytics using machine learning. *Nature Communications*, *14*(1), 3445. Advance online publication. DOI: 10.1038/s41467-023-39120-1

Barros, R. S., Queiroz, L. A. D., Assis, J. B., Pantoja, K. C., Bustia, S. X., Sousa, E. S. A., Rodrigues, S. F., Akamine, E. H., Sá-Nunes, A., & Martins, J. O. (2024). Effects of low-dose rapamycin on lymphoid organs of mice prone and resistant to accelerated senescence. *Frontiers in Immunology*, *15*, 1310505. DOI: 10.3389/fimmu.2024.1310505 PMID: 38515742

Benhamú, B., Martín-Fontecha, M., Vázquez-Villa, H., López-Rodríguez, M. L., & Ortega-Gutiérrez, S. (2022). New trends in aging drug discovery. *Biomedicines*, *10*(8), 2006. DOI: 10.3390/biomedicines10082006 PMID: 36009552

Brittain, H. K., Scott, R., & Thomas, E. (2017). The rise of the genome and personalised medicine. *Clinical Medicine*, *17*(6), 545–551. DOI: 10.7861/clinmedicine.17-6-545 PMID: 29196356

Brown, G. C. (2015). Living too long: The current focus of medical research on increasing the quantity, rather than the quality, of life is damaging our health and harming the economy. *EMBO Reports*, *16*(2), 137–141. DOI: 10.15252/embr.201439518 PMID: 25525070

Chang, N., Li, J., Lin, S., Zhang, J., Zeng, W., Ma, G., & Wang, Y. (2024). Emerging roles of SIRT1 activator, SRT2104, in disease treatment. *Scientific Reports*, *14*(1), 5521. DOI: 10.1038/s41598-024-55923-8 PMID: 38448466

Cohen, A. A. (2018). Aging across the tree of life: The importance of a comparative perspective for the use of animal models in aging. Biochimica et Biophysica Acta (BBA) -. *Biochimica et Biophysica Acta. Molecular Basis of Disease*, *1864*(9, 9, Part A), 2680–2689. DOI: 10.1016/j.bbadis.2017.05.028 PMID: 28690188

Cortial, L., Montero, V., Tourlet, S., Del Bano, J., & Blin, O. (2024). Artificial intelligence in drug repurposing for rare diseases: A mini-review. *Frontiers in Medicine*, *11*, 1404338. DOI: 10.3389/fmed.2024.1404338 PMID: 38841574

da Costa, J. P., Vitorino, R., Silva, G. M., Vogel, C., Duarte, A. C., & Rocha-Santos, T. (2016). A synopsis on aging—Theories, mechanisms and future prospects. *Ageing Research Reviews*, *29*, 90–112. DOI: 10.1016/j.arr.2016.06.005 PMID: 27353257

Domaszewska-Szostek, A., Puzianowska-Kuźnicka, M., & Kuryłowicz, A. (2021). Flavonoids in skin senescence prevention and treatment. *International Journal of Molecular Sciences*, *22*(18), 6814. DOI: 10.3390/ijms22136814 PMID: 34201952

Dönertaş, H. M., Fuentealba, M., Partridge, L., & Thornton, J. M. (2019). Identifying potential aging-modulating drugs in silico. *Trends in Endocrinology and Metabolism*, *30*(2), 118–131. DOI: 10.1016/j.tem.2018.11.005 PMID: 30581056

Dorling, J. L., Martin, C. K., & Redman, L. M. (2020). Calorie restriction for enhanced longevity: The role of novel dietary strategies in the present obesogenic environment. *Ageing Research Reviews*, *64*, 101038. DOI: 10.1016/j.arr.2020.101038 PMID: 32109603

Du, N., Yang, R., Jiang, S., Niu, Z., Zhou, W., Liu, C., Gao, L., & Sun, Q. (2024). Anti-aging drugs and the related signal pathways. *Biomedicines*, *12*(1), 127. DOI: 10.3390/biomedicines12010127 PMID: 38255232

Du, P. Y., Gandhi, A., Bawa, M., & Gromala, J. (2023). The ageing immune system as a potential target of senolytics. *Oxford Open Immunology*, *4*(1), iqad004. Advance online publication. DOI: 10.1093/oxfimm/iqad004 PMID: 37255929

Falshaw, N., Sagner, M., & Siow, R. C. (2024). The Longevity Med Summit: Insights on healthspan from cell to society. *Frontiers in Aging*, *5*, 1417455. DOI: 10.3389/fragi.2024.1417455 PMID: 39081393

Fialová, D., Kummer, I., Držaić, M., & Leppee, M. (2018). Ageism in medication use in older patients. In Ayalon, L., & Tesch-Römer, C. (Eds.), *Contemporary perspectives on ageism* (pp. 187–198). Springer., DOI: 10.1007/978-3-319-73820-8_14

Folch, J., Busquets, O., Ettcheto, M., Sánchez-López, E., Pallàs, M., Beas-Zarate, C., Marin, M., Casadesus, G., Olloquequi, J., Auladell, C., & Camins, A. (2018). Experimental models for aging and their potential for novel drug discovery. *Current Neuropharmacology*, *16*(10), 1466–1483. DOI: 10.2174/1570159X15666170707155345 PMID: 28685671

Gebremariam, K. M., & Sadana, R. (2019). On the ethics of healthy ageing: Setting impermissible trade-offs relating to the health and well-being of older adults on the path to universal health coverage. *International Journal for Equity in Health*, *18*(1), 140. DOI: 10.1186/s12939-019-0997-z PMID: 31488220

Goel, S., Singh, R., Singh, V., Singh, H., Kumari, P., Chopra, H., Sharma, R., Nepovimova, E., Valis, M., Kuca, K., & Emran, T. B. (2022). Metformin: Activation of 5′ AMP-activated protein kinase and its emerging potential beyond anti-hyperglycemic action. *Frontiers in Genetics*, *13*, 1022739. DOI: 10.3389/fgene.2022.1022739 PMID: 36386794

Guarente, L., Sinclair, D. A., & Kroemer, G. (2024). Human trials exploring anti-aging medicines. *Cell Metabolism*, *36*(2), 354–376. DOI: 10.1016/j.cmet.2023.12.007 PMID: 38181790

Guo, J., Huang, X., Dou, L., Yan, M., Shen, T., Tang, W., & Li, J. (2022). Aging and aging-related diseases: From molecular mechanisms to interventions and treatments. *Signal Transduction and Targeted Therapy*, *7*(1), 391. DOI: 10.1038/s41392-022-01251-0 PMID: 36522308

Hoang, D. M., Pham, P. T., Bach, T. Q., Ngo, A. T. L., Nguyen, Q. T., Phan, T. T. K., Nguyen, G. H., Le, P. T. T., Hoang, V. T., Forsyth, N. R., Heke, M., & Nguyen, L. T. (2022). Stem cell-based therapy for human diseases. *Signal Transduction and Targeted Therapy*, *7*(1), 272. DOI: 10.1038/s41392-022-01134-4 PMID: 35933430

Hsu, S. K., Cheng, K. C., Mgbeahuruike, M. O., Lin, Y. H., Wu, C. Y., Wang, H. D., Yen, C. H., Chiu, C. C., & Sheu, S. J. (2021). New insight into the effects of metformin on diabetic retinopathy, aging and cancer: Nonapoptotic cell death, immunosuppression, and effects beyond the AMPK pathway. *International Journal of Molecular Sciences*, *22*(17), 9453. DOI: 10.3390/ijms22179453 PMID: 34502359

Huard, C. A., Gao, X., Dey Hazra, M. E., Dey Hazra, R. O., Lebsock, K., Easley, J. T., Millett, P. J., & Huard, J. (2023). Effects of fisetin treatment on cellular senescence of various tissues and organs of old sheep. *Antioxidants*, *12*(8), 1646. DOI: 10.3390/antiox12081646 PMID: 37627641

Ineichen, B. V., Furrer, E., Grüninger, S. L., Zürrer, W. E., & Macleod, M. R. (2024). Analysis of animal-to-human translation shows that only 5% of animal-tested therapeutic interventions obtain regulatory approval for human applications. *PLoS Biology*, *22*(6), e3002667. DOI: 10.1371/journal.pbio.3002667 PMID: 38870090

Islam, M. T., Tuday, E., Allen, S., Kim, J., Trott, D. W., Holland, W. L., Donato, A. J., & Lesniewski, L. A. (2023). Senolytic drugs, dasatinib and quercetin, attenuate adipose tissue inflammation and ameliorate metabolic function in old age. *Aging Cell*, *22*(2), e13767. DOI: 10.1111/acel.13767 PMID: 36637079

Ji, S., Xiong, M., Chen, H., Liu, Y., Zhou, L., Hong, Y., Wang, M., Wang, C., Fu, X., & Sun, X. (2023). Cellular rejuvenation: Molecular mechanisms and potential therapeutic interventions for diseases. *Signal Transduction and Targeted Therapy*, *8*(1), 116. DOI: 10.1038/s41392-023-01343-5 PMID: 36918530

Kane, A. E., & Sinclair, D. A. (2018). Sirtuins and NAD+ in the development and treatment of metabolic and cardiovascular diseases. *Circulation Research*, *123*(7), 868–885. DOI: 10.1161/CIRCRESAHA.118.312498 PMID: 30355082

Kirkland, J. L., & Tchkonia, T. (2020). Senolytic drugs: From discovery to translation. *Journal of Internal Medicine*, *288*(5), 518–536. DOI: 10.1111/joim.13141 PMID: 32686219

Koushki, M., Amiri-Dashatan, N., Ahmadi, N., Abbaszadeh, H. A., & Rezaei-Tavirani, M. (2018). Resveratrol: A miraculous natural compound for diseases treatment. *Food Science & Nutrition*, *6*(8), 2473–2490. DOI: 10.1002/fsn3.855 PMID: 30510749

Krishnakumar, I. M., Jaja-Chimedza, A., Joseph, A., Balakrishnan, A., Maliakel, B., & Swick, A. (2022). Enhanced bioavailability and pharmacokinetics of a novel hybrid-hydrogel formulation of fisetin orally administered in healthy individuals: A randomised double-blinded comparative crossover study. *Journal of Nutritional Science*, *11*, e74. DOI: 10.1017/jns.2022.72 PMID: 36304817

Kulkarni, A. S., Gubbi, S., & Barzilai, N. (2020). Benefits of metformin in attenuating the hallmarks of aging. *Cell Metabolism*, *32*(1), 15–30. DOI: 10.1016/j.cmet.2020.04.001 PMID: 32333835

Kurczewska-Michalak, M., Lewek, P., Jankowska-Polańska, B., Giardini, A., Granata, N., Maffoni, M., Costa, E., Midão, L., & Kardas, P. (2021). Polypharmacy management in older adults: A scoping review of available interventions. *Frontiers in Pharmacology*, *12*, 734045. DOI: 10.3389/fphar.2021.734045 PMID: 34899294

Lambona, C., Zwergel, C., Valente, S., & Mai, A. (2024). SIRT3 activation: A promise in drug development? New insights into SIRT3 biology and its implications on the drug discovery process. *Journal of Medicinal Chemistry*, *67*(3), 1662–1689. DOI: 10.1021/acs.jmedchem.3c01979 PMID: 38261767

Lamming, D. W. (2016). Inhibition of the mechanistic target of rapamycin (mTOR)-Rapamycin and beyond. *Cold Spring Harbor Perspectives in Medicine*, *6*(5), a025924. DOI: 10.1101/cshperspect.a025924 PMID: 27048303

Lee, D. J. W., Hodzic Kuerec, A., & Maier, A. B. (2024). Targeting ageing with rapamycin and its derivatives in humans: A systematic review. *The Lancet. Healthy Longevity*, *5*(2), e152–e162. DOI: 10.1016/S2666-7568(23)00258-1 PMID: 38310895

Lelarge, V., Capelle, R., Oger, F., Mathieu, T., & Le Calvé, B. (2024). Senolytics: From pharmacological inhibitors to immunotherapies, a promising future for patients' treatment. *NPJ Aging*, *10*(1), 12. DOI: 10.1038/s41514-024-00138-4 PMID: 38321020

Li, Y., Tian, X., Luo, J., Bao, T., Wang, S., & Wu, X. (2024). Molecular mechanisms of aging and anti-aging strategies. *Cell Communication and Signaling : CCS*, *22*(1), 285. DOI: 10.1186/s12964-024-01663-1 PMID: 38790068

Li, Y. H., Li, Y. L., Wei, M. Y., & Li, G.-Y. (2024). Innovation and challenges of artificial intelligence technology in personalized healthcare. *Scientific Reports*, *14*(1), 18994. DOI: 10.1038/s41598-024-70073-7 PMID: 39152194

Liu, J. K. (2022). Antiaging agents: Safe interventions to slow aging and healthy lifespan extension. *Natural Products and Bioprospecting*, *12*(1), 18. DOI: 10.1007/s13659-022-00339-y PMID: 35534591

López-Gil, L., Pascual-Ahuir, A., & Proft, M. (2023). Genomic instability and epigenetic changes during aging. *International Journal of Molecular Sciences*, *24*(18), 14279. DOI: 10.3390/ijms241814279 PMID: 37762580

López-Otín, C., Blasco, M. A., Partridge, L., Serrano, M., & Kroemer, G. (2023). Hallmarks of aging: An expanding universe. *Cell*, *186*(2), 243–278. DOI: 10.1016/j.cell.2022.11.001 PMID: 36599349

Lv, Z., & Guo, Y. (2020). Metformin and its benefits for various diseases. *Frontiers in Endocrinology*, *11*, 191. DOI: 10.3389/fendo.2020.00191 PMID: 32425881

Madeo, F., Bauer, M. A., Carmona-Gutierrez, D., & Kroemer, G. (2019). Spermidine: A physiological autophagy inducer acting as an anti-aging vitamin in humans? *Autophagy*, *15*(1), 165–168. DOI: 10.1080/15548627.2018.1530929 PMID: 30306826

Madreiter-Sokolowski, C. T., Hiden, U., Krstic, J., Panzitt, K., Wagner, M., Enzinger, C., Khalil, M., Abdellatif, M., Malle, E., Madl, T., Osto, E., Schosserer, M., Binder, C. J., & Olschewski, A. (2024). Targeting organ-specific mitochondrial dysfunction to improve biological aging. *Pharmacology & Therapeutics*, *262*, 108710. DOI: 10.1016/j.pharmthera.2024.108710 PMID: 39179117

Mannick, J. B., & Lamming, D. W. (2023). Targeting the biology of aging with mTOR inhibitors. *Nature Aging*, *3*(6), 642–660. DOI: 10.1038/s43587-023-00416-y PMID: 37142830

Mao, B., Zhang, Q., Ma, L., Zhao, D.-S., Zhao, P., & Yan, P. (2022). Overview of research into mTOR inhibitors. *Molecules (Basel, Switzerland)*, *27*(16), 5295. DOI: 10.3390/molecules27165295 PMID: 36014530

Marafie, S. K., Al-Mulla, F., & Abubaker, J. (2024). mTOR: Its critical role in metabolic diseases, cancer, and the aging process. *International Journal of Molecular Sciences*, *25*(11), 6141. DOI: 10.3390/ijms25116141 PMID: 38892329

Martel, J., Chang, S.-H., Wu, C.-Y., Peng, H.-H., Hwang, T.-L., Ko, Y.-F., Young, J. D., & Ojcius, D. M. (2021). Recent advances in the field of caloric restriction mimetics and anti-aging molecules. *Ageing Research Reviews*, *66*, 101240. DOI: 10.1016/j.arr.2020.101240 PMID: 33347992

Martens, C. R., Wahl, D., & LaRocca, T. J. (2023). Personalized medicine: Will it work for decreasing age-related morbidities? In Oliveira, P. J., & Malva, J. O. (Eds.), *Aging* (pp. 683–700). Academic Press., DOI: 10.1016/B978-0-12-823761-8.00013-6

Mas-Bargues, C., & Alique, M. (2023). Extracellular vesicles as "very important particles" (VIPs) in aging. *International Journal of Molecular Sciences*, *24*(4), 4250. DOI: 10.3390/ijms24044250 PMID: 36835661

Mohammed, I., Hollenberg, M. D., Ding, H., & Triggle, C. R. (2021). A critical review of the evidence that metformin is a putative anti-aging drug that enhances healthspan and extends lifespan. *Frontiers in Endocrinology*, *12*, 718942. DOI: 10.3389/fendo.2021.718942 PMID: 34421827

Moqri, M., Herzog, C., Poganik, J. R., Justice, J. N., Belsky, D. W., Higgins-Chen, A. T., Chen, B. H., Cohen, A. A., Fuellen, G., Marioni, R. E., Fortney, K., Fedichev, P. O., Zhavoronkov, A., Barzilai, N., Lasky-Su, J., Kiel, D. P., Kennedy, B. K., & Ferrucci, L. (2024). Validation of biomarkers of aging. *Nature Medicine*, *30*(2), 360–372. DOI: 10.1038/s41591-023-02784-9 PMID: 38355974

Nadeeshani, H. J., Li, J., Ying, T., Zhang, B., & Lu, J. (2022). Nicotinamide mononucleotide (NMN) as an anti-aging health product – Promises and safety concerns. *Journal of Advanced Research*, *37*, 267–278. DOI: 10.1016/j.jare.2021.08.003 PMID: 35499054

Nagarajan, S., Mohandas, S., Ganesan, K., Xu, B., & Ramkumar, K. M. (2022). New insights into dietary pterostilbene: Sources, metabolism, and health promotion effects. *Molecules (Basel, Switzerland)*, *27*(19), 6316. DOI: 10.3390/molecules27196316 PMID: 36234852

Nambiar, A., Kellogg, D.III, Justice, J., Goros, M., Gelfond, J., Pascual, R., Hashmi, S., Masternak, M., Prata, L., LeBrasseur, N., Limper, A., Kritchevsky, S., Musi, N., Tchkonia, T., & Kirkland, J. (2023). Senolytics dasatinib and quercetin in idiopathic pulmonary fibrosis: Results of a phase I, single-blind, single-center, randomized, placebo-controlled pilot trial on feasibility and tolerability. *EBioMedicine*, *90*, 104481. DOI: 10.1016/j.ebiom.2023.104481 PMID: 36857968

Ni, Y. Q., & Liu, Y. S. (2021). New insights into the roles and mechanisms of spermidine in aging and age-related diseases. *Aging and Disease*, *12*(8), 1948–1963. DOI: 10.14336/AD.2021.0603 PMID: 34881079

Nieto-Torres, J. L., & Hansen, M. (2021). Macroautophagy and aging: The impact of cellular recycling on health and longevity. *Molecular Aspects of Medicine*, *82*, 101020. DOI: 10.1016/j.mam.2021.101020 PMID: 34507801

Novelle, M. G., Ali, A., Diéguez, C., Bernier, M., & de Cabo, R. (2016). Metformin: A hopeful promise in aging research. *Cold Spring Harbor Perspectives in Medicine*, *6*(3), a025932. DOI: 10.1101/cshperspect.a025932 PMID: 26931809

Palavra, F., Robalo, C., & Reis, F. (2017). Recent advances and challenges of mTOR inhibitors use in the treatment of patients with tuberous sclerosis complex. *Oxidative Medicine and Cellular Longevity*, *9820181*(1), 9820181. Advance online publication. DOI: 10.1155/2017/9820181 PMID: 28386314

Pan, H., & Finkel, T. (2017). Key proteins and pathways that regulate lifespan. *The Journal of Biological Chemistry*, *292*(16), 6452–6460. DOI: 10.1074/jbc.R116.771915 PMID: 28264931

Panwar, V., Singh, A., Bhatt, M., Tonk, R. K., Azizov, S., Raza, A. S., Sengupta, S., Kumar, D., & Garg, M. (2023). Multifaceted role of mTOR (mammalian target of rapamycin) signaling pathway in human health and disease. *Signal Transduction and Targeted Therapy*, *8*(1), 375. DOI: 10.1038/s41392-023-01608-z PMID: 37779156

Park, K., & Lee, M.-S. (2022). Current status of autophagy enhancers in metabolic disorders and other diseases. *Frontiers in Cell and Developmental Biology*, *10*, 811701. DOI: 10.3389/fcell.2022.811701 PMID: 35237600

Penella, G. M. (2024). Should the European Medicines Agency consider ageing a disease? *Bioethics*, *38*(5), 431–437. DOI: 10.1111/bioe.13265 PMID: 38165401

Pereira, B., Correia, F. P., Alves, I. A., Costa, M., Gameiro, M., Martins, A. P., & Saraiva, J. A. (2024). Epigenetic reprogramming as a key to reverse ageing and increase longevity. *Ageing Research Reviews*, *95*, 102204. DOI: 10.1016/j.arr.2024.102204 PMID: 38272265

Pijnenburg, M. A., & Leget, C. (2007). Who wants to live forever? Three arguments against extending the human lifespan. *Journal of Medical Ethics*, *33*(10), 585–587. DOI: 10.1136/jme.2006.017822 PMID: 17906056

Podyacheva, E., & Toropova, Y. (2023). The role of NAD+, SIRTs interactions in stimulating and counteracting carcinogenesis. *International Journal of Molecular Sciences*, *24*(9), 7925. DOI: 10.3390/ijms24097925 PMID: 37175631

Polidori, M. C. (2024). Aging hallmarks, biomarkers, and clocks for personalized medicine: (Re)positioning the limelight. *Free Radical Biology & Medicine*, *215*, 48–55. DOI: 10.1016/j.freeradbiomed.2024.02.012 PMID: 38395089

Qureshi, R., Irfan, M., Gondal, T. M., Khan, S., Wu, J., Hadi, M. U., Heymach, J., Le, X., Yan, H., & Alam, T. (2023). AI in drug discovery and its clinical relevance. *Heliyon*, *9*(7), e17575. DOI: 10.1016/j.heliyon.2023.e17575 PMID: 37396052

Raffaele, M., & Vinciguerra, M. (2022). The costs and benefits of senotherapeutics for human health. *The Lancet. Healthy Longevity*, *3*(1), e67–e77. DOI: 10.1016/S2666-7568(21)00300-7 PMID: 36098323

Ram, W. S. (2019). Patents on natural products for diagnosing/preventing/treating Alzheimer's disease. In Rahman, A. (Ed.), *Studies in Natural Products Chemistry* (Vol. 61, pp. 85–141). Elsevier., DOI: 10.1016/B978-0-444-64183-0.00003-8

Rao, S., He, Z., Wang, Z., Yin, H., Hu, X., Tan, Y., Wan, T., Zhu, H., Luo, Y., Wang, X., Li, H., Wang, Z., Hu, X., Hong, C., Wang, Y., Luo, M., Du, W., Qian, Y., Tang, S., & Chen, C. (2024). Extracellular vesicles from human urine-derived stem cells delay aging through the transfer of PLAU and TIMP1. *Acta Pharmaceutica Sinica. B*, *14*(3), 1166–1186. DOI: 10.1016/j.apsb.2023.12.009 PMID: 38487008

Rattan, S. I. S. (2014). Aging is not a disease: Implications for intervention. *Aging and Disease*, *5*(3), 196–202. DOI: 10.14336/ad.2014.0500196 PMID: 24900942

Rattan, S. I. S. (2018). Biogerontology: Research status, challenges and opportunities. *Acta Biomedica*, *89*(2), 291–301. DOI: 10.23750/abm.v89i2.7403 PMID: 29957767

Reisman N.R., (2004). Anti-aging medicine: The legal issues: Legal issues associated with the current and future practice of anti-aging medicine. The Journals of Gerontology: Series A, 59(7), B674–B681. https://doi.org/.DOI: 10.1093/gerona/59.7.B674

Rivera, V. M. M., Tlacuahuac Juárez, J. R., Murillo Melo, N. M., Leyva Garcia, N., Magaña, J. J., Cordero Martínez, J., & Jiménez Gutierrez, G. E. (2024). Natural autophagy activators to fight age-related diseases. *Cells*, *13*(19), 1611. DOI: 10.3390/cells13191611 PMID: 39404375

Robbins, P. D., Jurk, D., Khosla, S., Kirkland, J. L., LeBrasseur, N. K., Miller, J. D., Passos, J. F., Pignolo, R. J., Tchkonia, T., & Niedernhofer, L. J. (2021). Senolytic drugs: Reducing senescent cell viability to extend health span. *Annual Review of Pharmacology and Toxicology*, *61*(1), 779–803. DOI: 10.1146/annurev-pharmtox-050120-105018 PMID: 32997601

Rolland, Y., Sierra, F., Ferrucci, L., Barzilai, N., De Cabo, R., Mannick, J., Oliva, A., Evans, W., Angioni, D., De Souto Barreto, P., Raffin, J., Vellas, B., Kirkland, J. L., Andrieu, S., Bacqueville, D., Bischoff-Ferrari, H., Blivet, G., Cash, T., Cuervo, A.-M., & Zhavoronkov, A. (2023). Challenges in developing geroscience trials. *Nature Communications*, *14*(1), 5038. DOI: 10.1038/s41467-023-39786-7 PMID: 37598227

Sadria, M., & Layton, A. T. (2021). Interactions among mTORC, AMPK and SIRT: A computational model for cell energy balance and metabolism. *Cell Communication and Signaling : CCS*, *19*(1), 57. DOI: 10.1186/s12964-021-00706-1 PMID: 34016143

Sarubbo, F., Esteban, S., Miralles, A., & Moranta, D. (2018). Effects of resveratrol and other polyphenols on SIRT1: Relevance to brain function during aging. *Current Neuropharmacology*, *16*(2), 126–136. DOI: 10.2174/1570159X15666170703113212 PMID: 28676015

Schumacher, B., Pothof, J., Vijg, J., & Hoeijmakers, J. H. J. (2021). The central role of DNA damage in the ageing process. *Nature*, *592*(7856), 695–703. DOI: 10.1038/s41586-021-03307-7 PMID: 33911272

Serrano, D. R., Luciano, F. C., Anaya, B. J., Ongoren, B., Kara, A., Molina, G., Ramirez, B. I., Sánchez-Guirales, S. A., Simon, J. A., Tomietto, G., Rapti, C., Ruiz, H. K., Rawat, S., Kumar, D., & Lalatsa, A. (2024). Artificial Intelligence (AI) applications in drug discovery and drug delivery: Revolutionizing personalized medicine. *Pharmaceutics*, *16*(10), 1328. DOI: 10.3390/pharmaceutics16101328 PMID: 39458657

Sharma, A., Anand, S. K., Singh, N., Dwivedi, U. N., & Kakkar, P. (2023). AMP-activated protein kinase: An energy sensor and survival mechanism in the reinstatement of metabolic homeostasis. *Experimental Cell Research*, *428*(1), 113614. DOI: 10.1016/j.yexcr.2023.113614 PMID: 37127064

Shayan, F. N., Mohabbati-Kalejahi, N., Alavi, S., & Zahed, M. A. (2022). Sustainable Development Goals (SDGs) as a framework for corporate social responsibility (CSR). *Sustainability (Basel)*, *14*(3), 1222. DOI: 10.3390/su14031222

Shenoy, P., & Harugeri, A. (2015). Elderly patients' participation in clinical trials. *Perspectives in Clinical Research*, *6*(4), 184–189. DOI: 10.4103/2229-3485.167099 PMID: 26623388

Snell, T. W., Johnston, R. K., Srinivasan, B., Zhou, H., Gao, M., & Skolnick, J. (2016). Repurposing FDA-approved drugs for anti-aging therapies. *Biogerontology, 17*(5–6), 907–920. DOI: 10.1007/s10522-016-9660-x PMID: 27484416

Son, D. H., Park, W. J., & Lee, Y. J. (2019). Recent advances in anti-aging medicine. *Korean Journal of Family Medicine, 40*(5), 289–296. DOI: 10.4082/kjfm.19.0087 PMID: 31558007

Subbiah, V., Coleman, N., Piha-Paul, S. A., Tsimberidou, A. M., Janku, F., Rodon, J., Pant, S., Dumbrava, E. E. I., Fu, S., Hong, D. S., Zhang, S., Sun, M., Jiang, Y., Roszik, J., Song, J., Yuan, Y., Meric-Bernstam, F., & Naing, A. (2024). Phase I study of mTORC1/2 inhibitor sapanisertib (CB-228/TAK-228) in combination with metformin in patients with mTOR/AKT/PI3K pathway alterations and advanced solid malignancies. *Cancer Research Communications, 4*(2), 378–387. DOI: 10.1158/2767-9764.CRC-22-0260 PMID: 38126764

Tao, X., Zhu, Z., Wang, L., Li, C., Sun, L., Wang, W., & Gong, W. (2024). Biomarkers of aging and relevant evaluation techniques: A comprehensive review. *Aging and Disease, 15*(3), 977–1005. DOI: 10.14336/AD.2023.00808-1 PMID: 37611906

Tenchov, R., Sasso, J. M., Wang, X., & Zhou, Q. A. (2024). Antiaging strategies and remedies: A landscape of research progress and promise. *ACS Chemical Neuroscience, 15*(3), 408–446. DOI: 10.1021/acschemneuro.3c00532 PMID: 38214973

Tenchov, R., Sasso, J. M., Wang, X., & Zhou, Q. A. (2024). Aging hallmarks and progression and age-related diseases: A landscape view of research advancement. *ACS Chemical Neuroscience, 15*(1), 1–30. DOI: 10.1021/acschemneuro.3c00531 PMID: 38095562

Tian, E., Sharma, G., & Dai, C. (2023). Neuroprotective properties of berberine: Molecular mechanisms and clinical implications. *Antioxidants, 12*(10), 1883. DOI: 10.3390/antiox12101883 PMID: 37891961

Veerman, G. D. M., Hussaarts, K. G. A. M., Jansman, F. G. A., Koolen, S. W. L., van Leeuwen, R. W. F., & Mathijssen, R. H. J. (2020). Clinical implications of food–drug interactions with small-molecule kinase inhibitors. *The Lancet. Oncology, 21*(5), e265–e279. DOI: 10.1016/S1470-2045(20)30069-3 PMID: 32359502

Waldner, M., Fantus, D., Solari, M., & Thomson, A. W. (2016). New perspectives on mTOR inhibitors (rapamycin, rapalogs and TORKinibs) in transplantation. *British Journal of Clinical Pharmacology, 82*(5), 1158–1170. DOI: 10.1111/bcp.12893 PMID: 26810941

Wang, J., Yuan,S., Tu, Y., Lv, Z., Cheng, H., and Ding, X. (2024). Extracellular vesicles in skin health, diseases, and aging., Interdisciplinary Medicine, 2, 3, 2024, e202400112024 https://doi.org/.DOI: 10.1002/INMD.20240011

Wang, L., Qiu, Q., Yang, D., Cao, C., Lu, Y., Zeng, Y., Jiang, W., Shen, Y., & Ye, Y. (2024). Clinical research progress of ridaforolimus (AP23573, MK8668) over the past decade: A systemic review. *Frontiers in Pharmacology, 15*, 1173240. DOI: 10.3389/fphar.2024.1173240 PMID: 38584599

Wolff, C. A., Reid, J. J., Musci, R. V., Linden, M. A., Konopka, A. R., Peelor, F. F., Miller, B. F., Hamilton, K. L., & Bruns, D. R. (2020). Differential effects of rapamycin and metformin in combination with rapamycin on mechanisms of proteostasis in cultured skeletal myotubes. *The Journals of Gerontology. Series A, Biological Sciences and Medical Sciences*, *75*(1), 32–39. DOI: 10.1093/gerona/glz058 PMID: 30820523

Woo, J., Archard, D., Au, D., Bergstresser, S., Erler, A., Kwok, T., Newman, J., Tong, R., & Walker, T. (2019). Ethical perspectives on advances in biogerontology. *Aging Medicine (Milton, N.S.W.)*, *2*(2), 99–103. DOI: 10.1002/agm2.12061 PMID: 31942520

Wu, Q. J., Zhang, T. N., Chen, H. H., Yu, X.-F., Lv, J.-L., Liu, Y.-Y., Liu, Y.-S., Zheng, G., Zhao, J.-Q., Wei, Y.-F., Guo, J.-Y., Liu, F.-H., Chang, Q., Zhang, Y.-X., Liu, C.-G., & Zhao, Y.-H. (2022). The sirtuin family in health and disease. *Signal Transduction and Targeted Therapy*, *7*(1), 402. DOI: 10.1038/s41392-022-01257-8 PMID: 36581622

Xiaoran, L., Yang, C., Liang, L., Hu, G., Zhong, Z., & Jiang, Z. (2024). Artificial intelligence for optimizing recruitment and retention in clinical trials: A scoping review. *Journal of the American Medical Informatics Association : JAMIA*, *31*(11), 2749–2759. DOI: 10.1093/jamia/ocae243 PMID: 39259922

Xie, J., Wang, X., & Proud, C. G. (2016). mTOR inhibitors in cancer therapy. F1000Research, 5, F1000 Faculty Rev-2078. https://doi.org/DOI: 10.12688/f1000research.9207.1

Xu, T., Li, H., Dai, Z., Lau, G. K., Li, B., Zhu, W., Liu, X., Liu, H., Cai, W., Huang, S., Wang, Q., & Zhang, S. (2020). Spermidine and spermine delay brain aging by inducing autophagy in SAMP8 mice. *Aging (Albany NY)*, *12*(7), 6401–6414. DOI: 10.18632/aging.103035 PMID: 32268299

Yu, J., Li, T., & Zhu, J. (2023). Gene therapy strategies targeting aging-related diseases. *Aging and Disease*, *14*(2), 398–417. DOI: 10.14336/AD.2022.00725 PMID: 37008065

Zakrzewski, W., Dobrzyński, M., Szymonowicz, M., & Rybak, Z. (2019). Stem cells: Past, present, and future. *Stem Cell Research & Therapy*, *10*(1), 68. DOI: 10.1186/s13287-019-1165-5 PMID: 30808416

Zhang, C., Meng, Y., & Han, J. (2024). Emerging roles of mitochondrial functions and epigenetic changes in the modulation of stem cell fate. *Cellular and Molecular Life Sciences : CMLS*, *81*(26), 26. Advance online publication. DOI: 10.1007/s00018-023-05070-6 PMID: 38212548

Zhang, Y., & Zhou, Y. (2024). Advances in targeted therapies for age-related osteoarthritis: A comprehensive review of current research. *Biomedicine and Pharmacotherapy*, *179*, 117314. DOI: 10.1016/j.biopha.2024.117314 PMID: 39167845

Zhang, Z., Yang, R., Zi, Z., & Liu, B. (2024). A new clinical age of aging research. *Trends in Endocrinology and Metabolism*. Advance online publication. DOI: 10.1016/j.tem.2024.08.004 PMID: 39227191

Zhao, H., Song, G., Zhu, H., Qian, H., Pan, X., Song, X., Xie, Y., & Liu, C. (2023). Pharmacological effects of urolithin A and its role in muscle health and performance: Current knowledge and prospects. *Nutrients*, *15*(20), 4441. DOI: 10.3390/nu15204441 PMID: 37892516

Zhavoronkov, A., Mamoshina, P., Vanhaelen, Q., Scheibye-Knudsen, M., Moskalev, A., & Aliper, A. (2019). Artificial intelligence for aging and longevity research: Recent advances and perspectives. *Ageing Research Reviews*, *49*, 49–66. DOI: 10.1016/j.arr.2018.11.003 PMID: 30472217

Zhou, Z., Slattum, P. W., Ke, A., & Zhang, L. (2023). Managing Drug–Drug Interactions in Older Adults. *Journal of Clinical Pharmacology*, *63*(10), 1083–1090. DOI: 10.1002/jcph.2299 PMID: 37408371

Zhu, Y. (2022). Advances in CRISPR/Cas9. *BioMed Research International*, *2022*(1), 9978571. Advance online publication. DOI: 10.1155/2022/9978571 PMID: 36193328

Chapter 5
Gene Therapy Against Age-Related Diseases

Riya Rameshwar Rai
Amity University, Panvel, India

Sagar Barage
https://orcid.org/0000-0003-0752-6948
Amity University, Panvel, India

Rajshri Singh
https://orcid.org/0000-0001-5748-5799
Amity University, Panvel, India

ABSTRACT

Aging is a natural process characterized by the gradual decline of cellular function and increased susceptibility to diseases. Gene therapy offers a promising approach to combat age-related diseases by targeting and modifying specific longevity-associated genes with aging processes such as mitochondrial dysfunction and telomere shortening. Recent advancements have shown that modifying specific genes can slow down or reverse certain aspects of aging, potentially extending healthy lifespan. Gene-editing technologies like CRISPR and AAV-based antiaging gene therapies have shown success in treating conditions such as cardiovascular disease, neurodegeneration, and metabolic disorders. Experimental research indicates that improving DNA repair pathways and lowering oxidative stress may be able to reverse aging characteristics. This chapter explores the current advancements, challenges, and future prospects of gene therapy as a therapeutic strategy for age-related diseases.

INTRODUCTION

Aging is a universal and complex biological process that leads to the progressive decline of physiological functions, ultimately increasing susceptibility to disease and mortality (Lopez-Otín et al., 2013). While a natural part of life, this process involves intricate molecular, cellular, and systemic changes that gradually deteriorate the body's capacity to maintain homeostasis and respond to external stresses (Kirkwood, 2005). The definition of aging encompasses not only the physical manifestations observed

DOI: 10.4018/979-8-3693-9730-5.ch005

at an organismal level but also the biochemical, genetic, and environmental factors that influence the aging process at cellular and molecular levels.

From a biological standpoint, aging is marked by the gradual buildup of cellular damage over time, resulting in the compromised function of tissues and organs. Cellular damage occurs as a result of metabolic processes, exposure to environmental factors, and genetic predisposition, all of which interact and compound over time. This accumulation of damage disrupts normal cellular function and accelerates the breakdown of bodily systems (Campisi et al., 2019). Cellular senescence is the irreversible termination of cell division and an antagonistic marker of aging. Cellular senescence occurs when cells cease to divide permanently and it process cannot be reversed. It is like a "brake" on cell growth that is triggered to prevent damaged or old cells from continuing to divide and potentially causing harm, such as becoming cancerous. While this is beneficial in certain contexts, over time, the accumulation of these non-dividing cells contributes to the aging process and aging related disorders by causing inflammation and interfering with normal tissue function. Therefore, cellular senescence acts as both a protective mechanism and a sign of aging. As cells divide, telomeres—protective caps on the ends of chromosomes—shorten, eventually reaching a critical length that signals cells to stop dividing. This mechanism, though crucial for protecting genomic integrity, leads to a gradual reduction in tissue regenerative capacity, contributing to aging (Blackburn et al., 2015).

The aging process is regulated by both genetic and epigenetic factors, which influence the rate and progression of cellular and systemic decline (Sen et al., 2016). Genes associated with longevity, such as *FOXO* and *SIRT1*, play significant roles in pathways related to DNA repair, metabolic control, and stress resistance. Certain epigenetic factors, such as DNA methylation and histone modifications, regulate gene expression without changing the DNA sequence, affecting cellular aging and organismal lifespan. Environmental factors, including lifestyle, diet, and exposure to toxins, further interact with genetic as well as epigenetic factors, contributing to the variability in aging and susceptibility to aging related diseases across individuals. This interaction of intrinsic and extrinsic factors underscores the complex and multidimensional aspect of aging.

The study of aging biology seeks to elucidate the mechanisms that underpin these processes to identify potential interventions that can mitigate the adverse effects of aging. With advances in biotechnology and genomics, scientists are beginning to unravel the molecular pathways involved in aging and explore therapeutic avenues, such as gene therapy, to counteract age-related degeneration and improve healthspan and lifespan (Vijg& Campisi, 2008). To better understand the process of aging and its consequences for age-related diseases, researchers have identified key biological markers known as the "hallmarks of aging" (López-Otín et al., 2013). These hallmarks represent several distinct but interrelated processes that collectively drive aging and its associated pathologies. These hallmarks provide a structural framework in order to understand the root causes of cellular and molecular aging and form the basis for developing targeted interventions, including gene therapy, to address age-related decline.

GENOMIC INSTABILITY

One of the primary hallmarks of aging is genomic instability, which is the accumulation of DNA damage over time (Lombard et al., 2005). This damage can result from endogenous factors like reactive oxygen species (ROS) produced during cellular metabolism, or exogenous factors like UV radiation and chemical exposure. Accumulation of DNA damage leads to mutations and chromosomal aberrations, which compromise genomic integrity and cellular function. In the context of age-related diseases, genomic instability contributes to cancer, where uncontrolled cell proliferation is driven by accumulated mutations, and neurodegenerative diseases, where DNA damage affects the function of neurons.

Telomere Attrition

Telomeres are the protective caps at the ends of chromosomes and shorten with each cell division because of the end-replication problem, which causes incomplete replication of linear DNA molecules during replication. Short telomeres lead to cellular senescence and death, reducing tissue regeneration. Telomere shortening is closely associated with aging and has been linked to age-related conditions such as cardiovascular disease, where shorter telomeres correlate with increased disease risk (Cawthon et al., 2003).

Epigenetic Alterations

Epigenetic changes, including histone modification, DNA methylation, and chromatin remodeling, play a key role in regulating gene expression. As cells age, their epigenetic landscape changes, leading to dysfunction of genes involved in cellular repair, metabolism, and stress response (Zhang et al., 2023).

Loss of Proteostasis

Proteostasis, or protein homeostasis, is the cell's ability to maintain the stability and functionality of its proteins. Aging is associated with a decline in proteostasis, resulting in the accumulation of damaged or misfolded proteins which disrupt cellular function (Hipp et al., 2019).

Mitochondrial Dysfunction

Mitochondria, essential for energy production, experience functional decline with age, reducing cellular energy output and increasing oxidative stress through reactive oxygen species (ROS). This dysregulation is linked to aging related diseases like cardiovascular disease and neurodegeneration. Therapies focusing on mitochondrial function, including caloric restriction and compounds like resveratrol, have shown potential to reduce oxidative stress and enhance mitochondrial biogenesis, potentially mitigating some effects of aging (Somasundaram et al., 2024).

Cellular Senescence

Cellular senescence is essentially characterized by an irreversible cell-cycle arrest, which leads to the secretion of pro-inflammatory factors that promote tissue damage and age-related diseases like fibrosis and osteoarthritis. Senolytic therapies, which selectively remove senescent cells, have demonstrated promising results in preclinical studies by alleviating age-related symptoms and improving tissue health (Kirkland &Tchkonia, 2017).

Stem Cell Exhaustion

Aging affects the regenerative capacity of stem cells, leading to stem cell exhaustion, which limits tissue repair and contributes to conditions like sarcopenia and osteoporosis. Increased oxidative stress plays a role in this decline, as shown in models like mitochondrial mutator mice, which exhibit neural and hematopoietic stem cell dysfunction (Trifunovic et al., 2004).

Altered Intercellular Communication

Aging is accompanied by changes in the way cells communicate with each other, often leading to increased inflammation (known as "inflammaging"). This chronic, low-grade inflammation contributes to various of age-related diseases, including diabetes and cardiovascular disease. Modulating intercellular communication to reduce inflammation and restore healthy cellular interactions is a promising area of anti-aging research (Franceschi et al., 2018).

Deregulated Nutrient Sensing

Cellular pathways that sense and respond to nutrient availability, such as insulin/IGF-1 signaling (IIS), mTOR, and AMPK pathways, are central to metabolic regulation and longevity. Aging is associated with a deregulation of these pathways, leading to metabolic dysfunction and increased susceptibility to diseases like diabetes and obesity. Caloric restriction and pharmacological interventions targeting nutrient-sensing pathways, such as mTOR inhibitors, have shown promise in extending lifespan and reducing age-related disease risk in animal models (Templeman & Murphy, 2018; Kenyon, 2010). Understanding the intricate biological mechanisms of aging and its associated hallmarks has provided a robust framework for identifying potential therapeutic interventions.

These hallmarks—ranging from genomic instability and telomere attrition to proteostasis decline and mitochondrial dysfunction—highlight critical pathways that contribute to aging and aging related diseases. Advances in biotechnology, including the development of gene therapy, offer innovative strategies to target these pathways and potentially reverse or delay the adverse effects of aging. Existing studies on age-related diseases are constrained by their focus on symptomatic management (e.g., anti-inflammatory drugs, antioxidants) rather than addressing root causes such asmitochondrial dysfunction, genomic instability, and epigenetic dysregulation (López-Otín et al., 2013). Traditional therapies often exhibit short-term efficacy, off-target effects, and inability to simultaneously target multiple aging hallmarks, leading to suboptimal outcomes (Campisi et al., 2019). Gene therapy emerges as a superior alternative by directly correcting genetic and epigenetic drivers of aging. For instance, CRISPR-Cas9 systems enable precise editing of longevity-associated genes like APOE4 and TERT to mitigate Alzheimer's risk and telomere attrition, respectively (Doudna & Charpentier, 2014; Bernardes de Jesus et al., 2012), while adeno-associated viruses (AAVs) deliver Klotho or SIRT1 to enhance stress resistance and cognitive function with sustained effects (Leon et al., 2017; Dubal et al., 2015). Furthermore, combinatorial approaches, such as co-delivering FGF21 and sTGFβR2, address interconnected pathways like metabolic decline and fibrosis, outperforming single-target drugs (Davidsohn et al., 2019). Innovations in tissue-specific vectors (e.g., AAV9 for cardiac targeting) and non-viral systems (e.g., lipid nanoparticles for NLRP3 siRNA) further enhance precision and reduce systemic toxicity compared to conventional therapies (Meumann et al., 2023; Sung & Kim, 2019). By leveraging these advancements, gene therapy offers transformative potential to delay or reverse aging processes, as evidenced by preclinical successes in lifespan extension and disease mitigation (Yang et al., 2023). Gene therapy, in particular, holds promise as a transformative tool, enabling precise modifications to genetic and epigenetic regulators of aging. The next section will explore gene therapy as a strategic intervention, delving into its mechanisms, including gene replacement, editing, and epigenetic modification, alongside the viral and non-viral delivery systems that make these approaches feasible. By leveraging these technologies, researchers aim to move closer to mitigating the challenges of aging and extending healthspan.

MOLECULAR BASIS OF AGING

Cellular aging, also known as senescence, is a feature of the aging process in which cell division is permanently stopped in response to numerous stresses such as DNA damage, replicative exhaustion, oxidative stress or oncogene activation. Senescent cells have a complicated phenotype that involves gradual telomere attrition, activation of DNA damage response pathways, and long-term expression of cyclin-dependent kinase inhibitors, including the p53-p21^{cip1} and p16^{INK4a} pathways. These molecular events converge to enforce an irreversible cell cycle arrest, even in the presence of mitogenic signals (Hayflick and Moorhead, 1961; Serrano et al., 1997; Acosta et al., 2013). Beyond proliferative arrest, senescent cells acquire a distinct secretory profile, termed the senescence-associated secretory phenotype (SASP), which is comprised of growth factors, chemokines, matrix metalloproteinases, and pro-inflammatory cytokines. The SASP contributes to tissue remodeling, immune cell recruitment, and, paradoxically, both tumor suppression and promotion depending on the context and chronicity of its activation (Kirkland &Tchkonia, 2017). Concurrently, senescent cells exhibit higher senescence-associated β-galactosidase (SA-β-gal) activity, a widely used histochemical biomarker, along with epigenetic remodeling including the formation of senescence-associated heterochromatin foci (SAHF), global changes in DNA methylation patterns, and histone post-translational modifications (Olan et al., 2023; Crouch et al., 2022).

Senolytics

The functional distinction between acute and chronic senescence is significant, with the former aiding in tissue repair and tumor suppression via transient cellular responses, while the latter, driven by prolonged stress and diminished immune clearance, leads to accumulation of senescent cells, chronic inflammation, and age-related diseases such as osteoarthritis, neurodegeneration, and cardiovascular conditions (Jaul and Barron, 2017). Aging manifests heterogeneously across tissues, as transcriptomic studies reveal differential expression of aging-related genes (e.g., VCAM1, FGF10, GFAP, IGJ), and the senescence marker p16^INK4a shows tissue-specific patterns correlating with disease susceptibility and regenerative decline (Schaum et al., 2020; Safwan-Zaiter et al., 2022; Strzyz, 2022; Yun et al., 2023). Senolytic drugs, which eliminate senescent cells by targeting their anti-apoptotic pathways, have shown promise in preclinical models—examples include dasatinib (targeting progenitor cells), quercetin and fisetin (broad activity), and navitoclax (BCL-2 inhibition), though some face limitations such as toxicity (Zhu et al., 2015; Chaib et al., 2022; Tao et al., 2014; Zhu et al., 2017; Triana-Martinez et al., 2019). Additional strategies involve inhibiting HSP90 and mTOR pathways to compromise senescent cell survival and SASP production, though systemic side effects remain a barrier (Fuhrmann-Stroissnigg et al., 2017; Iida et al., 2020). Consequently, combination approaches with senomorphics, antioxidants, or immune modulators, along with targeted delivery systems like nanoparticles or prodrugs, are being explored to enhance efficacy and reduce toxicity, underscoring the potential but also the complexity of translating senolytics into effective clinical therapies (Saccon et al., 2021; Hense et al., 2022).

Beyond conventional pharmacological approaches, gene therapy provides a highly specific strategy for senescent cell clearance. Recent advances have demonstrated that the delivery of suicide genes or cytotoxic effectors under the control of senescence-associated promoters, such as CDKN2A/p16INK4a or CDKN1A/p21, enables the selective removal of senescent cells in vivo (Demaria et al., 2014; Childs et al., 2018). For example, the p16-3MR transgenic system utilizes the full p16INK4a promoter to express a triple fusion of luciferase, red fluorescent protein, and HSV-thymidine kinase, allowing for targeted ablation of senescent cells upon ganciclovir administration (Demaria et al., 2014). This approach has been successfully applied to reduce tumor burden and age-related tissue dysfunction. Such strategies offer significant advantages over small-molecule senolytics in terms of specificity and durability. Incorporating senolytic mechanisms into gene therapy constructs represents a critical frontier in the treatment of age-related diseases and the extension of healthspan.Emerging senotherapeutic strategies likeFOXO4-DRI, a synthetic peptide, designed to selectively induce apoptosis in senescent cells by disrupting the interaction between FOXO4 and p53, thereby freeing p53 to activate the apoptotic program. In the foundational study by Baar et al. (2017), FOXO4-DRI successfully cleared senescent cells both in vitro and in vivo, leading to improved tissue homeostasis, enhanced physical fitness, and better organ function in aged and chemotherapy-damaged mice without harming non-senescent cells. Building on this, Huang et al. (2021) demonstrated that FOXO4-DRI selectively eliminated senescent human chondrocytes expanded in vitro, significantly reducing senescence-associated markers while preserving healthy cell populations, suggesting its potential for improving regenerative therapies like cartilage repair. Together, these studies highlight FOXO4-DRI as a promising senolytic agent for both aging-related and regenerative medicine applications.

GENE THERAPY AS A STRATEGY

Gene therapy holds transformative potential for treating age-related diseases by addressing the root genetic and cellular processes that contribute to aging and degenerative conditions. Unlike conventional therapies that primarily target symptoms, gene therapy allows for the correction of genetic defects, the enhancement of protective cellular functions, and the alteration of gene expression to prevent disease progression. This strategy encompasses several mechanisms—gene replacement, gene editing, and epigenetic modification—each with unique applications and technological requirements. Additionally, the effective delivery of therapeutic genes relies on viral vectors like adeno-associated viruses (AAVs) and lentiviral vectors, which have been engineered to safely and precisely insert therapeutic genes into target cells (Yu et al., 2023).

Mechanisms of Gene Therapy

Gene therapy mechanisms vary depending on the desired cellular outcome, such as replacing dysfunctional genes, editing specific DNA sequences, or modifying gene expression through epigenetic pathways. Each approach addresses different cellular challenges associated with aging, offering distinct pathways for therapeutic intervention.

Gene Replacement Therapy

Gene replacement therapy focuses on introducing functional copies of defective or absent genes to restore normal cellular function. This method is particularly relevant for monogenic diseases—those caused by a single gene mutation—where the introduction of a healthy gene can counteract the effects of the defective one. In the context of aging, gene replacement therapy is used to address genetic deficiencies that exacerbate cellular aging and tissue degeneration (Yu et al., 2023). The procedure uses viral or non-viral vectors to deliver a functioning gene copy to target cells. The new gene enters the cell and either integrates into the genome or exists as an extrachromosomal element, enabling it to produce the necessary proteins or enzymes. For example, SIRT1 and FOXO3 are genes that enhance cellular repair and resilience against stress; their overexpression via gene replacement has shown promising outcomes in preclinical animals for reducing the ill-effects of oxidative stress and enhancing longevity (Guarente, 2013; Lombard et al., 2005). SIRT1 has been shown to play a vital role in protecting against DNA damage and promoting cell survival under stress, making it an attractive candidate for gene replacement therapy in aging models (Houtkooper et al., 2012). Similarly, FOXO3 has been implicated in being resistant to oxidative stress and increased lifespan, providing a potential therapeutic target to slow aging processes (Willcox et al., 2008). In neurodegenerative diseases, the replacement of alleles like APOE2, which has been linked to reduced Alzheimer's disease risk, offers promise for delaying disease progression and enhancing cognitive resilience (Corder et al., 1993). Challenges in gene replacement therapy include managing immune responses and minimizing insertional mutagenesis, which can disrupt other essential genes. Advances in vector design and precision targeting are gradually improving the safety of this approach.

Gene Editing Therapy

Gene editing offers a targeted approach for modifying specific DNA sequences within cells, allowing for precise interventions that correct genetic mutations or enhance protective genes associated with aging. CRISPR-Cas9, a widely used gene-editing tool, allows researchers to cut DNA at specific regions, facilitating the insertion, deletion, or modification of genes. This precision has significant implications for age-related diseases, particularly those driven by mutations or genetic variability. CRISPR-Cas9 works by directing the Cas9 enzyme binds to a specific DNA sequence, resulting in a double-stranded break. The natural repair processes of the cell can then rejoin the DNA, either through non-homologous end joining (NHEJ), which may introduce tiny insertions or deletions, or homology-directed repair (HDR), which uses a template for precise editing (Doudna & Charpentier, 2014; Hsu et al., 2014). This precision allows scientists to make beneficial modifications, such as correcting mutations in the *APOE4 variant* linked to Alzheimer's disease. Gene editing has also shown potential in telomere maintenance through modifications to the *TERT* gene, which encodes telomerase, an enzyme that extends telomeres and maintains chromosomal stability (Shay & Wright, 2011). Activating or upregulating *TERT* in high-turnover cells, such as skin and blood cells, offers the prospect of delaying cellular senescence and extending cell lifespan, contributing to enhanced healthspan and reduced age-related decline. Additionally, modifying genes associated with DNA repair, such as *SIRT6* and *FOXO*, has shown promise in preclinical models; enhanced DNA repair and stress resistance in these cases lead to greater resilience against age-related cellular damage. Despite its potential, gene editing encounters challenges, notably off-target effects, where unintended sequences may be edited, disrupting essential genes or regulatory regions. To address this, scientists are advancing next-generation CRISPR systems with improved fidelity and specificity, minimizing off-target effects and enhancing the safety of gene editing for therapeutic applications in aging (Guo et al., 2023).

Epigenetic Modification Therapy

Epigenetic modification therapy aims to adjust gene expression by altering the epigenome, rather than the DNA sequence itself. As mentioned earlier, DNA methylation and histone modifications, are integral to regulating gene activity and undergo age-related shifts that contribute to aging and age-associated diseases (Horvath, 2013). Epigenetic therapies may reactivate silenced genes associated with longevity, such as Klotho and FOXO3, which decline in activity with age. Targeting these genes for epigenetic modulation has shown promise in restoring youthful gene expression profiles in aged tissues (Dubal et al., 2015). In neurodegenerative diseases, abnormal methylation patterns exacerbate neuron loss and cognitive decline. Epigenetic reprogramming might even have the ability to restore normal gene function, reduce inflammation, and slow disease progression in these contexts. Though largely experimental, epigenetic modification therapy is advancing with research into more targeted epigenetic agents, providing hope for non-invasive rejuvenation strategies (Berdasco& Esteller, 2019). This approach also has potential in combating neurodegenerative diseases, where abnormal epigenetic patterns contribute to neuronal death and cognitive decline. In Alzheimer's disease, for instance, hypermethylation of genes associated with synaptic function and memory can exacerbate disease progression. By modifying the epigenetic state of these genes, epigenetic therapy can help restore normal cellular functioning and slow progression of disease. However, epigenetic modification therapies are still mostly experimental, and more research is required to ensure that targeted epigenetic changes are sustained and do not inadvertently disrupt other gene networks essential for cell health.

Introducing the transcription factors Oct4, Sox2, and Klf4 (collectively known as OSK) into mouse retinal ganglion cells can restore youthful patterns of DNA methylation and gene expression. This process supports the regeneration of axons after injury and reverses vision loss in both a mouse model of glaucoma and naturally aged mice. These positive outcomes rely on the presence of DNA demethylating enzymes TET1 and TET2. It appears that mammalian tissues retain epigenetic markers of youth—partially stored through DNA methylation—that can be reactivated to enhance tissue function and regeneration. The researchers suggest that epigenetic reprogramming, potentially via gene therapy, could help repair tissues and counteract age-related decline in humans. Importantly, OSK expression can rejuvenate the epigenome without compromising a cell's identity, offering a promising strategy to reverse aging effects in the central nervous system, particularly in retinal ganglion cells. This youthful epigenetic information may be stored through mechanisms such as covalent DNA changes, DNA-binding proteins, RNA-directed chromatin modifiers, and RNA-DNA hybrids established early in development (Lu et al., 2020).

CAR-T Cells for Cancer Treatment

Cells are essential to adaptive immunity, using diverse surface markers to recognize foreign invaders known as antigens. Scientists have engineered T cells to specifically target cancer cells (Brentjens et al., 2007; Kershaw et al., 2006; Gross et al., 1989). One such innovation is Chimeric Antigen Receptors (CARs). These are synthetic receptors that equip T cells to identify and bind to antigens present on tumor cells (Di Stasi et al., 2009; Hong et al., 2020; Milone et al., 2009). A prime example is

CD19, a surface protein consistently found on B cells and commonly involved in B-cell cancers. CAR-T cells targeting CD19 have shown strong clinical success in treating chronic lymphocytic leukemia and acute lymphoblastic leukemia, resulting in FDA approval (Maude et al., 2015). Beyond CD19, other targets like BCMA, CD20 (for B cells), and CD5 and CD7 (for T cells) have been developed to treat conditions like multiple myeloma (Bailey & Maus, 2019). For glioblastoma, a highly aggressive age-related brain cancer, emerging therapies like CAR-T cells targeting tumor-specific antigens (e.g., EGFRvIII) are being explored, though challenges such as tumor heterogeneity and the blood-brain barrier remain significant hurdles (Khiabani et al., 2024). To enhance their cancer-fighting abilities, engineered T cells have been further modified to overcome challenges like T cell exhaustion and tumor-induced immunosuppression, and to reprogram the immune environment (Rafiq et al., 2020; Roybal et al., 2016). For example, anti-apoptotic genes such as BCL-XL and BCL-2 are introduced to help T cells resist cell death and extend their lifespan (Kershaw et al., 2013).

To counteract immunosuppressive signals within tumors, Synthetic Notch (SynNotch) receptors have been added to T cells to modulate immune responses and alter the tumor microenvironment (Roybal et al., 2016). In addition, CAR-T cells have been engineered to release human anti-PD-L1 antibodies or PD-1-blocking scFvs, enhancing their activity (Rafiq et al., 2018; Suarez et al., 2016). Overexpression of Interleukin-12 in T cells has also been explored to boost their proliferation, influence regulatory immune cells like myeloid cells, and make tumors more responsive to immune attack (Chinnasamy et al., 2012).

Viral Vectors Used in Gene Therapy

Efficient delivery of therapeutic genes to target cells and tissues is essential for successful gene therapy. Viral vectors, which harness the natural ability of viruses to insert genetic material into cells, are commonly used in gene therapy due to their high efficiency and specificity. Among the viral vectors available, adeno-associated viruses (AAVs) and lentiviruses are particularly suited for age-related therapies due to their unique characteristics and compatibility with long-term gene expression.

Adeno-Associated Viruses (AAVs) in Therapeutic Delivery

Adeno-associated viruses (AAVs) are small (~25 nm), non-enveloped viruses with a single-stranded DNA genome (~4.7 kb) widely used in gene therapy due to their low immunogenicity, non-pathogenic nature, and ability to transduce both dividing and non-dividing cells. Their tropism for post-mitotic tissues, such as neurons and muscle, makes them particularly suited for treating age-related diseases. AAVs are best for brain/heart delivery (e.g., AAV-BDNF in Alzheimer's trials) to enhance DNA repair and oxidative stress resistance, or *VEGF* to promote angiogenesis in ischemic aging tissues. Different AAV serotypes offer tissue-specific targeting—AAV9 for cardiac tissue and AAV2 for liver—enabling more precise intervention. However, AAVs are limited by their small packaging capacity, which restricts delivery to relatively small transgenes. Current research is focused on engineering variants with enhanced efficiency and expanded cargo capacity to overcome these limitations in the context of aging therapeutics (Zincarelli et al., 2008).

Lentiviral Vectors for Genetic Modification

Lentiviral vectors are ~100 nm enveloped viruses with a single-stranded RNA genome (~9.7 kb) that, upon reverse transcription, integrate into the host genome, enabling stable, long-term transgene expression—particularly in dividing cells (Naldini, 2015). Their relatively large cargo capacity (~8–10 kb) surpasses that of adeno-associated viruses, allowing delivery of complex or multiple therapeutic genes. In aging research, lentiviral vectors have been effective for hematopoietic stem cell rejuvenation (e.g., SIRT6 overexpression) and other genes which are involved in telomere maintenance, DNA repair, and stress resistance, respectively (Tasselli et al., 2017; Hsu et al., 2014; Miyoshi et al., 1998). This makes them particularly effective for targeting stem cells and regenerating tissues with age-related decline. Their capacity for stable integration ensures sustained expression in proliferative tissues like bone marrow and muscle, offering a promising strategy for long-term regenerative gene therapy in aging models.

Non-Viral Delivery Methods: Lipid Nanoparticles and Electroporation

Non-viral delivery systems are emerging as promising alternatives to viral vectors for gene therapy due to their potential for reduced immunogenicity, enhanced safety, and scalable manufacturing. Among these, lipid nanoparticles (LNPs) and electroporation have gained significant attention for their capacity to deliver nucleic acids and therapeutic genes effectively. These methods are particularly relevant in the context of aging-related diseases, where precise and safe delivery to specific tissues is critical.

Table 1. Different vectors offer unique advantages and challenges for aging-related applications

Vector	Advantages	Limitations	Relevance to Aging
AAVs	- Low immunogenicity - Tissue-specific targeting - Long-term expression	- Small cargo capacity (~4.7 kb) - Pre-existing immunity in some populations	Ideal for chronic aging conditions (e.g., neurodegeneration, cardiovascular aging). Example: AAV-Klotho for cognitive decline.
Lentiviruses	- Large cargo capacity - Stable integration into genome	- Risk of insertional mutagenesis - Inflammatory responses	Suitable for ex vivo stem cell modifications (e.g., TERT delivery to hematopoietic stem cells).
LNPs	- Scalable production - Low immunogenicity - mRNA delivery capability	- Transient expression - Limited tissue penetration	Optimal for transient interventions (e.g., siRNA silencing of NLRP3 to reduce inflammaging).
Electroporation	- Non-viral - Direct delivery of CRISPR components	- Cell damage risk - Limited to accessible tissues	Useful for ex vivo editing (e.g., enhancing FOXO3 in patient-derived cells).

(Zincarelli et al., 2008; Naldini, 2015; Tasselli et al., 2017; Hsu et al., 2014; Kowalski et al., 2019; Jyotsana et al., 2019; Young & Dean, 2015; Whitehead et al., 2009; Mingozzi& High, 2011; Wang, Tai, & Gao, 2019)

Note. This table summarizes key characteristics of commonly used gene delivery systems in aging-related gene therapy. Each vector system offers distinct advantages and challenges depending on therapeutic goals, such as duration of gene expression, immune profile, and target tissue. Their selection must align with the nature of the aging pathology and the specific gene targets involved. Adapted from and supported by findings from Zincarelli et al. (2008), Naldini (2015), Tasselli et al. (2017), Hsu et al. (2014), Kowalski et al. (2019), Jyotsana et al. (2019), Young and Dean (2015), Whitehead, Langer, & Anderson (2009), Mingozzi and High (2011), and Wang, Tai, and Gao (2019).

Lipid Nanoparticles (LNPs)

Lipid nanoparticles (LNPs) are non-viral vectors that encapsulate nucleic acids—such as mRNA, plasmid DNA, or siRNA—within a lipid bilayer, offering a safe and flexible platform for age-related gene therapy. Measuring ~80–100 nm in size, LNPs protect cargo from enzymatic degradation and enable efficient cellular uptake via endocytosis, with subsequent endosomal release into the cytoplasm (Kowalski et al., 2019). In aging models, LNPs have been considered promising for transient anti-inflammatory therapies (e.g., IL-10 mRNA for atherosclerosis) and for mRNA encoding *TERT* to enhance telomerase activity and delay senescence, and siRNA targeting inflammatory genes like *NLRP3* to reduce age-associated chronic inflammation (Jyotsana et al., 2019). Unlike viral vectors, LNPs are biodegradable, less immunogenic, and amenable to repeat dosing. Their surface can be engineered with ligands to selectively target senescent or stem cells, making them especially promising for aging tissues such as the brain, liver, and skeletal muscle. Ongoing advances aim to improve tissue specificity and intracellular delivery efficiency, addressing current limitations and expanding their potential in regenerative aging therapies.

Electroporation

Electroporation, non-viral gene delivery method, creates transient pores in the cellular membranes using short electrical pulses, enabling direct intracellular delivery of large nucleic acids such as plasmid DNA or CRISPR components. It is especially effective in ex vivo applications, such as engineering patient-derived stem cells to express longevity-associated genes like SIRT1 and FOXO3, which support DNA repair and oxidative stress resistance in aging tissues (Young & Dean, 2015). Electroporation enables delivery without viral carriers and generally results in transient gene expression, reducing risks linked to genomic integration. While simple and scalable, its in vivo use is limited by potential cell damage, prompting ongoing optimization and integration with gene editing tools for safer, targeted aging therapies.

In vivo gene therapy has been studied using a variety of methods, including viral vectors like AAV and lentiviral vectors, as well as non-viral alternatives such lipid nanoparticles and electroporation. Viral vectors improve transduction efficiency and transgenic expression, but each approach has unique risks and benefits. Lentiviral vectors can integrate into the host's genome and accommodate larger pay-loads but carry a risk of insertional mutagenesis and may provoke more pronounced immune responses (Naldini, 2015). In contrast, non-viral methods offer improved safety by avoiding viral components, yet they often suffer from transient expression and lower overall efficiency in vivo (Whitehead, Langer, & Anderson, 2009). Among these modalities, AAV vectors are widely regarded as superior for clinical applications because they combine high in vivo transduction efficiency with a low immunogenic profile and the capacity to transduce both non-dividing and dividing cells, despite having a more limited cargo capacity (Mingozzi& High, 2011; Wang, Tai, & Gao, 2019).

TARGET GENES AND THEIR PRE-CLINICAL APPLICATIONS

Aging is fundamentally driven by complex molecular and genetic mechanisms that lead to progressive functional decline. Targeted gene therapies have shown potential in slowing or reversing some of these processes by addressing key molecular pathways involved in cellular aging. Pre-clinical applications of gene therapy have focused on the SIRT family for their roles in DNA repair and stress resistance, Klotho

(KL), FOXO, and VEGF genes for their contributions to cellular resilience and longevity, and TERT and APOE genes for their influence on telomere maintenance and cholesterol metabolism.

Role of SIRT Genes in DNA Repair and Stress Resistance

A family of proteins known as sirtuins is essential for controlling cellular metabolism and the stress response. The SIRT (Sirtuin) family, particularly SIRT1, SIRT3, and SIRT6, are critical in aging and longevity, functioning as nicotinamide adenine dinucleotide (NAD+)-dependent deacetylases involved in regulating metabolic homeostasis, DNA repair, and cellular stress response.

SIRT1

SIRT1 has gained considerable interest for its role in DNA repair and regulation of cellular stress responses, such as oxidative stress, inflammation, and cell death. It supports cell survival by deacetylating proteins like the tumor suppressor p53, which controls apoptosis, thereby contributing to genomic stability (Houtkooper et al., 2012). Preclinical research suggests that activating SIRT1 can extend lifespan by lowering reactive oxygen species (ROS) and enhancing mitochondrial function—key factors in combating age-related conditions like cardiovascular disease and neurodegeneration. In mouse studies, increased SIRT1 levels have been linked to delayed development of age-related illnesses and longer lifespans, highlighting its therapeutic promise for aging-related disorders. Interestingly, in mice fed a high-fat diet, overexpressing SIRT1—particularly in skeletal muscle—has been shown to reverse insulin resistance. While AAV1-Sirt1 treatment alone did not prevent obesity and insulin resistance caused by the high-fat diet, it did lead to higher levels of phosphorylated AMPK and genes involved in fatty acid β-oxidation. Additionally, skeletal muscle SIRT1 overexpression boosted baseline AKT phosphorylation. In another study, intravitreal delivery of SIRT1 in rats with diabetic retinopathy led to improved visual function (Kitaeva et al., 2024).

SIRT3

SIRT3, found in the mitochondria, plays a vital role in managing cellular energy metabolism and defending against oxidative stress. As mitochondria are the main source of reactive oxygen species (ROS), SIRT3 helps counteract this damage by activating antioxidant enzymes such as superoxide dismutase 2 (SOD2) and enhancing the efficiency of mitochondrial oxidative phosphorylation. Animal studies have demonstrated that activating SIRT3 can delay mitochondrial aging, improve heart function, and reduce damage associated with neurodegenerative diseases—conditions often linked to mitochondrial dysfunction (Someya et al., 2010). Research involving Sirt3-deficient mice shows that the loss of SIRT3 contributes to chronic liver inflammation, while restoring its expression can reduce liver inflammation and prevent cardiovascular damage (Gao et al., 2022). Additionally, the Receptor Activator of NF-κB Ligand (RANKL) boosts Sirt3 expression, promoting the formation and function of osteoclasts, which are involved in bone resorption. Conversely, SIRT3 deficiency impairs mitochondrial function in osteoclasts, limiting their activity and helping maintain bone mass in mice (Ling et al., 2021). Furthermore, reduced SIRT3 activity in heart cells leads to increased lactate dehydrogenase release, lower ATP production, disrupted mitochondrial membrane potential, and heightened oxidative stress. SIRT3 deficiency is also linked to increased expression of necroptosis-associated proteins and inflammation-related genes in both laboratory and live models (Song et al., 2021).

SIRT6

As outlined in Table 2, SIRT6 plays a key role in DNA repair processes, including base excision repair and maintaining chromatin stability. It also helps regulate inflammation by suppressing the NF-κBsignaling pathway, which tends to become hyperactive with age and is linked to chronic inflammatory conditions. In preclinical studies, boosting SIRT6 expression has been associated with better metabolic function, extended lifespan, and enhanced DNA repair, especially in metabolically active tissues like the brain and liver (Mostoslavsky et al., 2006). SIRT6 overexpression supports telomere maintenance, slows cellular aging, lowers the production of inflammatory cytokines linked to senescence, and protects against age-related metabolic shifts in vascular smooth muscle cells. However, a mutated form of the gene, SIRT6H133Y, was found to reduce the lifespan of both human and mouse vascular smooth muscle cells (Kitaeva et al., 2024; Grootaert et al., 2021). In atherosclerosis, SIRT6 promotes new blood vessel formation in plaques by increasing hypoxia-inducible factor 1α (HIF-1α) levels under low-oxygen conditions. Yet, it can also lead to damage in these vessels due to oxidative stress and the production of reactive oxygen species, which has been linked to carotid plaque hemorrhaging (Yang et al., 2021).

KL, FOXO, and VEGF Genes as Potential Targets

The Klotho (KL), FOXO, and VEGF genes have been recognized for their influence on cellular health, resilience, and longevity. Each of these genes contributes uniquely to processes associated with aging, from antioxidant responses and growth factor regulation to tissue repair.

Klotho (KL)

The Klotho gene encodes a transmembrane protein with anti-aging properties, particularly in modulating calcium-phosphate metabolism, oxidative stress, and inflammation. Klotho expression declines with age, and reduced Klotho levels are linked to age-related disorders like osteoporosis, chronic kidney disease, and cardiovascular disease. In pre-clinical studies, restoring Klotho levels in aging mice has shown protective effects on cognitive function, bone density, and cardiovascular health. The neuroprotective properties of Klotho have positioned it as a therapeutic target for neurodegenerative diseases, and gene therapies delivering Klotho have shown promise in improving cognitive resilience and reducing vascular calcification in pre-clinical trials (Leon et al., 2017). Klotho is a well-characterized aging-suppressor gene with demonstrated associations to longevity across multiple animal models (Yamazaki et al., 2010). Its expression exhibits a decline with advancing age in both murine and human systems, whereas upregulation of Klotho has been shown to attenuate or reverse age-related phenotypes (Gao et al., 2020; Chen et al., 2022). Reduced expression of Klotho has been observed in patients with chronic kidney disease (CKD), correlating with systemic degenerative manifestations such as vascular calcification, osteoporosis, and cutaneous atrophy (Gao et al., 2020). Genetic variants or deficiencies in Klotho function are linked to accelerated aging phenotypes and impaired mineral metabolism (Gao et al., 2020). Murine models with Klotho haploinsufficiency exhibit compromised renal function, while complete Klotho deficiency results in early-onset multisystemic degeneration, including cardiac dysfunction (Kurosu et al., 2005; Gao et al., 2020; Chen et al., 2022).

Therapeutic restoration of Klotho expression via gene transfer has demonstrated promising outcomes in preclinical settings. Intra-articular administration of plasmid DNA encoding α-Klotho has been shown to enhance local Klotho protein synthesis and delay cartilage degeneration in osteoarthritis models (Roig-Soriano et al., 2023; Chuchana et al., 2018). More advanced strategies using adeno-associated virus (AAV) vectors have facilitated region-specific delivery and sustained expression. For example, bilateral hippocampal injection of AAV-Klotho in rodent models of temporal lobe epilepsy resulted in significant overexpression of Klotho in the hippocampus, ameliorating cognitive deficits and exerting neuroprotective effects through modulation of oxidative stress and glutathione metabolism (Xiang et al., 2021; Xiang et al., 2022). AAV-mediated Klotho gene delivery has also demonstrated efficacy in attenuating hippocampal neurodegeneration, reducing arterial remodeling, and preserving renal architecture in models of spontaneous hypertension (Wang & Sun, 2009; Roig-Soriano et al., 2022). Notably, systemic administration of AAV9-Klotho in progeroid mouse models restored aspects of the epigenetic landscape, suppressed inflammatory markers, and conferred neuroprotective and anti-aging benefits (Roig-Soriano et al., 2022). Soluble Klotho delivered via AAVs has also been shown to reduce vascular stiffness, restore B-cell populations, normalize serum IgG levels, and mitigate age-associated vascular inflammation (Fan et al., 2022).

FOXO

Forkhead box O (FOXO) transcription factors, particularly FOXO3, play a pivotal role in maintaining cellular homeostasis by regulating genes involved in DNA damage repair, apoptosis, cell cycle arrest, oxidative stress resistance, and metabolism (Calnan & Brunet, 2008). Among the FOXO family (FOXO1, FOXO3, FOXO4, and FOXO6), FOXO3 has been most strongly associated with human longevity; several FOXO3 gene variants correlate with exceptional lifespan across multiple populations (Willcox et al., 2008; Li et al., 2009).Mechanistically, FOXO3 upregulates the expression of antioxidant enzymes, such as superoxide dismutase 2 (SOD2) and catalase, and DNA repair proteins like GADD45, thereby mitigating oxidative damage and preserving genomic integrity (van der Horst &Burgering, 2007). It also induces transient cell cycle arrest under stress via p27^Kip1^ and p21^Cip1^, allowing for DNA repair before cellular division (Greer & Brunet, 2005). These actions position FOXO3 as a central regulator of cellular stress responses, particularly in long-lived postmitotic cells like neurons and cardiomyocytes.

In animal models, enhanced FOXO3 activity improved oxidative stress resistance, promote autophagy, and extend lifespan (Martins et al., 2016). For instance, overexpression of FOXO transcription factors in C. elegans (the ortholog daf-16) significantly prolongs lifespan, while FOXO3 knockdown accelerates aging phenotypes in mammals (Murphy et al., 2003; Paik et al., 2007).Recent gene therapy approaches have sought to exploit FOXO3's protective functions. AAV-mediated delivery of constitutively active FOXO3 in aged mice led to reduced oxidative damage in cardiac tissue and improved cardiac function (Donato et al., 2015). Similarly, lentiviral vectors expressing FOXO3 in neural tissues have demonstrated neuroprotective effects in models of neurodegenerative disease (Zhang et al., 2022). These findings suggest that gene therapy targeting FOXO3 could become a promising strategy to counteract degenerative diseases, enhance tissue resilience, and promote healthy aging.Thus, integrating FOXO3 modulation into gene therapy platforms holds substantial therapeutic potential, bridging stress resistance mechanisms with regenerative medicine approaches.

Table 2. Genes involved in aging and their pre-clinical applications

Target Gene	Role/Function	Pre-clinical Applications	Impact on Aging/Diseases
SIRT1	DNA repair, stress response	Activation promotes longevity, reduces ROS, improves mitochondrial function	Delays age-related diseases, enhances genomic stability
SIRT3	Mitochondrial energy metabolism	Activation protects against oxidative damage, improves cardiac function	Delays mitochondrial aging, reduces neurodegenerative damage
SIRT6	DNA repair, inflammation modulation	Overexpression linked to improved metabolic health, increased lifespan	Maintains genomic integrity, counters age-related tissue damage
Klotho (KL)	Calcium-phosphate metabolism, oxidative stress moderation	Restoring Klotho levels shows protective effects on cognitive function and cardiovascular health	Potential target for neurodegenerative diseases, protects against age-related disorders
FOXO	Regulates apoptosis, DNA repair, oxidative stress response	Enhancing FOXO3 activity improves survival in neurons and cardiac cells	Protects against neurodegenerative diseases and ischemic injuries
VEGF	Angiogenesis	Gene therapy increases VEGF expression, improving blood flow and tissue repair	Addresses vascular insufficiency and enhances muscle regeneration
TERT	Telomere maintenance	Activation extends telomeres, prolonging cellular lifespan	Delays senescence, enhances tissue regeneration, improves function in aging cells
APOE	Lipid metabolism	Gene therapies targeting APOE reduce amyloid burden and improve cholesterol metabolism	Reduces risk of Alzheimer's disease and cardiovascular disease
NLRP3	Inflammatory responses	CRISPR to knock out NLRP3 reduces systemic inflammation	May alleviate atherosclerosis and Alzheimer's disease
IL-1β	Pro-inflammatory cytokine	AAV delivery of IL-1Ra reduces inflammation in pre-clinical models	Improves outcomes in arthritis and myocardial infarction
IL-10	Anti-inflammatory cytokine	Gene delivery reduces liver fibrosis and atherosclerosis	Promotes tissue repair, counters chronic inflammation
IL-6	Immune defense mediator	CRISPR modulation reduces IL-6 levels, alleviating inflammation	Preserves muscle mass, counters sarcopenia in aging

(Houtkooper et al., 2012; Kitaeva et al., 2024; Someya et al., 2010; Gao et al., 2022; Ling et al., 2021; Song et al., 2021; Mostoslavsky et al., 2006; Grootaert et al., 2021; Yang et al., 2021; Leon et al., 2017; Yamazaki et al., 2010; Gao et al., 2020; Chen et al., 2022; Roig-Soriano et al., 2023; Chuchana et al., 2018; Xiang et al., 2021; Xiang et al., 2022; Wang & Sun, 2009; Roig-Soriano et al., 2022; Fan et al., 2022; Willcox et al., 2008; Shay & Wright, 2011; Bernardes de Jesus et al., 2012; Mahley & Rall, 2000; Liang et al., 2022; Kaverina et al., 2023; Evans, 2018; Kamaly et al., 2016; Pototschnig et al., 2023; Volpatti et al., 2024)

Note. This table provides a concise overview of key genes implicated in aging and age-related diseases, summarizing their molecular roles, observed pre-clinical therapeutic applications, and their broader impact on aging phenotypes. These genes have been targeted in experimental gene therapy strategies due to their functions in genomic stability, metabolic regulation, inflammation modulation, angiogenesis, and telomere maintenance. The therapeutic potential of modulating these targets underscores the relevance of personalized and pathway-specific approaches in age-related intervention research.

VEGF (Vascular Endothelial Growth Factor)

Vascular endothelial growth factor (VEGF) is a critical regulator of angiogenesis, a process that diminishes with age, leading to impaired tissue perfusion, cardiovascular diseases, and delayed wound healing. Age-associated reductions in VEGF activity contribute to vascular insufficiency, muscle atrophy, and compromised regenerative capacity (Ferrara, 2004). Gene therapies aimed at increasing VEGF expression have demonstrated improvements in blood flow, tissue repair, and muscle regeneration in preclinical models.For instance, in a study by Messina et al. (2007), intramuscular administration of recombinant adeno-associated virus (rAAV) encoding VEGF in mdx mice, a model for Duchenne muscular dystrophy, resulted in enhanced VEGF expression, increased capillary density, and improved muscle regeneration. This treatment led to a significant increase in forelimb strength and a reduction in necrotic muscle fibers, indicating the therapeutic potential of VEGF gene delivery in muscular disorders. Similarly, Arsic et al. (2004) demonstrated that delivery of VEGF via AAV vectors in mouse skeletal muscle not only promoted angiogenesis but also stimulated muscle fiber regeneration. Their findings revealed that VEGF expression led to the appearance of regenerating muscle fibers characterized by central nuclei and increased muscle fiber cross-sectional area, suggesting a direct role of VEGF in muscle repair mechanisms. Furthermore, in a rabbit model of acute limb trauma, VEGF administration improved muscle force restoration and reduced connective tissue deposition, highlighting its role in enhancing muscle regeneration and functional recovery post-injury(Frey et al., 2012). A study by Zeng et al. (2024) utilized genome editing of VEGFA to prevent corneal neovascularization in vivo, demonstrating the therapeutic potential of precise VEGF modulation in ocular diseases.Administering this dual AAV-SpCas9/sgRNA-VEGFA system via subconjunctival injection effectively suppressed the suture-triggered upregulation of VEGFA, CD31, and α-smooth muscle actin, along with inhibiting corneal neovascularization in mice.These studies collectively underscore the therapeutic potential of VEGF-based gene therapies in mitigating age-related vascular and muscular degeneration by promoting angiogenesis, enhancing tissue perfusion, and facilitating muscle regeneration.

TERT AND APOE IN TELOMERE EXTENSION AND CHOLESTEROL METABOLISM

TERT and APOE are two genes with well-documented roles in cellular aging through their effects on telomere maintenance and lipid metabolism, respectively.

TERT (Telomerase Revesrse Transcriptase)

TERT is the enzyme component of telomerase that plays a key role in preserving the length of telomeres. As cells divide, telomeres gradually shorten, and when they reach a critically short length, the cell enters a state known as senescence. Telomerase activity is primarily limited to stem cells and certain immune cells, with most somatic cells experiencing gradual telomere shortening. However, telomerase activation through TERT has shown potential to reverse cellular aging by extending telomeres, thereby prolonging cellular lifespan and improving tissue regeneration capacity. Pre-clinical studies have shown that TERT expression in aging cells can delay senescence and reduce markers of cellular aging, providing a promising strategy for anti-aging therapies. For instance, TERT overexpression in animal models has improved liver function, enhanced cardiac regeneration, and reduced neurodegenerative decline (Shay & Wright, 2011).

A telomerase gene therapy was evaluated in adult (1-year-old) and aged (2-year-old) mice using a broadly tropic AAV vector encoding catalytically active mouse telomerase (mTERT). The treatment yielded significant improvements in molecular aging biomarkers and overall physiological health in both age groups. Importantly, there was no increase in tumor incidence among mTERT-treated mice compared to controls, suggesting that telomerase-associated tumorigenicity is markedly reduced when administered later in life. Moreover, median lifespan was seen to have a surge by 24% in adult mice and 13% in old mice, effects that were not replicated by control vectors expressing either eGFP or a catalytically inactive TERT variant, underscoring the necessity of enzymatically active telomerase for therapeutic efficacy (Bernardes de Jesus et al., 2012).

APOE (Apolipoprotein E)

APOE is a critical gene in lipid metabolism, with three main allelic forms (E2, E3, and E4)(Mahley & Rall, 2000). Recent experimental studies underscore the therapeutic potential of targeting APOE alleles to mitigate neurodegenerative and cardiovascular pathology. For instance, Jackson et al. (2024) demonstrated that gene therapy delivering the protective APOE2 allele into the brains of APP/PS1 mice expressing human APOE4 significantly reduced amyloid-β plaque deposition, decreased microglial activation, and ameliorated synaptic loss, despite continued expression of APOE4. Similarly, Hudry et al. (2013) explored the effects of different human APOE isoforms on amyloid deposition and neurotoxicity in mouse brains. By using AAV vectors to express APOE2, APOE3, or APOE4 in the brains of APP/PS1 transgenic mice, they observed that APOE2 expression led to a reduction in amyloid-beta levels and plaque burden, while APOE4 expression had the opposite effect.Phase I/II LX1001 trial of CNS APOE2 gene therapy is the first-in-human study, APOE4 homozygous Alzheimer's patients received a single intraparenchymal infusion of AAVrh.10-APOE2. At 6-month follow-up, CSF APOE2 rose dose-dependently, CSF tau biomarkers decreased by ~15%, and tau PET signal trended downward—all with an excellent safety profile (Lexeo Therapeutics, 2024).

ANTI-INFLAMMATORY GENES: NLRP3 AND INTERLEUKIN MODULATION

Chronic inflammation is a hallmark of aging and significantly contributes to the onset of age-related diseases. This ongoing, mild inflammatory state—referred to as "inflammaging"—has been linked to various conditions, including cardiovascular disease, neurodegeneration, and metabolic imbalances. Emerging anti-inflammatory gene therapies that target critical molecular pathways, such as the NLRP3 inflammasome and various interleukins, show promise in reducing the harmful impact of inflammation associated with aging (Franceschi et al., 2018; Liang et al., 2022).

The NLRP3 Inflammasome and Its Role in Aging

The NLRP3 inflammasome is a protein complex crucial for initiating inflammation. It responds to indicators of cellular stress—like oxidative damage, mitochondrial dysfunction, and protein misfolding—that are often present in aging tissues. Upon activation, NLRP3 promotes the release of pro-inflammatory cytokines, such as interleukin-1β (IL-1β) and interleukin-18 (IL-18), which amplify inflammation and can lead to tissue damage (Kaverina et al., 2023). NLRP3 activation contributes to atherosclerosis by promoting macrophage recruitment and foam cell formation, leading to plaque instability. In Alzheimer's disease, NLRP3 activation enhances amyloid-beta deposition and neuroinflammation, accelerating cognitive decline. NLRP3 contributes to insulin resistance and type II diabetes by promoting inflammation in adipose tissue and pancreatic islets. Researchers are exploring CRISPR-Cas9 to knock out NLRP3 in animal models, reducing systemic inflammation without impairing immune function. siRNA-based therapies targeting NLRP3 mRNA have shown efficacy in reducing inflammatory markers in preclinical models of atherosclerosis and Alzheimer's disease (Liang et al., 2022).

Interleukin Modulation in Anti-Aging Therapy

Interleukins are key mediators of the immune response, and their dysregulation contributes to chronic inflammation in aging. Gene therapies focusing on modulating interleukins aim to restore balance in immune signalling pathways.

Interleukin-1β (IL-1β). Increased levels of IL-1β are linked to chronic inflammatory states, contributing to conditions like arthritis, cardiovascular diseases, and neurodegeneration. AAV-mediated delivery of IL-1 receptor antagonists (IL-1Ra) has the potential to reduce inflammation and improve outcomes in preclinical models of arthritis and myocardial infarction(Evans, 2018).

Interleukin-10 (IL-10). IL-10 is an anti-inflammatory cytokine that is known to suppress pro-inflammatory signals, promoting tissue repair and immune homeostasis. Gene therapy approaches include delivering IL10 genes using lipid nanoparticles or AAVs. In rodent models, IL-10 gene therapy significantly reduced liver fibrosis and atherosclerosis (Kamaly et al., 2016).

Interleukin-6 (IL-6). While IL-6 is essential for immune defense, chronic elevation of IL-6 in aging is associated with inflammaging and muscle wasting (sarcopenia). CRISPR-based modulation of IL6 expression has shown efficacy in preclinical models, where reducing IL-6 levels alleviated inflammation and preserved muscle mass in aging animals (Pototschnig et al., 2023).

Mice with genetically inactivated NLRP3 showed extended lifespan, reduced systemic inflammation, and improved metabolic function. In Alzheimer's models, NLRP3 knockout reduced amyloid-beta plaques and neuroinflammation, improving cognitive performance (Liang et al., 2022). In models of atherosclerosis, IL-10 delivery reduced plaque size and improved arterial health by suppressing macrophage activity. IL-10 therapy also demonstrated anti-fibrotic effects in models of liver aging, reducing collagen deposition and restoring liver function. The potential synergy of NLRP3 and IL-10 is supported conceptually. For example: NLRP3 Suppression reduces pro-inflammatory cytokines like IL-1β and IL-18. IL-10 Therapy counters inflammation by modulating immune responses and suppressing cytokine overproduction (Volpatti et al., 2024).

RESULTS FROM EXPERIMENTAL STUDIES

KAT7 as a Therapeutic Target for Cellular Senescence and Lifespan Extension

A CRISPR-Cas9 screen in human mesenchymal precursor cells (hMPCs) from premature aging models identified the histone acetyltransferase KAT7 as a key regulator of cellular senescence. Inactivating KAT7 reduced histone H3 lysine 14 acetylation (H3K14ac), suppressed the senescence-related gene $p15^{INK4b}$, and reversed senescence markers in progeroid hMPCs. This included increased cell proliferation, fewer SA-β-gal positive cells, reduced expression of $p16^{INK4A}$ and $p21^{CIP1}$, and lower levels of SASP factors. Furthermore, in vivo gene therapy targeting Kat7 extended lifespan in both naturally aged and progeroid mice, demonstrating its therapeutic potential in combating age-related decline through modulation of the H3K14ac-$p15^{INK4b}$ senescence pathway (Wang et al., 2021).

Transcriptomic Modulation in Canine Models

This study identifies 61 age-associated genes (A-AGs) in domestic dogs, predominantly linked to metabolic regulation and immune function, indicating their potential as key molecular biomarkers of canine aging. To assess anti-aging interventions, aged dogs were treated with canine mesenchymal stem cells (cMSCs), rapamycin (Rapa), and nicotinamide mononucleotide (NMN). Among these, cMSC therapy yielded the most pronounced effects, significantly improving cardiac function and reducing pro-inflammatory cytokines IL-6 and TNF-α, while NMN and Rapa also attenuated inflammation but to a lesser extent. Transcriptomic analyses revealed that cMSC treatment modulated pathways involved in cell cycle regulation, myeloid cell differentiation, and immune cell function, suggesting that its therapeutic effects are mediated through mechanisms targeting cellular senescence and immune remodeling. These findings support the utility of domestic dogs as a translational model for studying the interplay between inflammation, metabolism, and aging, and position cMSCs as a promising intervention for age-associated physiological decline (Zeng et al., 2024).

Inducible OSK Gene Therapy Extends Lifespan

A gene therapy approach using adeno-associated viruses (AAVs) to deliver an inducible OSK (OCT4, SOX2, KLF4) system can significantly extend lifespan and improve health parameters in extremely aged (124-week-old) wild-type mice. The resesrchers found that the OSK treatment led to a 109% increase in median remaining lifespan compared to control mice, as well as a significant reduction in a frailty index score, indicating an overall improvement in health and function. Further, the authors showed that exogenous expression of OSK in human keratinocytes resulted in profound epigenetic age reversal, suggesting that partial reprogramming can restore a more youthful cellular state. This provides a potential mechanistic explanation for how the OSK treatment was able to reverse age-related changes and extend lifespan in the aged mice. Extended partial reprogramming resulted in transcriptomic alterations characterized by decreased expression of genes linked to inflammation, cellular aging, and stress response mechanisms. Complementary metabolomic and lipidomic analyses showed that this intervention reversed age-related alterations in systemic metabolism and lipid profiles. Functionally, it enhanced skin wound healing by promoting epidermal cell proliferation and reducing fibrosis. In contrast, short-term reprogramming (one month) had minimal effects, indicating a potential "window of opportunity" for effective rejuvenation. These findings support partial reprogramming as a promising and safe approach to mitigate aging phenotypes in wild-type mice (Browder et al., 2022). In the pancreas, where OSKM factors are strongly expressed, just one cycle of temporary OSKM activation was enough to reverse age-associated alterations in DNA methylation and gene expression, especially in pathways related to mTOR signaling, DNA repair, and collagen synthesis.Serum metabolomic analysis further revealed reversal of age-altered metabolites—4-hydroxyproline, thymine, trimethyl-lysine, and indole-3-propionic acid—highlighting systemic rejuvenation. Overall, transient OSKM expression can induce epigenetic, transcriptomic, and metabolic shifts toward a more youthful state across multiple tissues and in the bloodstream, though additional studies are needed to clarify the underlying mechanisms (Chondronasiou et al., 2022).

FGF and sTGFβR2 in Multiple Diseases

In preclinical studies, gene therapy targeting longevity-associated pathways using Fibroblast Growth Factor 21 (FGF21) and soluble TGFβ receptor 2 (sTGFβR2) has demonstrated significant potential in mitigating multiple age-related disorders and extending healthspan in mice. Specifically, FGF21 has been shown to improve metabolic function by enhancing insulin sensitivity, lowering blood glucose levels, and reducing lipid accumulation in models of type II diabetes (Kharitonenkov et al., 2005; Zhang et al., 2012). Its additional benefits on hepatic function and inflammation reduction further underscore its therapeutic potential in metabolic aging. When combined with sTGFβR2, which inhibits pro-fibrotic TGFβ signaling, FGF21 therapy has also led to substantial improvements in kidney atrophy by preserving renal architecture, reducing fibrosis, and lowering inflammatory markers (Davidsohn et al., 2019). Moreover, this dual therapy has shown broad-spectrum efficacy in addressing various aging hallmarks, such as mitochondrial dysfunction, chronic inflammation, and cellular senescence. For instance, in neurodegenerative models, FGF21 enhances synaptic plasticity and reduces oxidative stress, while sTGFβR2 dampens neuroinflammation (Hsuchou et al., 2007). The combination also improves cardiovascular health by modulating lipid metabolism and vascular inflammation, leading to reduced atherosclerotic lesions and improved vascular function (Tezze et al., 2019). These findings collectively demonstrate that FGF21 and sTGFβR2 therapies not only target individual age-related conditions but offer a systemic approach to delaying aging processes and improving healthspan in mammalian models.

Clinical Trials and Case Studies

Gene therapy has become a groundbreaking method for treating neurodegenerative disorders by directly targeting their molecular and genetic roots. Recent case studies have demonstrated notable progress in conditions like Alzheimer's, Parkinson's disease, and frontotemporal dementia.

AAV2-shmTOR Gene Therapy in Macular Degeneration

A recent investigation explored CRG-01 (AAV2-shmTOR), a gene therapy designed to modulate mTOR signaling, for its potential to combat oxidative stress and inflammation in age-related macular degeneration (AMD). CRG-01 showed encouraging results, reducing inflammation in various cell types linked to AMD, indicating its potential as a viable treatment. Unlike conventional anti-VEGF therapies, which primarily address vascular issues, AAV2-shmTOR targets the underlying inflammatory and oxidative mechanisms that drive disease progression. It effectively reduced pro-inflammatory cytokines like IL-6 and IL-1β, suppressed NF-κB activity, and maintained the integrity of endothelial tight junctions in retinal cells under TNF-α-induced stress. The study emphasizes the benefits of AAV-based gene therapies, including sustained therapeutic effects and fewer required treatments. Early safety evaluations in non-human primates revealed promising outcomes, suggesting the approach is well-tolerated. Researchers also propose that AAV2-shmTOR could be adapted to treat other retinal diseases involving similar pathological features. Nonetheless, comprehensive clinical trials are necessary to fully establish its safety and therapeutic effectiveness in AMD (Kim et al., 2025).

Alzheimer's Disease: BDNF & APOE4-Targetted Gene Therapy

A pioneering Phase I clinical trial conducted at UC San Diego is exploring the application of adeno-associated virus (AAV)-based gene therapy to deliver brain-derived neurotrophic factor (BDNF) as a potential treatment for Alzheimer's disease (AD). BDNF, critical for neuronal survival and synaptic function, is delivered directly to the entorhinal cortex and hippocampus—regions severely affected in AD. Preclinical studies in aged rats and amyloid-mouse models demonstrated that BDNF delivery preserved neuronal connections and reduced degeneration. Initial clinical results are focused on assessing safety, with hopes to rebuild neural circuits and slow cognitive decline. The trial seeks to assess whether delivering BDNF can safeguard neurons, maintain synaptic function, and potentially slow or stop the progression of early-stage Alzheimer's disease. BDNF is a naturally produced protein that plays a vital role in promoting neuron survival, development, and synaptic adaptability. Its levels are significantly reduced in Alzheimer's, contributing to cognitive decline. By reintroducing BDNF via gene therapy, the approach hopes to restore these essential functions. Prior studies in aged rodents and non-human primates demonstrated that BDNF delivery preserved brain volume, improved synaptic activity, and showed potential for neuroprotection, laying the groundwork for this human trial. Unlike traditional Alzheimer's treatments, which target symptoms or specific pathologies (e.g., amyloid plaques), this gene therapy aims to regenerate neural connections and directly address neuronal health. If successful, this trial could set a precedent for using gene therapy in treating other neurodegenerative diseases and highlight the therapeutic potential of neurotrophic factors (LaFee, 2021). As of October 2024, preliminary findings shared at the Clinical Trials on Alzheimer's Disease (CTAD) conference revealed that four participants had successfully received the gene therapy treatment—two with unilateral and two with bilateral infusions. MRI scans confirmed accurate targeting and appropriate vector distribution. No significant adverse events, including seizures, were reported up to 15 months post-treatment. Notably, in the first participant assessed with FDG-PET imaging, there was a 14% increase in metabolic activity on the treated side of the brain, suggesting potential functional improvements (Alzforum, 2024; UC San Diego Health, 2021). The trial is expected to complete the surgical interventions for AD patients by December 2024, with the MCI cohort's treatments anticipated to conclude in 2025. Final study completion is projected for October 2027 (Tuszynski, n.d.).

Preliminary findings from a Phase 1/2 clinical trial of LX1001, an AAV-delivered gene therapy designed to introduce APOE2 into the central nervous system of patients with Alzheimer's disease who are APOE4 homozygous, demonstrated a favorable safety profile and dose-dependent APOE2 expression. The therapy led to reductions in CSF tau biomarkers and tau PET signal in most participants, with no serious adverse events or amyloid-related imaging abnormalities. These findings suggest LX1001 may offer a novel, targeted approach to modifying disease progression in a high-risk AD population currently lacking approved therapies (Meglio, 2024).

Glutamic Acid Decarboxylase (GAD) Therapy for Parkinson's Disease

GAD therapy utilizes adeno-associated virus serotype 2 (AAV2) to introduce the GAD gene into the subthalamic nucleus of the brain. This gene produces an enzyme responsible for converting glutamate into gamma-aminobutyric acid (GABA), a key neurotransmitter involved in regulating motor function. By restoring GABAergic activity, the therapy aims to rebalance the overactive neural circuits contributing to Parkinson's disease symptoms. Clinical trials demonstrated that patients receiving GAD gene therapy showed significant improvements in motor functions, including reduced tremors and rigidity, compared to control groups. Beyond symptomatic relief, GAD therapy also exhibits potential for protecting dopaminergic neurons, slowing the progression of Parkinson's disease. Trials have consistently shown that AAV2-GAD therapy is well-tolerated, with minimal adverse effects, making it a viable candidate for broader clinical applications. This therapy is particularly promising for patients who are resistant to conventional treatments, such as levodopa. It provides a novel mechanism to enhance dopamine activity indirectly by modulating GABAergic pathways, highlighting its potential as a non-invasive and durable treatment option (Niethammer et al., 2017).

Trials investigating Age-Related Macular Degeneration (AMD)

Multiple early-stage clinical trials are currently in progress to assess the safety and effectiveness of gene therapy treatments for nAMD. One such approach involves the intravitreal injection of AAV2-sFLT01, which delivers a gene encoding an anti-angiogenic fusion protein designed to neutralize VEGF-A. This approach was found to be safe but did not show significant anatomical or functional improvements (Heier et al., 2017). Subretinal injection of AAV (rAAV).sFLT-1 vector encoding the natural soluble FLT-1 protein that neutralizes VEGF-A. This was also found to be safe but did not show significant improvements (Rakoczy et al., 2015; Rakoczy et al., 2019; Constable et al., 2017). Adeno-associated virus (AAV) delivers eNdi1, a modified NADH dehydrogenase gene, to enhance mitochondrial oxidative phosphorylation (OXPHOS) in retinal ganglion cells (RGCs) and retinal pigment epithelium (RPE). This reduces reactive oxygen species (ROS) and improves ATP synthesis. Restored RGC function in murine glaucoma models (intraocular pressure reduction: 25%) and improved RPE survival in dry AMD models. Phase I/II trials are planned by Vzarii Therapeutics for glaucoma and AMD (NCT05678945) (Millington-Ward et al., 2024). Intravitreal injection of ADVM-022, an AAV-based aflibercept gene therapy. This showed promising results in maintaining visual acuity and reducing the need for rescue treatment, but was later discontinued due to safety concerns in a separate trial for diabetic macular edema. Subretinal injection of RGX-314, an AAV-based gene therapy encoding a soluble anti-VEGF monoclonal antibody fragment. This demonstrated a good safety profile and sustained expression of the therapeutic protein, with some improvements in visual acuity and reduced need for rescue treatment. Subretinal injection of RetinoStat, a lentiviral vector encoding endostatin and angiostatin. This was found to be safe and well-tolerated, with sustained expression of the anti-angiogenic proteins, but did not show significant functional improvements. Gene silencing approaches using small interfering RNA (siRNA) targeting VEGF or its receptors have been explored, but have not advanced beyond early clinical trials due to limitations like short-term effects and potential off-target effects. Gene editing technologies like CRISPR-Cas9 are being investigated for their potential in treating nAMD, but clinical trials are still lacking (Finocchio et al., 2023).

CRISPR-Edited Allogeneic CAR-T (CTX130) for T Cell Lymphoma

CRISPR-Cas9 disrupts CD70 (tumor antigen) and PD-1 (immune checkpoint) in donor T cells, enhancing antitumor activity against CD70+ lymphomas common in elderly patients. In individuals with T-cell lymphoma who have undergone extensive prior treatment, CTX130 demonstrated a manageable safety profile and a promising rate of objective responses. Allogeneic CAR T cells, which are easily accessible, can be administered safely to patients with relapsed or refractory T-cell lymphoma. Regarding safety concerns, no graft-vs-host disease (GvHD) observed due to TRAC locus knockout. Additionally, a next-generation CAR T-cell therapy featuring enhanced potency gene modifications (CTX131) is currently in clinical trials (Iyer et al., 2025).

Clonal Hematopoiesis in ADA-SCID Gene Therapy

While ADA-SCID is not considered an age-related condition, it typically appears in newborns and infants, with gene therapy becoming a key early intervention to address the root genetic defect. Adenosine deaminase severe combined immunodeficiency (ADA-SCID) is a rare inherited disorder of the immune system, caused by mutations in the ADA gene, which result in the buildup of toxic metabolites and impaired development of immune cells. Participants who undergo gene therapy for ADA-SCID may not have any detectable clonal hematopoiesis (CHIP) mutations, as none were found in the 10 ADA-SCID participants evaluated. However, one participant did show a significant decrease in telomere length after the gene therapy, suggesting potential cellular aging effects. Further studies are needed to fully assess the risk of malignancy in gene therapy patients, as some participants may have underlying germline genetic variants that could increase cancer risk (White et al., 2022).

Table 3. Case studies for gene therapy in various aging-related diseases, including successes, failures, and mixed results

Disease	Gene Therapy	Study Design	Outcomes	Source
Alzheimer's Disease	NGF Gene Therapy (Nerve Growth Factor)	Phase I trial in AD patients (n=8). NGF delivered intraventricularly	- Cognitive improvement in some patients - Severe adverse effects (back pain, weight loss)	PMC: Gene Therapy in Alzheimer's Disease
Alzheimer's Disease	Lanabecestat (BACE Inhibitor)	Phase II/III trials (n=2,200+ AD patients)	- Reduced amyloid-β (Aβ) levels - No cognitive or functional improvement; trials terminated	SAGE: Key Insights from Clinical Trial Failures
Parkinson's Disease	AAV-GAD (Glutamic Acid Decarboxylase)	Phase I trial (n=12 PD patients). GAD delivered to the subthalamic nucleus via AAV	- Improved motor function (UPDRS ↓25%) - No major side effects	Weill Cornell: Parkinson's Gene Therapy Trial
Parkinson's Disease	VY-AADC01 (Aromatic L-Amino Acid Decarboxylase)	Phase Ib trial (n=15 PD patients). AADC delivered via AAV2 to striatum.	- Stabilized motor function. - Reduced levodopa requirements by 21–30%.	Neurology: Safety of AADC Gene Therapy
Cancer	HSV-TK + Ganciclovir	Phase I trials for prostate cancer and glioma.	- Tumor regression in some patients. - Chemoresistance developed in others	PMC: Gene Therapies for Cancer
Cancer	CAR-T Therapy (CRISPR-edited anti-CD19 CAR-T with PD-1 Knockout)	Phase I/II trial for non-Hodgkin lymphoma (n=16)	- 44% complete remission at 6+ months - No graft-vs-host disease due to TRAC knockout	The Lancet: Gene therapy targeting tau pathology

(Nilsson et al., 2010; Kim et al., 2022; Kaplitt, 2007; Christine et al., 2022; Das et al., 2015; Hu et al., 2023)

Note. The table categorizes therapies by disease type, therapy mechanism, study design, outcomes, and success/failure status. It highlights both successful and failed attempts, providing a balanced view of gene therapy progress for aging-related diseases.

Huntington's Disease (HD) and HTT Gene

Gene therapy strategies for Huntington's disease (HD) aim to lower levels of the mutant Huntingtin (HTT) protein, which builds up in the brain and leads to neurodegeneration. Recent research has investigated the use of RNA interference (RNAi) techniques delivered via adeno-associated virus (AAV) vectors to achieve this reduction.

Artificial MicroRNA (miRNA) Delivery via AAV Vectors. Researchers utilized AAV5 to deliver miRNAs that selectively target the mutant HTT allele while sparing the wild-type allele. This specificity reduces the risk of silencing normal HTT functions, which are essential for cellular health. Preclinical studies in HD mouse models have shown a significant reduction in mutant HTT protein levels, improved motor function, and reduced neurodegeneration (Miniarikova et al., 2017).

Short Hairpin RNA (shRNA) Therapy. Another approach involves embedding shRNA sequences into a miRNA scaffold for delivery via AAVs. This method enables sustained silencing of mutant HTT alleles with minimal off-target effects. Studies reported long-lasting therapeutic effects, including decreased neuronal cell death and improved behavioral outcomes in rodent HD models. AAV vectors offer high transduction efficiency in the brain and long-term gene expression with low immunogenicity. Serotypes like AAV5 and AAV9 are particularly effective in delivering therapies to the striatum, a brain region heavily affected in HD (Aguiar, van der Gaag, & Cortese, 2017).

Applications in Cardiovascular Aging and Repair

Cardiovascular aging contributes to conditions such as atherosclerosis, heart failure, and arterial stiffness. Gene therapy offers new opportunities to mitigate these issues by targeting molecular pathways involved in vascular repair and cardiac function.

VEGF-Based Angiogenesis for Ischemic Heart Disease

Vascular endothelial growth factor (VEGF) gene therapy has been applied to stimulate angiogenesis in ischemic tissues. Preclinical studies using AAV vectors delivering VEGF have shown improved blood vessel formation and tissue perfusion in animal models. Clinical applications aim to restore oxygen supply in patients with coronary artery disease, with ongoing trials evaluating its efficacy in reducing myocardial infarction risk (Florek, Mendyka, & Gomułka, 2024).

SDF-1 Gene Therapy for Heart Regeneration

Stromal cell-derived factor-1 (SDF-1) plays an important role in recruiting progenitor cells to damaged cardiac tissue. Gene therapies utilizing plasmid-based delivery of SDF-1 have shown potential in enhancing cardiac repair post-myocardial infarction. These approaches aim to improve heart function and reduce scar formation, addressing a major cause of heart failure in aging populations (Sundararaman et al., 2011).

Anti-Fibrotic Gene Therapy

Cardiac fibrosis is a hallmark of aging and heart disease, characterized by excess extracellular matrix deposition that stiffens the heart muscle. Gene editing tools like CRISPR-Cas9 are being explored to target genes involved in fibrotic pathways, such as TGF-β. Early preclinical studies indicate reduced fibrosis and improved cardiac compliance, making this a promising avenue for managing cardiovascular aging (Biernacka &Frangogiannis, 2011).

Telomere Therapy in Vascular Aging

Shortened telomeres are associated with vascular aging and endothelial dysfunction. Therapies aimed at upregulating telomerase activity (via TERT gene delivery) are under investigation to enhance endothelial health and prevent arterial stiffening. These interventions focus on maintaining vascular elasticity, potentially reducing hypertension and age-related cardiovascular complications. These advancements in gene therapy for neurodegenerative and cardiovascular diseases highlight the versatility of this technology in addressing complex age-related conditions. While challenges remain, such as delivery efficiency and long-term safety, ongoing research underscores the transformative potential of gene therapy in extending healthspan and treating aging-associated disorders (Shay & Wright, 2011). In the case of Liz Parrish, CEO of BioViva, she received both TERT and Follistatin gene therapies simultaneously. TERT was for Improved regenerative capacity and possibly longer lifespan (shown in animal models). Follistatin inhibits myostatin, a protein that limits muscle growth. It increases muscle mass and strength, combating sarcopenia (age-related muscle loss) (Regalado, 2015).

There are no mainstream, FDA-approved gene therapies currently in real-world use specifically for age-related diseases, except for Luxturna, which is technically for a rare inherited retinal condition but shows crossover into age-related vision therapy tech. Luxturna employs an adeno-associated viral vector to introduce a working version of the RPE65 gene into retinal cells, allowing them to produce the essential protein for vision and thereby restoring the visual cycle. Unofficial therapies (TERT, Follistatin) have been used in real people via experimental clinics, but not through official medical systems.

ETHICAL CONSIDERATIONS IN HUMAN TRIALS

Gene therapy for aging introduces a variety of ethical concerns, from questions about long-term societal impacts to issues surrounding access, safety, and consent in older populations.

Defining "Normal Aging" vs. Disease

One central ethical question is the distinction between treating a disease and modifying the natural aging process. While certain aspects of aging overlap with pathologies, such as cognitive decline or weakened immune function, other aspects are part of "normal" aging. Defining the line between these two raises ethical concerns regarding the extent of intervention allowed. If aging is targeted as a "disease," this may pressure society to pursue anti-aging interventions, leading to potential overmedicalization.

Equity and Accessibility

Gene therapies, particularly those targeting aging, could be prohibitively expensive. This raises questions about equitable access and whether such therapies would be available to only a privileged few. High costs may deepen health disparities and present ethical dilemmas regarding who gets access to potentially life-extending treatments. Public funding or regulatory policies promoting universal access could help mitigate these disparities but require careful planning to ensure resource allocation benefits society as a whole (Parens, 2015).

Informed Consent in Aging Populations

Gene therapy trials often require comprehensive informed consent due to the experimental nature and associated risks. For elderly participants, cognitive decline or impaired decision-making capabilities can complicate the consent process. Ensuring that participants fully understand the potential risks, benefits, and uncertainties of gene therapy for aging is essential but challenging. This requires rigorous ethical oversight, including third-party assessments and additional safeguards to confirm participants' comprehension and voluntariness.

Long-Term Societal and Environmental Impacts

If gene therapy for aging becomes successful and widely accessible, it could lead to a significant increase in life expectancy, which would have implications for social and environmental systems. Extended human lifespans could strain resources, healthcare, and social security systems. Additionally, prolonging life without corresponding enhancements in healthspan could lead to prolonged periods of morbidity. Ethical discussions must address these broader societal impacts, taking a holistic view of the potential ramifications of widespread gene therapy for aging (Post & Binstock, 2004).

TECHNICAL LIMITATIONS IN TARGETED GENE DELIVERY

Successful gene therapy depends on the precise delivery of therapeutic genes to specific cells or tissues, which presents unique challenges in the context of aging.

Targeting Specific Cell Types

Aging affects various tissues, including muscle, brain, skin, and immune cells, each with unique gene expression profiles and cellular environments. Delivering genes specifically to target cells without affecting surrounding tissues is difficult. Current viral vectors may lack the specificity needed to target only the intended cells, leading to potential off-target effects that increase the risk of side effects. New approaches, such as cell-specific promoters or tissue-targeting peptides, are being developed to enhance delivery specificity (Mendell et al., 2017).

Crossing the Blood-Brain Barrier (BBB)

Many age-related diseases, such as Alzheimer's, require therapeutic gene delivery to the brain. However, the blood-brain barrier (BBB) inhibits most therapeutic drugs from reaching brain tissues. Overcoming this barrier without invasive procedures is a major challenge in targeting neurological aspects of aging. Advanced techniques, such as focused ultrasound and nanoparticle-mediated delivery, are being explored to temporarily open the BBB or facilitate crossing for gene therapy applications in neurodegenerative diseases.

Limited Gene Payload Capacity

Viral vectors like AAVs have limited capacity for carrying therapeutic genes, restricting the types and number of genes that can be delivered in a single treatment. This is particularly challenging for aging, where multiple genes may need to be targeted simultaneously. Lentiviral vectors offer greater payload capacity, but they have integration risks, potentially causing insertional mutagenesis. Scientists are exploring non-viral delivery methods like nanoparticles or combining smaller gene therapies in tandem to address this limitation (Schlimgen et al., 2016).

Controlled and Sustained Gene Expression

Aging therapies may require long-term gene expression, especially for genes involved in cellular repair and resilience. However, achieving sustained expression without continuous intervention is challenging. Viral vectors may result in transient expression due to immune responses, while integrated vectors like lentiviruses have a risk of unwanted insertional effects. Researchers are investigating "on-demand" expression systems using inducible promoters, allowing gene expression to be activated only when needed, thus offering more control over therapeutic effects.

Off-Target Effects and Genomic Instability

Off-target effects continue to pose a challenge, especially with gene-editing tools like CRISPR-Cas9. Unintended edits to genes or regulatory regions can result in unpredictable consequences, including the disruption of vital cellular activities or the initiation of tumor formation. To address these risks, scientists are advancing next-generation CRISPR systems with greater accuracy and are exploring alternative editing technologies like base editors and prime editors, which allow for more precise genetic alterations with fewer potential side effects (Hsu et al., 2014).

Delivery Challenges and Tissue Specificity

Achieving efficient, cell-type-specific delivery while avoiding off-target transduction remains a major hurdle. Some tissues (e.g., the brain, skeletal muscle, or aged organs with reduced vascularization) are poorly accessible to current delivery systems, even with engineered viral vectors or lipid nanoparticles (Wang et al., 2019).

Immunogenicity of Vectors

Pre-existing immunity to viral vectors like AAVs or strong host immune responses can neutralize therapeutic vectors or lead to inflammatory complications, limiting repeat dosing or long-term expression (Mingozzi& High, 2011).

Durability and Regulation of Expression

Aging-related therapies often require long-term or tightly controlled gene expression, yet current vectors may offer only transient activity or lack inducible systems. Unregulated expression of genes like TERT or OSK can cause unwanted cell proliferation or dedifferentiation (Lu et al., 2020).

Scalability and Manufacturing Complexities

The production of clinical-grade vectors or delivery systems at scale, with consistent quality and batch-to-batch reproducibility, remains a logistical and regulatory bottleneck (Naldini, 2015).

SOCIETAL AND ECONOMIC CHALLENGES IN THERAPY ACCESSIBILITY

Gene therapies, including those targeting aging and age-related diseases, have shown transformative potential. However, their accessibility is fraught with significant societal and economic challenges. These barriers must be addressed to ensure equitable distribution and implementation of these life-extending treatments.

High Costs of Development and Treatment

One of the primary obstacles to therapy accessibility is the immense cost of development, clinical trials, and subsequent treatment. Gene therapies are inherently expensive due to:

Research and Development Costs. Developing a single gene therapy requires billions of dollars over decades. For example, the clinical development of therapies like Zolgensma for spinal muscular atrophy reportedly cost $2.1 million per patient due to the complexity of production and individualized dosing strategies. Gene therapies often require personalized approaches, such as custom viral vector production, which adds to the cost burden. Scaled-up manufacturing remains a challenge, further increasing the price tag(Cohen, 2019).

Regulatory and Approval Costs. Extensive preclinical testing, regulatory reviews, and post-market surveillance add financial strain. Small biotech companies often struggle to balance profitability with accessibility, leading to exorbitant pricing.

Socioeconomic Disparities

Gene therapies are not equally accessible to all socioeconomic groups. Economic disparities manifest in various ways:

Income Inequality. High-income individuals and countries are more likely to access cutting-edge therapies, while low-income populations are excluded due to financial constraints.

Insurance Gaps. Even in developed countries, access often depends on whether insurers cover these therapies. Gene therapies' high upfront costs make insurers reluctant to cover them, leaving uninsured or underinsured patients without options.

Global Disparities. While gene therapy trials and treatments are concentrated in wealthier nations, developing countries struggle to adopt these innovations due to infrastructure limitations and financial constraints.

Ethical and Societal Resistance

Gene therapies raise ethical concerns, such as:

Equity and Fairness. Critics argue that life-extending therapies could exacerbate societal inequalities, as only wealthy individuals might benefit from longer lifespans.

Cultural Perceptions. In some cultures, genetic manipulation is viewed with skepticism or outright opposition, leading to resistance against these treatments.

Risk of Exploitation. There are concerns about exploitative practices, such as clinical trials targeting vulnerable populations who may not benefit directly from the research findings.

Sustainability of Health

The introduction of high-cost gene therapies places immense pressure on public healthcare systems:

Budget Constraints. Governments face challenges in prioritizing funding for gene therapies over other essential healthcare services.

Long-Term Commitments. Many gene therapies promise lifelong benefits but require substantial upfront investment, posing financial sustainability issues for insurers and public health systems.

Lack of Public Awareness and Education. Public understanding of gene therapy remains limited, hindering its acceptance:

Misinformation. Myths and misconceptions about gene editing and genetic modification can deter adoption.

Limited Outreach. Insufficient patient education initiatives fail to inform the public about the benefits and limitations of gene therapies, leading to hesitancy.

Strategies to Address Accessibility

Policy and Pricing Innovations

Outcome-Based Pricing Models. Linking payment to therapeutic success could make treatments more affordable while ensuring cost-effectiveness.

Government Subsidies: Increased funding for gene therapy development can lower costs and improve accessibility.

Expanding Global Access. Encouraging technology transfer to developing countries can help establish local manufacturing and reduce dependency on imports.

International organizations could play a role in financing and distributing these therapies globally.

Strengthening Healthcare Infrastructure. Investments in treatment facilities, logistics, and training programs can enable broader delivery of gene therapies.

Public Engagement. Comprehensive education campaigns can dispel myths, address ethical concerns, and build societal trust in gene therapies.

Ethical Frameworks. Developing global ethical guidelines can ensure equitable access and prevent exploitation.

The World Health Organization (WHO) launched the "Decade of Healthy Ageing (2021–2030)" as a comprehensive global initiative aimed at improving the lives of older people, their families, and the communities in which they live. Recognizing the rapid increase in the aging population worldwide, WHO emphasizes that aging should not be seen solely as a medical issue, but as a multidimensional challenge involving health systems, social structures, and community support networks. The initiative defines "healthy ageing" as "the process of developing and maintaining the functional ability that enables well-being in older age." This goes beyond just the absence of disease and includes aspects like mobility, mental well-being, social participation, and access to supportive environments. The WHO urges global societies to move away from ageist attitudes and stereotypes. This involves promoting inclusive narratives that value the contribution of older adults. Health systems are encouraged to shift from disease-based models to person-centered care, including chronic disease management, long-term care, and rehabilitative services. The WHO promotes equitable access to quality long-term care, especially for those with significant functional declines, ensuring dignity and support for caregivers. The Decade of Healthy Ageing aligns with the UN Sustainable Development Goals (SDGs), particularly those related to health (SDG 3), inequality (SDG 10), and sustainable cities (SDG 11). It also provides a policy roadmap for national governments, researchers, and health practitioners to design and implement aging interventions at both the individual and systemic levels. This initiative underscores the holistic nature of aging interventions—they are not limited to biomedical solutions but include social policies, infrastructure, caregiver support, and public awareness. For scientists and healthcare professionals, this opens up interdisciplinary pathways for intervention design and collaborative research (World Health Organization, 2020).

When it comes to the development and approval of aging-related interventions, regulatory pathways differ significantly across countries, particularly between the FDA in the United States and the EMA in the European Union. These differences can influence how quickly therapies reach the public, how they are evaluated for efficacy and safety, and even how "aging" is conceptualized in terms of disease. Traditionally, the FDA does not recognize aging itself as a disease. This presents a regulatory challenge for companies developing anti-aging drugs or interventions aimed purely at life extension. As a result, many developers focus on specific age-related diseases (e.g., Alzheimer's, sarcopenia) to gain approval. Similarly, the EMA does not currently recognize aging as a disease, but it has shown more flexibility in considering biomarkers of aging in the evaluation of geriatric medicines, especially in the context of orphan drugs and complex therapies. FDA offers pathways such as Fast Track, Breakthrough Therapy, and Regenerative Medicine Advanced Therapy (RMAT) designations, which can accelerate development if an intervention addresses a serious or life-threatening condition. EMA provides designations like PRIME (PRIorityMEdicines) and Accelerated Assessment, which similarly aim to support innovative therapies. However, EMA tends to emphasize post-marketing safety and real-world data more strongly than the FDA. FDA typically requires larger, more standardized randomized controlled trials (RCTs) to demonstrate efficacy and safety, with strict endpoints. EMA may accept adaptive trial designs and has, in some cases, shown more openness to surrogate endpoints, especially for geriatric indications or where long-term data is difficult to obtain due to population age. The U.S. framework is more driven by innovation and private-sector investment, often leading to quicker but more fragmented regulatory responses. The EU framework, represented by the EMA, tends to balance innovation with social equity and cost-effectiveness, as health systems are publicly funded in most member states.

While gene therapies offer unparalleled promise in combating aging and extending healthspan, their societal and economic challenges demand urgent attention. By addressing issues of cost, infrastructure, and equity, stakeholders can ensure these life-changing therapies are accessible to all, regardless of socioeconomic status or geographic location. Collaborative efforts among governments, industries, and global organizations will be crucial to overcoming these barriers and fulfilling the potential of gene therapy for aging and other diseases.

CHALLENGES AND FUTURE PERSPECTIVES

Gene therapy has shown promise in addressing age-related conditions, but the transition from preclinical research to practical application is challenging. Aging poses specific obstacles for gene therapy, including immunogenicity, ethical considerations, and technical limitations. The following is an in-depth examination of the challenges and their potential impact on the future development of anti-aging gene therapies. One of the primary obstacles is the immune response, which poses a significant risk, particularly when using viral vectors for gene delivery. While viral vectors such as adeno-associated viruses (AAVs) and lentiviruses are highly efficient at transporting genetic material into target cells, they can also trigger immune reactions that may compromise the safety and efficacy of the treatment. However, they can provoke an immune response that reduces therapeutic efficacy and introduces risks of inflammation and toxicity. Many individuals have pre-existing immunity to certain viral vectors, especially AAVs, due to prior exposure. The immune system may recognize the vector as foreign, triggering an immune reaction that can neutralize the therapy before it reaches target cells (Mingozzi& High, 2013). This is particularly challenging for aging populations who may have higher levels of immunity from lifelong viral exposures. Research is ongoing to modify viral vectors to evade the immune system, such as by using capsid variants that reduce immunogenicity or by developing synthetic vectors that minimize immune recognition.

Once viral vectors enter the cells, the body's cytotoxic T cells may attack the infected cells as they would with viral infections, potentially leading to chronic inflammation. Chronic inflammation can exacerbate age-related decline and increase the risk of further complications. Long-term exposure to viral vectors is also linked to complications like hepatotoxicity, particularly in cases where the liver is involved as a primary organ for gene therapy. Strategies like short-term immunosuppressive regimens and localized delivery approaches are being tested to reduce these risks. The immune system's response can reduce the duration of gene expression, requiring repeated administrations of viral vectors. Each administration risks an increased immune response, making gene therapy less effective over time. Approaches to address this include non-viral delivery systems and transient immunosuppression protocols designed to increase tolerance to viral vectors. While oncolytic viruses show promise, their efficacy in aging populations may be limited by pre-existing antiviral immunity and immunosuppressive tumor microenvironments (Santos Apolonio et al., 2021). Overcoming these barriers—for instance, by engineering viruses to evade neutralization—will be crucial for advancing this modality in older patients.

Anti-VEGF therapy is the primary treatment for neovascular age-related macular degeneration (nAMD), but it involves repeated intravitreal injections, which can be inconvenient and challenging for patients(Kaiser et al., 2021). Gene therapy offers the potential for sustained release of therapeutic proteins, possibly improving visual outcomes with just a single treatment (Finocchio et al., 2023).

On June 6, 2024, the U.S. FDA approved imetelstat (Rytelo, developed by Geron Corporation), a first-in-class oligonucleotide telomerase inhibitor, for adults with low- to intermediate-1 risk myelodysplastic syndromes (MDS) who have transfusion-dependent anemia and are either unresponsive to, no longer benefit from, or cannot receive erythropoiesis-stimulating agents. This approval was supported by results from the Phase 3 IMerge trial (NCT02598661), a randomized, double-blind, placebo-controlled study involving 178 patients. Imetelstat significantly outperformed placebo, with 39.8% of patients achieving red blood cell transfusion independence (RBC-TI) for at least 8 weeks and 28% for at least 24 weeks, versus 15% and 3.3% in the placebo group (both $p < 0.001$). Common side effects included cytopenias, elevated liver enzymes, fatigue, musculoskeletal pain, and infections. The treatment is administered via intravenous infusion at 7.1 mg/kg every four weeks. The FDA's Assessment Aid pathway helped expedite the approval process.

Gene therapy holds immense potential for addressing aging and age-related diseases, offering opportunities to extend healthspan and improve the quality of life in older individuals. As advancements in molecular biology, genomics, and biotechnology converge, the future of gene therapy in gerontology appears promising. This section explores key areas of innovation and future directions, including CRISPR-based gene editing and its potential human applications, while also expanding on additional topics such as epigenetic rejuvenation, multi-gene delivery systems, and the integration of artificial intelligence in gene therapy research.

CRISPR-Based Gene Editing for Aging-Related Genes

CRISPR-Cas9 technology has revolutionized the field of genetic engineering, enabling precise editing of DNA sequences to correct mutations, enhance protective genes, or deactivate deleterious genes. In the context of aging, CRISPR-based approaches are being developed to target genes associated with longevity and cellular repair, offering a pathway for addressing the molecular drivers of aging.Aging is often accompanied by the accumulation of somatic mutations that impair cellular function. CRISPR-Cas9 can be employed to correct these mutations in genes such as APOE4 (associated with Alzheimer's disease), TERT (linked to telomere maintenance), and FOXO3 (involved in stress resistance). Correcting these mutations in preclinical models has demonstrated significant improvements in cellular resilience and organ function (Doudna & Charpentier, 2014).

Beyond editing specific DNA sequences, CRISPR-based tools such as CRISPR activation (CRISPRa) and interference (CRISPRi) can modulate gene expression without altering the genome. These tools can be used to upregulate longevity-associated genes like SIRT6 or downregulate pro-aging genes such as p16INK4a. Epigenetic-focused CRISPR systems, such as Cas9 fused with histone-modifying enzymes, have the potential to reverse age-associated epigenetic changes, promoting rejuvenation in tissues such as skin and muscle (Liu et al., 2021). CRISPR technologies are being applied to tackle major hallmarks of aging, such as genomic instability, telomere shortening, and mitochondrial dysfunction. For instance, by editing genes involved in DNA repair pathways (e.g., SIRT1 and BRCA1), CRISPR can enhance genomic stability, reducing mutation rates and delaying the onset of age-related diseases. Targeting mitochondrial genes, such as SIRT3 and POLG, may improve energy production and reduce oxidative stress, contributing to healthier aging (Houtkooper et al., 2012).

Potential for Human Applications in Gerontology

As preclinical research continues to yield promising results, the transition to human applications in gerontology presents significant opportunities and challenges. Gene therapies targeting specific aging-related conditions, such as neurodegeneration and cardiovascular disease, are beginning to enter clinical trials. For example, therapies focused on APOE4 modification in Alzheimer's disease patients aim to reduce amyloid plaque deposition and slow cognitive decline. Similarly, gene therapies enhancing VEGF expression are being tested for improving vascular health and reducing ischemic damage in older adults.

While most current trials focus on treating age-associated diseases, the prospect of directly targeting aging processes to extend human lifespan is gaining attention. Gene therapies aimed at upregulating Klotho, FOXO3, or SIRT1 could be employed as preventative measures, delaying the onset of multiple age-related diseases simultaneously. Preclinical studies in mice have shown that such interventions can significantly extend healthspan, raising the possibility of future applications in human populations (Dubal et al., 2015). Translating gene therapy to humans poses ethical, technical, and regulatory challenges. Ensuring safety, minimizing off-target effects, and achieving efficient gene delivery are critical for success. Additionally, issues such as equitable access to therapies, public perception of "anti-aging" treatments, and long-term societal impacts must be carefully considered. Ongoing research aims to address these challenges through innovations in delivery systems, such as lipid nanoparticles and tissue-specific promoters, which improve the precision and efficacy of gene therapy in humans (Naldini, 2015).

Epigenetic modifications play an important role in aging by influencing gene expression without altering DNA sequences. Reversing age-associated epigenetic changes through gene therapy is an emerging area of interest. Studies using Yamanaka factors (Oct4, Sox2, Klf4, and c-Myc) have shown that partial reprogramming can rejuvenate cells without compromising their identity. This technique has been applied in mice to reverse age-related tissue damage and extend lifespan (Ocampo et al., 2016). Future gene therapies may employ similar strategies to reset epigenetic markers in human cells, promoting systemic rejuvenation. Age-related hypermethylation of tumor suppressor genes and hypomethylation of pro-inflammatory genes contribute to the progression of aging. CRISPR-based epigenetic editing offers the ability to selectively modulate these methylation patterns, restoring a youthful epigenetic landscape. Such approaches can potentially treat conditions like cancer and immune dysfunction in older populations (Horvath, 2013). Addressing the multifaceted nature of aging requires interventions targeting multiple genes and pathways simultaneously. Multi-gene delivery systems are being developed to achieve this goal. Aging involves interconnected processes, including mitochondrial dysfunction, inflammation, and telomere shortening (Wiley et al., 2016). Combining therapies that target different pathways, such as SIRT1, FOXO3, and TERT, can produce synergistic effects. Preclinical studies in mice have demonstrated that multi-gene delivery significantly improves lifespan and reduces age-related decline compared to single-gene therapies (Shay & Wright, 2011).

Current approaches for reversing aging, treating injuries, and curing age-related diseases largely depend on delivering genetic material, such as DNA via adeno-associated viral (AAV) vectors or RNA using lipid nanoparticles (Yang et al., 2023; Lu et al., 2020; Sung & Kim, 2019). However, these genetic methods come with challenges, including high costs and safety concerns regarding the introduction of genetic material into the body. Developing chemical alternatives to mimic the rejuvenating effects of OSK (OCT4, SOX2, KLF4) factors could help reduce costs and speed up progress in regenerative medicine (Macip et al., 2023; Liuyang et al., 2023; Hu et al., 2023; Guan et al., 2022; Hou et al., 2013). Inducing OSK for four days led to a 43.2% reduction in the expression of age-upregulated genes and a 65.3% increase in the expression of age-downregulated genes, partially reversing age-related changes associated with cellular senescence. Using the nucleocytoplasmic compartmentalization (NCC) reporter system, OSK treatment restored NCC integrity in senescent cells to levels comparable to quiescent, non-senescent cells. Researchers identified six chemical cocktails capable of restoring NCC integrity in senescent cells, a key marker of age reversal. After just four days of treatment, these cocktails significantly reduced the estimated chronological age of senescent cells by several years. Gene expression analysis revealed that the chemical cocktails broadly improved features of senescence, influencing pathways related to inflammation, mitochondrial metabolism, and cell cycle regulation (Yang et al., 2023). This chemical approach could provide a method for treating various medical conditions and potentially even support whole-body rejuvenation (An et al., 2020; Du et al., 2022).

Current gene therapy approaches for aging like AAV delivery of longevity genes (e.g., TERT, Klotho) and partial reprogramming techniques using Yamanaka factors—face several limitations that challenge their clinical translation. These include difficulties achieving precise, tissue-specific, and temporally controlled gene expression, which is critical given the heterogeneity of aging processes across different organs; potential off-target effects and genomic instability that raise concerns about long-term safety and tumorigenicity (Ocampo et al., 2016; Lu et al., 2020); and immune responses associated with viral vectors that can limit therapeutic efficacy (de Magalhães, Stevens, & Thornton, 2019). Furthermore, the risk of inadvertent overexpression of target genes, such as the oncogenic potential inherent in unregulated telomerase activity, underscores the need for sophisticated regulatory mechanisms. In light of these challenges, alternative strategies—including senolytic drugs and novel biomaterial-based delivery systems—are being explored to provide safer, more controlled interventions that alleviate cellular senescence without the drawbacks of traditional gene therapy (Kirkland et al., 2017; Justice et al., 2019). Overall, while gene therapy remains a promising avenue to address the molecular underpinnings of aging, its current limitations highlight the necessity for further refinements in delivery, specificity, and safety to achieve effective, long-term clinical outcomes.

Advances in Delivery Platforms

New vector systems capable of carrying multiple genes, such as modified lentiviral vectors and lipid nanoparticles, are being designed to enhance payload capacity and tissue targeting. These innovations aim to deliver a combination of therapeutic genes to specific tissues, such as the brain, liver, or heart, where aging processes are most pronounced (Kotterman & Schaffer, 2014).

Integration of Artificial Intelligence in Gene Therapy Research

The incorporation of artificial intelligence (AI) into gene therapy research offers a powerful tool for accelerating discovery and optimizing therapeutic strategies.

AI-Driven Target Identification

AI algorithms can analyze genomic and transcriptomic data to identify novel aging-related genes and regulatory networks. Machine learning models have been used to predict gene-gene interactions and prioritize targets for intervention, enabling more efficient discovery of therapeutic candidates (Angermueller et al., 2016).

Optimizing Delivery Systems

AI is being applied to design improved viral and non-viral delivery vectors with enhanced specificity and reduced immunogenicity. Computational models simulate interactions between vectors and tissues, guiding the development of optimized delivery platforms for gene therapy (Erzurumluoglu et al., 2019).

Personalized Gene Therapy

AI tools are facilitating the development of personalized therapies by integrating individual genomic, epigenomic, and clinical data. This approach allows for tailored interventions that account for a person's unique genetic profile, ensuring maximum efficacy and minimal risk.

The future of gene therapy in aging is filled with exciting possibilities, driven by advancements in CRISPR-based editing, epigenetic rejuvenation, multi-gene delivery systems, and AI integration. These innovations hold the potential to revolutionize gerontology, offering not just treatments for age-related diseases but also interventions to delay or reverse the aging process itself. Overcoming current challenges and ethical considerations will be crucial to realizing these transformative therapies, paving the way for a new era of healthy aging and extended human lifespan.

Gene therapy for aging populations raises several pressing socioethical concerns, including issues of equity, consent, safety, and broader societal implications. One of the foremost concerns is the potential for unequal access, where only affluent individuals or countries may afford life-extending therapies, exacerbating global health disparities and creating a "longevity divide" (Cornetta et al., 2018). Informed consent in aging individuals—particularly those with cognitive impairments—adds another layer of complexity, as does the potential societal pressure to pursue such treatments to avoid perceived burdensomeness (Altawalbeh et al., 2020). Long-term safety remains uncertain, especially given the risks of tumorigenesis, immune reactions, or off-target effects from gene editing technologies such as CRISPR

(Cyranoski, 2019; Lander et al., 2019). If germline cells are affected, intergenerational consequences raise ethical questions about the autonomy of future individuals. Additionally, the resource-intensive nature of these therapies may strain healthcare systems and divert funding from more universally beneficial interventions (Hogle, 2005). Philosophical concerns about "playing God" and altering the natural course of life are echoed in cultural critiques, which question whether aging should be pathologized at all (Faragher, 2015). Social and psychological consequences—such as disrupted intergenerational dynamics, shifts in family structures, and increased population pressure—also warrant attention. As life extension challenges traditional notions of aging, identity, and mortality, some worry about the psychological toll of an extended but possibly directionless lifespan (Daniels, 2007). Regulatory gaps further complicate matters, as inconsistent oversight may lead to unethical experimentation or commercial exploitation of vulnerable populations (Kimmelman, 2012). The distinction between therapeutic use and human enhancement remains contentious, particularly when interventions shift from treating disease to optimizing traits like cognition or stamina (Buchanan, 2011). Addressing these socioethical challenges requires inclusive public discourse, strong regulatory frameworks, and international cooperation to ensure that gene therapy is applied equitably and responsibly.

CONCLUSION

Gene therapy has emerged as a promising frontier in combating age-related diseases, offering innovative solutions that target the underlying genetic and molecular causes of aging and its associated pathologies. This paper highlights significant advancements in gene-editing technologies, including CRISPR-Cas9, viral and non-viral delivery systems, and personalized therapeutic approaches, which collectively enhance the precision and efficacy of treatment strategies. Key findings underscore the therapeutic potential of addressing genetic defects, epigenetic dysregulation, and cellular senescence, with encouraging results demonstrated in preclinical and clinical studies for diseases such as Alzheimer's, cardiovascular disorders, and macular degeneration. Despite these advancements, several challenges persist, including the risks of off-target effects, immunogenicity, and the limited longevity of therapeutic effects. Ethical considerations and regulatory barriers also require careful navigation to ensure equitable and safe application of gene therapy in diverse populations.

Looking ahead, the field of gene therapy for age-related diseases should focus on several critical areas. Optimization of Delivery Systems. Developing safer and more efficient delivery vehicles, including non-viral nanoparticles and exosome-based systems, to minimize immune reactions and enhance tissue specificity. Addressing Longevity and Safety. Investigating long-term safety profiles and durable therapeutic outcomes through advanced genome-editing tools, such as base editing and prime editing. Integrative Approaches. Combining gene therapy with regenerative medicine, stem cell technologies, and pharmaceutical interventions to tackle the multifactorial nature of aging. Personalized Therapies. Expanding the use of omics technologies to design patient-specific interventions, ensuring optimal treatment responses and minimizing adverse effects. Ethical and Regulatory Frameworks. Strengthening policies to address ethical concerns, including access and affordability, while promoting international collaborations to streamline clinical translation. By addressing these areas, gene therapy holds immense potential to revolutionize the management of age-related diseases, improving not only the lifespan but also the quality of life in aging populations.

REFERENCES

Acosta, J. C., Banito, A., Wuestefeld, T., Georgilis, A., Janich, P., Morton, J. P., Athineos, D., Kang, T.-W., Lasitschka, F., Andrulis, M., Pascual, G., Morris, K. J., Khan, S., Jin, H., Dharmalingam, G., Snijders, A. P., Carroll, T., Capper, D., Pritchard, C., & Gil, J. (2013). A complex secretory program orchestrated by the inflammasome controls paracrine senescence. *Nature Cell Biology*, *15*(8), 978–990. DOI: 10.1038/ncb2784 PMID: 23770676

Aguiar, S., van der Gaag, B., & Cortese, F. A. B. (2017). RNAi mechanisms in Huntington's disease therapy: siRNA versus shRNA. *Translational Neurodegeneration*, *6*(1), 30. DOI: 10.1186/s40035-017-0101-9 PMID: 29209494

Altawalbeh, S. M., Alkhateeb, F. M., & Attarabeen, O. F. (2020). Ethical Issues in Consenting Older Adults: Academic Researchers and Community Perspectives. *Journal of Pharmaceutical Health Services Research*, *11*(1), 25–32. DOI: 10.1111/jphs.12327 PMID: 33042231

Alzforum. (2024). AAV2-BDNF. *Alzforum.* Available online: https://www.alzforum.org/therapeutics/aav2-bdnf

An, S., Cho, S. Y., Kang, J., Lee, S., Kim, H. S., Min, D. J., Son, E., & Cho, K. H. (2020). Inhibition of 3-phosphoinositide-dependent protein kinase 1 (PDK1) can revert cellular senescence in human dermal fibroblasts. *Proceedings of the National Academy of Sciences of the United States of America*, *117*(50), 31535–31546. DOI: 10.1073/pnas.1920338117 PMID: 33229519

Arsic, N., Zacchigna, S., Zentilin, L., Ramirez-Correa, G., Pattarini, L., Salvi, A., Sinagra, G., & Giacca, M. (2004). Vascular endothelial growth factor stimulates skeletal muscle regeneration in vivo. *Molecular Therapy : the Journal of the American Society of Gene Therapy*, *10*(5), 844–854. DOI: 10.1016/j.ymthe.2004.08.007 PMID: 15509502

Baar, M. P., Brandt, R. M. C., Putavet, D. A., Klein, J. D. D., Derks, K. W. J., Bourgeois, B. R. M., Stryeck, S., Rijksen, Y., van Willigenburg, H., Feijtel, D. A., van der Pluijm, I., Essers, J., van Cappellen, W. A., van IJcken, W. F., Houtsmuller, A. B., Pothof, J., de Bruin, R. W. F., Madl, T., Hoeijmakers, J. H. J., & de Keizer, P. L. J. (2017). Targeted Apoptosis of Senescent Cells Restores Tissue Homeostasis in Response to Chemotoxicity and Aging. *Cell*, *169*(1), 132–147.e16. DOI: 10.1016/j.cell.2017.02.031 PMID: 28340339

Berdasco, M., & Esteller, M. (2019). Clinical epigenetics: Seizing opportunities for translation. *Nature Reviews. Genetics*, *20*(2), 109–127. DOI: 10.1038/s41576-018-0074-2 PMID: 30479381

Bernardes de Jesus, B., Vera, E., Schneeberger, K., Tejera, A. M., Ayuso, E., Bosch, F., & Blasco, M. A. (2012). Telomerase gene therapy in adult and old mice delays aging and increases longevity without increasing cancer. *EMBO Molecular Medicine*, *4*(8), 691–704. DOI: 10.1002/emmm.201200245 PMID: 22585399

Biernacka, A., & Frangogiannis, N. G. (2011). Aging and Cardiac Fibrosis. *Aging and Disease*, *2*(2), 158–173. PMID: 21837283

Blackburn, E. H., Epel, E. S., & Lin, J. (2015). Human telomere biology: A contributory and interactive factor in aging, disease risks, and protection. *Science*, *350*(6265), 1193–1198. DOI: 10.1126/science.aab3389 PMID: 26785477

Brentjens, R. J., Santos, E., Nikhamin, Y., Yeh, R., Matsushita, M., La Perle, K., Quintás-Cardama, A., Larson, S. M., & Sadelain, M. (2007). Genetically targeted T cells eradicate systemic acute lymphoblastic leukemia xenografts. *Clinical Cancer Research*, *13*(18 Pt 1), 5426–5435. DOI: 10.1158/1078-0432.CCR-07-0674 PMID: 17855649

Browder, K. C., Reddy, P., Yamamoto, M., Haghani, A., Guillen, I. G., Sahu, S., Wang, C., Luque, Y., Prieto, J., Shi, L., Shojima, K., Hishida, T., Lai, Z., Li, Q., Choudhury, F. K., Wong, W. R., Liang, Y., Sangaraju, D., Sandoval, W., & Izpisua Belmonte, J. C. (2022). In vivo partial reprogramming alters age-associated molecular changes during physiological aging in mice. *Nature Aging*, *2*(3), 243–253. DOI: 10.1038/s43587-022-00183-2 PMID: 37118377

Buchanan, A. (2011). *Beyond Humanity?: The Ethics of Biomedical Enhancement.* Oxford University Press., DOI: 10.1093/acprof:oso/9780199587810.001.0001

Campisi, J., Kapahi, P., Lithgow, G. J., Melov, S., Newman, J. C., & Verdin, E. (2019). From discoveries in ageing research to therapeutics for healthy ageing. *Nature*, *571*(7764), 183–192. DOI: 10.1038/s41586-019-1365-2 PMID: 31292558

Cawthon, R. M., Smith, K. R., O'Brien, E., Sivatchenko, A., & Kerber, R. A. (2003). Association between telomere length in blood and mortality in people aged 60 years or older. *Lancet*, *361*(9355), 393–395. DOI: 10.1016/S0140-6736(03)12384-7 PMID: 12573379

Chaib, S., Tchkonia, T., & Kirkland, J. L. (2022). Cellular senescence and senolytics: The path to the clinic. *Nature Medicine*, *28*(8), 1556–1568. DOI: 10.1038/s41591-022-01923-y PMID: 35953721

Chen, K., Wang, S., & Sun, Z. (2022). In Vivo Cardiac-specific Expression of Adenylyl Cyclase 4 Gene Protects against Klotho Deficiency-induced Heart Failure. *Translational Research; the Journal of Laboratory and Clinical Medicine*, *244*, 101–113. DOI: 10.1016/j.trsl.2022.01.006 PMID: 35114419

Childs, B. G., Gluscevic, M., Baker, D. J., Laberge, R. M., Marquess, D., Dananberg, J., & van Deursen, J. M. (2017). Senescent cells: An emerging target for diseases of ageing. *Nature Reviews. Drug Discovery*, *16*(10), 718–735. DOI: 10.1038/nrd.2017.116 PMID: 28729727

Chinnasamy, D., Yu, Z., Kerkar, S. P., Zhang, L., Morgan, R. A., Restifo, N. P., & Rosenberg, S. A. (2012). Local delivery of interleukin-12 using T cells targeting VEGF receptor-2 eradicates multiple vascularized tumors in mice. *Clinical Cancer Research*, *18*(6), 1672–1683. DOI: 10.1158/1078-0432.CCR-11-3050 PMID: 22291136

Chondronasiou, D., Gill, D., Mosteiro, L., Urdinguio, R. G., Berenguer-Llergo, A., Aguilera, M., Durand, S., Aprahamian, F., Nirmalathasan, N., Abad, M., Martin-Herranz, D. E., Stephan-Otto Attolini, C., Prats, N., Kroemer, G., Fraga, M. F., Reik, W., & Serrano, M. (2022). Multi-omic rejuvenation of naturally aged tissues by a single cycle of transient reprogramming. *Aging Cell*, *21*(3), e13578. DOI: 10.1111/acel.13578 PMID: 35235716

Christine, C. W., Richardson, R. M., Van Laar, A. D., Thompson, M. E., Fine, E. M., Khwaja, O. S., Li, C., Liang, G. S., Meier, A., Roberts, E. W., Pfau, M. L., Rodman, J. R., Bankiewicz, K. S., & Larson, P. S. (2022). Safety of AADC Gene Therapy for Moderately Advanced Parkinson Disease: Three-Year Outcomes From the PD-1101 Trial. *Neurology*, *98*(1), e40–e50. DOI: 10.1212/WNL.0000000000012952 PMID: 34649873

Chuchana, P., Mausset-Bonnefont, A. L., Mathieu, M., Espinoza, F., Teigell, M., Toupet, K., Ripoll, C., Djouad, F., Noel, D., Jorgensen, C., & Apparailly, F. (2018). Secreted alpha-Klotho maintains cartilage tissue homeostasis by repressing NOS2 and ZIP8-MMP13 catabolic axis. *Aging (Albany NY)*, *10*(7), 1442–1453. DOI: 10.18632/aging.101481 PMID: 29920476

Cohen, J. P. (2019). At over $2 million Zolgensma is the world's most expensive therapy, yet relatively cost-effective. *Forbes.*Available online: https://www.forbes.com/sites/joshuacohen/2019/06/05/at-over-2-million-zolgensma-is-the-worlds-most-expensive-therapy-yet-relatively-cost-effective/

Constable, I. J., Lai, C. M., Magno, A. L., French, M. A., Barone, S. B., Schwartz, S. D., Blumenkranz, M. S., Degli-Esposti, M. A., & Rakoczy, E. P. (2017). Gene Therapy in Neovascular Age-related Macular Degeneration: Three-Year Follow-up of a Phase 1 Randomized Dose Escalation Trial. *American Journal of Ophthalmology*, *177*, 150–158. DOI: 10.1016/j.ajo.2017.02.018 PMID: 28245970

Corder, E. H., Saunders, A. M., Strittmatter, W. J., Schmechel, D. E., Gaskell, P. C., Small, G. W., Roses, A. D., Haines, J. L., & Pericak-Vance, M. A. (1993). Gene dose of apolipoprotein E type 4 allele and the risk of Alzheimer's disease in late onset families. *Science*, *261*(5123), 921–923. DOI: 10.1126/science.8346443 PMID: 8346443

Cornetta, K., Patel, K., Wanjiku, C. M., & Busakhala, N. (2018). Equitable Access to Gene Therapy: A Call to Action for the American Society of Gene and Cell Therapy. *Molecular Therapy : the Journal of the American Society of Gene Therapy*, *26*(12), 2715–2716. DOI: 10.1016/j.ymthe.2018.11.002 PMID: 30454956

Crouch, J., Shvedova, M., Thanapaul, R., Botchkarev, V., & Roh, D. (2022). Epigenetic Regulation of Cellular Senescence. *Cells*, *11*(4), 672. DOI: 10.3390/cells11040672 PMID: 35203320

Cyranoski, D. (2019). The CRISPR-baby scandal: What's next for human gene-editing. *Nature*, *566*(7745), 440–442. DOI: 10.1038/d41586-019-00673-1 PMID: 30809070

Daniels, N. (2007). *Just health: Meeting health needs fairly*. Cambridge University Press., DOI: 10.1017/CBO9780511809514

Das, S. K., Menezes, M. E., Bhatia, S., Wang, X. Y., Emdad, L., Sarkar, D., & Fisher, P. B. (2015). Gene Therapies for Cancer: Strategies, Challenges and Successes. *Journal of Cellular Physiology*, *230*(2), 259–271. DOI: 10.1002/jcp.24791 PMID: 25196387

Davidsohn, N., Pezone, M., Vernet, A., Graveline, A., Oliver, D., Slomovic, S., Punthambaker, S., Sun, X., Liao, R., Bonventre, J. V., & Church, G. M. (2019). A single combination gene therapy treats multiple age-related diseases. *Proceedings of the National Academy of Sciences of the United States of America*, *116*(47), 23505–23511. DOI: 10.1073/pnas.1910073116 PMID: 31685628 de Magalhães, J. P., Stevens, M., & Thornton, D. (2017). The Business of Anti-Aging Science. *Trends in Biotechnology*, *35*(11), 1062–1073. DOI: 10.1016/j.tibtech.2017.07.004 PMID: 28778607

Demaria, M., Ohtani, N., Youssef, S. A., Rodier, F., Toussaint, W., Mitchell, J. R., Laberge, R. M., Vijg, J., Van Steeg, H., Dollé, M. E., Hoeijmakers, J. H., de Bruin, A., Hara, E., & Campisi, J. (2014). An essential role for senescent cells in optimal wound healing through secretion of PDGF-AA. *Developmental Cell*, *31*(6), 722–733. DOI: 10.1016/j.devcel.2014.11.012 PMID: 25499914

Di Stasi, A., De Angelis, B., Rooney, C. M., Zhang, L., Mahendravada, A., Foster, A. E., Heslop, H. E., Brenner, M. K., Dotti, G., & Savoldo, B. (2009). T lymphocytes coexpressing CCR4 and a chimeric antigen receptor targeting CD30 have improved homing and antitumor activity in a Hodgkin tumor model. *Blood*, *113*(25), 6392–6402. DOI: 10.1182/blood-2009-03-209650 PMID: 19377047

Donato, A. J., Morgan, R. G., Walker, A. E., & Lesniewski, L. A. (2015). Cellular and molecular biology of aging endothelial cells. *Journal of molecular and cellular cardiology*, *89*(Pt B), 122–135. DOI: 10.1016/j.yjmcc.2015.01.021

Doudna, J. A., & Charpentier, E. (2014). Genome editing: The new frontier of genome engineering with CRISPR-Cas9. *Science*, *346*(6213), 1258096. DOI: 10.1126/science.1258096 PMID: 25430774

Du, J., Zheng, L., Gao, P., Yang, H., Yang, W. J., Guo, F., Liang, R., Feng, M., Wang, Z., Zhang, Z., Bai, L., Bu, Y., Xing, S., Zheng, W., Wang, X., Quan, L., Hu, X., Wu, H., Chen, Z., & Xiong, J.-W. (2022). A small-molecule cocktail promotes mammalian cardiomyocyte proliferation and heart regeneration. *Cell Stem Cell*, *29*(4), 545–558.e13. DOI: 10.1016/j.stem.2022.03.009 PMID: 35395187

Dubal, D. B., Zhu, L., Sanchez, P. E., Worden, K., Broestl, L., Johnson, E., Ho, K., Yu, G. Q., Kim, D., Betourne, A., & Kuro, O. (2015). Life extension factor klotho prevents mortality and enhances cognition in hAPP transgenic mice. *The Journal of Neuroscience : The Official Journal of the Society for Neuroscience*, *35*(6), 2358–2371. DOI: 10.1523/JNEUROSCI.5791-12.2015 PMID: 25673831

Evans, C. (2018). Editorial: Arthritis Gene Therapy Using Interleukin-1 Receptor Antagonist. *Arthritis & Rheumatology (Hoboken, N.J.)*, *70*(11), 1699–1701. DOI: 10.1002/art.40675 PMID: 30035385

Faragher, R. G. (2015). Should we treat aging as a disease? The consequences and dangers of miscategorisation. *Frontiers in Genetics*, *6*, 171. DOI: 10.3389/fgene.2015.00171 PMID: 26236330

Ferrara, N. (2004). Vascular endothelial growth factor: Basic science and clinical progress. *Endocrine Reviews*, *25*(4), 581–611. DOI: 10.1210/er.2003-0027 PMID: 15294883

Finocchio, L., Zeppieri, M., Gabai, A., Toneatto, G., Spadea, L., & Salati, C. (2023). Recent Developments in Gene Therapy for Neovascular Age-Related Macular Degeneration: A Review. *Biomedicines*, *11*(12), 3221. DOI: 10.3390/biomedicines11123221 PMID: 38137442

Florek, K., Mendyka, D., & Gomułka, K. (2024). Vascular Endothelial Growth Factor (VEGF) and Its Role in the Cardiovascular System. *Biomedicines*, *12*(5), 1055. DOI: 10.3390/biomedicines12051055 PMID: 38791016

Franceschi, C., Garagnani, P., Parini, P., Giuliani, C., & Santoro, A. (2018). Inflammaging: A new immune-metabolic viewpoint for age-related diseases. *Nature Reviews. Endocrinology*, *14*(10), 576–590. DOI: 10.1038/s41574-018-0059-4 PMID: 30046148

Frey, S. P., Jansen, H., Raschke, M. J., Meffert, R. H., & Ochman, S. (2012). VEGF improves skeletal muscle regeneration after acute trauma and reconstruction of the limb in a rabbit model. *Clinical Orthopaedics and Related Research*, *470*(12), 3607–3614. DOI: 10.1007/s11999-012-2456-7 PMID: 22806260

Fuhrmann-Stroissnigg, H., Ling, Y. Y., Zhao, J., McGowan, S. J., Zhu, Y., Brooks, R. W., Grassi, D., Gregg, S. Q., Stripay, J. L., Dorronsoro, A., Corbo, L., Tang, P., Bukata, C., Ring, N., Giacca, M., Li, X., Tchkonia, T., Kirkland, J. L., Niedernhofer, L. J., & Robbins, P. D. (2017). Identification of HSP90 inhibitors as a novel class of senolytics. *Nature Communications*, *8*(1), 422. DOI: 10.1038/s41467-017-00314-z PMID: 28871086

Gao, D., Wang, S., Lin, Y., & Sun, Z. (2020). In vivo AAV delivery of glutathione reductase gene attenuates anti-aging gene klotho deficiency-induced kidney damage. *Redox Biology*, *37*, 101692. DOI: 10.1016/j.redox.2020.101692 PMID: 32863229

Gao, P., You, M., Li, L., Zhang, Q., Fang, X., Wei, X., Zhou, Q., Zhang, H., Wang, M., Lu, Z., Wang, L., Sun, F., Liu, D., Zheng, H., Yan, Z., Yang, G., & Zhu, Z. (2022). Salt-Induced Hepatic Inflammatory Memory Contributes to Cardiovascular Damage Through Epigenetic Modulation of SIRT3. *Circulation*, *145*(5), 375–391. DOI: 10.1161/CIRCULATIONAHA.121.055600 PMID: 35100024

Greer, E. L., & Brunet, A. (2005). FOXO transcription factors at the interface between longevity and tumor suppression. *Oncogene*, *24*(50), 7410–7425. DOI: 10.1038/sj.onc.1209086 PMID: 16288288

Grootaert, M. O. J., Finigan, A., Figg, N. L., Uryga, A. K., & Bennett, M. R. (2021). SIRT6 Protects Smooth Muscle Cells From Senescence and Reduces Atherosclerosis. *Circulation Research*, *128*(4), 474–491. DOI: 10.1161/CIRCRESAHA.120.318353 PMID: 33353368

Gross, G., Waks, T., & Eshhar, Z. (1989). Expression of immunoglobulin-T-cell receptor chimeric molecules as functional receptors with antibody-type specificity. *Proceedings of the National Academy of Sciences of the United States of America*, *86*(24), 10024–10028. DOI: 10.1073/pnas.86.24.10024 PMID: 2513569

Guan, J., Wang, G., Wang, J., Zhang, Z., Fu, Y., Cheng, L., Meng, G., Lyu, Y., Zhu, J., Li, Y., Wang, Y., Liuyang, S., Liu, B., Yang, Z., He, H., Zhong, X., Chen, Q., Zhang, X., Sun, S., & Deng, H. (2022). Chemical reprogramming of human somatic cells to pluripotent stem cells. *Nature*, *605*(7910), 325–331. DOI: 10.1038/s41586-022-04593-5 PMID: 35418683

Guarente, L. (2013). Calorie restriction and sirtuins revisited. *Genes & Development*, *27*(19), 2072–2085. DOI: 10.1101/gad.227439.113 PMID: 24115767

Guo, C., Ma, X., Gao, F., & Guo, Y. (2023). Off-target effects in CRISPR/Cas9 gene editing. *Frontiers in Bioengineering and Biotechnology*, *11*, 1143157. DOI: 10.3389/fbioe.2023.1143157 PMID: 36970624

Hayflick, L., & Moorhead, P. S. (1961). The serial cultivation of human diploid cell strains. *Experimental Cell Research*, *25*(3), 585–621. DOI: 10.1016/0014-4827(61)90192-6 PMID: 13905658

Heier, J. S., Kherani, S., Desai, S., Dugel, P., Kaushal, S., Cheng, S. H., Delacono, C., Purvis, A., Richards, S., Le-Halpere, A., Connelly, J., Wadsworth, S. C., Varona, R., Buggage, R., Scaria, A., & Campochiaro, P. A. (2017). Intravitreous injection of AAV2-sFLT01 in patients with advanced neovascular age-related macular degeneration: A phase 1, open-label trial. *Lancet, 390*(10089), 50–61. DOI: 10.1016/S0140-6736(17)30979-0 PMID: 28526489

Hense, J. D., Garcia, D. N., Isola, J. V., Alvarado-Rincón, J. A., Zanini, B. M., Prosczek, J. B., Stout, M. B., Mason, J. B., Walsh, P. T., Brieño-Enríquez, M. A., Schadock, I., Barros, C. C., Masternak, M. M., & Schneider, A. (2022). Senolytic treatment reverses obesity-mediated senescent cell accumulation in the ovary. *GeroScience, 44*(3), 1747–1759. DOI: 10.1007/s11357-022-00573-9 PMID: 35460445

Hipp, M. S., Kasturi, P., & Hartl, F. U. (2019). The proteostasis network and its decline in ageing. *Nature Reviews. Molecular Cell Biology, 20*(7), 421–435. DOI: 10.1038/s41580-019-0101-y PMID: 30733602

Hoeijmakers, J. H. (2009). DNA damage, aging, and cancer. *The New England Journal of Medicine, 361*(15), 1475–1485. DOI: 10.1056/NEJMra0804615 PMID: 19812404

Hogle, L. F. (2005). Enhancement technologies and the body. *Annual Review of Anthropology, 34*(1), 695–716. DOI: 10.1146/annurev.anthro.33.070203.144020

Hong, M., Clubb, J. D., & Chen, Y. Y. (2020). Engineering CAR-T Cells for Next-Generation Cancer Therapy. *Cancer Cell, 38*(4), 473–488. DOI: 10.1016/j.ccell.2020.07.005 PMID: 32735779

Hou, P., Li, Y., Zhang, X., Liu, C., Guan, J., Li, H., Zhao, T., Ye, J., Yang, W., Liu, K., Ge, J., Xu, J., Zhang, Q., Zhao, Y., & Deng, H. (2013). Pluripotent stem cells induced from mouse somatic cells by small-molecule compounds. *Science, 341*(6146), 651–654. DOI: 10.1126/science.1239278 PMID: 23868920

Houtkooper, R. H., Pirinen, E., & Auwerx, J. (2012). Sirtuins as regulators of metabolism and healthspan. *Nature Reviews. Molecular Cell Biology, 13*(4), 225–238. DOI: 10.1038/nrm3293 PMID: 22395773

Hsu, P. D., Lander, E. S., & Zhang, F. (2014). Development and applications of CRISPR-Cas9 for genome engineering. *Cell, 157*(6), 1262–1278. DOI: 10.1016/j.cell.2014.05.010 PMID: 24906146

Hsuchou, H., Pan, W., & Kastin, A. J. (2007). The fasting polypeptide FGF21 can enter brain from blood. *Peptides, 28*(12), 2382–2386. DOI: 10.1016/j.peptides.2007.10.007 PMID: 17996984

Hu, Y., Yang, Y., Tan, P., Zhang, Y., Han, M., Yu, J., Zhang, X., Jia, Z., Wang, D., Yao, K., Pang, H., Hu, Z., Li, Y., Ma, T., Liu, K., & Ding, S. (2023). Induction of mouse totipotent stem cells by a defined chemical cocktail. *Nature, 617*(7960), 792–797. DOI: 10.1038/s41586-022-04967-9 PMID: 35728625

Hu, Y., Zu, C., Zhang, M., Wei, G., Li, W., Fu, S., Hong, R., Zhou, L., Wu, W., Cui, J., Wang, D., Du, B., Liu, M., Zhang, J., & Huang, H. (2023). Safety and efficacy of CRISPR-based non-viral PD1 locus specifically integrated anti-CD19 CAR-T cells in patients with relapsed or refractory Non-Hodgkin's lymphoma: A first-in-human phase I study. *EClinicalMedicine, 60*, 102010. DOI: 10.1016/j.eclinm.2023.102010 PMID: 37251628

Huang, Y., He, Y., Makarcyzk, M. J., & Lin, H. (2021). Senolytic Peptide FOXO4-DRI Selectively Removes Senescent Cells From *in vitro* Expanded Human Chondrocytes. *Frontiers in Bioengineering and Biotechnology, 9*, 677576. DOI: 10.3389/fbioe.2021.677576 PMID: 33996787

Hudry, E., Dashkoff, J., Roe, A. D., Takeda, S., Koffie, R. M., Hashimoto, T., Scheel, M., Spires-Jones, T., Arbel-Ornath, M., Betensky, R., Davidson, B. L., & Hyman, B. T. (2013). Gene transfer of human Apoe isoforms results in differential modulation of amyloid deposition and neurotoxicity in mouse brain. *Science Translational Medicine*, *5*(212), 212ra161. Advance online publication. DOI: 10.1126/scitranslmed.3007000 PMID: 24259049

Iida, Y., Okamoto, A., Hollis, R. L., Gourley, C., & Herrington, C. S. (2021). Clear cell carcinoma of the ovary: A clinical and molecular perspective. *International Journal of Gynecological Cancer : Official Journal of the International Gynecological Cancer Society*, *31*(4), 605–616. DOI: 10.1136/ijgc-2020-001656 PMID: 32948640

Iyer, S. P., Sica, R. A., Ho, P. J., Prica, A., Zain, J., Foss, F. M., Hu, B., Beitinjaneh, A., Weng, W. K., Kim, Y. H., Khodadoust, M. S., Huen, A. O., Williams, L. M., Ma, A., Huang, E., Ganpule, A., Nagar, S. D., Sripakdeevong, P., Cullingford, E. L., & Horwitz, S. M. (2025). Safety and activity of CTX130, a CD70-targeted allogeneic CRISPR-Cas9-engineered CAR T-cell therapy, in patients with relapsed or refractory T-cell malignancies (COBALT-LYM): A single-arm, open-label, phase 1, dose-escalation study. *The Lancet. Oncology*, *26*(1), 110–122. DOI: 10.1016/S1470-2045(24)00508-4 PMID: 39617017

Jackson, R. J., Keiser, M. S., Meltzer, J. C., Fykstra, D. P., Dierksmeier, S. E., Hajizadeh, S., Kreuzer, J., Morris, R., Melloni, A., Nakajima, T., Tecedor, L., Ranum, P. T., Carrell, E., Chen, Y., Nishtar, M. A., Holtzman, D. M., Haas, W., Davidson, B. L., & Hyman, B. T. (2024). APOE2 gene therapy reduces amyloid deposition and improves markers of neuroinflammation and neurodegeneration in a mouse model of Alzheimer disease. *Molecular Therapy : the Journal of the American Society of Gene Therapy*, *32*(5), 1373–1386. DOI: 10.1016/j.ymthe.2024.03.024 PMID: 38504517

Jaul, E., & Barron, J. (2017). Age-Related Diseases and Clinical and Public Health Implications for the 85 Years Old and Over Population. *Frontiers in Public Health*, *5*, 335. DOI: 10.3389/fpubh.2017.00335 PMID: 29312916

Justice, J. N., Nambiar, A. M., Tchkonia, T., LeBrasseur, N. K., Pascual, R., Hashmi, S. K., Prata, L., Masternak, M. M., Kritchevsky, S. B., Musi, N., & Kirkland, J. L. (2019). Senolytics in idiopathic pulmonary fibrosis: Results from a first-in-human, open-label, pilot study. *EBioMedicine*, *40*, 554–563. DOI: 10.1016/j.ebiom.2018.12.052 PMID: 30616998

Justice, J. N., Nambiar, A. M., Tchkonia, T., LeBrasseur, N. K., Pascual, R., Hashmi, S. K., Prata, L., Masternak, M. M., Kritchevsky, S. B., Musi, N., & Kirkland, J. L. (2019). Senolytics in idiopathic pulmonary fibrosis: Results from a first-in-human, open-label, pilot study. *EBioMedicine*, *40*, 554–563. DOI: 10.1016/j.ebiom.2018.12.052 PMID: 30616998

Jyotsana, N., Sharma, A., Chaturvedi, A., Budida, R., Scherr, M., Kuchenbauer, F., Lindner, R., Noyan, F., Sühs, K. W., Stangel, M., Grote-Koska, D., Brand, K., Vornlocher, H. P., Eder, M., Thol, F., Ganser, A., Humphries, R. K., Ramsay, E., Cullis, P., & Heuser, M. (2019). Lipid nanoparticle-mediated siRNA delivery for safe targeting of human CML in vivo. *Annals of Hematology*, *98*(8), 1905–1918. DOI: 10.1007/s00277-019-03713-y PMID: 31104089

Kaiser, S. M., Arepalli, S., & Ehlers, J. P. (2021). Current and Future Anti-VEGF Agents for Neovascular Age-Related Macular Degeneration. *Journal of Experimental Pharmacology*, *13*, 905–912. DOI: 10.2147/JEP.S259298 PMID: 34616189

Kamaly, N., Fredman, G., Fojas, J. J., Subramanian, M., Choi, W. I., Zepeda, K., Vilos, C., Yu, M., Gadde, S., Wu, J., Milton, J., Carvalho Leitao, R., Rosa Fernandes, L., Hasan, M., Gao, H., Nguyen, V., Harris, J., Tabas, I., & Farokhzad, O. C. (2016). Targeted Interleukin-10 Nanotherapeutics Developed with a Microfluidic Chip Enhance Resolution of Inflammation in Advanced Atherosclerosis. *ACS Nano, 10*(5), 5280–5292. DOI: 10.1021/acsnano.6b01114 PMID: 27100066

Kanekiyo, T., Xu, H., & Bu, G. (2014). ApoE and Aβ in Alzheimer's disease: Accidental encounters or partners? *Neuron, 81*(4), 740–754. DOI: 10.1016/j.neuron.2014.01.045 PMID: 24559670

Kaplitt, M. (2007, June 21). Promising results from first gene therapy clinical trial for Parkinson's disease reported in The Lancet. *The Lancet.* Available online: https://www.thelancet.com/journals/lancet/article/PIIS0140-6736(07)61250-4/fulltext

Kaverina, N., Schweickart, R. A., Chan, G. C., Maggiore, J. C., Eng, D. G., Zeng, Y., McKinzie, S. R., Perry, H. S., Ali, A., O'Connor, C., Pereira, B. M. V., Theberge, A. B., Vaughan, J. C., Loretz, C. J., Chang, A., Hukriede, N. A., Bitzer, M., Pippin, J. W., Wessely, O., & Shankland, S. J. (2023). Inhibiting NLRP3 signaling in aging podocytes improves their life- and health-span. *Aging (Albany NY), 15*(14), 6658–6689. DOI: 10.18632/aging.204897 PMID: 37487005

Kenyon, C. J. (2010). The genetics of ageing. *Nature, 464*(7288), 504–512. DOI: 10.1038/nature08980 PMID: 20336132

Kershaw, M. H., Westwood, J. A., Parker, L. L., Wang, G., Eshhar, Z., Mavroukakis, S. A., White, D. E., Wunderlich, J. R., Canevari, S., Rogers-Freezer, L., Chen, C. C., Yang, J. C., Rosenberg, S. A., & Hwu, P. (2006). A phase I study on adoptive immunotherapy using gene-modified T cells for ovarian cancer. *Clinical Cancer Research, 12*(20 Pt 1), 6106–6115. DOI: 10.1158/1078-0432.CCR-06-1183 PMID: 17062687

Kharitonenkov, A., Shiyanova, T. L., Koester, A., Ford, A. M., Micanovic, R., Galbreath, E. J., Sandusky, G. E., Hammond, L. J., Moyers, J. S., Owens, R. A., Gromada, J., Brozinick, J. T., Hawkins, E. D., Wroblewski, V. J., Li, D. S., Mehrbod, F., Jaskunas, S. R., & Shanafelt, A. B. (2005). FGF-21 as a novel metabolic regulator. *The Journal of Clinical Investigation, 115*(6), 1627–1635. DOI: 10.1172/JCI23606 PMID: 15902306

Khiabani, N. A., Doustvandi, M. A., Story, D., Nobari, S. A., Hajizadeh, M., Petersen, R., Dunbar, G., & Rossignol, J. (2024). Glioblastoma therapy: State of the field and future prospects. *Life Sciences, 359*, 123227. DOI: 10.1016/j.lfs.2024.123227 PMID: 39537100

Kim, C. K., Lee, Y. R., Ong, L., Gold, M., Kalali, A., & Sarkar, J. (2022). Alzheimer's Disease: Key Insights from Two Decades of Clinical Trial Failures. *Journal of Alzheimer's Disease, 87*(1), 83–100. DOI: 10.3233/JAD-215699 PMID: 35342092

Kim, J., Moon, S. Y., Kang, H. G., Kim, H. J., Choi, J. S., Lee, S. H. S., Park, K., & Won, S. Y. (2025). Therapeutic potential of AAV2-shmTOR gene therapy in reducing retinal inflammation and preserving endothelial Integrity in age-related macular degeneration. *Scientific Reports, 15*(1), 9517. DOI: 10.1038/s41598-025-93993-4 PMID: 40108376

Kimmelman, J. (2012). *Gene transfer and the ethics of first-in-human research: Lost in translation*. Cambridge University Press., DOI: 10.1017/CBO9780511642364

Kirkland, J. L., & Tchkonia, T. (2017). Cellular Senescence: A Translational Perspective. *EBioMedicine, 21*, 21–28. DOI: 10.1016/j.ebiom.2017.04.013 PMID: 28416161

Kirkland, J. L., Tchkonia, T., Zhu, Y., Niedernhofer, L. J., & Robbins, P. D. (2017). The Clinical Potential of Senolytic Drugs. *Journal of the American Geriatrics Society, 65*(10), 2297–2301. DOI: 10.1111/jgs.14969 PMID: 28869295

Kirkwood, T. B. (2005). Understanding the odd science of aging. *Cell, 120*(4), 437–447. DOI: 10.1016/j.cell.2005.01.027 PMID: 15734677

Kitaeva, K. V., Solovyeva, V. V., Blatt, N. L., & Rizvanov, A. A. (2024). Eternal Youth: A Comprehensive Exploration of Gene, Cellular, and Pharmacological Anti-Aging Strategies. *International Journal of Molecular Sciences, 25*(1), 643. DOI: 10.3390/ijms25010643 PMID: 38203812

Kotterman, M. A., & Schaffer, D. V. (2014). Engineering adeno-associated viruses for clinical gene therapy. *Nature Reviews. Genetics, 15*(7), 445–451. DOI: 10.1038/nrg3742 PMID: 24840552

Kowalski, P. S., Rudra, A., Miao, L., & Anderson, D. G. (2019). Delivering the Messenger: Advances in Technologies for Therapeutic mRNA Delivery. *Molecular Therapy : the Journal of the American Society of Gene Therapy, 27*(4), 710–728. DOI: 10.1016/j.ymthe.2019.02.012 PMID: 30846391

Kurosu, H., Yamamoto, M., Clark, J. D., Pastor, J. V., Nandi, A., Gurnani, P., McGuinness, O. P., Chikuda, H., Yamaguchi, M., Kawaguchi, H., Shimomura, I., Takayama, Y., Herz, J., Kahn, C. R., Rosenblatt, K. P., & Kuro-o, M. (2005). Suppression of aging in mice by the hormone Klotho. *Science, 309*(5742), 1829–1833. DOI: 10.1126/science.1112766 PMID: 16123266

LaFee, S. (2021). First-in-human clinical trial to assess gene therapy for Alzheimer's disease. *UC San Diego Health.* Available online: https://health.ucsd.edu/news/press-releases/2021-02-18-first-in-human-clinical-trial-to-assess-gene-therapy-for-alzheimers-disease/

Lander, E. S., Baylis, F., Zhang, F., Charpentier, E., Berg, P., Bourgain, C., Friedrich, B., Joung, J. K., Li, J., Liu, D., Naldini, L., Nie, J. B., Qiu, R., Schoene-Seifert, B., Shao, F., Terry, S., Wei, W., & Winnacker, E. L. (2019). Adopt a moratorium on heritable genome editing. *Nature, 567*(7747), 165–168. DOI: 10.1038/d41586-019-00726-5 PMID: 30867611

Leon, J., Moreno, A. J., Garay, B. I., Chalkley, R. J., Burlingame, A. L., Wang, D., & Dubal, D. B. (2017). Peripheral elevation of a klotho fragment enhances brain function and resilience in young, aging, and α synuclein transgenic mice. *Cell Reports, 20*(6), 1360–1371. DOI: 10.1016/j.celrep.2017.07.024 PMID: 28793260

Lexeo Therapeutics. (2024).Lexeo Therapeutics announces positive interim data for LX1001, first-ever gene therapy to impact the underlying genetic cause of APOE4-associated Alzheimer's disease, at the Clinical Trials on Alzheimer's Disease (CTAD) Conference. *Lexeo Therapeutics. Available online:*https://ir.lexeotx.com/news-releases/news-release-details/lexeo-therapeutics-announces-positive-interim-data-lx1001-first

Liang, T., Zhang, Y., Wu, S., Chen, Q., & Wang, L. (2022). The role of NLRP3 inflammasome in Alzheimer's disease and potential therapeutic targets. *Frontiers in Pharmacology, 13*, 845185. DOI: 10.3389/fphar.2022.845185 PMID: 35250595

Ling, W., Krager, K., Richardson, K. K., Warren, A. D., Ponte, F., Aykin-Burns, N., Manolagas, S. C., Almeida, M., & Kim, H. N. (2021). Mitochondrial Sirt3 contributes to the bone loss caused by aging or estrogen deficiency. *JCI Insight, 6*(10), e146728. DOI: 10.1172/jci.insight.146728 PMID: 33878033

Liuyang, S., Wang, G., Wang, Y., He, H., Lyu, Y., Cheng, L., Yang, Z., Guan, J., Fu, Y., Zhu, J., Zhong, X., Sun, S., Li, C., Wang, J., & Deng, H. (2023). Highly efficient and rapid generation of human pluripotent stem cells by chemical reprogramming. *Cell Stem Cell, 30*(3), 450–459.e9. DOI: 10.1016/j.stem.2023.02.008 PMID: 36944335

Lombard, D. B., Chua, K. F., Mostoslavsky, R., Franco, S., Gostissa, M., & Alt, F. W. (2005). DNA repair, genome stability, and aging. *Cell, 120*(4), 497–512. DOI: 10.1016/j.cell.2005.01.028 PMID: 15734682

López-Otín, C., Blasco, M. A., Partridge, L., Serrano, M., & Kroemer, G. (2013). The hallmarks of aging. *Cell, 153*(6), 1194–1217. DOI: 10.1016/j.cell.2013.05.039 PMID: 23746838

Lu, Y., Brommer, B., Tian, X., Krishnan, A., Meer, M., Wang, C., Vera, D. L., Zeng, Q., Yu, D., Bonkowski, M. S., Yang, J. H., Zhou, S., Hoffmann, E. M., Karg, M. M., Schultz, M. B., Kane, A. E., Davidsohn, N., Korobkina, E., Chwalek, K., & Sinclair, D. A. (2020). Reprogramming to recover youthful epigenetic information and restore vision. *Nature, 588*(7836), 124–129. DOI: 10.1038/s41586-020-2975-4 PMID: 33268865

Macip, C. C., Hasan, R., Hoznek, V., Kim, J., Metzger, L. E.IV, Sethna, S., & Davidsohn, N. (2023). Gene therapy mediated partial reprogramming extends lifespan and reverses age-related changes in aged mice. *bioRxiv.* DOI: 10.1101/2023.01.04.522507

Mahley, R. W., & Rall, S. C.Jr. (2000). Apolipoprotein E: Far more than a lipid transport protein. *Annual Review of Genomics and Human Genetics, 1*(1), 507–537. DOI: 10.1146/annurev.genom.1.1.507 PMID: 11701639

Martins, R., Lithgow, G. J., & Link, W. (2016). Long live FOXO: Unraveling the role of FOXO proteins in aging and longevity. *Aging Cell, 15*(2), 196–207. DOI: 10.1111/acel.12427 PMID: 26643314

Maude, S. L., Teachey, D. T., Porter, D. L., & Grupp, S. A. (2015). CD19-targeted chimeric antigen receptor T-cell therapy for acute lymphoblastic leukemia. *Blood, 125*(26), 4017–4023. DOI: 10.1182/blood-2014-12-580068 PMID: 25999455

Meglio, M. (2024, November 4). Lexeo Therapeutics' gene therapy LX1001 increases APOE2 expression in patients with Alzheimer disease. *NeurologyLive.* Available online: https://www.neurologylive.com/view/lexeo-therapeutics-gene-therapy-lx1001-increases-apoe2-expression-patients-alzheimer-disease

Mendell, J. R., Al Zaidy, S., Shell, R., Arnold, W. D., Rodino Klapac, L. R., Prior, T. W., Lowes, L., Alfano, L., Berry, K., Church, K., Kissel, J. T., Nagendran, S., L'Italien, J., Sproule, D. M., Wells, C., Cardenas, J. A., Heitzer, M. D., Kaspar, A., Corcoran, S., & Kaspar, B. K. (2017). Single dose gene replacement therapy for spinal muscular atrophy. *The New England Journal of Medicine, 377*(18), 1713–1722. DOI: 10.1056/NEJMoa1706198 PMID: 29091557

Messina, S., Mazzeo, A., Bitto, A., Aguennouz, M., Migliorato, A., De Pasquale, M. G., Minutoli, L., Altavilla, D., Zentilin, L., Giacca, M., Squadrito, F., & Vita, G. (2007). VEGF overexpression via adeno-associated virus gene transfer promotes skeletal muscle regeneration and enhances muscle function in mdx mice. *The FASEB Journal*, *21*(13), 3737–3746. DOI: 10.1096/fj.07-8459com PMID: 17575261

Meumann, N., Cabanes Creus, M., Ertelt, M., Navarro, R. G., Lucifora, J., Yuan, Q., Nien Huber, K., Abdelrahman, A., Vu, X. K., Zhang, L., Franke, A. C., Schmithals, C., Piiper, A., Vogt, A., Gonzalez Carmona, M., Frueh, J. T., Ullrich, E., Meuleman, P., Talbot, S. R., & Büning, H. (2023). Adeno associated virus serotype 2 capsid variants for improved liver directed gene therapy. *Hepatology (Baltimore, Md.)*, *77*(3), 802–815. DOI: 10.1002/hep.32733 PMID: 35976053

Millington-Ward, S., Palfi, A., Shortall, C., Finnegan, L. K., Bargroff, E., Post, I. J. M., Maguire, J., Irnaten, M. O., Brien, C., Kenna, P. F., Chadderton, N., & Farrar, G. J. (2024). AAV-NDI1 Therapy Provides Significant Benefit to Murine and Cellular Models of Glaucoma. *International Journal of Molecular Sciences*, *25*(16), 8876. DOI: 10.3390/ijms25168876 PMID: 39201561

Milone, M. C., Fish, J. D., Carpenito, C., Carroll, R. G., Binder, G. K., Teachey, D., Samanta, M., Lakhal, M., Gloss, B., Danet-Desnoyers, G., Campana, D., Riley, J. L., Grupp, S. A., & June, C. H. (2009). Chimeric receptors containing CD137 signal transduction domains mediate enhanced survival of T cells and increased antileukemic efficacy in vivo. *Molecular Therapy : the Journal of the American Society of Gene Therapy*, *17*(8), 1453–1464. DOI: 10.1038/mt.2009.83 PMID: 19384291

Mingozzi, F., & High, K. A. (2013). Immune responses to AAV vectors: Overcoming barriers to successful gene therapy. *Blood*, *122*(1), 23–36. DOI: 10.1182/blood-2013-01-306647 PMID: 23596044

Miniarikova, J., Zimmer, V., Martier, R., Brouwers, C. C., Pythoud, C., Richetin, K., Rey, M., Lubelski, J., Evers, M. M., van Deventer, S. J., Petry, H., Déglon, N., & Konstantinova, P. (2017). AAV5-miHTT gene therapy demonstrates suppression of mutant huntingtin aggregation and neuronal dysfunction in a rat model of Huntington's disease. *Gene Therapy*, *24*(10), 630–639. DOI: 10.1038/gt.2017.71 PMID: 28771234

Miyoshi, H., Blömer, U., Takahashi, M., Gage, F. H., & Verma, I. M. (1998). Development of a self inactivating lentivirus vector. *Journal of Virology*, *72*(10), 8150–8157. DOI: 10.1128/JVI.72.10.8150-8157.1998 PMID: 9733856

Mostoslavsky, R., Chua, K. F., Lombard, D. B., Pang, W. W., Fischer, M. R., Gellon, L., Liu, P., Mostoslavsky, G., Franco, S., Murphy, M. M., Mills, K. D., Patel, P., Hsu, J. T., Hong, A. L., Ford, E., Cheng, H. L., Kennedy, C., Nunez, N., Bronson, R., & Alt, F. W. (2006). Genomic instability and aging like phenotype in the absence of mammalian SIRT6. *Cell*, *124*(2), 315–329. DOI: 10.1016/j.cell.2005.11.044 PMID: 16439206

Murphy, C. T., McCarroll, S. A., Bargmann, C. I., Fraser, A., Kamath, R. S., Ahringer, J., Li, H., & Kenyon, C. (2003). Genes that act downstream of DAF-16 to influence the lifespan of Caenorhabditis elegans. *Nature*, *424*(6946), 277–283. DOI: 10.1038/nature01789 PMID: 12845331

Niethammer, M., Tang, C. C., LeWitt, P. A., Rezai, A. R., Leehey, M. A., Ojemann, S. G., Flaherty, A. W., Eskandar, E. N., Kostyk, S. K., Sarkar, A., Siddiqui, M. S., Tatter, S. B., Schwalb, J. M., Poston, K. L., Henderson, J. M., Kurlan, R. M., Richard, I. H., Sapan, C. V., Eidelberg, D., & Feigin, A. (2017). Long-term follow-up of a randomized AAV2-GAD gene therapy trial for Parkinson's disease. *JCI Insight*, *2*(7), e90133. DOI: 10.1172/jci.insight.90133 PMID: 28405611

Nilsson, P., Iwata, N., Muramatsu, S., Tjernberg, L. O., Winblad, B., & Saido, T. C. (2010). Gene therapy in Alzheimer's disease - potential for disease modification. *Journal of Cellular and Molecular Medicine*, *14*(4), 741–757. DOI: 10.1111/j.1582-4934.2010.01038.x PMID: 20158567

Ocampo, A., Reddy, P., Martinez-Redondo, P., Platero-Luengo, A., Hatanaka, F., Hishida, T., Li, M., Lam, D., Kurita, M., Beyret, E., Araoka, T., Vazquez-Ferrer, E., Donoso, D., Roman, J. L., Xu, J., Rodriguez Esteban, C., Nuñez, G., Nuñez Delicado, E., Campistol, J. M., & Izpisua Belmonte, J. C. (2016). In Vivo Amelioration of Age-Associated Hallmarks by Partial Reprogramming. *Cell*, *167*(7), 1719–1733.e12. DOI: 10.1016/j.cell.2016.11.052 PMID: 27984723

Olan, I., Handa, T., & Narita, M. (2023). Beyond SAHF: An integrative view of chromatin compartmentalization during senescence. *Current Opinion in Cell Biology*, *83*, 102206. DOI: 10.1016/j.ceb.2023.102206 PMID: 37451177

Paik, J. H., Kollipara, R., Chu, G., Ji, H., Xiao, Y., Ding, Z., Miao, L., Tothova, Z., Horner, J. W., Carrasco, D. R., Jiang, S., Gilliland, D. G., Chin, L., Wong, W. H., Castrillon, D. H., & DePinho, R. A. (2007). FoxOs are lineage-restricted redundant tumor suppressors and regulate endothelial cell homeostasis. *Cell*, *128*(2), 309–323. DOI: 10.1016/j.cell.2006.12.029 PMID: 17254969

Post, S. G., & Binstock, R. H. (2004). *The fountain of youth: Cultural, scientific, and ethical perspectives on a biomedical goal*. Oxford University Press., DOI: 10.1093/oso/9780195170085.001.0001

Pototschnig, I., Feiler, U., Diwoky, C., Vesely, P. W., Rauchenwald, T., Paar, M., Bakiri, L., Pajed, L., Hofer, P., Kashofer, K., Sukhbaatar, N., Schoiswohl, G., Weichhart, T., Hoefler, G., Bock, C., Pichler, M., Wagner, E. F., Zechner, R., & Schweiger, M. (2023). Interleukin-6 initiates muscle- and adipose tissue wasting in a novel C57BL/6 model of cancer-associated cachexia. *Journal of Cachexia, Sarcopenia and Muscle*, *14*(1), 93–107. DOI: 10.1002/jcsm.13109 PMID: 36351437

Rafiq, S., Yeku, O. O., Jackson, H. J., Purdon, T. J., van Leeuwen, D. G., Drakes, D. J., Song, M., Miele, M. M., Li, Z., Wang, P., Yan, S., Xiang, J., Ma, X., Seshan, V. E., Hendrickson, R. C., Liu, C., & Brentjens, R. J. (2018). Targeted delivery of a PD-1-blocking scFv by CAR-T cells enhances anti-tumor efficacy in vivo. *Nature Biotechnology*, *36*(9), 847–856. DOI: 10.1038/nbt.4195 PMID: 30102295

Rakoczy, E. P., Lai, C. M., Magno, A. L., Wikstrom, M. E., French, M. A., Pierce, C. M., Schwartz, S. D., Blumenkranz, M. S., Chalberg, T. W., Degli-Esposti, M. A., & Constable, I. J. (2015). Gene therapy with recombinant adeno-associated vectors for neovascular age-related macular degeneration: 1 year follow-up of a phase 1 randomised clinical trial. *Lancet*, *386*(10011), 2395–2403. DOI: 10.1016/S0140-6736(15)00345-1 PMID: 26431823

Rakoczy, E. P., Magno, A. L., Lai, C. M., Pierce, C. M., Degli-Esposti, M. A., Blumenkranz, M. S., & Constable, I. J. (2019). Three-Year Follow-Up of Phase 1 and 2a rAAV.sFLT-1 Subretinal Gene Therapy Trials for Exudative Age-Related Macular Degeneration. *American Journal of Ophthalmology, 204*, 113–123. DOI: 10.1016/j.ajo.2019.03.006 PMID: 30878487

Regalado, A. (2015). A tale of do-it-yourself gene therapy. *MIT Technology Review.* Available online: https://www.technologyreview.com/2015/10/14/166211/a-tale-of-do-it-yourself-gene-therapy/

Roig-Soriano, J., Grinan-Ferre, C., Espinosa-Parrilla, J. F., Abraham, C. R., Bosch, A., Pallas, M., & Chillon, M. (2022). AAV-mediated expression of secreted and transmembrane alphaKlotho isoforms rescues relevant aging hallmarks in senescent SAMP8 mice. *Aging Cell, 21*(5), e13581. DOI: 10.1111/acel.13581 PMID: 35274439

Roig-Soriano, J., Sanchez-de-Diego, C., Esandi-Jauregui, J., Verdes, S., Abraham, C. R., Bosch, A., Ventura, F., & Chillon, M. (2023). Differential toxicity profile of secreted and processed alpha-Klotho expression over mineral metabolism and bone microstructure. *Scientific Reports, 13*(1), 4211. DOI: 10.1038/s41598-023-31117-6 PMID: 36918615

Roybal, K. T., Williams, J. Z., Morsut, L., Rupp, L. J., Kolinko, I., Choe, J. H., Walker, W. J., McNally, K. A., & Lim, W. A. (2016). Engineering T Cells with Customized Therapeutic Response Programs Using Synthetic Notch Receptors. *Cell, 167*(2), 419–432.e16. DOI: 10.1016/j.cell.2016.09.011 PMID: 27693353

Saccon, T. D., Nagpal, R., Yadav, H., Cavalcante, M. B., Nunes, A. D. C., Schneider, A., Gesing, A., Hughes, B., Yousefzadeh, M., Tchkonia, T., Kirkland, J. L., Niedernhofer, L. J., Robbins, P. D., & Masternak, M. M. (2021). Senolytic Combination of Dasatinib and Quercetin Alleviates Intestinal Senescence and Inflammation and Modulates the Gut Microbiome in Aged Mice. *The Journals of Gerontology. Series A, Biological Sciences and Medical Sciences, 76*(11), 1895–1905. DOI: 10.1093/gerona/glab002 PMID: 33406219

Safwan-Zaiter, H., Wagner, N., & Wagner, K. D. (2022). Dynamic Spatiotemporal Expression Pattern of the Senescence-Associated Factor p16Ink4a in Development and Aging. *Cells, 11*(3), 541. DOI: 10.3390/cells11030541 PMID: 35159350

Santos Apolonio, J., Lima de Souza Gonçalves, V., Cordeiro Santos, M. L., Silva Luz, M., Silva Souza, J. V., Rocha Pinheiro, S. L., de Souza, W. R., Sande Loureiro, M., & de Melo, F. F. (2021). Oncolytic virus therapy in cancer: A current review. *World Journal of Virology, 10*(5), 229–255. DOI: 10.5501/wjv.v10.i5.229 PMID: 34631474

Schaum, N., Lehallier, B., Hahn, O., Pálovics, R., Hosseinzadeh, S., Lee, S. E., Sit, R., Lee, D. P., Losada, P. M., Zardeneta, M. E., Fehlmann, T., Webber, J. T., McGeever, A., Calcuttawala, K., Zhang, H., Berdnik, D., Mathur, V., Tan, W., Zee, A., & Wyss-Coray, T. (2020). Ageing hallmarks exhibit organ-specific temporal signatures. *Nature, 583*(7817), 596–602. DOI: 10.1038/s41586-020-2499-y PMID: 32669715

Schlimgen, R., Howard, J., Wooley, D., Thompson, M., Baden, L. R., Yang, O. O., Christiani, D. C., Mostoslavsky, G., Diamond, D. V., Duane, E. G., Byers, K., Winters, T., Gelfand, J. A., Fujimoto, G., Hudson, T. W., & Vyas, J. M. (2016). Risks associated with lentiviral vector exposures and prevention strategies. *Journal of Occupational and Environmental Medicine*, *58*(12), 1159–1166. DOI: 10.1097/JOM.0000000000000879 PMID: 27930472

Sen, P., Shah, P. P., Nativio, R., & Berger, S. L. (2016). Epigenetic mechanisms of longevity and aging. *Cell*, *166*(4), 822–839. DOI: 10.1016/j.cell.2016.07.050 PMID: 27518561

Serrano, M., Lin, A. W., McCurrach, M. E., Beach, D., & Lowe, S. W. (1997). Oncogenic ras provokes premature cell senescence associated with accumulation of p53 and p16INK4a. *Cell*, *88*(5), 593–602. DOI: 10.1016/S0092-8674(00)81902-9 PMID: 9054499

Shay, J. W., & Wright, W. E. (2011). Role of telomeres and telomerase in cancer. *Seminars in Cancer Biology*, *21*(6), 349–353. DOI: 10.1016/j.semcancer.2011.10.001 PMID: 22015685

Somasundaram, I., Jain, S. M., Blot-Chabaud, M., Pathak, S., Banerjee, A., Rawat, S., Sharma, N. R., & Duttaroy, A. K. (2024). Mitochondrial dysfunction and its association with age-related disorders. *Frontiers in Physiology*, *15*, 1384966. DOI: 10.3389/fphys.2024.1384966 PMID: 39015222

Someya, S., Yu, W., Hallows, W. C., Xu, J., Vann, J. M., Leeuwenburgh, C., Tanokura, M., Denu, J. M., & Prolla, T. A. (2010). Sirt3 mediates reduction of oxidative damage and prevention of age related hearing loss under caloric restriction. *Cell*, *143*(5), 802–812. DOI: 10.1016/j.cell.2010.10.002 PMID: 21094524

Song, S., Ding, Y., Dai, G. L., Zhang, Y., Xu, M. T., Shen, J. R., Chen, T. T., Chen, Y., & Meng, G. L. (2021). Sirtuin 3 deficiency exacerbates diabetic cardiomyopathy via necroptosis enhancement and NLRP3 activation. *Acta Pharmacologica Sinica*, *42*(2), 230–241. DOI: 10.1038/s41401-020-0490-7 PMID: 32770173

Strzyz, P. (2022). Senescent fibroblasts support lung repair. *Nature Reviews. Molecular Cell Biology*, *23*(12), 775. DOI: 10.1038/s41580-022-00559-7 PMID: 36329214

Suarez, E. R., Chang, D.-K., Sun, J., Sui, J., Freeman, G. J., Signoretti, S., Zhu, Q., & Marasco, W. A. (2016). Chimeric antigen receptor T cells secreting anti-PD-L1 antibodies more effectively regress renal cell carcinoma in a humanized mouse model. *Oncotarget*, *7*(23), 34341–34355. DOI: 10.18632/oncotarget.9114 PMID: 27145284

Sundararaman, S., Miller, T. J., Pastore, J. M., Kiedrowski, M., Aras, R., & Penn, M. S. (2011). Plasmid-based transient human stromal cell-derived factor-1 gene transfer improves cardiac function in chronic heart failure. *Gene Therapy*, *18*(9), 867–873. DOI: 10.1038/gt.2011.18 PMID: 21472007

Sung, Y. K., & Kim, S. W. (2019). Recent advances in the development of gene delivery systems. *Biomaterials Research*, *23*(1), 8. DOI: 10.1186/s40824-019-0156-z PMID: 30915230

Tao, Z. F., Hasvold, L., Wang, L., Wang, X., Petros, A. M., Park, C. H., Boghaert, E. R., Catron, N. D., Chen, J., Colman, P. M., Czabotar, P. E., Deshayes, K., Fairbrother, W. J., Flygare, J. A., Hymowitz, S. G., Jin, S., Judge, R. A., Koehler, M. F., Kovar, P. J., & Souers, A. J. (2014). Discovery of a Potent and Selective BCL-XL Inhibitor with in Vivo Activity. *ACS Medicinal Chemistry Letters*, *5*(10), 1088–1093. DOI: 10.1021/ml5001867 PMID: 25313317

Templeman, N. M., & Murphy, C. T. (2018). Regulation of reproduction and longevity by nutrient-sensing pathways. *The Journal of Cell Biology*, *217*(1), 93–106. DOI: 10.1083/jcb.201707168 PMID: 29074705

Tezze, C., Romanello, V., & Sandri, M. (2019). FGF21 as modulator of metabolism in health and disease. *Frontiers in Physiology*, *10*, 419. DOI: 10.3389/fphys.2019.00419 PMID: 31057418

Triana-Martínez, F., Picallos-Rabina, P., Da Silva-Álvarez, S., Pietrocola, F., Llanos, S., Rodilla, V., Soprano, E., Pedrosa, P., Ferreirós, A., Barradas, M., Hernández-González, F., Lalinde, M., Prats, N., Bernadó, C., González, P., Gómez, M., Ikonomopoulou, M. P., Fernández-Marcos, P. J., García-Caballero, T., & Collado, M. (2019). Identification and characterization of Cardiac Glycosides as senolytic compounds. *Nature Communications*, *10*(1), 4731. DOI: 10.1038/s41467-019-12888-x PMID: 31636264

Trifunovic, A., Wredenberg, A., Falkenberg, M., Spelbrink, J. N., Rovio, A. T., Bruder, C. E., & Bohlooly, Y. (2004). Premature ageing in mice expressing defective mitochondrial DNA polymerase. *Nature*, *429*(6990), 417–423. DOI: 10.1038/nature02517 PMID: 15164064

Tuszynski, M. (n.d.). AAV2-BDNF for Alzheimer's disease and mild cognitive impairment (NCT05040217). *UC San Diego Clinical Trials.* Available online: https://clinicaltrials.ucsd.edu/trial/NCT05040217

van der Horst, A., & Burgering, B. M. (2007). Stressing the role of FoxO proteins in lifespan and disease. *Nature Reviews. Molecular Cell Biology*, *8*(6), 440–450. DOI: 10.1038/nrm2190 PMID: 17522590

Vijg, J., & Campisi, J. (2008). Puzzles, promises and a cure for ageing. *Nature*, *454*(7208), 1065–1071. DOI: 10.1038/nature07216 PMID: 18756247

Volpatti, L. R., de Matos, S. N., Borjas, G., Reda, J., Watkins, E. A., Zhou, Z., Nguyen, M., Solanki, A., Fang, Y., & Hubbell, J. A. (2024). LDL-Binding IL-10 Reduces Vascular Inflammation in Atherosclerotic Mice. *bioRxiv,* 2024.03.04.582839. DOI: 10.1101/2024.03.04.582839

Wang, D., Tai, P. W. L., & Gao, G. (2019). Adeno-associated virus vector as a platform for gene therapy delivery. *Nature Reviews. Drug Discovery*, *18*(5), 358–378. DOI: 10.1038/s41573-019-0012-9 PMID: 30710128

Wang, W., Zheng, Y., Sun, S., Li, W., Song, M., Ji, Q., Wu, Z., Liu, Z., Fan, Y., Liu, F., Li, J., Esteban, C. R., Wang, S., Zhou, Q., Belmonte, J. C. I., Zhang, W., Qu, J., Tang, F., & Liu, G. H. (2021). A genome-wide CRISPR-based screen identifies KAT7 as a driver of cellular senescence. *Science Translational Medicine*, *13*(575), eabd2655. Advance online publication. DOI: 10.1126/scitranslmed.abd2655 PMID: 33408182

Wang, Y., & Sun, Z. (2009). Klotho gene delivery prevents the progression of spontaneous hypertension and renal damage. *Hypertension*, *54*(4), 810–817. DOI: 10.1161/HYPERTENSIONAHA.109.134320 PMID: 19635988

White, S. L., Lee, T. D., Toy, T., Carroll, J. E., Polsky, L., Campo Fernandez, B., Davila, A., Kohn, D. B., & Chang, V. Y. (2022). Evaluation of clonal hematopoiesis in pediatric ADA-SCID gene therapy participants. *Blood Advances*, *6*(21), 5732–5736. DOI: 10.1182/bloodadvances.2022007803 PMID: 35914227

Whitehead, K. A., Langer, R., & Anderson, D. G. (2009). Knocking down barriers: Advances in siRNA delivery. *Nature Reviews. Drug Discovery*, *8*(2), 129–138. Advance online publication. DOI: 10.1038/nrd2742 PMID: 19180106

Wiley, C. D., Velarde, M. C., Lecot, P., Liu, S., Sarnoski, E. A., Freund, A., Shirakawa, K., Lim, H. W., Davis, S. S., Ramanathan, A., Gerencser, A. A., Verdin, E., & Campisi, J. (2016). Mitochondrial dysfunction induces senescence with a distinct secretory phenotype. *Cell Metabolism*, *23*(2), 303–314. DOI: 10.1016/j.cmet.2015.11.011 PMID: 26686024

Willcox, B. J., Donlon, T. A., He, Q., Chen, R., Grove, J. S., Yano, K., Masaki, K. H., Willcox, D. C., Rodriguez, B., & Curb, J. D. (2008). FOXO3A genotype is strongly associated with human longevity. *Proceedings of the National Academy of Sciences of the United States of America*, *105*(37), 13987–13992. DOI: 10.1073/pnas.0801030105 PMID: 18765803

World Health Organization. (2020). Decade of healthy ageing: baseline report. *World Health Organization.* Available online: https://www.who.int/publications/i/item/9789240017900

Xiang, T., Luo, X., Ye, L., Huang, H., & Wu, Y. (2022). Klotho alleviates NLRP3 inflammasome-mediated neuroinflammation in a temporal lobe epilepsy rat model by activating the Nrf2 signaling pathway. *Epilepsy & Behavior*, *128*, 108509. DOI: 10.1016/j.yebeh.2021.108509 PMID: 35104732

Xiang, T., Luo, X., Zeng, C., Li, S., Ma, M., & Wu, Y. (2021). Klotho ameliorated cognitive deficits in a temporal lobe epilepsy rat model by inhibiting ferroptosis. *Brain Research*, *1772*, 147668. DOI: 10.1016/j.brainres.2021.147668 PMID: 34592245

Yamazaki, Y., Imura, A., Urakawa, I., Shimada, T., Murakami, J., Aono, Y., Hasegawa, H., Yamashita, T., Nakatani, K., Saito, Y., Okamoto, N., Kurumatani, N., Namba, N., Kitaoka, T., Ozono, K., Sakai, T., Hataya, H., Ichikawa, S., Imel, E. A., & Nabeshima, Y. (2010). Establishment of sandwich ELISA for soluble alpha-Klotho measurement: Age-dependent change of soluble alpha-Klotho levels in healthy subjects. *Biochemical and Biophysical Research Communications*, *398*(3), 513–518. DOI: 10.1016/j.bbrc.2010.06.110 PMID: 20599764

Yang, J. H., Hayano, M., Griffin, P. T., Amorim, J. A., Bonkowski, M. S., Apostolides, J. K., Salfati, E. L., Blanchette, M., Munding, E. M., Bhakta, M., Chew, Y. C., Guo, W., Yang, X., Maybury-Lewis, S., Tian, X., Ross, J. M., Coppotelli, G., Meer, M. V., Rogers-Hammond, R., & Sinclair, D. A. (2023). Loss of epigenetic information as a cause of mammalian aging. *Cell*, *186*(2), 305–326.e27. DOI: 10.1016/j.cell.2022.12.027 PMID: 36638792

Yang, J. H., Petty, C. A., Dixon-McDougall, T., Lopez, M. V., Tyshkovskiy, A., Maybury-Lewis, S., Tian, X., Ibrahim, N., Chen, Z., Griffin, P. T., Arnold, M., Li, J., Martinez, O. A., Behn, A., Rogers-Hammond, R., Angeli, S., Gladyshev, V. N., & Sinclair, D. A. (2023). Chemically induced reprogramming to reverse cellular aging. *Aging (Albany NY)*, *15*(13), 5966–5989. DOI: 10.18632/aging.204896 PMID: 37437248

Yang, Z., Huang, Y., Zhu, L., Yang, K., Liang, K., Tan, J., & Yu, B. (2021). SIRT6 promotes angiogenesis and hemorrhage of carotid plaque via regulating HIF-1α and reactive oxygen species. *Cell Death & Disease*, *12*(1), 77. DOI: 10.1038/s41419-020-03372-2 PMID: 33436551

Young, J. L., & Dean, D. A. (2015). Electroporation-mediated gene delivery. *Advances in Genetics*, *89*, 49–88. DOI: 10.1016/bs.adgen.2014.10.003 PMID: 25620008

Yu, J., Li, T., & Zhu, J. (2023). Gene Therapy Strategies Targeting Aging-Related Diseases. *Aging and Disease*, *14*(2), 398–417. DOI: 10.14336/AD.2022.00725 PMID: 37008065

Yun, J., Hansen, S., Morris, O., Madden, D. T., Libeu, C. P., Kumar, A. J., Wehrfritz, C., Nile, A. H., Zhang, Y., Zhou, L., Liang, Y., Modrusan, Z., Chen, M. B., Overall, C. C., Garfield, D., Campisi, J., Schilling, B., Hannoush, R. N., & Jasper, H. (2023). Senescent cells perturb intestinal stem cell differentiation through Ptk7 induced noncanonical Wnt and YAP signaling. *Nature Communications*, *14*(1), 156. DOI: 10.1038/s41467-022-35487-9 PMID: 36631445

Zeng, M., Zhou, T., Li, Z., Li, G., Zhang, S., Wang, L., Huang, Q. G., Li, J. D., Samarawickrama, P. N., He, Y., & Wang, G. D. (2024). Transcriptomic and intervention evidence reveals domestic dogs as a promising model for anti-inflammatory investigation. *Aging Cell*, *23*(5), e14127. DOI: 10.1111/acel.14127 PMID: 38426629

Zeng, Z., Li, S., Ye, X., Wang, Y., Wang, Q., Chen, Z., Wang, Z., Zhang, J., Wang, Q., Chen, L., Zhang, S., Zou, Z., Lin, M., Chen, X., Zhao, G., McAlinden, C., Lei, H., Zhou, X., & Huang, J. (2024). Genome Editing VEGFA Prevents Corneal Neovascularization In Vivo. *Advanced Science (Weinheim, Baden-Wurttemberg, Germany)*, *11*(25), e2401710. DOI: 10.1002/advs.202401710 PMID: 38582513

Zhang, S., Lu, Y., Shi, W., Ren, Y., Xiao, K., Chen, W., Li, L., & Zhao, J. (2022). SIRT1/FOXO1 Axis-Mediated Hippocampal Angiogenesis is Involved in the Antidepressant Effect of ChaihuShugan San. *Drug Design, Development and Therapy*, *16*, 2783–2801. DOI: 10.2147/DDDT.S370825 PMID: 36039087

Zhang, Y., Xie, Y., Berglund, E. D., Coate, K. C., He, T. T., Katafuchi, T., Xiao, G., Potthoff, M. J., Wei, W., Wan, Y., Yu, R. T., Evans, R. M., Kliewer, S. A., & Mangelsdorf, D. J. (2012). The starvation hormone, fibroblast growth factor 21, extends lifespan in mice. *eLife*, *1*, e00065. DOI: 10.7554/eLife.00065 PMID: 23066506

Zhang, Y., Zhang, Q., Zhang, Y., & Han, J. (2023). The role of histone modification in DNA replication coupled nucleosome assembly and cancer. *International Journal of Molecular Sciences*, *24*(5), 4939. DOI: 10.3390/ijms24054939 PMID: 36902370

Zhu, Y., Doornebal, E. J., Pirtskhalava, T., Giorgadze, N., Wentworth, M., Fuhrmann-Stroissnigg, H., Niedernhofer, L. J., Robbins, P. D., Tchkonia, T., & Kirkland, J. L. (2017). New agents that target senescent cells: The flavone, fisetin, and the BCL-X_L inhibitors, A1331852 and A1155463. *Aging (Albany NY)*, *9*(3), 955–963. DOI: 10.18632/aging.101202 PMID: 28273655

Zhu, Y., Tchkonia, T., Pirtskhalava, T., Gower, A. C., Ding, H., Giorgadze, N., Palmer, A. K., Ikeno, Y., Hubbard, G. B., Lenburg, M., O'Hara, S. P., LaRusso, N. F., Miller, J. D., Roos, C. M., Verzosa, G. C., LeBrasseur, N. K., Wren, J. D., Farr, J. N., Khosla, S., & Kirkland, J. L. (2015). The Achilles' heel of senescent cells: From transcriptome to senolytic drugs. *Aging Cell*, *14*(4), 644–658. DOI: 10.1111/acel.12344 PMID: 25754370

Zincarelli, C., Soltys, S., Rengo, G., & Rabinowitz, J. E. (2008). Analysis of AAV serotypes 1–9 mediated gene expression and tropism in mice after systemic injection. *Molecular Therapy : the Journal of the American Society of Gene Therapy*, *16*(6), 1073–1080. DOI: 10.1038/mt.2008.76 PMID: 18414476

KEY TERMS AND DEFINITIONS

Gene Therapy: A medical technique that involves modifying or manipulating an individual's genes to treat or prevent disease. This is often done by introducing a functional gene into cells to replace a faulty or missing one.

Aging-Related Diseases: Diseases whose incidence or severity increases with age. Examples include Alzheimer's disease, cardiovascular disorders, and certain types of cancer. These conditions are often linked to the biological processes that occur during aging.

CRISPR-Cas9: A revolutionary genome-editing tool that uses a guide RNA to locate a specific DNA sequence and the Cas9 enzyme to make precise cuts in the DNA. This technology allows scientists to add, remove, or alter genetic material with high accuracy.

Epigenetic Regulation: The process by which the expression of genes is controlled without changing the underlying DNA sequence. This is typically achieved through chemical modifications such as DNA methylation or histone modification, which influence how genes are turned on or off.

Cellular Senescence: A state in which cells permanently stop dividing and enter a stable growth-arrest phase without dying. While this can serve as a protective mechanism against cancer, the accumulation of senescent cells is also associated with aging and tissue dysfunction.

Mitochondrial Dysfunction: A condition in which the mitochondria—the cell's energy-producing organelles—fail to function properly. This can lead to reduced energy production, increased production of harmful reactive oxygen species, and has been implicated in aging and various diseases.

Neurodegenerative Disorders: A group of conditions characterized by the progressive degeneration or death of nerve cells (neurons), leading to impairments in motor skills, memory, or cognitive functions. Common examples include Alzheimer's disease, Parkinson's disease, and Huntington's disease.

Regenerative Medicine: A field of medicine focused on repairing, replacing, or regenerating damaged tissues and organs to restore normal function. This often involves the use of stem cells, tissue engineering, and gene therapy to harness the body's natural healing abilities.

Genomic Stability: The maintenance of the correct structure and sequence of an organism's genome over time. High genomic stability is essential for preventing mutations that can lead to diseases such as cancer, and it relies on robust DNA repair and cell cycle control mechanisms.

Targeted Delivery Systems: Technologies or methods designed to deliver therapeutic agents—such as drugs, genes, or proteins—directly to specific cells or tissues. This approach aims to maximize treatment efficacy while minimizing side effects by ensuring that the therapy acts only on the intended target.

Longevity: The duration of an individual's life or the ability to live a long life. In research, longevity is often studied in the context of factors that extend lifespan and delay the onset of age-related diseases.

Oxidative Stress: A state in which there is an imbalance between the production of reactive oxygen species (free radicals) and the body's ability to detoxify them or repair the resulting damage. This imbalance can damage cells, proteins, and DNA, and is associated with aging and various diseases.

Chapter 6
Stem-Cell Therapy for Anti-Aging

Tharani Sureshkumar
https://orcid.org/0009-0000-9898-3225
PSGR Krishnammal College for Women, India

Krishnasreya Mohandas
https://orcid.org/0009-0001-3311-6638
PSGR Krishnammal College for Women, India

Elakkiya Maruthamuthu Rathinam
https://orcid.org/0009-0004-8001-3203
PSGR Krishnammal College for Women, India

Chitra Devi Balasundaram Saraswathy
https://orcid.org/0000-0002-6205-9556
PSGR Krishnammal College for Women, India

Sarmad Moin
https://orcid.org/0000-0003-2521-2731
Suresh Gyan Vihar University, India

ABSTRACT

Stem-cell therapy is a promising approach to combating aging by targeting cellular degeneration and tissue repair. This chapter provides a comprehensive overview of advancements in stem-cell therapy for anti-aging, examining how stem cells can reverse or slow age-related changes at molecular and tissue levels. We explore various stem cell types used in anti-aging therapies, including mesenchymal stem cells (MSCs), induced pluripotent stem cells (iPSCs), and embryonic stem cells (ESCs), highlighting their roles in tissue regeneration, immune enhancement, and cellular rejuvenation. Additionally, this chapter discusses recent clinical trials, potential applications for age-related diseases, and key ethical and safety considerations in stem-cell-based anti-aging treatments. As the field progresses, we examine emerging trends and challenges, including regulatory hurdles and the need for robust clinical evidence. This chapter provides a balanced, up-to-date perspective on stem-cell therapy's potential to revolutionize anti-aging interventions and enhance longevity.

DOI: 10.4018/979-8-3693-9730-5.ch006

1. INTRODUCTION

Aging is a complex, time-dependent process characterized by irreversible changes at molecular, cellular, and organ levels, leading to a decline in biological functions (Stanić & Matić, 2019). It results from cumulative damage to proteins and DNA, disrupting homeostasis and increasing disease susceptibility (Pyo, Yun, Yoon, Choi, & Lee, 2020). Key biological mechanisms include oxidative stress, telomere shortening, and mitochondrial dysfunction, which contribute to age-related changes (Namita, Mondal, & Bandhu, 2021). Metabolomics has emerged as a valuable tool for identifying biomarkers of aging, revealing alterations in metabolites related to amino acids, lipids, and carbohydrates (Srivastava, 2019). The interplay of genetic, environmental, and lifestyle factors further complicates the understanding of aging mechanisms (Srivastava, 2019). Overall, the study of aging encompasses various theories and mechanisms, highlighting the need for continued research to unravel its complexities (Namita et al., 2021; Stanić & Matić, 2019).

Anti-aging interventions aim to extend both lifespan and healthspan in humans by targeting the biological processes of aging. Caloric restriction has shown promise in animal models, leading to the development of more feasible dietary approaches like intermittent fasting (Ros & Carrascosa, 2020). Pharmacological interventions targeting molecular effectors involved in nutrient sensing pathways and longevity are being explored (Gonzalez-Freire et al., 2020; Ros & Carrascosa, 2020). These include drugs targeting mTOR, sirtuins, and senescent cells (Nielsen, Bakula, & Scheibye-Knudsen, 2022). Clinical trials are underway to evaluate the efficacy of various interventions, such as GlyNAC supplementation, dietary restriction, and exercise training (Parker, 2022). However, translating results from animal studies to humans remains challenging due to species heterogeneity and the lack of reliable biomarkers for aging (Gonzalez-Freire et al., 2020; Nielsen et al., 2022). Future research will focus on larger-scale clinical trials to assess the safety and effectiveness of these interventions in humans.

Stem cell therapy shows promise for treating age-related disorders and promoting healthy aging. Stem cells play crucial roles in tissue development, homeostasis, and regeneration (B. Liu, Qu, Zhang, Belmonte, & Liu, 2022). However, aging negatively impacts stem cell function, reducing their regenerative potential (El Assaad et al., 2024; Narbonne, 2018). Aging affects various aspects of stem cells, including epigenetic changes, protein homeostasis, and systemic factors like chronic inflammation and metabolic disorders (B. Liu et al., 2022). Despite these challenges, stem cell therapies offer potential for mitigating neurological symptoms in age-related diseases such as Parkinson's, Huntington's, and stroke (Nguyen et al., 2019). Mesenchymal stem cells, in particular, have attracted attention for their immunomodulatory and tissue regeneration properties (El Assaad et al., 2024). While using young donor stem cells or rejuvenating aged patient-derived stem cells may help, the success of transplantation in aged patients remains problematic due to unsupportive extrinsic factors (Narbonne, 2018).

2. THE BIOLOGY OF AGING

2.1. Cellular Senescence and Its Role in Aging

Cellular senescence, a state of permanent cell cycle arrest, plays a crucial role in aging and age-related diseases (Wei & Ji, 2018). Senescent cells accumulate damage and develop a senescence-associated secretory phenotype (SASP), contributing to chronic inflammation and tissue dysfunction (Calcinotto et al.,

2019; Ogrodnik, Salmonowicz, & Gladyshev, 2019). While senescence serves as a defense mechanism against cancer and aids in embryonic development and tissue repair, its accumulation over time leads to various pathological conditions, including nonalcoholic fatty liver disease, obesity, and pulmonary hypertension (Calcinotto et al., 2019; Wei & Ji, 2018). Recent research has focused on developing senotherapeutics, including senolytics to eliminate senescent cells and senomorphics to suppress the SASP (L. Zhang et al., 2022). These interventions have shown promise in preclinical studies and small clinical trials, demonstrating the potential to alleviate age-related disorders and improve healthspan (L. Zhang et al., 2022). Consequently, targeting cellular senescence has emerged as a key therapeutic approach in aging research and disease treatment.

2.2. Telomere Shortening and Genomic Instability

Telomere shortening is a key driver of genomic instability, contributing to cancer development and embryonic abnormalities. Critically short telomeres can lead to chromosomal fusion, aneuploidy, and other genetic alterations (Forood, 2024; Keefe, 2020). In embryonic stem cells, telomere attrition promotes retrotransposon activation and increased chromatin accessibility, resulting in elevated mutations and copy number variations (Zhao et al., 2023). During early embryo development, telomere dynamics differ between sexes, with oocytes having shorter telomeres than sperm, potentially contributing to meiotic dysfunction and embryonic genomic instability (Keefe, 2020). Cancer cells maintain telomere length through telomerase reactivation or the Alternative Lengthening of Telomeres (ALT) pathway, which can be targeted for therapeutic interventions (Forood, 2024). Recent research has also highlighted the role of retrotransposons in regulating genome stability through interactions with telomeres, offering new perspectives on telomere-related genomic instability mechanisms (Lu & Liu, 2024).

2.3. Mitochondrial Dysfunction and Oxidative Stress

Mitochondrial dysfunction and oxidative stress play crucial roles in various age-related neurodegenerative diseases and heart failure (Elfawy & Das, 2019; Kiyuna, e Albuquerque, Chen, Mochly-Rosen, & Ferreira, 2018). These conditions are characterized by impaired bioenergetics, increased reactive oxygen species (ROS) production, and alterations in mitochondrial dynamics and quality control mechanisms (Misrani, Tabassum, & Yang, 2021). The imbalance between ROS production and oxidation affects mitochondrial function, leading to cellular damage and death (Elfawy & Das, 2019). Targeting mitochondrial detoxification systems and enhancing antioxidant bioavailability have shown promise in preventing or treating these disorders (Kiyuna et al., 2018). Astaxanthin, a carotenoid with anti-oxidative properties, has demonstrated potential in maintaining mitochondrial integrity under pathological conditions (S. H. Kim & Kim, 2018). Additionally, lifestyle interventions such as physical exercise and antioxidant-rich diets may help restore mitochondrial function and slow disease progression (Misrani et al., 2021). These findings highlight the importance of addressing mitochondrial dysfunction and oxidative stress in age-related diseases.

2.4. Stem Cell Exhaustion and Tissue Degeneration

Stem cell exhaustion is a hallmark of aging that contributes to tissue degeneration and functional decline. Research has revealed various mechanisms underlying this process. In hair follicles, epithelial cells escape from the stem cell compartment, leading to miniaturization and hair loss (C. Zhang et al., 2021). Mesenchymal stem cells undergo senescence and exhibit a senescence-associated secretory phenotype, accelerating tissue aging and inflammation (Y. Liu & Chen, 2020). Epigenetic changes in adult stem cells impair their differentiation and self-renewal capabilities, further contributing to aging-related tissue dysfunction (Kosan, Heidel, Godmann, & Bierhoff, 2018). Experimental depletion of Sox2+ stem cells in mice results in premature aging symptoms, including kyphosis, hair graying, and reduced fat mass, as well as cellular senescence in various tissues (Vilas et al., 2018). These findings collectively demonstrate that stem cell exhaustion is a key driver of tissue degeneration and aging, highlighting the importance of maintaining stem cell function for healthy aging.

3. ROLE OF STEM CELLS IN AGING AND REGENERATION

3.1. Types of Stem Cells

3.1.1. Embryonic Stem Cells (ESCs)

Embryonic stem cells (ESCs), derived from the inner cell mass of blastocysts, possess unique properties of self-renewal and pluripotency (Hassani, Moradi, Taleahmad, Braun, & Baharvand, 2019; Raščanin, Rančić, Dragović, & Jovanović, 2019; Varzideh, Gambardella, Kansakar, Jankauskas, & Santulli, 2023). These characteristics are regulated by complex networks involving epigenetic modifications, transcription factors, signaling pathways, and histone modifications (Hassani et al., 2019; Varzideh et al., 2023). ESCs have potential applications in regenerative medicine, transplantation, disease modeling, and treatment of various conditions (Raščanin et al., 2019). Different culture media have been developed to maintain ESCs in a state of naïve pluripotency and preserve genomic stability (Hassani et al., 2019). While ESCs represent the gold standard for pluripotency in vitro, induced pluripotent stem cells (iPSCs) offer advantages in autologous transplantation and avoid ethical concerns (Raščanin et al., 2019). Ongoing research focuses on understanding the molecular mechanisms underlying ESC pluripotency and self-renewal in both murine and human models (Varzideh et al., 2023).

3.1.2. Induced Pluripotent Stem Cells (iPSCs)

Induced Pluripotent Stem Cells (iPSCs) are reprogrammed somatic cells that possess pluripotency, capable of self-renewal and differentiation into various cell types (Rančić, Rascanin, Miljkovic, & Jovanovic, 2020). They offer significant potential in regenerative medicine, disease modeling, and drug discovery (Karagiannis, Nakauchi, & Yamanaka, 2018). iPSCs are generated through the forced expression of specific transcription factors, providing a powerful tool for studying cell fate decisions and human development (Cerneckis, Cai, & Shi, 2024; Moradi et al., 2019). While similar to embryonic stem cells, iPSCs present fewer ethical concerns and can be patient-specific, reducing the risk of tissue rejection (Rančić et al., 2020). The technology has advanced rapidly, with ongoing clinical studies using iPSC-based cell therapies and drug screening (Karagiannis et al., 2018). However, legal and ethical considerations must be addressed to fully exploit iPSCs' potential while minimizing abuse (Moradi et al., 2019). The versatility of iPSCs extends to creating complex 3D organoids and modeling various diseases, including neurological disorders and COVID-19 (Cerneckis et al., 2024).

3.1.3. Mesenchymal Stem Cells (MSCs)

Mesenchymal stem cells (MSCs) are multipotent adult stem cells capable of differentiating into various mesodermal lineages (P. Li, Gong, Shultz, & Ren, 2019; Timaner, Tsai, & Shaked, 2020). Originally identified in bone marrow, MSCs have since been isolated from numerous tissues, including adipose tissue, dental pulp, and birth-derived tissues (Akhlaq, 2022; Berebichez-Fridman & Montero-Olvera, 2018). These cells possess low immunogenicity, strong immunomodulatory potential, and the ability to secrete cytokines and extracellular vesicles (Akhlaq, 2022). MSCs play crucial roles in wound healing and cancer progression, influencing processes such as angiogenesis, metastasis, and therapy resistance (P. Li et al., 2019; Timaner et al., 2020). Their multilineage potential, immunomodulatory properties, and capacity for tissue repair have led to numerous clinical applications, including cartilage and bone repair, neuronal regeneration, and treatment of immune disorders (Akhlaq, 2022; Berebichez-Fridman & Montero-Olvera, 2018). MSCs from different sources possess distinct characteristics, influencing their suitability for specific clinical applications in regenerative medicine and tissue engineering (Berebichez-Fridman & Montero-Olvera, 2018).

3.1.4. Hematopoietic Stem Cells (HSCs)

Hematopoietic stem cells (HSCs) are multipotent adult stem cells capable of self-renewal and differentiation into various blood cell lineages (Gilchrist, Lee, Hu, & Harley, 2019). They play a crucial role in hematopoiesis and have been extensively studied for clinical applications, including bone marrow transplantation (Yamamoto, Wilkinson, & Nakauchi, 2018). Recent research has revealed the importance of metabolic activity in HSC function, with dysregulation potentially leading to hematological disorders (Wilkinson & Yamazaki, 2018). HSCs undergo functional changes throughout an organism's lifetime, transitioning from expansion during fetal development to quiescence in adulthood and decline with aging (Kasbekar, Mitchell, Proven, & Passegué, 2023). These age-related changes involve alterations in cell cycle regulation, inflammatory response pathways, epigenetics, and metabolism (Kasbekar et al., 2023). Understanding these processes is crucial for developing strategies to rejuvenate aged HSCs and improve clinical outcomes in stem cell therapies (Kasbekar et al., 2023; Yamamoto et al., 2018) (Table 1).

Table 1. Comparison of different stem cell types in anti-aging therapy

Stem Cell Type	Key Characteristics and Benefits	Challenges and Considerations	References
Adipose-Derived Stem Cells (ADSCs)	- High accessibility and abundance. - Promote mitophagy, improving mitochondrial quality and delaying aging. - Enhance collagen synthesis and angiogenesis in skin.	- Variability in differentiation capacity among donors. - Potential contamination with fibroblasts.	(Brohem et al., 2013; J.-H. Kim, Jung, Kim, Kim, & Choi, 2011; Lv et al., 2021; Mohamed-Ahmed et al., 2018)
Bone Marrow Mesenchymal Stem Cells (BMSCs)	- Higher osteogenic and chondrogenic capacity compared to ADSCs. - Participate in tissue homeostasis and have anti-inflammatory effects.	- Aging affects their regenerative capacity and increases pro-inflammatory features. - Require careful donor matching to avoid variability.	(Fraile, Eiro, Costa, Martín, & Vizoso, 2022; Mohamed-Ahmed et al., 2018; Y. Zhang, Ravikumar, Ling, Nurcombe, & Cool, 2021)
Human Mesenchymal Stem Cells (hMSCs)	- Unique immunomodulatory properties extend therapeutic potential beyond tissue regeneration. - Can be rejuvenated or replaced to combat aging.	- In vitro aging leads to diminished therapeutic efficacy and increased pro-inflammatory phenotype.	(Fraile et al., 2022; Y. Zhang et al., 2021)
General Adult Stem Cells	- Low risk of teratomas and ethical concerns. - Can be preconditioned to enhance therapeutic outcomes.	- Aging and environmental factors decrease stem cell functionality over time. - Require optimization of cell preparation and delivery methods.	(Goodell & Rando, 2015; S. Liu et al., 2016)

3.2. Stem Cell Decline With Aging

Stem cell decline with aging is a critical factor in tissue degeneration and reduced regenerative capacity (De, Karmakar, & Bhattacharya, 2021; B. Liu et al., 2022). This decline is characterized by epigenetic changes, loss of protein homeostasis, and systemic influences such as chronic inflammation and metabolic disorders (B. Liu et al., 2022). Skeletal muscle stem cells, or satellite cells, exemplify this age-related dysfunction, failing to maintain muscle regeneration in advanced age (Muñoz-Cánoves, Neves, & Sousa-Victor, 2020). However, emerging research suggests that manipulating epigenetic factors can potentially reverse aging-associated stem cell decline (D. Chen & Kerr, 2019). This aligns with the stem cell theory of aging, which posits that aging results from the inability of tissue-specific stem cells to replenish tissues with functional cells (D. Chen & Kerr, 2019). Recent advances in single-cell technologies offer new opportunities to understand stem cell aging mechanisms and develop interventions to promote healthy aging and combat age-related diseases (D. Chen & Kerr, 2019; B. Liu et al., 2022).

3.3. Mechanisms of Stem Cell-Mediated Tissue Regeneration

Stem cell-mediated tissue regeneration involves complex mechanisms, including differentiation, immunomodulation, and paracrine activities (Fan, Zhang, Li, & Fu, 2020). Mesenchymal stem cells (MSCs) exert therapeutic effects through direct cell-cell contact, mitochondrial transfer, and extracellular vesicle secretion (X.-L. Fan et al., 2020). The biophysical and biomechanical properties of the cellular environment significantly influence stem cell behavior, including migration, self-renewal, proliferation, and differentiation (Naqvi & McNamara, 2020). Biomaterials play a crucial role in enhancing stem cell functionality by providing appropriate mechanical cues and improving cell-cell and cell-extracellular matrix interactions (Shafiq, Ali, Han, & Kim, 2021). Various biomaterial-based platforms, such as nanoparticles, hydrogels, and scaffolds, can be utilized to spatiotemporally present bioactive cues to stem cells, enhancing their immunomodulatory properties and improving engraftment and retention at target sites (Shafiq et al., 2021). Understanding these mechanisms is essential for developing effective regenerative medicine approaches and tissue engineering strategies.

4. STEM-CELL THERAPY APPROACHES FOR ANTI-AGING

4.1. Autologous vs. Allogeneic Stem Cell Therapy

Stem cell therapy shows promise for various conditions, with both autologous and allogeneic sources being investigated. For intrauterine adhesions, autologous stem cells demonstrated better outcomes in endometrial thickness and pregnancy rates compared to allogeneic cells (J.-m. Chen, Huang, Chen, Lin, & Shi, 2022). In mesenchymal stem cell applications, autologous and allogeneic sources each have advantages and disadvantages, with donor variability and microenvironment interactions influencing outcomes (C. Li, Zhao, Cheng, & Wang, 2021). For knee osteoarthritis, both autologous and allogeneic mesenchymal stem cell injections showed potential for improving pain and function, though direct comparisons are lacking (Mautner, Carr, Whitley, & Bowers, 2019). In treating refractory or relapsed peripheral T-cell lymphoma, allogeneic hematopoietic stem cell transplantation may offer better effectiveness but with higher transplant-related mortality compared to autologous transplantation (Du, Yu, Han, Zhu, & Huang, 2021). Overall, the choice between autologous and allogeneic stem cell therapy depends on the specific condition and considerations of efficacy, safety, and practical factors.

4.2. Exogenous Stem Cell Transplantation

Exogenous stem cell transplantation offers promising therapeutic potential for various diseases and tissue regeneration. Xenogeneic stem cells can treat end-stage organ failures and other conditions by replacing dysfunctional cells or improving the regenerative environment (Jiang, Li, & Liu, 2021). Recent research suggests a synergistic relationship between transplanted and endogenous stem cells, which could enhance therapeutic outcomes (Madhavan & Collier, 2010). Transplanted cells may act as initiators, triggering endogenous stem cell-mediated tissue repair (Dong & Caplan, 2012). This process involves complex homing mechanisms, essential for successful engraftment in hematopoietic stem cell transplantation and potentially important for mesenchymal stem cell recruitment to injury sites (Liesveld, Sharma, & Aljitawi, 2020). Challenges include insufficient endogenous stem cell pools, aging-related dysfunction, and hostile microenvironments (Dong & Caplan, 2012). Xenogeneic stem cell transplantation has shown significant therapeutic effects in treating conditions such as liver failure and myocardial infarction (Jiang et al., 2021). Understanding and manipulating stem cell homing processes may enhance engraftment potential and improve overall treatment efficacy (Liesveld et al., 2020).

4.2.1. MSCs for Skin Rejuvenation and Wound Healing

Mesenchymal stromal cells (MSCs) show significant potential for skin rejuvenation and wound healing. MSCs promote cell migration, angiogenesis, epithelialization, and granulation tissue formation, accelerating wound closure (Hu, Borrelli, Lorenz, Longaker, & Wan, 2018). They enhance re-epithelialization, proliferation, neovascularization, and wound contraction, while reducing inflammation (Martinello et al., 2018). In skin rejuvenation, MSCs stimulate collagen and elastic fiber production, inhibit metalloproteinase activation, and protect against UV-induced senescence (Jo et al., 2021). Despite their therapeutic promise, challenges remain regarding MSC survival and homing capacity post-administration (Liubaviciute, Ivaskiene, & Biziuleviciene, 2020). To address this, researchers are developing strategies to improve MSC efficacy, including novel bioengineering approaches for cell delivery (Hu et al., 2018). Additionally, induced pluripotent stem cell (iPSC)-derived MSCs are emerging as an advanced alternative for cell therapy in skin regeneration and rejuvenation (Jo et al., 2021).

4.2.2. HSC Transplantation for Immune System Rejuvenation

Hematopoietic stem cell (HSC) transplantation has emerged as a promising approach for immune system rejuvenation and potentially extending healthy lifespan. Heterochronous autologous HSC transplantation (haHSCT) involves collecting and cryopreserving young HSCs for later reinfusion in older age (Rožman, 2018, 2020). This method has shown promise in animal studies, extending longevity and improving immune function (Rožman, 2018). Research demonstrates that aging-associated immune remodeling is primarily driven by changes in HSC function, with aged HSCs reconstituting distinct T- and B-cell subsets mirroring aged immune systems (Leins et al., 2018). Importantly, rejuvenation of aged HSCs through inhibition of Cdc42 activity can reestablish a young-like immune system capable of mounting strong responses to vaccination (Leins et al., 2018). However, translating these findings to humans remains complex, and systemic approaches addressing inflamm-aging may be necessary for effective immune rejuvenation (Pishel, 2023; Rožman, 2020)

4.3. Endogenous Stem Cell Stimulation

4.3.1. Use of Growth Factors and Small Molecules

Recent research has focused on stimulating endogenous stem cells for tissue regeneration using small molecules and growth factors. This approach offers advantages over stem cell transplantation, potentially avoiding integration issues (Um, Lee, Jung, & Williams, 2018). Small molecules and growth factors can modulate key signaling pathways to derive endothelial cells from dental stem cells, offering a promising alternative for vascularization in bioengineered dental pulp constructs (Yi, Dissanayaka, & Zhang, 2020). Chemical reprogramming using small molecules and growth factors presents a safer alternative to traditional viral-based reprogramming methods for generating induced pluripotent stem cells and direct cell conversion (Y. Kim, Jeong, & Choi, 2020). In skin regeneration, understanding the role of endogenous stem cells and factors like the TGF-β pathway could lead to scar-free healing treatments (Giri, Machens, & Bader, 2019). These approaches show potential for treating degenerative diseases and promoting tissue regeneration, with some compounds already transitioning to clinical use (Um et al., 2018).

4.3.2. Paracrine Effects and Exosome-Based Therapy

Extracellular vesicles (EVs), including exosomes, play a crucial role in paracrine signaling and cell-to-cell communication, particularly in cardiac repair and regeneration (Bollini, Smits, Balbi, Lazzarini, & Ameri, 2018). Stem cell-derived EVs, especially from mesenchymal stem cells (MSCs) and induced pluripotent stem cells (iPSCs), have shown promising therapeutic potential in various disease models (Bruno, Kholia, Deregibus, & Camussi, 2019; C. Fan et al., 2020). These EVs can modulate key cellular processes such as proliferation, angiogenesis, and inflammation, contributing to tissue repair and regeneration (Bruno et al., 2019). In the context of cardiac repair, EVs from exogenous stem cells have been demonstrated to regulate cell apoptosis, proliferation, and fibrosis in the infarcted heart (C. Fan et al., 2020). Moreover, EVs mediate communication between different cardiac cell types, including cardiomyocytes, fibroblasts, and cardiac progenitor cells, influencing cardiac homeostasis and regeneration (Bollini et al., 2018). The therapeutic potential of MSC-derived exosomes is being explored for various diseases, including cancer (Xunian & Kalluri, 2020).

4.4. Gene Editing and Reprogramming

4.4.1. Role of CRISPR and Epigenetic Modifications

Recent advances in CRISPR technologies have opened new avenues for stem cell engineering and regenerative medicine. CRISPR/Cas9 systems can be used for genome editing, gene activation (CRISPRa), and gene interference (CRISPRi) in stem cells (Hsu et al., 2019). These techniques offer promising approaches for combating aging-related diseases by genetically enhancing therapeutic cells, such as mesenchymal and neural stem cells (Cai et al., 2022). CRISPR tools can be applied to investigate stem cell gene functions, modify DNA and RNA nucleotides, and regulate gene expression (Mollashahi et al., 2023). Additionally, epitranscriptomic modifications, particularly N6-methyladenosine and 5-(hydroxy-) methylcytosine, play crucial roles in stem cell differentiation and brain development (Noack & Calegari, 2018). The combination of CRISPR-based editing platforms and RNA modifying enzymes provides opportunities to explore the functional significance of these epitranscriptome changes in stem cell reprogramming and tissue regeneration (Noack & Calegari, 2018).

4.4.2. iPSC-Based Rejuvenation Strategies

Recent research has explored partial reprogramming as a promising strategy for cell rejuvenation and generation of induced somatic cells without full dedifferentiation to pluripotency (Lehmann et al., 2019). This approach involves transient expression of pluripotency genes, particularly the Yamanaka factors (OSKM), to achieve rejuvenation while maintaining cell identity (Simpson, Olova, & Chandra, 2021). Induced pluripotent stem cells (iPSCs) offer potential for patient-specific cell replacement therapies and can be combined with gene editing techniques like CRISPR/Cas9 for treating genetic and degenerative diseases (Al Abbar, Ngai, Nograles, Alhaji, & Abdullah, 2020). Reprogramming-induced rejuvenation strategies, which aim to separate the rejuvenative properties of reprogramming from complete dedifferentiation, are emerging as promising anti-aging approaches (Simpson et al., 2021). These techniques have shown success in both in vitro and in vivo models, offering potential to improve healthspan and longevity (Alle, Le Borgne, Milhavet, & Lemaitre, 2021). However, further research is needed to fully understand and optimize these rejuvenation strategies.

5. CLINICAL APPLICATIONS AND EVIDENCE

Stem cell therapy shows promise for anti-aging applications, particularly in addressing physical frailty and facial skin aging. Mesenchymal stem cells (MSCs) have demonstrated positive results in clinical trials, with intravenous Lomecel-B and umbilical cord-derived stem cells showing potential for reducing frailty (R. P. Garay, 2023). Adipose-derived stem cells have yielded encouraging outcomes for facial skin rejuvenation (Zarei & Abbaszadeh, 2019). The anti-aging effects of stem cells are attributed to their multipotency, immunomodulation, and secretion of paracrine factors and extracellular vesicles (El Assaad et al., 2024). Various stem cell sources, including bone marrow-derived and umbilical cord blood cells, have been explored for treating aging-related disorders such as Parkinson's disease, vascular dementia, and Alzheimer's disease (Borlongan et al., 2021). While stem cell therapy shows promise, further research is needed to fully understand its mechanisms and long-term effects in anti-aging applications (Table 2).

Table 2. Current clinical trials on stem-cell therapy for anti-aging

Clinical Trial Focus	Description	Key Findings	References
Skin Aging	Several clinical trials have focused on stem cell-derived cell-free therapies, which include secretomes and extracellular vesicles (EVs) to prevent skin aging. These therapies target multiple regenerative pathways, regulate oxidative stress, prevent ECM degradation, and modulate inflammatory pathways.	Improvements have been observed in wrinkles, elasticity, hydration, pores, and pigmentation	(Chou, Alfarafisa, Ikezawa, & Khairani, 2023)
Physical Frailty and Facial Skin Aging	Mesenchymal stem cell interventions are being tested for their efficacy in slowing or reversing aging processes, particularly in physical frailty and facial skin aging. Positive results have been reported in phase II studies with intravenous Lomecel-B and autologous adipose-derived stem cells.	Sixteen clinical trials are currently underway, with promising results in increasing healthy life expectancy and reducing public health costs.	(R. Garay, 2023)
Aging Frailty	A phase II randomized, double-blind, placebo-controlled clinical trial tested allogeneic mesenchymal stem cells (allo-hMSCs) for aging frailty. The study focused on physical performance and immune markers.	No therapy-related serious adverse events were reported, and significant improvements in physical performance and inflammatory biomarkers were observed.	(Tompkins et al., 2017)
Conditioned Medium for Skin Aging	Research on stem cell-conditioned media has shown success in reducing risk factors for skin aging. This approach is being explored in various in vitro, in vivo, and clinical trials.	Conditioned media from stem cells has demonstrated potential in reducing skin aging risk factors.	(Alquraisy et al., 2024)

6. ETHICAL AND REGULATORY CONSIDERATIONS

Stem cell therapy for anti-aging presents both promising potential and significant ethical and regulatory challenges. While stem cells offer regenerative capabilities and potential tissue repair benefits (El Assaad et al., 2024), concerns persist regarding inadequate characterization, poor adverse effect disclosure, and unorthodox marketing practices (Piuzzi, Emara, Chahla, & Mandelbaum, 2020). Regulatory frameworks vary across countries, with efforts to develop comprehensive guidelines for safety and ethical integrity (Khabade, Agarwal, Mahajan, & Mandlik, 2024). However, loopholes in regulations and unclear efficacy reports impede value-based assessments (Piuzzi et al., 2020). The rapid proliferation of stem cell clinics globally reflects public interest in potential benefits for incurable diseases, necessitating careful policy-making and oversight by regulatory bodies (Sharma, 2019). To address these challenges, a multidisciplinary approach involving legislative and medical professional societies is recommended to advance regulations governing stem cell interventions and ensure ethical integration with evidence-based benefits and risks (Piuzzi et al., 2020).

7. FUTURE PERSPECTIVES AND CHALLENGES

Stem cell therapy has emerged as a promising approach to combat aging and age-related disorders. Mesenchymal stem cells, with their multipotency and immunomodulatory properties, show potential for tissue regeneration and anti-aging effects (El Assaad et al., 2024). Various stem cell types and their applications have been explored, including the use of graphene scaffolds and extracellular vesicle-based therapies (Zakrzewski, Dobrzyński, Szymonowicz, & Rybak, 2019). Researchers have investigated mechanisms of stem cell senescence, such as mitochondrial dysfunction and epigenetic alterations, leading to proposed rejuvenation strategies like pharmaceutical interventions and cellular reprogramming (Larijani et al., 2021). Stem cells' plasticity, self-renewal, and multidirectional differentiation potential make them promising candidates for reversing aging and addressing age-related tissue degeneration (Chang, Fan, Pan, & Zhu, 2022). However, challenges remain in developing effective stem cell therapies for widespread clinical use, necessitating further research and quality control (El Assaad et al., 2024; Zakrzewski et al., 2019).

8. CONCLUSION

Stem-cell therapy holds great potential for mitigating age-related decline and promoting longevity by targeting key mechanisms of aging, including cellular senescence, mitochondrial dysfunction, and stem cell exhaustion. Various stem cell types, including mesenchymal, hematopoietic, and induced pluripotent stem cells, have shown promise in tissue regeneration, immune system rejuvenation, and neuroprotection. Emerging approaches such as gene editing, exosome therapy, and personalized regenerative medicine continue to refine stem-cell-based anti-aging strategies. However, challenges related to safety, ethical concerns, and clinical translation must be addressed to ensure the widespread application of stem-cell therapy in aging interventions. Future research and advancements in biotechnology will be crucial in unlocking the full potential of stem cells for extending health span and lifespan.

REFERENCES

Akhlaq, S. (2022). Journey of mesenchymal stem cells in biomedical research: Current aspects and scenario.

Al Abbar, A., Ngai, S. C., Nograles, N., Alhaji, S. Y., & Abdullah, S. (2020). Induced pluripotent stem cells: Reprogramming platforms and applications in cell replacement therapy. *BioResearch Open Access*, *9*(1), 121–136. DOI: 10.1089/biores.2019.0046 PMID: 32368414

Alle, Q., Le Borgne, E., Milhavet, O., & Lemaitre, J.-M. (2021). Reprogramming: Emerging strategies to rejuvenate aging cells and tissues. *International Journal of Molecular Sciences*, *22*(8), 3990. DOI: 10.3390/ijms22083990 PMID: 33924362

Alquraisy, A., Wilar, G., Mohammed, A., El-Rayyes, A., Suhandi, C., & Wathoni, N. (2024). A Comprehensive Review of Stem Cell Conditioned Media Role for Anti-Aging on Skin. *Stem Cells and Cloning : Advances and Applications*, *17*, 5–19. DOI: 10.2147/SCCAA.S480437 PMID: 39310304

Berebichez-Fridman, R., & Montero-Olvera, P. R. (2018). Sources and clinical applications of mesenchymal stem cells: State-of-the-art review. *Sultan Qaboos University Medical Journal*, *18*(3), e264–e277. DOI: 10.18295/squmj.2018.18.03.002 PMID: 30607265

Bollini, S., Smits, A. M., Balbi, C., Lazzarini, E., & Ameri, P. (2018). Triggering endogenous cardiac repair and regeneration via extracellular vesicle-mediated communication. *Frontiers in Physiology*, *9*, 1497. DOI: 10.3389/fphys.2018.01497 PMID: 30405446

Borlongan, M. C., Farooq, J., Sadanandan, N., Wang, Z.-J., Cozene, B., Lee, J.-Y., & Steinberg, G. K. (2021). Stem cells for aging-related disorders. *Stem Cell Reviews and Reports*, *17*(6), 2054–2058. DOI: 10.1007/s12015-021-10222-x PMID: 34374944

Brohem, C., Carvalho, C., Radoski, C., Santi, F., Baptista, M., Swinka, B., & Lorencini, M. (2013). Comparison between fibroblasts and mesenchymal stem cells derived from dermal and adipose tissue. *International Journal of Cosmetic Science*, *35*. Advance online publication. DOI: 10.1111/ics.12064 PMID: 23651429

Bruno, S., Kholia, S., Deregibus, M. C., & Camussi, G. (2019). The role of extracellular vesicles as paracrine effectors in stem cell-based therapies. *Stem cells: therapeutic applications*, 175-193.

Cai, Y., Ji, Z., Wang, S., Zhang, W., Qu, J., Belmonte, J. C. I., & Liu, G.-H. (2022). Genetic enhancement: An avenue to combat aging-related diseases. *Life Medicine*, *1*(3), 307–318. DOI: 10.1093/lifemedi/lnac054 PMID: 39872744

Calcinotto, A., Kohli, J., Zagato, E., Pellegrini, L., Demaria, M., & Alimonti, A. (2019). Cellular senescence: Aging, cancer, and injury. *Physiological Reviews*, *99*(2), 1047–1078. DOI: 10.1152/physrev.00020.2018 PMID: 30648461

Cerneckis, J., Cai, H., & Shi, Y. (2024). Induced pluripotent stem cells (iPSCs): Molecular mechanisms of induction and applications. *Signal Transduction and Targeted Therapy*, *9*(1), 112. DOI: 10.1038/s41392-024-01809-0 PMID: 38670977

Chang, L., Fan, W., Pan, X., & Zhu, X. (2022). Stem cells to reverse aging. *Chinese Medical Journal, 135*(08), 901–910. DOI: 10.1097/CM9.0000000000001984 PMID: 35089883

Chen, D., & Kerr, C. (2019). The epigenetics of stem cell aging comes of age. *Trends in Cell Biology, 29*(7), 563–568. DOI: 10.1016/j.tcb.2019.03.006 PMID: 31030975

Chen, J., Huang, Q.-y., Chen, W., Lin, S., & Shi, Q.-y. (2022). Clinical evaluation of autologous and allogeneic stem cell therapy for intrauterine adhesions: A systematic review and meta-analysis. *Frontiers in Immunology, 13*, 899666. DOI: 10.3389/fimmu.2022.899666 PMID: 35860277

Chou, Y., Alfarafisa, N., Ikezawa, M., & Khairani, A. (2023). Progress in the Development of Stem Cell-Derived Cell-Free Therapies for Skin Aging. *Clinical, Cosmetic and Investigational Dermatology, 16*, 3383–3406. DOI: 10.2147/CCID.S434439 PMID: 38021432

De, D., Karmakar, P., & Bhattacharya, D. (2021). *Stem cell aging and regenerative medicine. Cell Biology and Translational Medicine* (Vol. 12). Stem Cells in Development and Disease.

Dong, F., & Caplan, A. I. (2012). Cell transplantation as an initiator of endogenous stem cell-based tissue repair. *Current Opinion in Organ Transplantation, 17*(6), 670–674. DOI: 10.1097/MOT.0b013e328359a617 PMID: 23111645

Du, J., Yu, D., Han, X., Zhu, L., & Huang, Z. (2021). Comparison of allogeneic stem cell transplant and autologous stem cell transplant in refractory or relapsed peripheral T-cell lymphoma: A systematic review and meta-analysis. *JAMA Network Open, 4*(5), e219807–e219807. DOI: 10.1001/jamanetworkopen.2021.9807 PMID: 34042995

El Assaad, N., Chebly, A., Salame, R., Achkar, R., Atme, N. B., Akouch, K., & Ghosn, M. (2024). Anti-aging based on stem cell therapy: A scoping review. *World Journal of Experimental Medicine, 14*(3), 97233. DOI: 10.5493/wjem.v14.i3.97233 PMID: 39312703

Elfawy, H. A., & Das, B. (2019). Crosstalk between mitochondrial dysfunction, oxidative stress, and age related neurodegenerative disease: Etiologies and therapeutic strategies. *Life Sciences, 218*, 165–184. DOI: 10.1016/j.lfs.2018.12.029 PMID: 30578866

Fan, C., Zhang, E., Joshi, J., Yang, J., Zhang, J., & Zhu, W. (2020). Utilization of human induced pluripotent stem cells for cardiac repair. *Frontiers in Cell and Developmental Biology, 8*, 36. DOI: 10.3389/fcell.2020.00036 PMID: 32117968

Fan, X.-L., Zhang, Y., Li, X., & Fu, Q.-L. (2020). Mechanisms underlying the protective effects of mesenchymal stem cell-based therapy. *Cellular and Molecular Life Sciences : CMLS, 77*(14), 2771–2794. DOI: 10.1007/s00018-020-03454-6 PMID: 31965214

Forood, A. M. K. (2024). Mechanisms of telomere dysfunction in cancer from genomic instability to therapy: A.

Fraile, M., Eiro, N., Costa, L., Martín, A., & Vizoso, F. (2022). Aging and Mesenchymal Stem Cells: Basic Concepts, Challenges and Strategies. *Biology (Basel), 11*(11), 1678. Advance online publication. DOI: 10.3390/biology11111678 PMID: 36421393

Garay, R. (2023). Recent clinical trials with stem cells to slow or reverse normal aging processes. *Frontiers in Aging*, *4*, 1148926. Advance online publication. DOI: 10.3389/fragi.2023.1148926 PMID: 37090485

Garay, R. P. (2023). Recent clinical trials with stem cells to slow or reverse normal aging processes. *Frontiers in Aging*, *4*, 1148926. DOI: 10.3389/fragi.2023.1148926 PMID: 37090485

Gilchrist, A. E., Lee, S., Hu, Y., & Harley, B. A. (2019). Hematopoietic Stem Cells: Soluble Signals and Remodeling in a Synthetic Gelatin-Based Hematopoietic Stem Cell Niche (Adv. Healthcare Mater. 20/2019). *Advanced Healthcare Materials*, *8*(20), 1970080. DOI: 10.1002/adhm.201970080 PMID: 31532901

Giri, S., Machens, H.-G., & Bader, A. (2019). Therapeutic potential of endogenous stem cells and cellular factors for scar-free skin regeneration. *Drug Discovery Today*, *24*(1), 69–84. DOI: 10.1016/j.drudis.2018.10.014 PMID: 30408529

Gonzalez-Freire, M., Diaz-Ruiz, A., Hauser, D., Martinez-Romero, J., Ferrucci, L., Bernier, M., & de Cabo, R. (2020). The road ahead for health and lifespan interventions. *Ageing Research Reviews*, *59*, 101037. DOI: 10.1016/j.arr.2020.101037 PMID: 32109604

Goodell, M., & Rando, T. (2015). Stem cells and healthy aging. *Science*, *350*(6265), 1199–1204. DOI: 10.1126/science.aab3388 PMID: 26785478

Hassani, S.-N., Moradi, S., Taleahmad, S., Braun, T., & Baharvand, H. (2019). Transition of inner cell mass to embryonic stem cells: Mechanisms, facts, and hypotheses. *Cellular and Molecular Life Sciences : CMLS*, *76*(5), 873–892. DOI: 10.1007/s00018-018-2965-y PMID: 30420999

Hsu, M.-N., Chang, Y.-H., Truong, V. A., Lai, P.-L., Nguyen, T. K. N., & Hu, Y.-C. (2019). CRISPR technologies for stem cell engineering and regenerative medicine. *Biotechnology Advances*, *37*(8), 107447. DOI: 10.1016/j.biotechadv.2019.107447 PMID: 31513841

Hu, M. S., Borrelli, M. R., Lorenz, H. P., Longaker, M. T., & Wan, D. C. (2018). Mesenchymal stromal cells and cutaneous wound healing: A comprehensive review of the background, role, and therapeutic potential. *Stem Cells International*, *2018*(1), 6901983. DOI: 10.1155/2018/6901983 PMID: 29887893

Jiang, L.-L., Li, H., & Liu, L. (2021). Xenogeneic stem cell transplantation: Research progress and clinical prospects. *World Journal of Clinical Cases*, *9*(16), 3826–3837. DOI: 10.12998/wjcc.v9.i16.3826 PMID: 34141739

Jo, H., Brito, S., Kwak, B. M., Park, S., Lee, M.-G., & Bin, B.-H. (2021). Applications of mesenchymal stem cells in skin regeneration and rejuvenation. *International Journal of Molecular Sciences*, *22*(5), 2410. DOI: 10.3390/ijms22052410 PMID: 33673711

Karagiannis, P., Nakauchi, A., & Yamanaka, S. (2018). Bringing induced pluripotent stem cell technology to the bedside. *JMA Journal*, *1*(1), 6–14. DOI: 10.31662/jmaj.2018-0005 PMID: 33748517

Kasbekar, M., Mitchell, C. A., Proven, M. A., & Passegué, E. (2023). Hematopoietic stem cells through the ages: A lifetime of adaptation to organismal demands. *Cell Stem Cell*, *30*(11), 1403–1420. DOI: 10.1016/j.stem.2023.09.013 PMID: 37865087

Keefe, D. L. (2020). Telomeres and genomic instability during early development. *European Journal of Medical Genetics*, *63*(2), 103638. DOI: 10.1016/j.ejmg.2019.03.002 PMID: 30862510

Khabade, A., Agarwal, S., Mahajan, H., & Mandlik, S. (2024). Navigating Regulatory requirements for Stem Cells Therapy- A review on Regulations of US, European Union, Japan and India. *International Journal of Drug Regulatory Affairs*, *12*(3), 66–81. DOI: 10.22270/ijdra.v12i3.704

Kim, J.-H., Jung, M., Kim, H.-S., Kim, Y.-M., & Choi, E. (2011). Adipose-derived stem cells as a new therapeutic modality for ageing skin. *Experimental Dermatology*, *20*(5), 383–387. Advance online publication. DOI: 10.1111/j.1600-0625.2010.01221.x PMID: 21355887

Kim, S. H., & Kim, H. (2018). Inhibitory effect of astaxanthin on oxidative stress-induced mitochondrial dysfunction-a mini-review. *Nutrients*, *10*(9), 1137. DOI: 10.3390/nu10091137 PMID: 30134611

Kim, Y., Jeong, J., & Choi, D. (2020). Small-molecule-mediated reprogramming: A silver lining for regenerative medicine. *Experimental & Molecular Medicine*, *52*(2), 213–226. DOI: 10.1038/s12276-020-0383-3 PMID: 32080339

Kiyuna, L. A., Albuquerque, R. P., Chen, C.-H., Mochly-Rosen, D., & Ferreira, J. C. B. (2018). Targeting mitochondrial dysfunction and oxidative stress in heart failure: Challenges and opportunities. *Free Radical Biology & Medicine*, *129*, 155–168. DOI: 10.1016/j.freeradbiomed.2018.09.019 PMID: 30227272

Kosan, C., Heidel, F. H., Godmann, M., & Bierhoff, H. (2018). Epigenetic erosion in adult stem cells: Drivers and passengers of aging. *Cells*, *7*(12), 237. DOI: 10.3390/cells7120237 PMID: 30501028

Larijani, B., Foroughi-Heravani, N., Alaei, S., Rezaei-Tavirani, M., Alavi-Moghadam, S., Payab, M., & Arjmand, B. (2021). *Opportunities and challenges in stem cell aging. Cell Biology and Translational Medicine* (Vol. 13). Stem Cells in Development and Disease.

Lehmann, M., Canatelli-Mallat, M., Chiavellini, P., Cónsole, G. M., Gallardo, M. D., & Goya, R. G. (2019). Partial reprogramming as an emerging strategy for safe induced cell generation and rejuvenation. *Current Gene Therapy*, *19*(4), 248–254. DOI: 10.2174/1566523219666190902154511 PMID: 31475896

Leins, H., Mulaw, M., Eiwen, K., Sakk, V., Liang, Y., Denkinger, M., Geiger, H., & Schirmbeck, R. (2018). Aged murine hematopoietic stem cells drive aging-associated immune remodeling. *Blood*, *132*(6), 565–576. DOI: 10.1182/blood-2018-02-831065 PMID: 29891535

Li, C., Zhao, H., Cheng, L., & Wang, B. (2021). Allogeneic vs. autologous mesenchymal stem/stromal cells in their medication practice. *Cell & Bioscience*, *11*(1), 1–21. DOI: 10.1186/s13578-021-00698-y PMID: 34727974

Li, P., Gong, Z., Shultz, L. D., & Ren, G. (2019). Mesenchymal stem cells: From regeneration to cancer. *Pharmacology & Therapeutics*, *200*, 42–54. DOI: 10.1016/j.pharmthera.2019.04.005 PMID: 30998940

Liesveld, J. L., Sharma, N., & Aljitawi, O. S. (2020). Stem cell homing: From physiology to therapeutics. *Stem Cells (Dayton, Ohio)*, *38*(10), 1241–1253. DOI: 10.1002/stem.3242 PMID: 32526037

Liu, B., Qu, J., Zhang, W., Belmonte, J. C. I., & Liu, G.-H. (2022). A stem cell aging framework, from mechanisms to interventions. *Cell Reports*, *41*(3), 111451. DOI: 10.1016/j.celrep.2022.111451 PMID: 36261013

Liu, S., Zhou, J., Zhang, X., Liu, Y., Chen, J., Hu, B., Song, J., & Zhang, Y. (2016). Strategies to Optimize Adult Stem Cell Therapy for Tissue Regeneration. *International Journal of Molecular Sciences, 17*(6), 982. Advance online publication. DOI: 10.3390/ijms17060982 PMID: 27338364

Liu, Y., & Chen, Q. (2020). Senescent mesenchymal stem cells: Disease mechanism and treatment strategy. *Current Molecular Biology Reports, 6*(4), 173–182. DOI: 10.1007/s40610-020-00141-0 PMID: 33816065

Liubaviciute, A., Ivaskiene, T., & Biziuleviciene, G. (2020). Modulated mesenchymal stromal cells improve skin wound healing. *Biologicals, 67*, 1–8. DOI: 10.1016/j.biologicals.2020.08.003 PMID: 32828641

Lu, X., & Liu, L. (2024). Genome stability from the perspective of telomere length. *Trends in Genetics, 40*(2), 175–186. DOI: 10.1016/j.tig.2023.10.013 PMID: 37957036

Lv, M., Zhang, S., Jiang, B., Cao, S., Dong, Y., Cao, L., & Guo, S. (2021). Adipose-derived stem cells regulate metabolic homeostasis and delay aging by promoting mitophagy. *The FASEB Journal, 35*(7). Advance online publication. DOI: 10.1096/fj.202100332R PMID: 34143518

Madhavan, L., & Collier, T. J. (2010). A synergistic approach for neural repair: Cell transplantation and induction of endogenous precursor cell activity. *Neuropharmacology, 58*(6), 835–844. DOI: 10.1016/j.neuropharm.2009.10.005 PMID: 19853620

Martinello, T., Gomiero, C., Perazzi, A., Iacopetti, I., Gemignani, F., DeBenedictis, G., & Brun, P. (2018). Allogeneic mesenchymal stem cells improve the wound healing process of sheep skin. *BMC Veterinary Research, 14*(1), 1–9. DOI: 10.1186/s12917-018-1527-8 PMID: 29940954

Mautner, K., Carr, D., Whitley, J., & Bowers, R. (2019). Allogeneic versus autologous injectable mesenchymal stem cells for knee osteoarthritis: Review and current status. *Techniques in Orthopaedics : TIO, 34*(4), 244–256. DOI: 10.1097/BTO.0000000000000357

Misrani, A., Tabassum, S., & Yang, L. (2021). Mitochondrial dysfunction and oxidative stress in Alzheimer's disease. *Frontiers in Aging Neuroscience, 13*, 617588. DOI: 10.3389/fnagi.2021.617588 PMID: 33679375

Mohamed-Ahmed, S., Fristad, I., Lie, S., Suliman, S., Mustafa, K., Vindenes, H., & Idris, S. (2018). Adipose-derived and bone marrow mesenchymal stem cells: A donor-matched comparison. *Stem Cell Research & Therapy, 9*(1), 168. Advance online publication. DOI: 10.1186/s13287-018-0914-1 PMID: 29921311

Mollashahi, B., Latifi-Navid, H., Owliaee, I., Shamdani, S., Uzan, G., Jamehdor, S., & Naserian, S. (2023). Research and therapeutic approaches in stem cell genome editing by CRISPR toolkit. *Molecules (Basel, Switzerland), 28*(4), 1982. DOI: 10.3390/molecules28041982 PMID: 36838970

Moradi, S., Mahdizadeh, H., Šarić, T., Kim, J., Harati, J., Shahsavarani, H., Greber, B., & Moore, J. B.IV. (2019). Research and therapy with induced pluripotent stem cells (iPSCs): Social, legal, and ethical considerations. *Stem Cell Research & Therapy, 10*(1), 1–13. DOI: 10.1186/s13287-019-1455-y PMID: 31753034

Muñoz-Cánoves, P., Neves, J., & Sousa-Victor, P. (2020). Understanding muscle regenerative decline with aging: New approaches to bring back youthfulness to aged stem cells. *The FEBS Journal*, *287*(3), 406–416. DOI: 10.1111/febs.15182 PMID: 31854082

Namita, M., Mondal, M., & Bandhu, B. (2021). Mechanism of Biological Aging-A Review. *International Journal of Physiology*, *9*(1), 23–29. DOI: 10.37506/ijop.v9i1.2607

Naqvi, S., & McNamara, L. (2020). Stem cell mechanobiology and the role of biomaterials in governing mechanotransduction and matrix production for tissue regeneration. *Frontiers in Bioengineering and Biotechnology*, *8*, 597661. DOI: 10.3389/fbioe.2020.597661 PMID: 33381498

Narbonne, P. (2018). The effect of age on stem cell function and utility for therapy. *Cell Medicine*, *10*, 2155179018773756. DOI: 10.1177/2155179018773756 PMID: 32634187

Nguyen, H., Zarriello, S., Coats, A., Nelson, C., Kingsbury, C., Gorsky, A., Rajani, M., Neal, E. G., & Borlongan, C. V. (2019). Stem cell therapy for neurological disorders: A focus on aging. *Neurobiology of Disease*, *126*, 85–104. DOI: 10.1016/j.nbd.2018.09.011 PMID: 30219376

Nielsen, J. L., Bakula, D., & Scheibye-Knudsen, M. (2022). Clinical trials targeting aging. *Frontiers in Aging*, *3*, 820215. DOI: 10.3389/fragi.2022.820215 PMID: 35821843

Noack, F., & Calegari, F. (2018). Epitranscriptomics: A new regulatory mechanism of brain development and function. *Frontiers in Neuroscience*, *12*, 85. DOI: 10.3389/fnins.2018.00085 PMID: 29515357

Ogrodnik, M., Salmonowicz, H., & Gladyshev, V. N. (2019). Integrating cellular senescence with the concept of damage accumulation in aging: Relevance for clearance of senescent cells. *Aging Cell*, *18*(1), e12841. DOI: 10.1111/acel.12841 PMID: 30346102

Pishel, I. (2023). Immune system rejuvenation—Approaches and real achievements. *Exploration of Immunology*, *3*(4), 325–340. DOI: 10.37349/ei.2023.00105

Piuzzi, N. S., Emara, A., Chahla, J., & Mandelbaum, B. R. (2020). Ethical and practical considerations for integrating cellular ("stem cell") therapy into clinical practice. *Current Reviews in Musculoskeletal Medicine*, *13*(4), 525–529. DOI: 10.1007/s12178-020-09647-7 PMID: 32468421

Pyo, I. S., Yun, S., Yoon, Y. E., Choi, J.-W., & Lee, S.-J. (2020). Mechanisms of aging and the preventive effects of resveratrol on age-related diseases. *Molecules (Basel, Switzerland)*, *25*(20), 4649. DOI: 10.3390/molecules25204649 PMID: 33053864

Rančić, N., Rascanin, S., Miljkovic, M., & Jovanovic, M. (2020). Induced pluripotent Stem Cells: Where we are currently? *Naučni časopis urgentne medicine-Halo 194, 26*(3), 153-161.

Raščanin, S., Rančić, N., Dragović, S., & Jovanović, M. (2019). Embryonic stem cells: Where do we stand at the moment. *Acta Medica Medianae*, *58*(3), 138–146. DOI: 10.5633/amm.2019.0320

Ros, M., & Carrascosa, J. M. (2020). Current nutritional and pharmacological anti-aging interventions. *Biochimica et Biophysica Acta (BBA)-. Biochimica et Biophysica Acta. Molecular Basis of Disease*, *1866*(3), 165612. DOI: 10.1016/j.bbadis.2019.165612 PMID: 31816437

Rožman, P. (2018). The potential of non-myeloablative heterochronous autologous hematopoietic stem cell transplantation for extending a healthy life span. *GeroScience*, *40*(3), 221–242. DOI: 10.1007/s11357-018-0027-x PMID: 29948868

Rožman, P. (2020). How could we slow or reverse the human aging process and extend the healthy life span with heterochronous autologous hematopoietic stem cell transplantation. *Rejuvenation Research*, *23*(2), 159–170. DOI: 10.1089/rej.2018.2164 PMID: 31203790

Shafiq, M., Ali, O., Han, S.-B., & Kim, D.-H. (2021). Mechanobiological strategies to enhance stem cell functionality for regenerative medicine and tissue engineering. *Frontiers in Cell and Developmental Biology*, *9*, 747398. DOI: 10.3389/fcell.2021.747398 PMID: 34926444

Simpson, D. J., Olova, N. N., & Chandra, T. (2021). Cellular reprogramming and epigenetic rejuvenation. *Clinical Epigenetics*, *13*(1), 1–10. DOI: 10.1186/s13148-021-01158-7 PMID: 34488874

Srivastava, S. (2019). Emerging insights into the metabolic alterations in aging using metabolomics. *Metabolites*, *9*(12), 301. DOI: 10.3390/metabo9120301 PMID: 31847272

Stanić, S., & Matić, S. (2019). The biology and t heories of aging. *Theoretical Biology Forum*, *112*, 79–89. DOI: 10.19272/201911402006 PMID: 32125352

Timaner, M., Tsai, K. K., & Shaked, Y. (2020). *The multifaceted role of mesenchymal stem cells in cancer.* Paper presented at the Seminars in cancer biology. DOI: 10.1016/j.semcancer.2019.06.003

Tompkins, B., Difede, D., Khan, A., Landin, A., Schulman, I., Pujol, M., Heldman, A. W., Miki, R., Goldschmidt-Clermont, P. J., Goldstein, B. J., Mushtaq, M., Levis-Dusseau, S., Byrnes, J. J., Lowery, M., Natsumeda, M., Delgado, C., Saltzman, R., Vidro-Casiano, M., Da Fonseca, M., & Hare, J. (2017). Allogeneic Mesenchymal Stem Cells Ameliorate Aging Frailty: A Phase II Randomized, Double-Blind, Placebo-Controlled Clinical Trial. *The Journals of Gerontology. Series A, Biological Sciences and Medical Sciences*, *72*(11), 1513–1522. DOI: 10.1093/gerona/glx137 PMID: 28977399

Um, J., Lee, J.-H., Jung, D.-W., & Williams, D. R. (2018). Re-education begins at home: An overview of the discovery of in vivo-active small molecule modulators of endogenous stem cells. *Expert Opinion on Drug Discovery*, *13*(4), 307–326. DOI: 10.1080/17460441.2018.1437140 PMID: 29421943

Varzideh, F., Gambardella, J., Kansakar, U., Jankauskas, S. S., & Santulli, G. (2023). Molecular mechanisms underlying pluripotency and self-renewal of embryonic stem cells. *International Journal of Molecular Sciences*, *24*(9), 8386. DOI: 10.3390/ijms24098386 PMID: 37176093

Vilas, J. M., Carneiro, C., Da Silva-Álvarez, S., Ferreirós, A., González, P., Gómez, M., & González-Barcia, M. (2018). Adult Sox2+ stem cell exhaustion in mice results in cellular senescence and premature aging. *Aging Cell*, *17*(5), e12834. DOI: 10.1111/acel.12834 PMID: 30129215

Wei, W., & Ji, S. (2018). Cellular senescence: Molecular mechanisms and pathogenicity. *Journal of Cellular Physiology*, *233*(12), 9121–9135. DOI: 10.1002/jcp.26956 PMID: 30078211

Wilkinson, A. C., & Yamazaki, S. (2018). The hematopoietic stem cell diet. *International Journal of Hematology*, *107*(6), 634–641. DOI: 10.1007/s12185-018-2451-1 PMID: 29605874

Xunian, Z., & Kalluri, R. (2020). Biology and therapeutic potential of mesenchymal stem cell-derived exosomes. *Cancer Science*, *111*(9), 3100–3110. DOI: 10.1111/cas.14563 PMID: 32639675

Yamamoto, R., Wilkinson, A. C., & Nakauchi, H. (2018). Changing concepts in hematopoietic stem cells. *Science*, *362*(6417), 895–896. DOI: 10.1126/science.aat7873 PMID: 30467158

Yi, B., Dissanayaka, W. L., & Zhang, C. (2020). Growth factors and small-molecule compounds in derivation of endothelial lineages from dental stem cells. *Journal of Endodontics*, *46*(9), S63–S70. DOI: 10.1016/j.joen.2020.06.024 PMID: 32950197

Zakrzewski, W., Dobrzyński, M., Szymonowicz, M., & Rybak, Z. (2019). Stem cells: Past, present, and future. *Stem Cell Research & Therapy*, *10*(1), 1–22. DOI: 10.1186/s13287-019-1165-5 PMID: 30808416

Zarei, F., & Abbaszadeh, A. (2019). Application of cell therapy for anti-aging facial skin. *Current Stem Cell Research & Therapy*, *14*(3), 244–248. DOI: 10.2174/1574888X13666181113113415 PMID: 30421684

Zhang, C., Wang, D., Wang, J., Wang, L., Qiu, W., Kume, T., Dowell, R., & Yi, R. (2021). Escape of hair follicle stem cells causes stem cell exhaustion during aging. *Nature Aging*, *1*(10), 889–903. DOI: 10.1038/s43587-021-00103-w PMID: 37118327

Zhang, L., Pitcher, L. E., Yousefzadeh, M. J., Niedernhofer, L. J., Robbins, P. D., & Zhu, Y. (2022). Cellular senescence: A key therapeutic target in aging and diseases. *The Journal of Clinical Investigation*, *132*(15), e158450. DOI: 10.1172/JCI158450 PMID: 35912854

Zhang, Y., Ravikumar, M., Ling, L., Nurcombe, V., & Cool, S. (2021). Age-Related Changes in the Inflammatory Status of Human Mesenchymal Stem Cells: Implications for Cell Therapy. *Stem Cell Reports*, *16*(4), 694–707. DOI: 10.1016/j.stemcr.2021.01.021 PMID: 33636113

Zhao, N., Yin, G., Liu, C., Zhang, W., Shen, Y., Wang, D., & Guo, R. (2023). Critically short telomeres derepress retrotransposons to promote genome instability in embryonic stem cells. *Cell Discovery*, *9*(1), 45. DOI: 10.1038/s41421-023-00538-y PMID: 37130870

Chapter 7
Epigenetics of Aging and Epigenetic Modifications of Aging-Associated Diseases

Tejasvini Ramesh
Amity Institute of Biotechnology, Amity University, Mumbai, India

Rajshri Singh
https://orcid.org/0000-0001-5748-5799
Amity Institute of Biotechnology, Amity University, Mumbai, India

Sagar H. Barage
https://orcid.org/0000-0003-0752-6948
Amity Institute of Biotechnology, Amity University, Mumbai, India

ABSTRACT

Aging is a complex process characterized by various biological, morphological, and anatomical changes. The epigenetic modifications include DNA methylation, histone modifications, and the action of non-coding RNA play essential roles in genes function as we age. With age, the cascade of epigenetic alterations can lead to genetic mutations and altered gene expression, contributing to a range of age-related diseases. Recent studies suggest that external factors such as climate change and environmental stressors disrupt these epigenetic mechanisms and trigger harmful epigenetic changes that lead to earlier onset of aging-related conditions. Further, this modification contributes to development of cardiovascular disease, neurodegenerative diseases, and metabolic syndromes, underscoring the importance for understanding the epigenetic aspects of these health issues. We have shed light on role of epigenetic factors and mechanisms involved in aging and the development of related diseases.

DOI: 10.4018/979-8-3693-9730-5.ch007

1. INTRODUCTION

1.1. What is Aging?

The gradual decline of physiological processes required for survival and reproduction of human beings is known as aging. Aging has a direct correlation to time. Thus, as we get older, with more time, there is an increased susceptibility to the deleterious effects of aging.

A typical trait of a species is its lifespan. It is the longest period of time a member of that species has ever lived. Although their exact lifespans are uncertain, lake trout and tortoises are thought to live for over 150 years. A lab mouse can live up to 4.5 years, but a domestic dog can live up to 20 years. Drosophila fruit flies have a maximum life span of three months if they make it to enclosure (nearly 90% of them die as larvae in the wild). (Gilbert SF, 2000)

Human Beings can live up to 121 years (Arking 1998). Before the foundation of modern nursing (1900s), early man used live for approximately (20 to 40) years old. After Florence Nightingale founded modern nursing in the 1910s, the average life expectancy increased to around (50-60) years old, according to a World Health Organization (WHO) report, 2024.

Aging can be also characterized as a change at the molecular and genetic level that expresses itself at the physiological and anatomical level.

1.2. Factors Affecting Aging

The way that aging appears in various species is greatly influenced by both biological and environmental variables. We can learn more about the aging process and investigate strategies to support lifespan and good health by looking at these factors.

1.2.a. Anatomical Factors Affecting Aging

Genetic composition is one of the main biological factors that determine aging. According to Levine et al. (2018), specific genes such as SIRT1 and FOXO3 play critical roles in oxidative stress management and DNA repair, two processes essential for longevity. Because genetic differences impact cellular functioning, different animals have different lifespans. Research shows that in humans, environmental variables and lifestyle choices account for 75% of lifespan variability, with genetics accounting for about 25%.(Borsoi et al., 2023)

Cellular senescence represents another significant facet of aging. As noted by Hannum et al. (2013), cells sustain damage from metabolic processes and external stimuli as they divide. Some cells eventually reach a state in which they cease to divide yet continue to function metabolically. Age-related illnesses and tissue malfunction may result from this buildup of senescent cells. It is interesting to note that different species exhibit different rates of cellular senescence; some long-lived species have lower rates.

Aging is also significantly influenced by an organism's metabolic rate. Arking (1998) explains that longer lifespans are typically exhibited by organisms with slower metabolic rates. For example, compared to smaller creatures like mice, larger animals like elephants and whales have slower metabolisms, which contributes to their longer lifespans. Furthermore, studies have demonstrated that calorie restriction can increase lifespan in a variety of animals by boosting cellular repair processes and stress resistance.

Another important biological component affecting aging is hormonal changes. Growth, metabolism, and reproduction are all significantly impacted by hormones including growth hormone, insulin-like growth factor (IGF), and sex hormones like oestrogen and testosterone. Hormonal changes as organisms age can affect longevity and general health.

1.2.b. Environmental Factors Affecting Aging

The aging process can be greatly impacted by a variety of external factors, including environmental influences. Pollution and air quality are two key issues. Numerous studies have established a strong connection between exposure to environmental contaminants and various health problems that may accelerate aging in all animals. For instance, research indicates that air pollution increases the risk of cardiovascular diseases in humans by approximately 30% and is also linked to cognitive impairment, with individuals living in polluted areas showing a 10-15% decline in cognitive function compared to those in cleaner environments.

The climate also has a significant impact on how organisms age. Serious health concerns can arise from extreme weather events, especially for populations that are already at risk. For example, severe cold can raise the risk of hypothermia by 50% among elderly individuals, while heatwaves can lead to heat stress or dehydration, which is responsible for 56 heat-related fatalities in India between March and May 2024 alone. This figure is likely an underestimation due to rural deaths often going unreported. (World Weather Attribution, 2024)

Another significant environmental component that supports health as we age is access to green spaces. Studies have shown that living close to parks or other natural areas improves mental health by reducing anxiety and depression symptoms by up to 30%, lowers stress levels, and promotes physical activity. Individuals living within a 1-kilometer radius of green spaces are 25% more likely to engage in regular physical activity compared to those who do not have such access (Carlos López-Otín • et al., 2013). These benefits are particularly important in urban areas where access to nature may be limited.

Additionally, the social environment plays a crucial role in how people age. Strong social ties can enhance an older person's quality of life by providing emotional support and reducing feelings of loneliness. Research shows that socially active seniors have a 50% lower risk of cognitive decline compared to their isolated counterparts (Patterson & Margolis, 2023). Conversely, social isolation can lead to higher stress levels and worse health outcomes, contributing to a decline in overall well-being.

Lastly, diet significantly influences how we age. Diets rich in vital nutrients such as vitamins, minerals, and antioxidants can combat inflammation and oxidative stress, two major contributors to aging. For example, diets high in fruits and vegetables are associated with a 20% reduction in the risk of developing chronic diseases like heart disease and diabetes (Di Giosia et al., 2022). Additionally, studies suggest that individuals following a Mediterranean diet which emphasizes whole grains, healthy fats, and lean proteins experience slower biological aging compared to those with less nutritious diets.

1.3. Aging in Humans

Aging is a natural part of life that affects all living organisms, particularly humans. It involves a range of changes at the physical, molecular, and biological levels. Understanding these aspects can help us develop strategies to promote healthy aging and mitigate age-related diseases. In this book chapter, we will explore the epigenetics of aging and aging associated diseases.

2. WHAT IS EPIGENETICS?

Epigenetics is a compelling field that studies how gene activity is regulated without changing the underlying DNA sequence. The term derives from the Greek prefix "epi," meaning "over" or "above," indicating that these modifications exist on top of the genetic code. Epigenetic changes involve chemical alterations to DNA and associated proteins, influencing whether genes are activated or silenced (Y. Li, 2021). This regulation is crucial for cellular function and has significant implications for development, health, and disease.

Key mechanisms of epigenetic regulation include DNA methylation, where methyl groups are added to DNA to silence genes, and histone modification, which alters how tightly DNA is packaged around histones, affecting gene accessibility and expression. Together, these modifications ensure that cells produce only the necessary proteins for their specific functions, enabling specialization among different cell types.

Epigenetic changes can be influenced by environmental factors such as diet, stress, and toxins. These modifications are important during development and can impact health throughout an individual's life. Certain epigenetic alterations have been linked to diseases like cancer, where abnormal gene activity leads to uncontrolled cell growth. Additionally, some epigenetic changes can be inherited, meaning parental experiences may affect their offspring's health.

The study of epigenetics offers new insights into biological processes and challenges the notion that genetics alone determines traits, highlighting the interplay between genes and the environment (Y. Li, 2021). As research advances, it promises innovative therapeutic strategies to reverse harmful epigenetic changes or enhance beneficial ones, ultimately improving health outcomes across generations.

2.1. Factors Affecting Epigenetics

Epigenetics is influenced by a myriad of factors that can significantly affect gene expression and, consequently, human health. These factors can be classified into internal and external categories, each contributing to the complex interplay of genetic regulation.

Figure 1. Factors affecting epigenetics

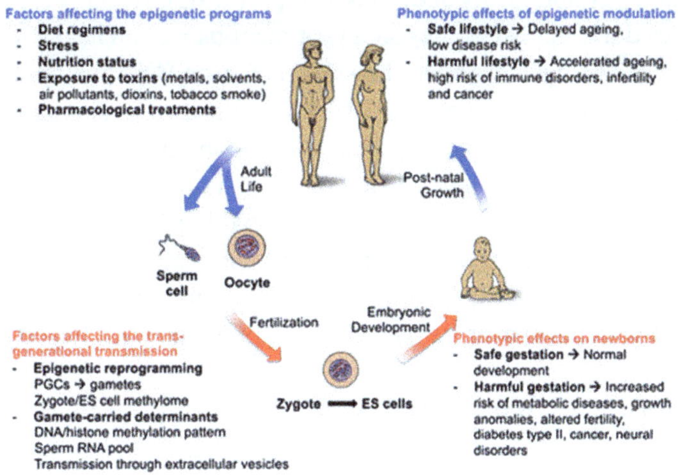

(Trerotola et al., 2015)

2.1.a. Internal Factors Affecting Epigeneticss

Internal factors primarily include genetic variability among individuals. Genetic differences can influence how epigenetic mechanisms operate, affecting susceptibility to diseases. For instance, variations in genes responsible for DNA methylation, such as MTHFR (methylenetetrahydrofolate reductase), can significantly alter an individual's risk for conditions such as cancer or metabolic disorders. Research indicates that individuals with certain polymorphisms in the MTHFR gene may have a 30-50% increased risk of developing colorectal cancer due to impaired folate metabolism and subsequent DNA hypomethylation (M. Ye et al., 2025). Understanding these genetic predispositions is essential for personalized medicine, as they help predict how individuals may respond to environmental influences. For example, studies have shown that individuals with specific genetic variants may respond differently to dietary changes, impacting their overall health and disease risk (Niforou et al., 2020)

2.2.a.(i) Developmental Stages

Another critical internal factor is the stage of development. The epigenome is particularly malleable during early life stages, including prenatal and early postnatal periods. Changes in the epigenome during these times can have profound effects on health throughout life. For example, research has demonstrated that maternal nutrition during pregnancy can lead to epigenetic modifications in the offspring that affect their risk of developing obesity and metabolic syndrome later in life (Şanlı & Kabaran, 2019). A study published in *Nature* found that children whose mothers experienced nutritional deficiencies during pregnancy had altered DNA methylation patterns associated with genes involved in metabolism and growth, potentially influencing their health trajectory(Abrishamcar et al., 2024). Furthermore, epigenetic modifications that occur during embryonic development can be passed down through generations, potentially influencing the health of descendants.

2.1.a.(ii) Hormonal and Physiological States

Hormonal changes and physiological conditions also play a significant role in epigenetic regulation. Fluctuations in hormones during puberty, pregnancy, or menopause can lead to changes in gene expression patterns. For instance, oestrogen has been shown to influence DNA methylation patterns associated with breast cancer risk; postmenopausal women with lower oestrogen levels exhibit different methylation profiles compared to premenopausal women (Gibney & Nolan, 2010). Additionally, metabolic states such as obesity, can induce specific epigenetic alterations that affect insulin sensitivity and inflammation. Research indicates that obesity is associated with global hypomethylation of DNA and increased expression of pro-inflammatory genes, which can exacerbate health outcomes related to diabetes and cardiovascular diseases (Vickers, 2014). A study found that individuals with obesity had significantly altered DNA methylation patterns at over 1,000 loci, many of which were linked to metabolic pathways.

2.1.b. External Factors Affecting Epigenetics:

2.1.b.(i) Environmental Exposures

Environmental factors encompass a wide range of influences that can modify the epigenome. Exposure to environmental toxins, such as heavy metals (e.g., lead, mercury) and air pollutants (e.g., particulate matter), has been shown to cause significant epigenetic changes. For instance, research has demonstrated that lead exposure can lead to increased DNA methylation at specific gene loci associated with neurodevelopmental disorders, potentially resulting in long-term cognitive deficits in children. A study found that children exposed to high levels of lead had a 7-point decrease in IQ compared to those with lower exposure levels(Larsen & Sánchez-Triana, 2023).Air pollution is another significant contributor to epigenetic alterations. Studies indicate that exposure to fine particulate matter (PM2.5) is associated with a 20% increase in the risk of developing cardiovascular diseases and a 10-15% decline in cognitive function among individuals living in polluted areas(Krittanawong et al., 2023). Furthermore, maternal exposure to pollutants during pregnancy can affect the foetal epigenome, leading to long-term health implications for offspring.

2.1.b.(ii) Diet and Nutrition

Diet is a prominent external factor affecting epigenetics. Nutritional components such as vitamins (e.g., folate), polyphenols found in fruits and vegetables, and fatty acids can influence DNA methylation and histone modifications. For instance, folate is critical for the synthesis of S-adenosylmethionine (SAM), a key methyl donor for DNA methylation processes. Insufficient folate intake has been associated with hypomethylation of tumour suppressor genes, increasing cancer risk by approximately 30% (M. Ye et al., 2025). Conversely, a balanced diet rich in antioxidants may promote beneficial epigenetic changes that support overall health. A study found that individuals consuming a Mediterranean diet rich in fruits, vegetables, whole grains, nuts, and healthy fats exhibited lower levels of DNA methylation at sites associated with inflammation and cancer risk compared to those following a Western diet(Niforou et al., 2020). Specifically, participants adhering to this diet showed a 30% reduction in biomarkers linked to oxidative stress.

2.1.b.(iii) Lifestyle Choices

Lifestyle choices significantly impact the epigenome as well. Physical activity has been linked to favourable epigenetic modifications in muscle and adipose tissues, enhancing metabolic health. For example, regular exercise has been shown to induce hypomethylation of genes associated with fat metabolism, improving insulin sensitivity and reducing obesity-related complications (Kumar et al., 2018). A recent study indicated that individuals who engage in moderate physical activity for at least 150 minutes per week had significantly improved epigenetic profiles compared to sedentary individuals. On the other hand, harmful behaviours such as smoking and excessive alcohol consumption can lead to detrimental changes in gene expression patterns associated with various diseases. Smoking is known to cause widespread DNA methylation changes, particularly hypermethylation of genes involved in lung function and cancer pathways; smokers exhibit an average of 1,000 differentially methylated regions compared to non-smokers(Hoang et al., 2024). Similarly, heavy alcohol consumption has been linked to altered histone modifications that contribute to liver disease and other metabolic disorders.

2.1.b.(iv) Psychological Stress

Psychological stress is another external factor that can influence the epigenome. Chronic stress has been shown to alter DNA methylation patterns related to genes involved in stress response and mental health. For instance, research indicates that individuals experiencing high levels of psychological stress exhibit increased methylation of the BDNF gene, which plays a crucial role in neuronal survival and plasticity; this alteration is associated with heightened risks for anxiety and depression (Zhu et al., 2023) The cumulative effects of stress over time may contribute to the development of conditions such as anxiety and depression by reshaping gene expression profiles. A longitudinal study found that participants who reported chronic stress had an average increase of 15% in DNA methylation levels at specific loci related to inflammatory responses over five years(Borsoi et al., 2023).

2.1.b.(v) Pharmacological Influences

Finally, pharmacological treatments can also affect epigenetic mechanisms. Certain medications have been found to induce changes in DNA methylation or histone modifications, potentially altering gene expression related to disease processes. For example, some cancer therapies utilize DNA methyltransferase inhibitors, which reverse aberrant hypermethylation patterns in tumour suppressor genes, thereby restoring their expression and inhibiting tumour growth (Hu et al., 2021). Understanding how these treatments interact with the epigenome is crucial for developing effective therapeutic strategies aimed at improving patient outcomes across various diseases. Recent advancements have highlighted the potential for combining traditional therapies with epigenetic modulators; studies suggest this approach could improve response rates by up to 40% in certain cancer types (Burford, 2023).

2.2. Epigenetic Clock

An epigenetic clock is a groundbreaking tool that estimates biological age by analysing specific patterns of DNA methylation in an individual's genome. Unlike chronological age, which simply counts the years since birth, biological age reflects the cumulative effects of various factors such as genetics, environmental influences, lifestyle choices, and overall health on an individual's cellular and molecular state. This innovative approach has garnered significant attention in the field of aging research, as it provides valuable insights into health risks and longevity. (Vasileva et al., 2023)

The functionality of epigenetic clocks is quite fascinating. These clocks are constructed using advanced machine learning algorithms that analyse DNA methylation data from particular sites known as CpG sites (de Lima Camillo et al., 2022). As people age, these sites undergo predictable changes, making them reliable indicators of biological age. Among the most recognized epigenetic clocks is Horvath's clock, developed by researcher Steve Horvath. This clock utilizes 353 DNA methylation sites and can predict biological age across various tissues and cell types. Other notable clocks include Hannum's clock, which focuses primarily on blood samples, and PhenoAge, which incorporates additional health-related biomarkers alongside DNA methylation data for a more comprehensive assessment.

Epigenetic clocks have a wide array of applications that extend beyond mere curiosity about aging. They serve as valuable biomarkers for assessing individual health risks and predicting the onset of age-related diseases. (Duan et al., 2022) Research has shown that individuals with higher discrepancies between their epigenetic age and chronological age known as epigenetic age acceleration (EAA) are at greater risk for conditions such as cardiovascular disease and certain types of cancer (Margiotti et al., 2023). Moreover, these clocks can be instrumental in evaluating the effectiveness of lifestyle interventions aimed at promoting healthy aging. For instance, positive changes in diet or exercise routines may lead to favourable shifts in biological age as measured by these clocks.

Despite their promise, there are limitations to the use of epigenetic clocks. Current models can be influenced by factors like immune cell composition, which varies with age and can impact predictions. Researchers are actively working to develop more refined clocks that account for these variables. One recent advancement is the IntrinClock, which aims to isolate intrinsic aging processes from those related to immune cell differentiation.

As research continues to evolve, integrating epigenetic clocks into clinical practice holds great potential for enhancing personalized medicine approaches. By providing a more nuanced understanding of biological aging, these tools can inform strategies for disease prevention and health promotion throughout a person's life. In essence, epigenetic clocks represent a significant leap forward in our understanding of aging biology, offering a powerful means to assess biological age and its implications for health and longevity.

3. MECHANISMS LEADING TO EPIGENETIC MODIFICATIONS AND AGING IN HUMAN BEINGS

3.1. DNA Methylation

DNA methylation involves the addition of a methyl group to the DNA molecule, typically at cytosine bases in CpG dinucleotides. This modification can regulate gene expression without altering the underlying DNA sequence, influencing various biological processes such as development, differentiation, and aging. (Horvath, 2013)

Figure 2. DNA methylation and epigenetics of aging

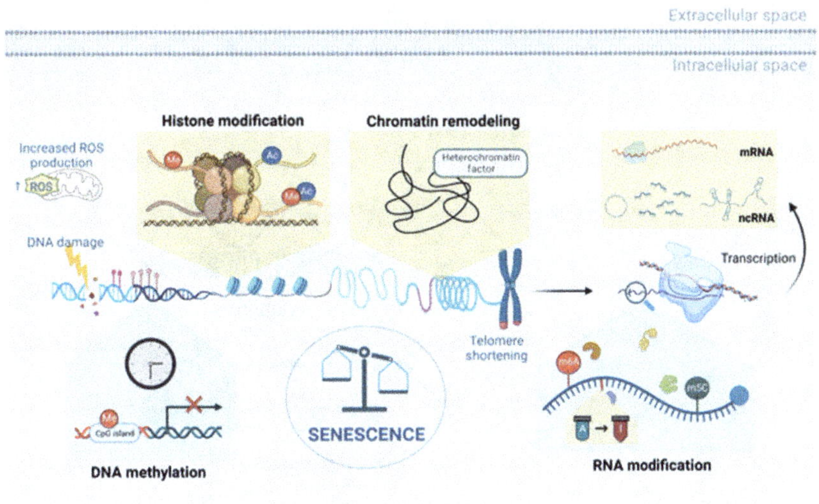

(K. Wang et al., 2022)

3.1.a. Chemical Process

In humans, DNA methylation involves the addition of a methyl group ($-CH_3$) to the 5' carbon of the cytosine ring in a CpG dinucleotide. This process is catalyzed by DNA methyltransferases (DNMTs), which are crucial for establishing and maintaining methylation patterns.(Kumar et al., 2018)

Figure 3. Process of chemical process of DNA methylation in humans and aging

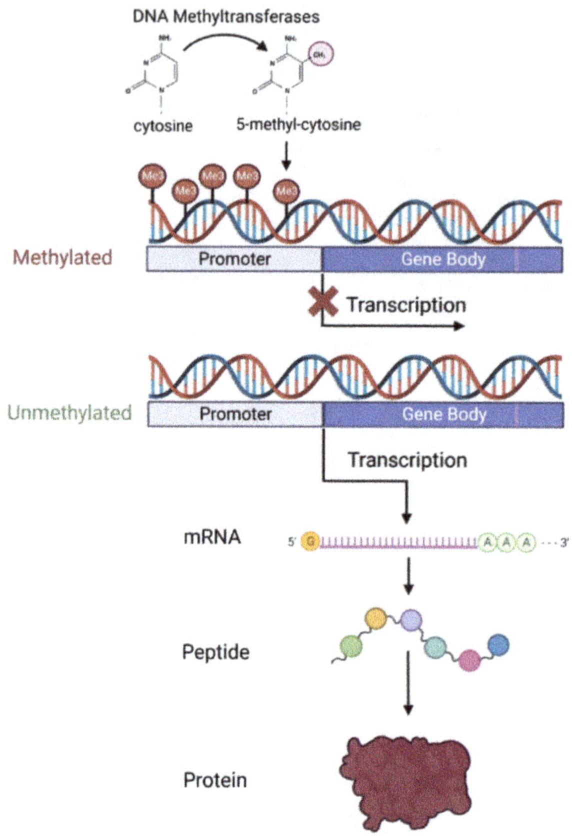

(S. S. Wang et al., 2023)

Human DNA contains approximately 28 million CpG sites, but only about 1-2% of these are located in CpG islands, which are often found in the promoter regions of genes. Methylation of these CpG islands is a key regulatory mechanism for gene expression (de Lima Camillo et al., 2022).

3.1.b. Types of DNA Methyltransferases in Humans:

3.1.b.(i). DNMT

This enzyme is primarily responsible for maintaining DNA methylation patterns during DNA replication. It recognizes hemi methylated DNA (where one strand is methylated and the other is not) and adds a methyl group to the unmethylated cytosine on the newly synthesized strand, ensuring that the methylation pattern is preserved in daughter cells (Ming et al., 2021).

3.1.b.(ii). DNMT3A and DNMT3B

These enzymes are involved in de novo methylation, establishing new methylation patterns on previously unmethylated DNA. They are particularly important during early development and in the differentiation of various cell types.

3.1.b.(iii). Recent Findings

Research has shown that DNMT1 can also participate in de novo methylation under certain conditions, while DNMT3A and DNMT3B can maintain methylation patterns, indicating a more complex interplay among these enzymes than previously understood. (Kumar et al., 2018)

3.1.c. Regulation of Gene Expression in Humans

3.1.c.(i). Transcriptional Silencing

In humans, when the promoter region of a gene is heavily methylated, it typically leads to transcriptional repression. This occurs because the methylation prevents the binding of transcription factors and the transcriptional machinery, effectively silencing the gene.

3.1.c.(ii). Methylation and Chromatin Structure

Methylation is associated with the recruitment of proteins that promote a closed chromatin conformation, further silencing gene expression. Methyl-binding domain proteins (MBDs) bind to methylated DNA and recruit histone deacetylases (HDACs) and other repressive complexes, leading to a more compact and transcriptionally inactive chromatin state(de Lima Camillo et al., 2022).

3.1.d. Aging and DNA Methylation Changes in Humans

As humans age, there is a general trend of decreased global DNA methylation levels. This hypomethylation can lead to genomic instability, increased expression of transposable elements, and activation of oncogenes, contributing to age-related diseases such as cancer.

Figure 4. Aging and DNA methylation

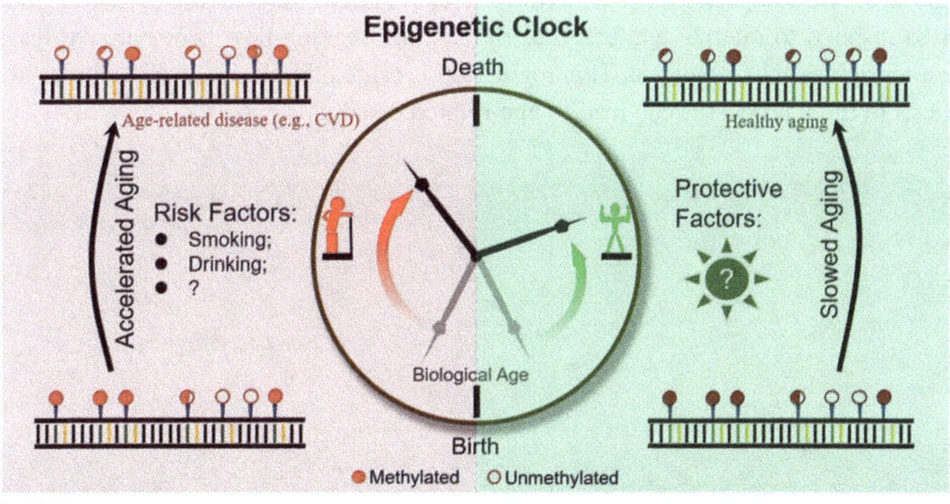

(Xiao et al., 2019)

In contrast to global hypomethylation, certain genes, particularly tumour suppressor genes, may become hypermethylated with age. This hypermethylation can silence protective genes, increasing the risk of age-related diseases, including various cancers.

The concept of epigenetic drift refers to the gradual changes in DNA methylation patterns over time, which can lead to altered gene expression profiles associated with aging and age-related pathologies. This drift can affect genes involved in critical processes such as inflammation, metabolism, and cell cycle regulation (Zhu et al., 2023).

3.1.e. Environmental Influences on DNA Methylation in Humans

3.1.e.(i). Lifestyle Factors

Environmental factors such as diet, physical activity, smoking, and exposure to pollutants can significantly influence DNA methylation patterns in humans. For example, studies have shown that dietary components like folate and other B vitamins can affect DNA methylation status, potentially impacting aging and disease risk. (Borsoi et al., 2023)

3.1.e.(ii). Transgenerational Effects

There is evidence that environmental stimuli can lead to heritable changes in DNA methylation, affecting not only the individual exposed but also their offspring. This suggests a mechanism by which lifestyle and environmental factors can influence aging across generations.

3.2. Histone Modifications

Histone modifications are fundamental to the field of epigenetics, particularly in understanding how gene expression is regulated during the aging process in humans. These modifications involve the addition or removal of various chemical groups to histone proteins, which are integral components of chromatin the structure that packages DNA in the nucleus. The dynamic nature of histone modifications allows cells to respond to internal and external signals, influencing how genes are expressed without altering the underlying DNA sequence. This regulation is critical for maintaining cellular homeostasis, and disruptions in these processes can lead to age-related diseases.

Figure 5. Histone modification and epigenetics of aging

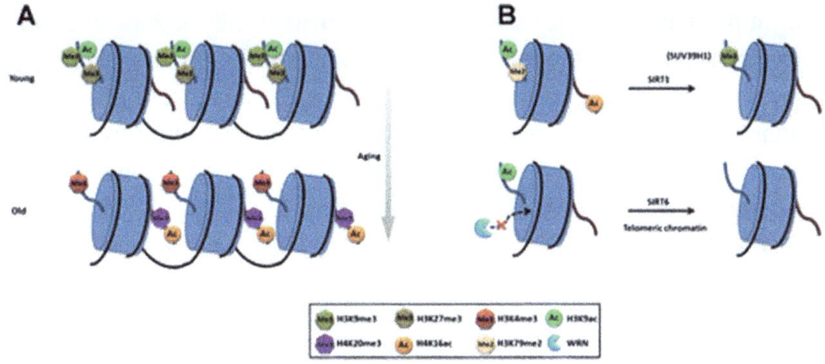

(Cheung et al., 2015)

3.2.a. Types of Histone Modifications

Histones can undergo numerous post-translational modifications, each affecting gene expression differently.

3.2.a.(i). Acetylation

This modification typically occurs on lysine residues and is associated with active transcription. Acetylation neutralizes the positive charge of histones, leading to a more relaxed chromatin structure that allows transcription factors and RNA polymerase to access DNA. For example, increased acetylation of histone H3 at lysine 9 (H3K9ac) is often found at actively transcribed genes. (Gates et al., 2017)

3.2.a.(ii). Methylation

Unlike acetylation, methylation can either activate or repress gene expression depending on the specific lysine residue modified and the number of methyl groups added (mono-, di-, or tri-methylation). For instance, trimethylation of H3K4 (H3K4me3) is generally associated with active promoters, while trimethylation of H3K27 (H3K27me3) is linked to gene repression (H. Wang & Helin, 2025). The balance between these opposing marks plays a critical role in determining gene expression profiles during aging.

3.2.a.(iii). Phosphorylation

Phosphorylation and epigenetic modifications play crucial roles in the aging process by influencing gene expression and cellular function. Epigenetics involves changes such as DNA methylation and histone modifications that do not alter the DNA sequence but affect how genes are expressed. As organisms age, global DNA hypomethylation and specific histone changes, including decreased acetylation and altered phosphorylation patterns, can lead to genomic instability and the activation of genes associated with aging and cellular senescence. These modifications collectively contribute to the decline in cellular function and increased susceptibility to age-related diseases. (Soto-Palma et al., 2022)

Phosphorylation, in particular, is vital for regulating chromatin dynamics and gene activity during aging. It can either promote or inhibit the recruitment of transcription factors necessary for gene expression related to stress responses and repair mechanisms. The accumulation of phosphorylated proteins is often linked to cellular senescence, a state where cells cease to divide but remain metabolically active, contributing to tissue dysfunction. Understanding these processes opens up potential avenues for interventions aimed at mitigating the effects of aging, such as lifestyle changes or pharmacological strategies that target epigenetic regulation.

3.2.a.(iv). Ubiquitination

The addition of ubiquitin molecules to histones can signal for either degradation or transcriptional activation, depending on the context. Ubiquitination is involved in various cellular processes, including DNA repair and cell cycle regulation.

3.2.b. Global Loss of Histone Proteins

One significant aspect of aging is the global loss of canonical histones across different tissues. This phenomenon has been linked to several factors, including decreased histone biosynthesis and increased degradation due to cellular stressors. As histone levels decline, genomic stability may be compromised, leading to altered chromatin structure and function. This loss can result in changes in nucleosome positioning, which affects how tightly DNA is wrapped around histones and consequently influences gene accessibility. (Soto-Palma et al., 2022)

Research has shown that this reduction in histone levels correlates with a decline in cellular function and an increase in age-related diseases. For example, studies have demonstrated that aged tissues exhibit a decrease in the overall abundance of specific histone modifications that promote active transcription, leading to a silencing of genes critical for stress responses and metabolic regulation (Yi & Kim, 2020).

3.2.c. Changes in Histone Modification Profiles

As individuals age, there are notable changes in the patterns of histone modifications. Increased levels of repressive marks such as H3K27me3 have been observed in aging tissues, indicating a shift toward a more repressed chromatin state that may silence genes important for maintaining cellular homeostasis. This epigenetic silencing can affect genes involved in critical processes such as inflammation, metabolism, and cellular repair mechanisms.

Conversely, while some active marks like H3K4me3 may increase at certain promoters during aging, they can become mislocalized or dysregulated. This dysregulation may lead to inappropriate expression of genes associated with inflammation or other age-related pathologies. The interplay between these active and repressive marks creates a complex regulatory landscape that influences overall gene expression profiles associated with aging.

3.2.d. Impact on Gene Expression

The alterations in histone modification patterns directly impact gene expression profiles that are characteristic of aging.

3.2.d.(i). Stress Response Genes

Genes involved in stress response mechanisms may become downregulated due to increased repressive histone marks. This down regulation can impair cellular resilience to oxidative stress and other damaging factors associated with aging (Yuan et al., 2023).

3.2.d.(ii). Inflammatory Pathways

On the other hand, genes related to inflammatory responses may be upregulated due to changes in active histone marks. Chronic low-grade inflammation is a hallmark of aging and contributes to various age-related diseases such as cardiovascular disease and neurodegenerative disorders. (López-Otín et al., 2013)

This imbalance in gene expression resulting from altered histone modifications underscores the complexity of aging biology and highlights potential therapeutic targets for interventions aimed at promoting healthy aging.

3.2.e. Role of Environmental Factors

Environmental factors significantly influence histone modifications throughout life. Nutritional habits play a crucial role; for example, certain dietary components such as polyphenols found in fruits and vegetables can enhance histone acetylation by activating specific enzymes (e.g., histone acetyltransferases). Conversely, diets high in saturated fats may lead to detrimental changes in histone modification patterns that promote inflammation and metabolic dysfunction.

Moreover, exposure to environmental toxins such as heavy metals or endocrine disruptors can induce harmful epigenetic alterations that increase disease risk as individuals age. Research has shown that lifestyle factors like smoking and physical inactivity are linked to increased epigenetic age acceleration (EAA), further emphasizing how external influences shape biological aging through their effects on histone modifications.

3.2.f. Histone Variants

In addition to canonical histones, variants such as H2A.Z and H3.3 play specialized roles in chromatin dynamics during aging (Yi & Kim, 2020). These variants can be incorporated into nucleosomes independently of DNA replication and are thought to modulate chromatin structure under stress conditions. The accumulation of certain histone variants has been linked to cellular senescence and age-related changes; for instance, H2A.Z has been shown to facilitate transcriptional activation under stressful conditions but may also contribute to senescence-associated changes when dysregulated.

3.2.g. Interplay with Other Epigenetic Mechanisms

Histone modifications do not act alone; they interact with other epigenetic mechanisms such as DNA methylation and non-coding RNAs (ncRNAs). Changes in DNA methylation patterns can influence the recruitment of histone-modifying enzymes, creating feedback loops that further propagate epigenetic changes during aging. Additionally, ncRNAs can modulate the expression of genes encoding histone-modifying enzymes, linking environmental signals directly to epigenetic regulation. (Pathania, 2023)

Figure 6. Histone modification

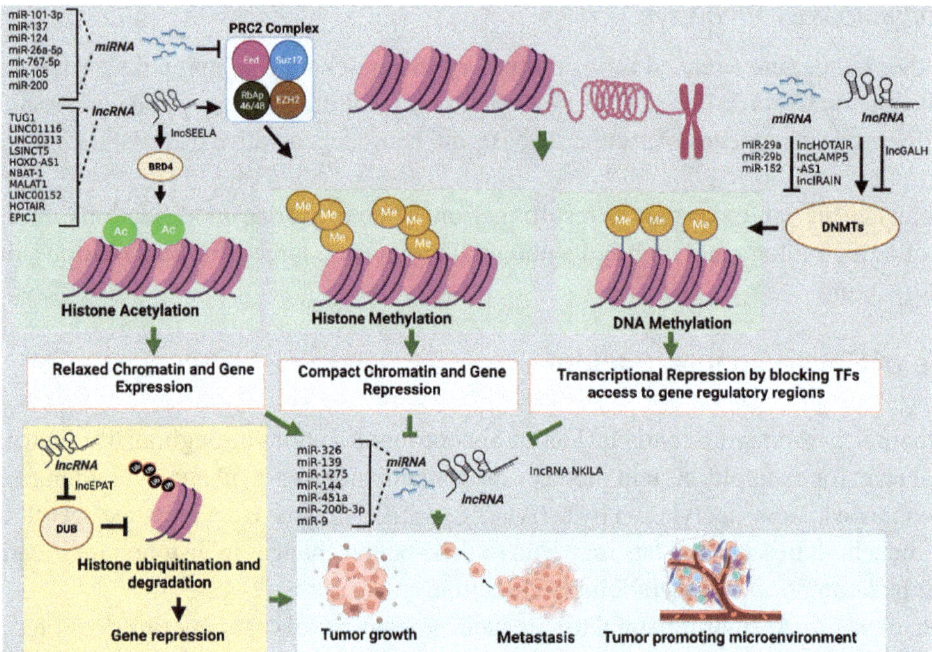

(Pathania, 2023)

3.3. Telomere Shortening

Telomere shortening is a fundamental mechanism associated with aging and plays a critical role in the epigenetic landscape of human cells. Telomeres are repetitive nucleotide sequences located at the ends of linear chromosomes, serving to protect chromosome integrity during cell division (Rossiello et al., 2022). Each time a cell divides, telomeres shorten due to the "end-replication problem," which occurs because DNA polymerases cannot fully replicate the ends of linear DNA strands. This gradual shortening acts as a biological clock that limits the number of times a cell can divide, ultimately leading to cellular senescence or apoptosis when telomeres reach a critically short length. The process of telomere shortening is primarily driven by several factors:

3.3.a. End-Replication Problem

During DNA replication, the enzymes responsible for copying DNA (DNA polymerases) cannot completely replicate the very ends of linear chromosomes. As a result, with each cell division, approximately 50 to 200 base pairs are lost from the telomeres. This phenomenon is known as the end-replication problem and contributes significantly to telomere attrition over time (Rossiello et al., 2022).

3.3.b. Oxidative Stress

Telomeric DNA is particularly susceptible to oxidative damage due to its high guanine content. Reactive oxygen species (ROS) generated from metabolic processes or environmental factors can cause damage to telomeric DNA, leading to further shortening and dysfunction. Oxidative stress can induce DNA damage responses that exacerbate telomere shortening and contribute to cellular senescence.

3.3.c. Cellular Stress and Inflammation

Chronic inflammation and cellular stress can accelerate telomere shortening. Inflammatory cytokines can activate signalling pathways that promote cellular senescence, leading to increased rates of telomere attrition. The accumulation of senescent cells can create a pro-inflammatory environment that further impacts neighbouring cells, perpetuating the cycle of aging.

3.3.d. Telomerase Activity

In most somatic cells, telomerase has low or absent activity. However, in certain cells such as germ cells, stem cells, and many cancer cells, telomerase is active and helps maintain telomere length by adding nucleotide repeats back to the ends of chromosomes. The lack of sufficient telomerase activity in somatic cells means that they are unable to counteract the effects of telomere shortening effectively.

3.3.e. Epigenetic Implications of Telomere Shortening

The shortening of telomeres has profound epigenetic implications that contribute to aging.

3.3.e.(i). Activation of DNA Damage Response (DDR)

When telomeres become critically short, they can no longer bind sufficient amounts of protective proteins, leading to their recognition as damaged DNA ends. This triggers the activation of DNA damage response pathways, which induce cell cycle inhibitors such as p21 and p16. These inhibitors arrest cell proliferation and promote cellular senescence, marking a significant shift in cellular function.

3.3.e.(ii). Cellular Senescence

Telomere shortening is one of the primary triggers for cellular senescence—a state where cells cease to divide but remain metabolically active. Senescent cells often exhibit altered gene expression profiles due to changes in histone modifications and DNA methylation patterns (Dasgupta et al., 2024).

This altered state contributes to age-related phenotypes and can influence tissue function by secreting inflammatory cytokines and other factors that affect neighbouring cells.

3.3.e.(iii). Impact on Gene Expression

The epigenetic changes associated with telomere shortening can lead to dysregulation of genes involved in critical processes such as inflammation, metabolism, and stress responses. For instance, genes that promote cell survival may be downregulated due to increased repressive histone marks at their promoters, while pro-inflammatory genes may become upregulated.

3.3.e.(iv). Cumulative Effects on Aging

The accumulation of short telomeres in tissues over time correlates with various age-related diseases such as cardiovascular disease, diabetes, and neurodegenerative disorders. As more cells enter senescence due to critically short telomeres, tissue function declines, contributing to the overall aging process.

3.4. Oxidative Stress

One of the primary contributors to aging is oxidative stress, which results from an imbalance between reactive oxygen species (ROS) production and the body's antioxidant defenses (Guillaumet-Adkins et al., 2017). This imbalance not only causes direct damage to cellular components but also triggers a series of epigenetic changes that significantly influence the aging process. Oxidative stress plays a significant role in the aging process by inducing epigenetic modifications that can alter gene expression and contribute to age-related decline.

Figure 7. Oxidative stress and epigenetics of aging

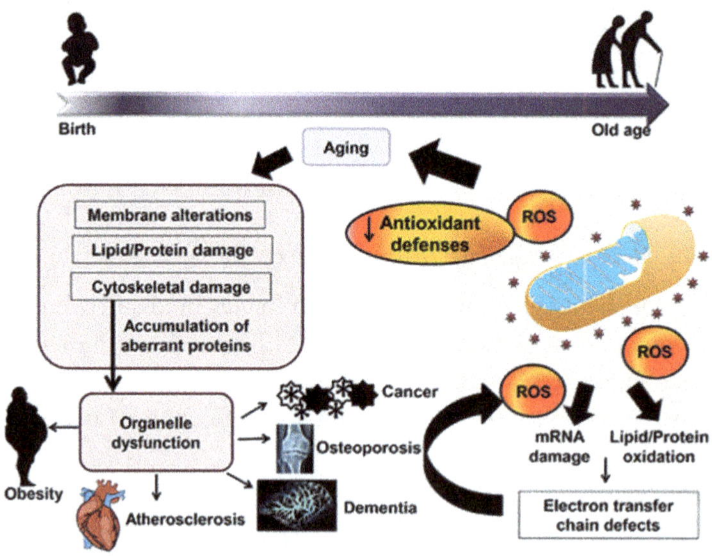

(Tan et al., 2018)

This relationship is complex and involves various mechanisms that affect cellular function and longevity. As individuals age, the accumulation of ROS leads to cellular damage, impacting DNA, proteins, and lipids. This damage is a key factor in the aging process and is linked to various age-related diseases, including neurodegenerative disorders and cardiovascular diseases.

3.4.a. Mechanism of Oxidative Stress in Relation to Epigenetic Modifications Speeding Aging in Humans

Oxidative stress influences various metabolic and cellular pathways that contribute to aging through epigenetic modifications.

3.4.a.(i). Mitochondrial Dysfunction and ROS Production

Mitochondria are the primary source of reactive oxygen species (ROS) during ATP production through oxidative phosphorylation. As individuals age, mitochondrial function tends to decline, leading to decreased efficiency in the electron transport chain. This inefficiency results in increased leakage of electrons and subsequent ROS generation. Elevated levels of ROS can damage mitochondrial DNA (mtDNA), proteins, and lipids, creating a feedback loop that further impairs mitochondrial function. The accumulation of oxidative damage in mitochondria is a significant contributor to the aging process, as it affects energy metabolism and promotes cellular senescence (Miwa et al., 2022). In addition to intrinsic mitochondrial sources, NADPH oxidase (NOX) enzymes also contribute to ROS production. These enzymes can be activated by various stimuli, including high glucose levels, particularly in conditions such as diabetes. The overactivity of NOX leads to increased oxidative stress, which can result in cellular damage and promote aging-related pathologies (Zilberter et al., 2023). This dual role of mitochondria and NOX in generating ROS underscores the complexity of oxidative stress in aging.

3.4.a.(ii) Polyol Pathway Activation

Under conditions of hyperglycaemia, excess glucose is diverted into the polyol pathway, where it is converted to sorbitol by the enzyme aldose reductase. This conversion utilizes NADPH, a critical cofactor for various antioxidant defence mechanisms. The depletion of NADPH reduces the cell's capacity to counteract oxidative stress effectively, leading to an increased burden of oxidative damage. Additionally, the accumulation of sorbitol can create osmotic pressure within cells, contributing to cellular dysfunction and damage. This pathway is particularly relevant in tissues sensitive to glucose fluctuations, such as the retina and kidneys. In these tissues, the activation of the polyol pathway due to chronic high glucose levels can lead to complications such as diabetic retinopathy and nephropathy (Zilberter et al., 2023). The interplay between hyperglycaemia, oxidative stress, and epigenetic modifications in these contexts highlights the importance of metabolic regulation in aging.

3.4.a.(iii). Protein Kinase C (PKC) Pathway

Oxidative stress can activate Protein Kinase C (PKC), a family of serine/threonine kinases that play a crucial role in various signalling pathways regulating cell growth and survival. Upon activation by ROS or other stimuli, PKC can enhance ROS production through the activation of NADPH oxidase (NOX). This creates a feedback loop where increased PKC activity leads to further oxidative stress. In vascular endothelial cells, for example, chronic PKC activation is associated with endothelial dysfunction, a hallmark of aging and cardiovascular disease. This dysfunction is characterized by impaired vasodilation and increased inflammation (Lu et al., 2022). By linking oxidative stress with PKC signalling pathways, we gain insight into how these mechanisms contribute to age-related vascular complications.

3.4.a.(iv). Advanced Glycation End Products (AGEs)

Elevated oxidative stress promotes the formation of Advanced Glycation End Products (AGEs), which arise from the non-enzymatic reaction between sugars and proteins or lipids. AGEs can modify cellular structures and activate inflammatory pathways via receptors for AGEs (RAGE). This interaction triggers a cascade of inflammatory responses that contribute to tissue damage and dysfunction (Luevano-Contreras & Chapman-Novakofski, 2010). The accumulation of AGEs is particularly relevant in age-related diseases such as diabetes and cardiovascular conditions. AGEs have been implicated in promoting vascular stiffness, enhancing inflammation, and accelerating atherosclerosis. Thus, understanding how oxidative stress facilitates AGE formation provides critical insights into its role in aging and related diseases.

3.4.a.(v). Nuclear Factor Erythroid 2–Related Factor 2 (Nrf2) Pathway

Nrf2 is a transcription factor that plays a pivotal role in regulating cellular responses to oxidative stress by activating genes involved in antioxidant defence mechanisms. Under normal conditions, Nrf2 is kept in the cytoplasm bound to its inhibitor Keap1. However, when cells experience oxidative stress, Nrf2 dissociates from Keap1 and translocates into the nucleus, where it binds to antioxidant response elements (AREs) in gene promoters. Chronic oxidative stress can lead to dysregulation of Nrf2 signalling pathways. For example, prolonged exposure to high levels of ROS may overwhelm Nrf2's protective capacity or lead to its degradation (Swamy et al., 2016). This impairment reduces the expression of key antioxidant enzymes and contributes to increased susceptibility to oxidative damage—an important factor in aging-related decline.

3.4.a.(vi). Sirtuin Pathway

Sirtuins are a family of NAD+-dependent deacetylases that play crucial roles in regulating cellular responses to stress and promoting longevity. Among them, SIRT1 is particularly well-studied for its involvement in mitigating oxidative stress effects through deacetylation of various target proteins, including p53 and histones. When NAD+ levels are sufficient, SIRT1 activity promotes cellular resilience by enhancing DNA repair mechanisms and regulating metabolic processes. However, oxidative stress can deplete NAD+ levels due to increased consumption during ATP production or other metabolic processes. Reduced SIRT1 activity leads to hyperacetylation of p53 and other proteins involved in cell cycle regulation and apoptosis, promoting senescence-like phenotypes in cells (Zhao et al., 2020). This decline in SIRT1 function underscores its critical role in maintaining cellular health during aging.

3.4.a.(vii). Cell Cycle Regulation Pathways

Oxidative stress has profound effects on key regulators of the cell cycle, particularly proteins such as p53 and p21. Increased ROS levels can lead to post-translational modifications of p53 that enhance its stability and transcriptional activity. Activated p53 induces the expression of p21, a cyclin-dependent kinase inhibitor that enforces cell cycle arrest. This mechanism serves as a protective response against DNA damage; however, chronic activation due to persistent oxidative stress can lead to irreversible cell cycle arrest or senescence (Soto-Palma et al., 2022). The accumulation of senescent cells contributes to tissue dysfunction and age-related decline by secreting pro-inflammatory cytokines which is a phenomenon known as the senescence-associated secretory phenotype (SASP).

3.4.a.(viii). Inflammatory Signalling Pathways

Oxidative stress plays a critical role in activating inflammatory signalling pathways, particularly through nuclear factor kappa B (NF-kB). Under normal conditions, NF-kB is sequestered in the cytoplasm by an inhibitor (IκB). However, oxidative stress can lead to IκB degradation or modification, resulting in NF-kB translocation into the nucleus where it activates genes involved in inflammation (X. Li et al., 2023a). Chronic activation of NF-kB due to persistent oxidative stress contributes significantly to age-related inflammation—a condition often referred to as "inflammaging." This state is characterized by elevated levels of pro-inflammatory cytokines that exacerbate tissue damage and promote various age-related diseases such as arthritis, cardiovascular disease, and neurodegeneration.

3.4.b. Impact of Oxidative Stress on Inducing Epigenetic Changes and Aging

Oxidative stress arises from an imbalance between the production of reactive oxygen species (ROS) and the body's antioxidant defences. This imbalance can lead to significant cellular damage, particularly affecting DNA and histones, which in turn influences gene expression.

One of the primary ways oxidative stress alters gene expression is through changes in DNA methylation patterns. Increased ROS levels can lead to both global hypomethylation and hypermethylation of specific genes. For instance, oxidative stress has been shown to enhance the activity of DNA methyltransferases (DNMTs), resulting in aberrant methylation that silences tumour suppressor genes while activating oncogenes (Tan et al., 2018). This dysregulation is critical as it can contribute to the development of age-related diseases such as cancer and neurodegenerative disorders.

Oxidative stress also impacts histone modifications, which are crucial for regulating chromatin structure and gene expression. Increased oxidative damage can lead to alterations in histone acetylation and methylation patterns. For example, oxidative stress has been shown to increase acetylation of histones associated with pro-inflammatory genes, promoting a chronic inflammatory state typical of aging.

Furthermore, the activity of sirtuins, NAD+-dependent deacetylases involved in histone modification, decreases with oxidative stress, further contributing to age-related changes in gene expression.

The expression of non-coding RNAs, particularly microRNAs (miRNAs), is also influenced by oxidative stress. Certain miRNAs are upregulated in response to ROS, leading to the downregulation of target genes involved in cell cycle regulation and apoptosis. For example, miR-34a has been implicated in promoting cellular senescence during aging by targeting genes that regulate cell proliferation (Zuccolo et al., 2020).

The dysregulation of miRNA expression due to oxidative stress may further exacerbate age-related decline by disrupting cellular homeostasis.

3.5. Inflammation

Inflammation is a critical biological response that protects the body from harmful stimuli, including pathogens, damaged cells, and irritants. However, chronic inflammation can have detrimental effects, particularly in the context of aging and epigenetic modifications(X. Li et al., 2023a). In humans, the interplay between inflammation, epigenetic changes, and aging is complex and multifaceted.

3.5.a. The Role of Inflammation in Epigenetic Modifications

Inflammation triggers a series of biological responses that can lead to significant epigenetic changes. These changes include DNA methylation, histone modifications, and alterations in non-coding RNA expression.

Inflammatory stimuli can induce changes in DNA methylation patterns. For instance, pro-inflammatory cytokines such as tumour necrosis factor-alpha (TNF-α) and interleukin-6 (IL-6) can lead to hypermethylation of specific gene promoters associated with inflammatory responses. This alteration can silence genes that regulate anti-inflammatory pathways or promote cell survival, thereby exacerbating chronic inflammation and contributing to age-related diseases such as diabetes and cardiovascular conditions.

Inflammation also affects histone modifications, which are crucial for regulating chromatin structure and gene expression. For example, the activation of nuclear factor kappa B (NF-κB) during inflammatory responses can recruit histone acetyltransferases (HATs) and histone deacetylases (HDACs), leading to changes in histone acetylation levels at inflammatory gene loci (Swaroop et al., 2021). This process can enhance the transcription of pro-inflammatory genes while repressing anti-inflammatory genes. Histone methylation changes have also been observed, where enzymes like Jmjd3 regulate histone marks that control inflammatory gene expression.

Inflammatory signals can modulate the expression of non-coding RNAs, particularly microRNAs (miRNAs). For instance, miRNAs such as miR-155 are upregulated during inflammatory responses and are involved in promoting inflammation by targeting genes that inhibit inflammatory pathways (Zuccolo et al., 2020). This dysregulation contributes to a feedback loop that perpetuates chronic inflammation.

3.5.b. Chronic Inflammation and Aging

Chronic inflammation is often referred to as "inflammaging," a term that describes the low-grade, systemic inflammation associated with aging. This state is characterized by elevated levels of pro-inflammatory cytokines and immune cell activation.

As individuals age, the levels of circulating pro-inflammatory cytokines such as IL-1β, TNF-α, and IL-6 increase (Tylutka et al., 2024). These cytokines contribute to the development of age-related diseases by promoting tissue damage and dysfunction. The persistent presence of these cytokines can lead to further epigenetic modifications that alter gene expression patterns associated with aging.

Aging is associated with epigenetic drift, where normal patterns of DNA methylation and histone modifications become disrupted (Yuan et al., 2023). Chronic inflammation accelerates this drift by inducing epigenetic changes that activate oncogenes or silence tumour suppressor genes. This dysregulation increases the risk of developing age-related diseases such as cancer.

3.6. Cellular Senescence

Cellular senescence is a state of irreversible cell cycle arrest that occurs in response to various stressors, including DNA damage, oxidative stress, and telomere shortening. It plays a crucial role in aging and age-related diseases by contributing to tissue dysfunction and promoting a pro-inflammatory environment. The mechanisms underlying cellular senescence are closely linked to epigenetic modifications, which can significantly impact gene expression and contribute to the aging process.

3.6.a. Induction of Cellular Senescence

Cellular senescence can be triggered by multiple factors, including accumulation of DNA damage, often due to oxidative stress or telomere shortening, activates the DDR. Key proteins involved in this response include p53 and ATM (Ataxia Telangiectasia Mutated), which stabilize p53 and promote its transcriptional activity. Activated p53 induces the expression of p21, a cyclin-dependent kinase inhibitor that enforces cell cycle arrest (Soto-Palma et al., 2022). This process is crucial for preventing the propagation of damaged cells, thereby acting as a tumour suppressive mechanism.

With each cell division, telomeres shorten. When they reach a critical length, they trigger a DDR that also leads to cellular senescence. This mechanism serves as a biological clock that limits the number of times a cell can divide.

3.6.b. Epigenetic Changes Associated with Cellular Senescence

The transition to a senescent state involves significant epigenetic alterations that regulate gene expression patterns essential for maintaining the senescent phenotype.

Senescent cells exhibit distinct changes in DNA methylation patterns compared to their proliferative counterparts. For example, hypermethylation often occurs at promoters of genes associated with cell proliferation and survival, effectively silencing them. Conversely, genes involved in inflammatory responses may become hypomethylated and activated, contributing to the senescence-associated secretory phenotype (SASP) (Zuccolo et al., 2020). These changes can lead to chronic inflammation and tissue dysfunction characteristic of aging.

Histone modifications are also crucial for establishing and maintaining the senescent state. In senescent cells, there is often an increase in histone acetylation at promoters of SASP-related genes, facilitating their expression. Additionally, repressive histone marks can accumulate at genes that promote cell cycle progression, effectively silencing them. The dynamic interplay between activating and repressive histone modifications is essential for regulating gene expression during senescence.

Non-coding RNAs, especially microRNAs (miRNAs), play significant roles in regulating cellular senescence. Certain miRNAs are upregulated in response to senescence signals and can target mRNAs of genes that inhibit senescence or promote proliferation. For instance, miR-34a promotes cellular senescence by targeting genes involved in cell cycle regulation. The dysregulation of non-coding RNAs during senescence contributes to the maintenance of the senescent phenotype.

3.6.c. Impact on Aging

The accumulation of senescent cells over time has profound implications for aging. Senescent cells secrete various pro-inflammatory cytokines, growth factors, and proteases collectively known as the SASP. This secretory profile alters the tissue microenvironment, promoting inflammation and influencing the behaviour of neighbouring cells. The persistent presence of SASP factors contributes to "inflammaging," a chronic low-grade inflammation associated with aging that exacerbates age-related diseases (Dasgupta et al., 2024).

Aging is associated with epigenetic drift. Cellular senescence accelerates this drift by inducing specific epigenetic changes that can lead to genomic instability and increased risk of age-related diseases such as cancer. The accumulation of these epigenetic alterations reflects a loss of epigenetic information necessary for maintaining normal cellular function.

3.7. Nutritional and Environmental Factors

Nutritional and environmental factors play a crucial role in shaping the epigenome, influencing gene expression, and contributing to the aging process in humans. These factors can induce significant epigenetic modifications, such as DNA methylation changes, histone modifications, and alterations in non-coding RNA expression. Nutrients derived from food can significantly alter epigenetic marks, impacting gene expression and cellular function throughout life. Key nutritional components include vitamins, minerals, and bioactive compounds.

3.7.a. Nutritional Influences on Epigenetic Modifications

Certain nutrients are also involved in the one-carbon metabolism pathway, which is essential for DNA methylation processes. For example, folate, vitamin B12, and methionine are critical for generating S-adenosylmethionine (SAM), a key methyl donor for DNA methylation. Diets rich in these methyl-donating nutrients can lead to increased DNA methylation, influencing gene expression patterns associated with development and aging(Maugeri & Barchitta, 2020). Conversely, deficiencies in these nutrients can result in global hypomethylation or hypermethylation of specific genes, potentially leading to age-related diseases such as cancer.

Nutritional factors influence histone modifications as well, which are critical for regulating chromatin structure and gene accessibility. For instance, histone acetylation is often enhanced by diets rich in fruits and vegetables that contain phytochemicals. These modifications can promote gene expression by making chromatin more accessible to transcription factors. In contrast, diets high in saturated fats may lead to dysregulation of histone acetylation and deacetylation processes, contributing to inflammation and metabolic dysfunction.

Nutritional components can modulate the expression of non-coding RNAs, particularly microRNAs (miRNAs), which play significant roles in post-transcriptional regulation of gene expression. For example, certain dietary fats have been shown to influence miRNA profiles that regulate lipid metabolism and inflammation. Dysregulation of miRNAs due to poor dietary choices may contribute to age-related diseases by altering the expression of genes involved in cellular repair and inflammation.

3.7.b. Environmental Influences on Epigenetic Modifications

Environmental factors such as pollutants, toxins, and lifestyle choices also significantly impact the epigenome.

3.7.b.(i). Chemical Exposures

Exposure to environmental toxins (e.g., heavy metals, pesticides) can lead to epigenetic alterations that affect gene expression. For instance, studies have shown that exposure to cadmium can induce DNA hypermethylation of tumor suppressor genes, promoting cancer development. Similarly, air pollution has been associated with changes in DNA methylation patterns linked to cardiovascular diseases.

3.7.b.(ii). Microbiome Interactions

The gut microbiome plays a pivotal role in modulating host epigenetics through the production of short-chain fatty acids (SCFAs) from dietary fibers (Silva et al., 2020). SCFAs can influence histone acetylation by inhibiting histone deacetylases (HDACs), leading to increased gene expression associated with anti-inflammatory responses (Licciardi et al., 2011). A diet low in fiber may reduce SCFA production, leading to altered epigenetic states that promote inflammation and metabolic disorders.

3.7.c. Implications for Aging

The cumulative effects of nutritional and environmental factors on the epigenome have significant implications for aging.

3.7.c.(i) Epigenetic Drift

Aging is characterized by epigenetic drift—changes in DNA methylation patterns that occur over time. Poor nutrition and adverse environmental exposures can accelerate this drift by inducing specific epigenetic changes that disrupt normal cellular functions. This drift may lead to the activation of oncogenes or silencing of tumour suppressor genes, increasing the risk of age-related diseases such as cancer.

3.7.c.(ii). Chronic Inflammation

Nutritional deficiencies and environmental stressors can contribute to chronic inflammation through their effects on the epigenome. For example, diets high in processed foods may promote a pro-inflammatory state by altering gene expression related to immune responses. Chronic inflammation is a hallmark of aging (inflammaging) and is associated with various age-related diseases.

3.8. Non-Coding RNA

Non-coding RNAs (ncRNAs) are a diverse class of RNA molecules that do not encode proteins but play critical roles in regulating gene expression and maintaining cellular homeostasis. In the context of aging, non-coding RNAs have emerged as significant epigenetic regulators that influence various biological processes, including cellular senescence, inflammation, and metabolic functions.

3.8.a. Types of Non-Coding RNAs Involved in Aging

Non-coding RNAs can be broadly categorized into two main types: microRNAs (miRNAs) and long non-coding RNAs (lncRNAs). Both types play essential roles in the regulation of gene expression and are implicated in the aging process.

3.8.a.(i). MicroRNAs (miRNAs)

These are short, typically 20-24 nucleotides long, and function by binding to complementary sequences on target messenger RNAs (mRNAs), leading to their degradation or inhibition of translation. miRNAs are involved in various cellular processes, including proliferation, differentiation, and apoptosis. Dysregulation of miRNA expression has been linked to age-related diseases, including cancer and neurodegenerative disorders. For instance, miR-34a is known to promote cellular senescence by targeting genes that regulate cell cycle progression and apoptosis (Zuccolo et al., 2020).

3.8.a.(ii). Long Non-Coding RNAs (lncRNAs)

These are longer than 200 nucleotides and play diverse roles in gene regulation. lncRNAs can modulate chromatin structure, interact with transcription factors, and influence mRNA stability. Certain lncRNAs have been identified as key regulators of aging. For example, the lncRNA PANDA (P21-associated non-coding RNA DNA damage-activated) is involved in mediating the response to DNA damage and has been shown to play a role in cellular senescence by sequestering transcription factors that promote proliferation (Puvvula, 2019).

3.8.b. Mechanisms of Action

Non-coding RNAs exert their effects on gene expression through various mechanisms that can influence aging. Non-coding RNAs can modulate the expression of genes involved in critical pathways related to aging. For instance, miRNAs can downregulate genes associated with cell proliferation and survival, leading to increased cellular senescence and reduced regenerative capacity. This regulation is crucial for maintaining tissue homeostasis but can contribute to age-related decline when dysregulated.

Figure 8. Non coding RNA

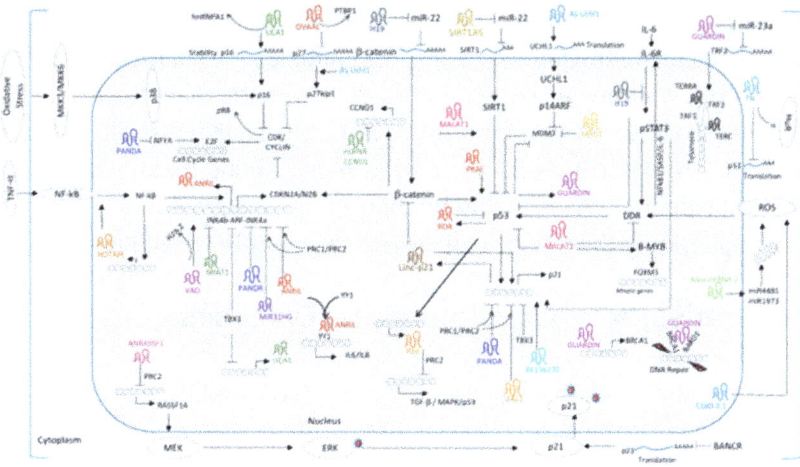

(Puvvula, 2019)

Non-coding RNAs can influence epigenetic modifications directly or indirectly. For example, some lncRNAs can recruit chromatin-modifying complexes to specific genomic loci, leading to changes in histone modifications or DNA methylation patterns. This recruitment can result in the silencing or activation of target genes associated with aging. The interplay between non-coding RNAs and epigenetic modifiers highlights their role as critical regulators of the epigenome.

In senescent cells, non-coding RNAs play a crucial role in regulating the senescence-associated secretory phenotype (SASP). The SASP comprises pro-inflammatory cytokines and growth factors that influence neighbouring cells and contribute to tissue dysfunction during aging. For example, certain miRNAs can modulate the expression of SASP factors, thereby impacting inflammation and tissue repair mechanisms associated with aging(Dasgupta et al., 2024).

4. DISEASES IN HUMANS

As individuals age, the accumulation of epigenetic alterations can disrupt normal gene regulation, contributing to the development of age-related diseases such as musculoskeletal disorders, neurodegenerative diseases, cancer, cardiovascular diseases, diabetes, chronic obstructive pulmonary disease (COPD), osteoporosis, and chronic inflammation. Understanding the interplay between aging and epigenetics is essential for identifying potential therapeutic strategies aimed at promoting healthier aging and reducing the burden of age-related diseases.

4.1. Musculoskeletal Diseases

Musculoskeletal diseases, including osteoarthritis (OA) and osteoporosis (OP), are prevalent in older adults. Osteoporosis affects approximately 200 million people worldwide, with an estimated 1 in 3 women and 1 in 5 men over the age of 50 experiencing a fracture due to osteoporosis (Shen et al., 2022). The aging process leads to changes in DNA methylation patterns in osteoblasts, where hypermethylation of genes like *Runx2* can impair bone formation. Histone modifications also play a role; increased histone acetylation can promote the expression of matrix metalloproteinases (MMPs) that degrade cartilage, contributing to OA.

Oxidative stress is another significant factor, as it can induce DNA damage and alter gene expression related to bone metabolism. Chronic inflammation associated with aging further exacerbates these epigenetic changes, leading to increased susceptibility to musculoskeletal disorders (Borsoi et al., 2023). A study published in the *Journal of Bone and Mineral Research* found that postmenopausal women with osteoporosis exhibited distinct DNA methylation changes in genes regulating bone density compared to healthy controls, emphasizing the role of epigenetics in musculoskeletal health (Chen et al., 2023).

4.2. Neurodegenerative/Neurodevelopmental Diseases

Neurodegenerative diseases such as Alzheimer's disease (AD) and Parkinson's disease (PD) are characterized by progressive neuronal loss and dysfunction, with prevalence rates rising dramatically with age (Borsoi et al., 2023). For example, approximately 6 million Americans are living with Alzheimer's disease, and this number is expected to rise to nearly 14 million by 2060 (Hajjo et al., 2022). Epigenetic modifications significantly influence these conditions; hypermethylation of the *APP* gene contributes to amyloid plaque formation in AD.

Histone modifications also play a crucial role; altered acetylation patterns can affect genes involved in neuronal survival. Non-coding RNAs such as miR-34a have been linked to neurodegeneration by promoting apoptosis in neurons (Ilieva, 2024). Increased oxidative stress leads to DNA damage and subsequent epigenetic alterations that exacerbate neurodegeneration.

4.3. Cancer

4.3.a. Colorectal Cancer

Colorectal cancer (CRC) is one of the most common cancers worldwide, with an estimated incidence of over 1.9 million new cases diagnosed globally in 2020. Age is a significant risk factor for CRC, as the majority of cases occur in individuals over 50 years old(WHO, 2023). Epigenetic modifications play a critical role; hypermethylation of tumour suppressor genes like *MLH1* can lead to microsatellite instability and increased cancer risk.

Altered histone acetylation levels can also affect oncogenes and tumour suppressor genes involved in colorectal carcinogenesis. The modification of histone deacetylases, such as HDAC3, through deubiquitination can upregulate cancer stem cell-related genes, contributing to the stemness and chemoresistance of colorectal cancer cells (Zhan et al., 2020). Additionally, histone deacetylase inhibitors have emerged as potential therapeutic agents that exert anti-tumour effects by regulating multiple cellular processes including cell cycle arrest, growth inhibition, and induction of apoptosis in colorectal cancer (Qin et al., 2020)

4.3.b. Leukaemia

Leukaemia is characterized by an overproduction of abnormal white blood cells, with acute myeloid leukaemia (AML) being one of the most common types among older adults. Acute myeloid leukaemia (AML), a hematologic malignancy marked by clonal expansion of undifferentiated myeloid precursors, demonstrates strong age-associated incidence patterns. While AML accounts for ~19,000 annual diagnoses in the U.S., its frequency rises exponentially after age 60, with median diagnosis at 68 years (J.-Y. Kim et al., 2025). This age dependence reflects accumulating epigenetic dysregulation, particularly in DNA methylation dynamics. Aging hematopoietic stem cells (HSCs) exhibit clonal expansion driven by mutations in *DNMT3A* and *IDH1/2* – epigenetic regulators that alter DNA methylation patterns at enhancers controlling hematopoietic differentiation genes like MYC and ETV6 (Wilson et al., 2022). These mutations create a premalignant state where HSCs show **accelerated epigenetic aging**, as evidenced by methylation clocks revealing epigenetic ages exceeding chronological age by ~8.5 years in adult AML and ~3.2 years in paediatric cases.

The disease is characterized by **focal CpG island hypermethylation** mediated by DNMT3A activity, which disrupts enhancer-driven transcriptional programs critical for normal haematopoiesis. Concurrently, genome-wide hypomethylation promotes genomic instability, while histone modification imbalances – particularly reduced H3K79me2 and H3K36me3 levels near transcription start sites – impair differentiation by silencing tumour suppressors and activating proto-oncogenes. This epigenetic landscape synergizes with aging-associated declines in DNA repair capacity, allowing survival of HSC clones primed for leukemic transformation through secondary mutations in proliferative pathways like *FLT3* or *NPM1*.

Therapeutic strategies targeting these age-related epigenetic mechanisms, including hypomethylating agents and histone deacetylase inhibitors, aim to restore differentiation capacity while mitigating chemotherapy resistance in elderly patients. However, AML's complex interplay between acquired epigenetic lesions and intrinsic aging processes remains a critical challenge for durable remissions.

4.3.c. Cancer of Reproductive Organs

Cancers affecting reproductive organs include breast cancer and prostate cancer, significantly influenced by age-related hormonal changes and epigenetics. Breast cancer remains the most common cancer among women, with about 1 in 8 women diagnosed during their lifetime. In breast cancer, aberrant methylation patterns can silence tumour suppressor genes like *BRCA1*, increasing cancer risk.

Non-coding RNAs have been implicated in regulating gene expression related to reproductive organ cancers through their interaction with chromatin-modifying complexes. Research published in *Nature Communications* identified lncRNAs that were upregulated due to oestrogen exposure, leading to altered gene expression profiles associated with cell proliferation (Liu et al., 2020).

4.4. Cardiovascular Diseases

Cardiovascular diseases (CVDs) remain the leading cause of death worldwide, with global deaths rising from 12.1 million in 1990 to 20.5 million in 2021, largely due to population aging and preventable risk factors like poor diet, smoking, and physical inactivity (World Heart Federation (WHF), 2023). Age is a significant risk factor for CVD, as cumulative damage from metabolic, environmental, and genetic factors contributes to conditions such as atherosclerosis and ischemic heart disease.

Epigenetic changes associated with aging play a critical role in CVD pathogenesis. Age-related alterations in DNA methylation affect genes involved in inflammation, lipid metabolism, and vascular homeostasis, promoting the development of atherosclerotic plaques (Di Cesare et al., 2024). Additionally, dysregulated histone acetylation influences the expression of inflammatory cytokines such as interleukin-6 (IL-6) and tumour necrosis factor-alpha (TNF-α), exacerbating vascular inflammation and endothelial dysfunction. Evidence suggests that dietary interventions like the Mediterranean diet can induce favourable epigenetic modifications at loci associated with cardiovascular health, potentially mitigating age-related CVD risks (Cardiology Magazine, JACC, 2023).

These findings underscore the importance of addressing modifiable risk factors and leveraging epigenetic insights to develop targeted prevention strategies for aging populations globally.

4.5. Diabetes

4.5.a. Type 2 Diabetes

Type 2 diabetes is characterized by insulin resistance and affects approximately 462 million individuals globally, corresponding to 6.28% of the world's population. Its prevalence increases significantly with age, with 15% of adults aged 50–69 and 22% of those aged 70 or older affected, highlighting the strong association between aging and diabetes risk (Khan et al., 2019). Epigenetic modifications significantly influence insulin signalling pathways critical for glucose metabolism; age-related changes often result in altered DNA methylation patterns affecting insulin receptor expression or downstream signalling molecules like IRS1.

4.5.b. Obesity and Diabetes

Obesity serves as a major risk factor for developing type 2 diabetes; it is characterized by excessive fat accumulation resulting from an imbalance between energy intake and expenditure. Globally, obesity has become a critical public health challenge, with its prevalence more than tripling since 1975. As of 2024, over one billion people worldwide are living with obesity, including 880 million adults and 159 million children and adolescents. The global prevalence of obesity is approximately 14% among men and 18.5% among women, with the highest rates observed in regions such as Polynesia, Micronesia, and parts of the Middle East and North Africa (WHO, 2024).

A case study published in *Springer* highlights the long-term metabolic impact of childhood obesity through epigenetic mechanisms. Researchers identified persistent DNA methylation changes at genes regulating energy homeostasis, which were linked to increased susceptibility to type 2 diabetes and other metabolic disorders in adulthood. These findings underscore how early-life obesity not only affects immediate health outcomes but also programs lifelong metabolic risks through epigenetic modifications (Koliaki et al., 2023).

4.6. Chronic Obstructive Pulmonary Disease (COPD)

Chronic obstructive pulmonary disease encompasses progressive lung diseases including emphysema and chronic bronchitis characterized by airflow obstruction primarily due environmental exposures such as smoking or air pollution. COPD affects approximately 16 million Americans but many more may have it without being diagnosed.

A case study published within *The American Journal of Respiratory and Critical Care Medicine* examined how cigarette smoke exposure led to distinct DNA methylation signatures within lung tissue samples from COPD patients compared healthy controls. These findings suggested specific gene silencing events mediated via aberrant methylation contributed towards impaired lung function observed amongst affected individuals.

4.7. Osteoporosis

Osteoporosis is characterized by decreased bone density resulting from an imbalance between bone resorption versus formation processes affecting approximately 10 million Americans aged over 50 years old while another estimated 44 million have low bone density placing them at risk for fractures.

Research published within *Bone* investigated how age-related changes impacted regulatory pathways governing osteoblast activity via alterations observed within histone acetylation states. Findings indicated specific histone modifications correlated directly with diminished osteoblast function contributing towards increased fracture risk observed amongst elderly populations.

4.8. Chronic Inflammation

Chronic inflammation refers broadly towards persistent low-grade inflammatory states often observed during aging termed inflammaging, which contributes towards multiple age-related diseases including cardiovascular disease, diabetes, and neurodegenerative disorders.

A case study published within *Nature Immunology* explored how chronic inflammation impacts systemic health across various populations revealing distinct profiles associated between cytokine production alongside corresponding shifts observed within DNA methylation signatures linked directly back towards underlying mechanisms driving these pathologies forward into advanced stages throughout lifespan.

5. TREATMENT OPTIONS

Various treatment options are emerging as promising strategies to mitigate the effects of aging and improve health outcomes. These options include pharmacological agents, gene therapy, lifestyle interventions, nutraceuticals and natural compounds, targeting inflammation, utilizing epigenetic biomarkers, and combination therapies. Each approach offers unique mechanisms to influence epigenetic regulation and address the underlying causes of age-related diseases.

5.1. Pharmacological Agents

Pharmacological agents designed to target epigenetic modifications involve using small molecules to influence the activity of enzymes that modify DNA and histones. These agents aim to restore normal gene expression patterns disrupted by aging (Macip et al., 2024).

Common pharmacological agents include histone deacetylase inhibitors (HDAC inhibitors), DNA methyltransferase inhibitors, and compounds like resveratrol that activate sirtuins. For example, HDAC inhibitors such as vorinostat and romidepsin are being explored for their potential in treating age-related diseases by promoting histone acetylation and enhancing the expression of neuroprotective genes (Blagosklonny, 2012).

The treatment typically involves administering these agents orally or intravenously, depending on the specific drug and condition being targeted. Clinical trials are ongoing to evaluate their safety and efficacy in various age-related conditions.

Pharmacological agents have shown promise in reversing some aspects of aging at the cellular level. For instance, HDAC inhibitors can promote neuroprotection in neurodegenerative diseases by enhancing synaptic plasticity and neuronal survival (Piskovatska et al., 2019). These agents work by modifying the epigenetic landscape of cells, thereby influencing gene expression patterns that are critical for maintaining cellular function during aging.

5.2. Gene Therapy

Gene therapy involves delivering genetic material into a patient's cells to correct or modify the expression of genes associated with aging and age-related diseases. This can include introducing genes that promote cellular rejuvenation or inhibit disease pathways.

Recent advancements have utilized adeno-associated viruses (AAVs) to deliver longevity-associated genes such as FGF21, sTGFβR2, and αKlotho. These genes have been shown to confer health benefits when expressed in animal models.

The procedure typically involves a single administration of the gene therapy vector, which carries the therapeutic genes into the target cells. Studies have demonstrated that this approach can dramatically improve or completely reverse multiple age-related conditions in mice (Macip et al., 2024). Gene therapy has shown potential in extending lifespan and improving health span by addressing multiple age-related diseases simultaneously. For example, a study indicated that delivering a combination of three longevity-associated genes improved heart function and reduced kidney atrophy in aged mice. This approach targets the epigenetic information loss during aging, effectively rejuvenating cellular functions.

Complementing these strategies, CRISPR-based epigenetic editing has emerged as a powerful tool for precise modulation of gene expression and chromatin states. CRISPR-Cas systems, including dCas9 fused to epigenetic modifiers, enable targeted alterations in DNA methylation or histone acetylation at specific loci, reactivating silenced genes critical for cellular health and reversing age-related epigenetic changes (Lau & Suh, 2017). This technology also holds promise for personalized medicine by tailoring interventions to an individual's unique genetic and epigenetic profile, potentially preventing or mitigating aging-related diseases (Kolanu, 2024)

5.3. Lifestyle Interventions

Lifestyle interventions focus on modifying daily habits to promote better health outcomes and mitigate the effects of aging. These interventions can include dietary changes, physical activity, stress management, and sleep optimization.

Key lifestyle changes include adopting a balanced diet rich in antioxidants (e.g., fruits, vegetables), engaging in regular aerobic exercise, practicing mindfulness or meditation, and ensuring adequate sleep quality (Ghodeshwar et al., 2023)

Implementing lifestyle interventions typically involves creating personalized plans that incorporate these elements into daily routines. Healthcare providers often work with patients to set achievable goals and monitor progress over time.

Research has shown that lifestyle interventions can lead to favourable epigenetic changes that enhance overall health and longevity. For instance, caloric restriction has been linked to reduced DNA methylation changes associated with aging, while regular exercise has been shown to improve metabolic health through beneficial epigenetic modifications (Zhai et al., 2023). These interventions work by enhancing cellular resilience against stressors associated with aging.

5.4. Nutraceuticals and Natural Compounds

Nutraceuticals are bioactive compounds found in foods that can influence health by modulating epigenetic mechanisms related to aging. They serve as adjunctive therapies to support overall well-being.

Common nutraceuticals include resveratrol (found in red wine), curcumin (found in turmeric), quercetin (found in fruits), and omega-3 fatty acids (found in fish oil). These compounds have been studied for their potential epigenetic effects.

Nutraceuticals can be consumed as part of a regular diet or taken as dietary supplements. Dosages vary based on individual needs and specific health goals.

Nutraceuticals have demonstrated potential in reversing epigenetic changes associated with aging. For example, curcumin has been shown to inhibit DNA methyltransferases and promote histone acetylation, leading to reactivation of tumour suppressor genes. These effects may help reduce the risk of age-related diseases such as cancer and cardiovascular conditions by restoring normal cellular functions (Hassan et al., 2019).

5.5. Targeting Inflammation

Targeting inflammation involves using pharmacological agents or lifestyle modifications to reduce chronic inflammation associated with aging. This approach aims to mitigate its impact on health span and reduce the risk of age-related diseases.

Anti-inflammatory drugs such as non-steroidal anti-inflammatory drugs (NSAIDs) are commonly used, along with lifestyle strategies like adopting an anti-inflammatory diet rich in omega-3 fatty acids and antioxidants (J. Ye & Ghosh, 2018).

The use of anti-inflammatory medications typically requires a prescription or over-the-counter purchase, while dietary changes involve incorporating specific foods into daily meals.

Reducing chronic inflammation through targeted therapies can lead to favourable epigenetic changes that improve health outcomes. Studies have shown that anti-inflammatory strategies can lower levels of pro-inflammatory cytokines associated with various age-related diseases, thereby enhancing overall health span by promoting a more balanced immune response (X. Li et al., 2023b).

5.6. Epigenetic Biomarkers

Utilizing epigenetic biomarkers involves identifying specific DNA methylation patterns or histone modifications that correlate with biological age or disease risk. This approach aids in early detection and monitoring of aging-related conditions.

Biomarkers such as Horvath's epigenetic clock or GrimAge are used to assess biological age based on DNA methylation profiles obtained from blood or tissue samples.

The process typically involves collecting biological samples from individuals followed by laboratory analysis using techniques like bisulfite sequencing or methylation arrays to determine epigenetic age (Bocklandt et al., 2011).

Recent advancements in artificial intelligence (AI) have revolutionized the discovery and validation of epigenetic biomarkers. Machine learning algorithms and deep learning models can analyse vast datasets from multi-omics studies, identifying novel DNA methylation sites and histone modification patterns associated with aging and age-related diseases. AI-driven approaches, such as explainable AI models, have been instrumental in refining epigenetic clocks and uncovering complex relationships between epigenetic changes and disease progression. For example, AI has enabled the integration of single-cell sequencing and spatial transcriptomics data to identify tissue-specific biomarkers of aging, enhancing the precision of biological age estimation (Marino et al., 2023).

Identifying epigenetic biomarkers allows for personalized interventions based on an individual's biological age rather than chronological age. This can lead to more targeted therapies aimed at reversing or slowing down the aging process by addressing specific epigenetic alterations identified through biomarker analysis. Furthermore, AI-driven biomarker discovery supports the development of therapeutic biomarkers that monitor responses to interventions such as geroprotective drugs or dietary modifications, offering a dynamic tool for tailoring treatments to individual needs (Lyu et al., 2024). Together, these advancements highlight the synergy between AI technologies and epigenetics in advancing personalized medicine for healthy aging.

5.7. Combination Therapies

Combination therapies integrate multiple treatment modalities—such as pharmacological agents, gene therapy, lifestyle interventions, and nutraceuticals—to address various pathways involved in aging simultaneously.

This approach may involve using HDAC inhibitors alongside lifestyle changes or combining gene therapy targeting multiple longevity-associated genes with dietary modifications rich in antioxidants.

Implementing combination therapies requires careful planning by healthcare providers who tailor treatments based on individual patient needs and disease profiles. Monitoring progress across different modalities is essential for optimizing outcomes.

Research suggests that combination therapies may enhance therapeutic efficacy compared to single-agent approaches by addressing multiple mechanisms underlying aging simultaneously. For example, combining senolytic drugs with lifestyle modifications has shown promise in improving overall health span while reducing the burden of age-related diseases more effectively than either strategy alone.

6. CONCLUSION

In this chapter, we have explored the intricate relationship between epigenetics and the aging process, emphasizing how non-coding RNAs, DNA methylation, and histone modifications contribute to the biological changes associated with aging in humans. As we age, the epigenetic mechanisms that regulate gene expression become increasingly vulnerable, leading to a cascade of alterations that can promote age-related diseases.

The evidence presented highlights that epigenetic drift, characterized by global changes in DNA methylation patterns and histone modifications, plays a critical role in the aging process. This drift not only affects gene regulation but also contributes to the development of various age-related conditions, including cardiovascular diseases, neurodegenerative disorders, and metabolic syndromes. Furthermore, external factors such as environmental stressors and nutritional influences can exacerbate these epigenetic changes, underscoring the importance of understanding the broader context in which aging occurs.

Recent research has illuminated potential therapeutic avenues aimed at reversing or mitigating the effects of aging through epigenetic interventions. Strategies targeting non-coding RNAs or restoring proper DNA methylation patterns hold promise for enhancing health span and reducing the burden of age-related diseases. By manipulating these epigenetic factors, we may be able to delay the onset of aging-related conditions and improve overall quality of life as we grow older.

However, despite these promising advances, significant challenges remain in the field of epigenetic research. The reversibility of age-related modifications is still poorly understood, raising questions about the long-term efficacy and safety of potential therapies. Additionally, variability in epigenetic markers across different populations complicates efforts to establish universal therapeutic targets, necessitating a more nuanced approach to treatment development that considers genetic diversity.

Ethical considerations also play a pivotal role in shaping the future of epigenetic therapies. Issues such as privacy, informed consent, and equitable access to treatments must be carefully addressed to prevent misuse or discrimination based on individual epigenetic information. Regulatory challenges further complicate clinical translation; establishing safety standards for somatic cell epigenetic editing and ensuring long-term efficacy remain critical hurdles that must be navigated before widespread clinical application can occur.

Moreover, AI-driven epigenetic biomarker discovery offers a powerful tool for overcoming some of these obstacles by enabling precise identification of age-related epigenetic changes and tailoring interventions to individual needs. This approach not only enhances our understanding of biological aging but also supports personalized medicine by integrating multi-omics data into therapeutic development.

In summary, this chapter emphasizes the critical role of epigenetics in aging and its implications for health. As our understanding deepens, addressing current scientific challenges alongside ethical and regulatory considerations will be essential for translating discoveries into impactful therapies that promote healthier aging globally. The integration of innovative technologies such as AI in biomarker discovery and therapeutic development will be crucial in paving the way for effective interventions that can meaningfully alter the trajectory of aging and improve quality of life for individuals across diverse populations. Ultimately, a collaborative effort among researchers, clinicians, ethicists, and policymakers will be vital in harnessing the potential of epigenetics to transform our approach to aging and age-related diseases.

REFERENCES

Abrishamcar, S., Zhuang, B. C., Thomas, M., Gladish, N., MacIsaac, J. L., Jones, M. J., Simons, E., Moraes, T. J., Mandhane, P. J., Brook, J. R., Subbarao, P., Turvey, S. E., Chen, E., Miller, G. E., Kobor, M. S., & Hüls, A. (2024). Association between maternal perinatal stress and depression and infant DNA methylation in the first year of life. *Translational Psychiatry*, *14*(1), 445. DOI: 10.1038/s41398-024-03148-8 PMID: 39438450

Blagosklonny, M. V. (2012). Prospective Treatment of Age-Related Diseases by Slowing Down Aging. *American Journal of Pathology*, *181*(4), 1142–1146. DOI: 10.1016/j.ajpath.2012.06.024 PMID: 22841821

Bocklandt, S., Lin, W., Sehl, M. E., Sánchez, F. J., Sinsheimer, J. S., Horvath, S., & Vilain, E. (2011). Epigenetic predictor of age. *PLoS One*, *6*(6), e14821. DOI: 10.1371/journal.pone.0014821 PMID: 21731603

Borsoi, F. T., Neri-Numa, I. A., de Oliveira, W. Q., de Araújo, F. F., & Pastore, G. M. (2023). Dietary polyphenols and their relationship to the modulation of non-communicable chronic diseases and epigenetic mechanisms: A mini-review. *Food Chemistry. Molecular Sciences*, *6*, 100155. DOI: 10.1016/j.fochms.2022.100155 PMID: 36582744

López-Otín, C., Blasco, M. A., Partridge, L., Serrano, M., & Kroemer, G. (2013). The hallmarks of aging. *Cell*, *153*(6), 1194–1217.

Chen, Y., Sun, Y., Xue, X., & Ma, H. (2023). Comprehensive analysis of epigenetics mechanisms in osteoporosis. *Frontiers in Genetics*, *14*, 1153585. Advance online publication. DOI: 10.3389/fgene.2023.1153585 PMID: 37056287

Cheung, H.-H., Pei, D., & Chan, W.-Y. (2015). Stem cell aging in adult progeria. *Cell Regeneration*, *4*(1), 4:6. DOI: 10.1186/s13619-015-0021-z

Dasgupta, N., Arnold, R., Equey, A., Gandhi, A., & Adams, P. D. (2024). The role of the dynamic epigenetic landscape in senescence: Orchestrating SASP expression. *NPJ Aging*, *10*(1), 48. DOI: 10.1038/s41514-024-00172-2 PMID: 39448585

de Lima Camillo, L. P., Lapierre, L. R., & Singh, R. (2022). A pan-tissue DNA-methylation epigenetic clock based on deep learning. *NPJ Aging*, *8*(1), 4. DOI: 10.1038/s41514-022-00085-y

Di Cesare, M., Perel, P., Taylor, S., Kabudula, C., Bixby, H., Gaziano, T. A., McGhie, D. V., Mwangi, J., Pervan, B., Narula, J., Pineiro, D., & Pinto, F. J. (2024). The Heart of the World. *Global Heart*, *19*(1), 11. Advance online publication. DOI: 10.5334/gh.1288 PMID: 38273998

Di Giosia, P., Stamerra, C. A., Giorgini, P., Jamialahamdi, T., Butler, A. E., & Sahebkar, A. (2022). The role of nutrition in inflammaging. *Ageing Research Reviews*, *77*, 101596. DOI: 10.1016/j.arr.2022.101596 PMID: 35219904

Duan, R., Fu, Q., Sun, Y., & Li, Q. (2022). Epigenetic clock: A promising biomarker and practical tool in aging. *Ageing Research Reviews*, *81*, 101743. DOI: 10.1016/j.arr.2022.101743 PMID: 36206857

Gates, L. A., Shi, J., Rohira, A. D., Feng, Q., Zhu, B., Bedford, M. T., Sagum, C. A., Jung, S. Y., Qin, J., Tsai, M.-J., Tsai, S. Y., Li, W., Foulds, C. E., & O'Malley, B. W. (2017). Acetylation on histone H3 lysine 9 mediates a switch from transcription initiation to elongation. *The Journal of Biological Chemistry, 292*(35), 14456–14472. DOI: 10.1074/jbc.M117.802074 PMID: 28717009

Ghodeshwar, G. K., Dube, A., & Khobragade, D. (2023). Impact of Lifestyle Modifications on Cardiovascular Health: A Narrative Review. *Cureus*. Advance online publication. DOI: 10.7759/cureus.42616 PMID: 37641769

Gilbert, S. F. (2000). Aging: The Biology of Senescence. In *Developmental Biology* (6th ed.).

Guillaumet-Adkins, A., Yañez, Y., Peris-Diaz, M. D., Calabria, I., Palanca-Ballester, C., & Sandoval, J. (2017). Epigenetics and Oxidative Stress in Aging. *Oxidative Medicine and Cellular Longevity, 2017*(1). DOI: 10.1155/2017/9175806

Hajjo, R., Sabbah, D. A., Abusara, O. H., & Al Bawab, A. Q. (2022). A Review of the Recent Advances in Alzheimer's Disease Research and the Utilization of Network Biology Approaches for Prioritizing Diagnostics and Therapeutics. *Diagnostics (Basel), 12*(12), 2975. DOI: 10.3390/diagnostics12122975 PMID: 36552984

Hassan, F., Rehman, M. S., Khan, M. S., Ali, M. A., Javed, A., Nawaz, A., & Yang, C. (2019). Curcumin as an Alternative Epigenetic Modulator: Mechanism of Action and Potential Effects. *Frontiers in Genetics, 10*, 514. Advance online publication. DOI: 10.3389/fgene.2019.00514 PMID: 31214247

Hoang, T. T., Lee, Y., McCartney, D. L., Kersten, E. T. G., Page, C. M., Hulls, P. M., Lee, M., Walker, R. M., Breeze, C. E., Bennett, B. D., Burkholder, A. B., Ward, J., Brantsæter, A. L., Caspersen, I. H., Motsinger-Reif, A. A., Richards, M., White, J. D., Zhao, S., Richmond, R. C., & London, S. J. (2024). Comprehensive evaluation of smoking exposures and their interactions on DNA methylation. *EBioMedicine, 100*, 104956. DOI: 10.1016/j.ebiom.2023.104956 PMID: 38199042

Horvath, S. (2013). DNA methylation age of human tissues and cell types. *Genome Biology, 14*(10), 3156. DOI: 10.1186/gb-2013-14-10-r115 PMID: 24138928

Hu, C., Liu, X., Zeng, Y., Liu, J., & Wu, F. (2021). DNA methyltransferase inhibitors combination therapy for the treatment of solid tumor: Mechanism and clinical application. *Clinical Epigenetics, 13*(1), 166. DOI: 10.1186/s13148-021-01154-x PMID: 34452630

Ilieva, M. S. (2024). Non-Coding RNAs in Neurological and Neuropsychiatric Disorders: Unraveling the Hidden Players in Disease Pathogenesis. *Cells, 13*(12), 1063. DOI: 10.3390/cells13121063 PMID: 38920691

Khan, M. A. B., Hashim, M. J., King, J. K., Govender, R. D., Mustafa, H., & Al Kaabi, J. (2019). Epidemiology of Type 2 Diabetes – Global Burden of Disease and Forecasted Trends. *Journal of Epidemiology and Global Health, 10*(1), 107. DOI: 10.2991/jegh.k.191028.001 PMID: 32175717

Kim, D.-H., Tang, Z., Shimada, M., Fierz, B., Houck-Loomis, B., Bar-Dagen, M., Lee, S., Lee, S.-K., Muir, T. W., Roeder, R. G., & Lee, J. W. (2013). Histone H3K27 Trimethylation Inhibits H3 Binding and Function of SET1-Like H3K4 Methyltransferase Complexes. *Molecular and Cellular Biology, 33*(24), 4936–4946. DOI: 10.1128/MCB.00601-13 PMID: 24126056

Kim, J.-Y., Vijayakumar, K. A., & Cho, G.-W. (2025). Exploring the impact of methylation aging on acute myeloid leukemia: Insights from the aging clock. *Leukemia Research*, *148*, 107620. DOI: 10.1016/j.leukres.2024.107620 PMID: 39550906

Kolanu, N. D. (2024). CRISPR–Cas9 Gene Editing: Curing Genetic Diseases by Inherited Epigenetic Modifications. *Global Medical Genetics*, *11*(01), 113–122. DOI: 10.1055/s-0044-1785234 PMID: 38560484

Koliaki, C., Dalamaga, M., & Liatis, S. (2023). Update on the Obesity Epidemic: After the Sudden Rise, Is the Upward Trajectory Beginning to Flatten? *Current Obesity Reports*, *12*(4), 514–527. DOI: 10.1007/s13679-023-00527-y PMID: 37779155

Krittanawong, C., Qadeer, Y. K., Hayes, R. B., Wang, Z., Thurston, G. D., Virani, S., & Lavie, C. J. (2023). PM2.5 and cardiovascular diseases: State-of-the-Art review. *International Journal of Cardiology. Cardiovascular Risk and Prevention*, *19*, 200217. DOI: 10.1016/j.ijcrp.2023.200217 PMID: 37869561

Kumar, S., Chinnusamy, V., & Mohapatra, T. (2018). Epigenetics of Modified DNA Bases: 5-Methylcytosine and Beyond. *Frontiers in Genetics*, *9*, 640. Advance online publication. DOI: 10.3389/fgene.2018.00640 PMID: 30619465

Larsen, B., & Sánchez-Triana, E. (2023). Global health burden and cost of lead exposure in children and adults: A health impact and economic modelling analysis. *The Lancet. Planetary Health*, *7*(10), e831–e840. DOI: 10.1016/S2542-5196(23)00166-3 PMID: 37714172

Lau, C.-H., & Suh, Y. (2017). Genome and Epigenome Editing in Mechanistic Studies of Human Aging and Aging-Related Disease. *Gerontology*, *63*(2), 103–117. DOI: 10.1159/000452972 PMID: 27974723

Li, X., Li, C., Zhang, W., Wang, Y., Qian, P., & Huang, H. (2023a). Inflammation and aging: Signaling pathways and intervention therapies. *Signal Transduction and Targeted Therapy*, *8*(1), 239. DOI: 10.1038/s41392-023-01502-8 PMID: 37291105

Li, Y. (2021). Modern epigenetics methods in biological research. *Methods (San Diego, Calif.)*, *187*, 104–113. DOI: 10.1016/j.ymeth.2020.06.022 PMID: 32645449

Licciardi, P. V., Ververis, K., & Karagiannis, T. C. (2011). Histone Deacetylase Inhibition and Dietary Short-Chain Fatty Acids. *ISRN Allergy*, *2011*, 1–8. DOI: 10.5402/2011/869647 PMID: 23724235

Liu, S., Lai, W., Shi, Y., Liu, N., Ouyang, L., Zhang, Z., Chen, L., Wang, X., Qian, B., Xiao, D., Yan, Q., Cao, Y., Liu, S., & Tao, Y. (2020). Annotation and cluster analysis of long noncoding RNA linked to male sex and estrogen in cancers. *NPJ Precision Oncology*, *4*(1), 5. DOI: 10.1038/s41698-020-0110-5 PMID: 32195358

Lu, W., Tang, S., Li, A., Huang, Q., Dou, M., Zhang, Y., Hu, X., Chang, R. C. C., Wong, G. T. C., & Huang, C. (2022). The role of PKC/PKR in aging, Alzheimer's disease, and perioperative neurocognitive disorders. *Frontiers in Aging Neuroscience*, *14*, 973068. Advance online publication. DOI: 10.3389/fnagi.2022.973068 PMID: 36172481

Luevano-Contreras, C., & Chapman-Novakofski, K. (2010). Dietary Advanced Glycation End Products and Aging. *Nutrients*, *2*(12), 1247–1265. DOI: 10.3390/nu2121247 PMID: 22254007

Lyu, Y.-X., Fu, Q., Wilczok, D., Ying, K., King, A., Antebi, A., Vojta, A., Stolzing, A., Moskalev, A., Georgievskaya, A., Maier, A. B., Olsen, A., Groth, A., Simon, A. K., Brunet, A., Jamil, A., Kulaga, A., Bhatti, A., Yaden, B., & Bakula, D. (2024). Longevity biotechnology: Bridging AI, biomarkers, geroscience and clinical applications for healthy longevity. *Aging (Albany NY)*, *16*(20), 12955–12976. DOI: 10.18632/aging.206135 PMID: 39418098

Macip, C. C., Hasan, R., Hoznek, V., Kim, J., Lu, Y. R., Metzger, L. E.IV, Sethna, S., & Davidsohn, N. (2024). Gene Therapy-Mediated Partial Reprogramming Extends Lifespan and Reverses Age-Related Changes in Aged Mice. *Cellular Reprogramming*, *26*(1), 24–32. DOI: 10.1089/cell.2023.0072 PMID: 38381405

Margiotti, K., Monaco, F., Fabiani, M., Mesoraca, A., & Giorlandino, C. (2023). Epigenetic Clocks: In Aging-Related and Complex Diseases. *Cytogenetic and Genome Research*, *163*(5–6), 247–256. DOI: 10.1159/000534561 PMID: 37899027

Marino, N., Putignano, G., Cappilli, S., Chersoni, E., Santuccione, A., Calabrese, G., Bischof, E., Vanhaelen, Q., Zhavoronkov, A., Scarano, B., Mazzotta, A. D., & Santus, E. (2023). Towards AI-driven longevity research: An overview. *Frontiers in Aging*, *4*, 1057204. DOI: 10.3389/fragi.2023.1057204 PMID: 36936271

Maugeri, A., & Barchitta, M. (2020). How Dietary Factors Affect DNA Methylation: Lesson from Epidemiological Studies. *Medicina*, *56*(8), 374. DOI: 10.3390/medicina56080374 PMID: 32722411

Ming, X., Zhu, B., & Li, Y. (2021). Mitotic inheritance of DNA methylation: More than just copy and paste. *Journal of Genetics and Genomics*, *48*(1), 1–13. DOI: 10.1016/j.jgg.2021.01.006 PMID: 33771455

Miwa, S., Kashyap, S., Chini, E., & von Zglinicki, T. (2022). Mitochondrial dysfunction in cell senescence and aging. *The Journal of Clinical Investigation*, *132*(13), e158447. Advance online publication. DOI: 10.1172/JCI158447 PMID: 35775483

Niforou, A., Konstantinidou, V., & Naska, A. (2020). Genetic Variants Shaping Inter-individual Differences in Response to Dietary Intakes—A Narrative Review of the Case of Vitamins. *Frontiers in Nutrition*, *7*, 558598. Advance online publication. DOI: 10.3389/fnut.2020.558598 PMID: 33335908

Pathania, A. S. (2023). Crosstalk between Noncoding RNAs and the Epigenetics Machinery in Pediatric Tumors and Their Microenvironment. *Cancers (Basel)*, *15*(10), 2833. DOI: 10.3390/cancers15102833 PMID: 37345170

Patterson, S. E., & Margolis, R. (2023). Family Ties and Older Adult Well-Being: Incorporating Social Networks and Proximity. *The Journals of Gerontology. Series B, Psychological Sciences and Social Sciences*, *78*(12), 2080–2089. DOI: 10.1093/geronb/gbad139 PMID: 37738615

Piskovatska, V., Strilbytska, O., Koliada, A., Vaiserman, A., & Lushchak, O. (2019). *Health Benefits of Anti-aging Drugs.*, DOI: 10.1007/978-981-13-3681-2_13

Puvvula, P. K. (2019). LncRNAs Regulatory Networks in Cellular Senescence. *International Journal of Molecular Sciences*, *20*(11), 2615. DOI: 10.3390/ijms20112615 PMID: 31141943

Qin, J., Wen, B., Liang, Y., Yu, W., & Li, H. (2020). Histone Modifications and their Role in Colorectal Cancer [Review]. *Pathology Oncology Research : POR*, *26*(4), 2023–2033. DOI: 10.1007/s12253-019-00663-8 PMID: 31055775

Rossiello, F., Jurk, D., Passos, J. F., & d'Adda di Fagagna, F. (2022). Telomere dysfunction in ageing and age-related diseases. *Nature Cell Biology*, *24*(2), 135–147. DOI: 10.1038/s41556-022-00842-x PMID: 35165420

Şanlı, E., & Kabaran, S. (2019). Maternal Obesity, Maternal Overnutrition and Fetal Programming: Effects of Epigenetic Mechanisms on the Development of Metabolic Disorders. *Current Genomics*, *20*(6), 419–427. DOI: 10.2174/1389202920666191030092225 PMID: 32476999

Shen, Y., Huang, X., Wu, J., Lin, X., Zhou, X., Zhu, Z., Pan, X., Xu, J., Qiao, J., Zhang, T., Ye, L., Jiang, H., Ren, Y., & Shan, P.-F. (2022). The Global Burden of Osteoporosis, Low Bone Mass, and Its Related Fracture in 204 Countries and Territories, 1990-2019. *Frontiers in Endocrinology*, *13*, 882241. Advance online publication. DOI: 10.3389/fendo.2022.882241 PMID: 35669691

Silva, Y. P., Bernardi, A., & Frozza, R. L. (2020). The Role of Short-Chain Fatty Acids From Gut Microbiota in Gut-Brain Communication. *Frontiers in Endocrinology*, *11*, 25. Advance online publication. DOI: 10.3389/fendo.2020.00025 PMID: 32082260

Soto-Palma, C., Niedernhofer, L. J., Faulk, C. D., & Dong, X. (2022). Epigenetics, DNA damage, and aging. *The Journal of Clinical Investigation*, *132*(16), e158446. Advance online publication. DOI: 10.1172/JCI158446 PMID: 35968782

Swamy, S. M., Rajasekaran, N. S., & Thannickal, V. J. (2016). Nuclear Factor–Erythroid-2–Related Factor 2 in Aging and Lung Fibrosis. *American Journal of Pathology*, *186*(7), 1712–1723. DOI: 10.1016/j.ajpath.2016.02.022 PMID: 27338106

Swaroop, S., Batabyal, A., & Bhattacharjee, A. (2021). HAT/HDAC: The epigenetic regulators of inflammatory gene expression [Review]. *International Journal of Epigenetics*, *1*(2), 5. DOI: 10.3892/ije.2021.5

Tan, B. L., Norhaizan, M. E., Liew, W.-P.-P., & Sulaiman Rahman, H. (2018). Antioxidant and Oxidative Stress: A Mutual Interplay in Age-Related Diseases. *Frontiers in Pharmacology*, *9*, 1162. Advance online publication. DOI: 10.3389/fphar.2018.01162 PMID: 30405405

Trerotola, M., Relli, V., Simeone, P., & Alberti, S. (2015). Epigenetic inheritance and the missing heritability. *Human Genomics*, *9*(1), 17. DOI: 10.1186/s40246-015-0041-3 PMID: 26216216

Tylutka, A., Walas, Ł., & Zembron-Lacny, A. (2024). Level of IL-6, TNF, and IL-1β and age-related diseases: A systematic review and meta-analysis. *Frontiers in Immunology*, *15*, 1330386. DOI: 10.3389/fimmu.2024.1330386 PMID: 38495887

Vasileva, D., Greenwood, C. M. T., & Daley, D. (2023). A Review of the Epigenetic Clock: Emerging Biomarkers for Asthma and Allergic Disease. *Genes*, *14*(9), 1724. DOI: 10.3390/genes14091724 PMID: 37761864

Vickers, M. (2014). Early Life Nutrition, Epigenetics and Programming of Later Life Disease. *Nutrients*, *6*(6), 2165–2178. DOI: 10.3390/nu6062165 PMID: 24892374

Wang, H., & Helin, K. (2025). Roles of H3K4 methylation in biology and disease. *Trends in Cell Biology*, *35*(2), 115–128. DOI: 10.1016/j.tcb.2024.06.001 PMID: 38909006

Wang, K., Liu, H., Hu, Q., Wang, L., Liu, J., Zheng, Z., Zhang, W., Ren, J., Zhu, F., & Liu, G.-H. (2022). Epigenetic regulation of aging: Implications for interventions of aging and diseases. *Signal Transduction and Targeted Therapy*, *7*(1), 374. DOI: 10.1038/s41392-022-01211-8 PMID: 36336680

Wang, S. S., Lewis, M. J., & Pitzalis, C. (2023). DNA Methylation Signatures of Response to Conventional Synthetic and Biologic Disease-Modifying Antirheumatic Drugs (DMARDs) in Rheumatoid Arthritis. *Biomedicines*, *11*(7), 1987. DOI: 10.3390/biomedicines11071987 PMID: 37509625

Wilson, E. R., Helton, N. M., Heath, S. E., Fulton, R. S., Payton, J. E., Welch, J. S., Walter, M. J., Westervelt, P., DiPersio, J. F., Link, D. C., Miller, C. A., Ley, T. J., & Spencer, D. H. (2022). Focal disruption of DNA methylation dynamics at enhancers in IDH-mutant AML cells. *Leukemia*, *36*(4), 935–945. DOI: 10.1038/s41375-021-01476-y PMID: 34873300

World Health Organization: WHO. (2024). *Ageing and health.*

Xiao, F.-H., Wang, H.-T., & Kong, Q.-P. (2019). Dynamic DNA Methylation During Aging: A "Prophet" of Age-Related Outcomes. *Frontiers in Genetics*, *10*, 107. Advance online publication. DOI: 10.3389/fgene.2019.00107 PMID: 30833961

Ye, J., & Ghosh, S. (2018). Omega-3 PUFA vs. NSAIDs for Preventing Cardiac Inflammation. *Frontiers in Cardiovascular Medicine*, *5*, 146. Advance online publication. DOI: 10.3389/fcvm.2018.00146 PMID: 30406113

Ye, M., Xu, G., Zhang, L., Kong, Z., & Qiu, Z. (2025). Meta Analysis of Methylenetetrahydrofolate Reductase (MTHFR) C677T polymorphism and its association with folate and colorectal cancer. *BMC Cancer*, *25*(1), 169. DOI: 10.1186/s12885-025-13546-w PMID: 39875876

Yi, S.-J., & Kim, K. (2020). New Insights into the Role of Histone Changes in Aging. *International Journal of Molecular Sciences*, *21*(21), 8241. DOI: 10.3390/ijms21218241 PMID: 33153221

Yuan, M., Yang, B., Rothschild, G., Mann, J. J., Sanford, L. D., Tang, X., Huang, C., Wang, C., & Zhang, W. (2023). Epigenetic regulation in major depression and other stress-related disorders: Molecular mechanisms, clinical relevance and therapeutic potential. *Signal Transduction and Targeted Therapy*, *8*(1), 309. DOI: 10.1038/s41392-023-01519-z PMID: 37644009

Zhai, J., Kongsberg, W. H., Pan, Y., Hao, C., Wang, X., & Sun, J. (2023). Caloric restriction induced epigenetic effects on aging. *Frontiers in Cell and Developmental Biology*, *10*, 1079920. Advance online publication. DOI: 10.3389/fcell.2022.1079920 PMID: 36712965

Zhan, W., Liao, X., Liu, J., Tian, T., Yu, L., & Li, R. (2020). USP38 regulates the stemness and chemoresistance of human colorectal cancer via regulation of HDAC3. *Oncogenesis*, *9*(5), 48. DOI: 10.1038/s41389-020-0234-z PMID: 32404892

Zhao, L., Cao, J., Hu, K., He, X., Yun, D., Tong, T., & Han, L. (2020). Sirtuins and their Biological Relevance in Aging and Age-Related Diseases. *Aging and Disease*, *11*(4), 927. DOI: 10.14336/AD.2019.0820 PMID: 32765955

Zhu, J. H., Bo, H. H., Liu, B. P., & Jia, C. X. (2023). The associations between DNA methylation and depression: A systematic review and meta-analysis. *Journal of Affective Disorders*, *327*, 439–450. DOI: 10.1016/j.jad.2023.01.079 PMID: 36717033

Zilberter, Y., Tabuena, D. R., & Zilberter, M. (2023). NOX-induced oxidative stress is a primary trigger of major neurodegenerative disorders. *Progress in Neurobiology*, *231*, 102539. DOI: 10.1016/j.pneurobio.2023.102539 PMID: 37838279

Zuccolo, E., Badi, I., Scavello, F., Gambuzza, I., Mancinelli, L., Macrì, F., Tedesco, C. C., Veglia, F., Bonfigli, A. R., Olivieri, F., & Raucci, A. (2020). The microRNA-34a-Induced Senescence-Associated Secretory Phenotype (SASP) Favors Vascular Smooth Muscle Cells Calcification. *International Journal of Molecular Sciences*, *21*(12), 4454. DOI: 10.3390/ijms21124454 PMID: 32585876

Chapter 8
Natural Antioxidants and Their Impact on Aging:
Insights Into Mechanisms for Extending Life Span

Saliya S. Bawani
https://orcid.org/0000-0003-3302-7704
Bangalore University, India

Rakesh Hanumanthappa
https://orcid.org/0009-0009-4936-4861
Bangalore University, India

Rizwan Sharief
https://orcid.org/0009-0006-6926-2895
Bangalore University, India

ABSTRACT

Aging is a complex process influenced by biological mechanisms, lifestyle choices, environmental factors, and genetic predispositions. Key biological hallmarks include genomic instability, mitochondrial dysfunction, and OS, which contribute to age-related diseases such as CVD, NDD and sarcopenia. Lifestyle factors like diet, physical activity, and sleep quality significantly impact health. Genetic variations and epigenetic modifications further modulate individual aging trajectories. OS driven by reactive oxygen species, plays a central role in aging, with antioxidants from natural sources offering protective benefits. This chapter deliberates the overview of the aging process with special emphases on OS and methods for mitigating its effects; it further highlights the necessity for individualized techniques like nutrigenomics and examines treatment approaches. Future studies should prioritize large-scale investigations and include genetic, environmental, and lifestyle factors to promote healthy aging and enhance quality of life.

DOI: 10.4018/979-8-3693-9730-5.ch008

INTRODUCTION

The Process of Aging

Aging is a complex interplay of various factors, including lifestyle choices, environmental influence, and genetic predispositions. Understanding the impact of these factors is essential for developing effective strategies to support healthy aging and improved quality of life in elderly individuals (Addo & Khan, 2024). Overall, general health and the quality of life of an individual is significantly improved by numerous physical, psychological, and social changes that precede aging (Anton et al., 2020).

The biological basis of aging involves multiple mechanisms that lead to progressive functional decline in different body systems; hence, it is important to understand its basic biogerontology mechanism. Recent research has identified the accumulation of DNA damage to be the primary cause of aging, highlighting genomic instability as an essential feature of this biological process. DNA accumulation promotes increased mutations, reduced efficiency in DNA repair mechanisms, and chromosomal aberrations, all contributing to aging (Lombard et al., 2005; Hoeijmakers, 2009; López-Otín et al., 2013). Aging is also significantly influenced by mitochondrial failure, telomere shortening, oxidative stress (OS), autophagy and cellular senescence. With every cell division, the telomere progressively gets shorter till it reaches the critical length, resulting in cellular senescence and altering its dynamics (Epel et al., 2006; Campisi & Robert, 2014; Blackburn et al., 2015).

There is an inherent connection between aging and metabolism, as evidenced by notable changes in body composition with aging, such as sarcopenia (muscle fat) and increasing central adiposity (visceral fat) (Palmer & Jensen, 2022). These metabolic alterations are influenced by both genetic factors and lifestyle choices, particularly physical activity levels and dietary habits. For instance, one of the primary concerns in the aging process is sarcopenia, characterized by progressive loss of muscle mass and function. According to current research, the prevalence of sarcopenia cases is expected to increase by 35% in older individuals by 2025 (Rogeri et al., 2021; Almohaisen et al., 2022). This condition is triggered by multiple factors, including improper nutrition, sedentary habits, negative protein balance, genetic predisposition, hormonal changes and inflammatory processes.

Lifestyle Factors Affecting Aging

Lifestyle factors play a significant role in shaping various aspects of the aging process, including factors like sedentary behavior, nutrition, and sleep quality. Sedentary behavior, characterized by minimal physical activity or no activity, whereas regular and consistent physical activity, are the key lifestyle elements that can greatly impact the rate and quality of aging (Tremblay et al., 2010). Engaging in moderate exercise has been shown to improve cardiovascular health, maintain muscle mass, enhance mobility and reduce the risk of chronic diseases (Polidori et al., 2000). However, many older individuals face barriers to physical activity, including mobility limitations and lack of motivation, due to environmental factors (such as unsafe neighborhoods) (Rasinaho et al., 2007). Besides this, nutrition also plays a pivotal role in aging. As individuals age, their nutritional needs change, often leading to a decline in dietary quality (Bloom et al., 2017). Older individuals frequently experience reduced intake of nutrient-dense foods, which results in deficiencies of essential vitamins and minerals (Bloom et al., 2017; Ortolá et al., 2019).

In addition to the physiological changes, factors such as decreased appetite, dental issues, and digestive discomfort are prevalent among older populations making it difficult to maintain the diet.

Alongside nutrition, sleep quality is another significant factor which is often compromised in older adults, leading to various health issues, including cognitive decline, mood disorders, and weakened immune function, irregular sleep patterns, sleep architecture as well as pre-existing medical conditions like stress are crucial factors contributing poor sleep quality involved in age related changes and maintaining the quality of life (Crowley, 2011).

To mitigate the above-mentioned challenges, it is essential to promote a balanced diet, quality sleep and regular physical activity, as all these contributing factors are interrelated in the wellness of an aging individual. Dietary modifications, specifically those that focus on increasing the intake of high-quality proteins, micronutrients and nutrient-dense foods are essential. Also, maintaining proper food habits and improving quality sleep can help counteract the effects of aging. Moreover, personalized lifestyle approaches tailored to individual needs and preferences can improve dietary adherence and thereby improve long term health outcomes (Trovato et al., 2012).

Environmental Factors Affecting Aging

Pollution is a significant environmental factor that adversely affects health, particularly in aging populations. As individuals age, their physiological systems become more vulnerable to external stressors, including various pollutants. Airborne pollutants, such as particulate matter (PM), nitrogen dioxide (NO_2), sulphur dioxide (SO_2), and carbon monoxide (CO), are prevalent in urban areas and have been linked to various health problems. Fine particulate matter (PM 2.5) can penetrate deep into the lungs and enter into the bloodstream, leading to systemic inflammation, exacerbating chronic conditions like asthma, chronic obstructive pulmonary disease (COPD), and cardiovascular diseases (CVD) (Fisher et al., 2016; To et al., 2016; Duan et al., 2020). In addition to air pollution, contaminants in drinking water like heavy metals, pesticides, and pathogens, pose a significant health risk. Older adults are particularly susceptible to waterborne diseases due to weakened immune system and pre-existing health conditions. Long-term exposure to contaminated water can lead to chronic health issues, including kidney damage and gastrointestinal disorders.

Additionally, soil contamination from industrial waste, agricultural chemicals, and heavy metals can affect food quality and safety (Barinova et al., 2020). Consuming such contaminated food can lead to various health problems, such as neurological disorders and increases the risk of cancer, particularly among individuals who may have compromised health. Pollutants can generate reactive oxygen species (ROS), which contribute to oxidative stress leading to cellular damage thereby accelerating the aging process and resulting in the development of various diseases. Chronic exposure to pollutants can also trigger systemic inflammation and immune-senescence (a decline in immune functions), promoting tissue damage, impairing immune responses and leading to dysfunction in multiple organ systems, making an individual more vulnerable to infections and chronic diseases (Fisher et al., 2016; Barinova et al., 2020).

On the social side, the social environment plays a crucial role in shaping health outcomes and influence the process of aging. Factors including socio-economic status, social support networks, and community engagement are key to determining the well-being of older individuals. Strong social support networks are consistently associated with better health outcomes. Emotional support from family and friends can mitigate stress and promote mental well-being. Studies have shown that older adults with robust social connections experience lower rates of depression and anxiety, improving overall health.

Conversely, loneliness can contribute to a decline in mental and physical health, increasing the risk of chronic diseases and mortality. Interventions aimed at reducing loneliness, such as community programs, active participation in social activities and volunteering at social clubs provide opportunities for social interactions, physical activities and a sense of purpose that can significantly enhance both mental and physical well-being and improve quality of life in older individual (McMaughan et al., 2020; Steptoe & Zaninotto, 2020).

Furthermore, the socio-economic status of older adults plays a significant role in their health outcomes. Those with higher income and education levels generally have better access to health care, nutritious food, and safe living conditions. In contrast, individuals from lower socio-economic backgrounds often encounter a barrier to these resources, contributing to poorer health. These disparities highlight the need for improved access to quality healthcare services to promote healthy aging, particularly in low-income communities (McMaughan et al., 2020; Steptoe & Zaninotto, 2020). The design of neighborhoods also impacts the overall well-being of older adults. A walkable neighborhood that provides access to parks, recreational facilities, and community centers encourages physical activity and fosters social engagement (Ramos et al., 2020). A safe living environment is essential for maintaining independence and participation in community activities; safety concerns can lead to social withdrawal and reduced physical activity. Additionally, access to reliable transportation is vital for older adults to engage in social activities and access healthcare services, enhancing their mobility and promoting healthier aging, this could also be achieved by using advanced technologies to monitor and assist the elderly population (Esposito et al., 2016). Community programs that encourage social interaction, such as group exercise classes and art workshops help reduce loneliness and improve mental health. At the same time, support services like meal delivery and home visits enable older adults to maintain their independence. Policymakers are encouraged to implement initiatives aimed at enhancing the social environment for older adults through funding for community centers, transportation services, and affordable housing options, ultimately improving their quality of life and health outcomes (Huxhold et al., 2014; Spulber, 2015; Willie-Tyndale et al., 2016).

THE ROLE OF GENETIC VARIATIONS IN AGING AND LONGEVITY

Genetic variations play a crucial role in determining individual differences in longevity and susceptibility to age-related diseases. These variations can manifest as single nucleotide polymorphisms (SNPs), copy number variations, and other genetic alterations that can influence the biological processes associated with aging. SNPs are the most common type of genetic variation linked to longevity, affecting metabolic pathways, inflammation, and cellular repair mechanisms. For instance, specific SNPs in genes related to the insulin/IGF-1 signaling pathway are associated with increased lifespan in various model organisms, including worms, flies, and mice (Ziv & Hu, 2011; Di Bona et al., 2014). SNPs are also associated with a reduced risk of age-related diseases such as CVD, diabetes, Alzheimer's disease (AD), and Parkinson's disease (PD) (Srivastava et al., 2015). For instance, variations in the APOE gene, particularly the APOE ε2 allele is associated with a lower risk of developing AD and increased longevity (Shinohara et al., 2020).

This highlights the importance of genetic predisposition in determining not only lifespan but also health span. While genetic variations significantly influence longevity, their effects are often modulated by environmental factors, which can either amplify or diminish the impact of genetic predispositions. For instance, a balanced diet and regular exercise may be more beneficial to people with specific genetic variations than to those without them (Hill & Mulder, 2010). This underscores the complex interplay between the genes and environmental factors in shaping longevity. Further, a sound understanding of these genetic factors or pathways is essential for regulating growth, metabolism, stress responses and longevity mechanisms.

One interesting example of this interplay is seen in populations with high longevity (high number of centenarians) in regions referred to as the Blue Zone. These populations often share specific genetic traits that interact positively with their lifestyle and environmental conditions. The Okinawan population in Japan has a genetic variation that, combined with their traditional diet and active lifestyle, contributes to their extended lifestyle (Willcox et al., 2006). In addition to the genetic variations, epigenetic modification and histone modification also play a significant role in longevity. Such modifications can be influenced by environmental factors such as diet, stress, and exposure to toxins. For instance, DNA methylation patterns change with age, and specific methylation profiles are associated with longevity (Gentilini et al., 2013). Some epigenetic modifications serve as biomarkers of biological age and provide valuable insights into an individual's aging process and longevity (Johnson et al., 2012; Salameh et al., 2020). Research indicates that individuals with favorable epigenetic profiles may have a lower risk of age-related diseases and a longer lifespan, suggesting that lifestyle interventions along with dietary modifications or pharmacological agents can extend lifespan and promote healthy aging (Peedicayil, 2006 & Abdul et al., 2017).

Building on this, the hallmarks of aging, a concept proposed by López-Otín et al. in 2013, highlights the biological process contributing to aging and age-related disease. These hallmarks include genomic instability, telomere attrition, epigenetic alterations, loss of proteostasis, deregulated nutrient sensing, mitochondrial dysfunction, cellular senescence, stem cell exhaustion, and altered intercellular communication. Genetic regulation of these processes is key to understanding their influence on aging. Genomic instability leads to the accumulation of mutations over time, accelerating aging process. Specific genes involved in DNA repair, such as BRCA1 and ATM have also been linked to longevity. Efficient DNA repair mechanisms further help in preventing accumulation of mutation, thereby reducing the risk of age-related diseases (Clarke & Mostoslavsky, 2022). The telomerase enzyme maintains the length of the telomere region in the chromosomes; genetic variation in this enzyme is associated with altered lifespan (Epel et al., 2006; Blackburn et al., 2015). Epigenetic alterations, including changes in DNA methylation and histone modifications, play a critical role in regulating aging process. Some epigenetic modifications have been identified as biomarkers of biological age, providing valuable insights into an individual's aging process and potential longevity (Johnson et al., 2012; Salameh et al., 2020). Interventions aimed at reversing epigenetic changes, such as dietary modifications or pharmacological agents, have shown promise in promoting healthy aging and extending lifespan (Peedicayil, 2006).

Cellular senescence is another process involved in aging, a state of irreversible cell cycle arrest that occurs due to DNA damage or telomere shortening. While senescence serves as a protective mechanism against cancer, the accumulation of senescent cells can contribute to tissue dysfunction and age-related diseases (Huang et al., 2022). Mutation in the cell cycle regulator gene p53 can influence premature senescence and increase the susceptibility to age-related diseases (Rufini et al., 2013). Emerging therapies targeting senescent cells through senolytics aim to selectively eliminate these cells, potentially promoting healthy aging (Gasek et al., 2021). While genetics plays a significant role in determining longevity and health span, many genetic factors are modifiable through lifestyle choices and environmental influences; for example, diet which can significantly influences health and longevity.

Dietary patterns such as the Mediterranean diet are linked to reduced risk of age-related diseases and increased lifespan. Moreover, genetic variations can affect how individuals respond to dietary interventions, highlighting the importance of personalized nutrition (Trichopoulou, 2004). Similarly, physical activity is crucial for longevity and lowering chronic diseases. Genetic factors such as ACTN3 (which influences muscle function) can modulate an individual's response to exercise, further emphasizing the role of personalized health strategies (Pickering & Kiely, 2017). Environmental factors such as exposure to pollutants also impact health, with genetic predispositions determining resilience or vulnerability to these exposures. These interactions underscore the importance of considering genetic-environment interactions for public health strategies aimed at promoting healthy aging.

INFLUENCE OF OXIDATIVE STRESS ON AGING

Reactive oxygen species (ROS) are chemically reactive molecules containing oxygen. They are a natural byproduct of oxygen metabolism and play a crucial role in various biological processes. ROS produced in excess can lead to oxidative stress (OS), a condition associated with aging and various conditions. ROS includes superoxide ions (O_2^-), hydroxyl radical (•OH), hydrogen peroxide (H_2O_2) and hypochlorous acid (HOCl), all of which act as secondary messengers in cellular processes like proliferation and differentiation (Halliwell, 2006). Under normal physiological conditions, minimal levels of ROS are beneficial for cell differentiation and intracellular signalling, as well as for defending against microorganisms (Koppenol et al., 1992; Mates, 2000). However, an overproduction of ROS can overwhelm the body's antioxidant defenses, resulting in oxidative damage to cells (Sharief & Mahaboob, 2020; Basha et al., 2021).

The generation of superoxide anions (O_2^-), a primary source of ROS, impedes the electron transport chain (ETC Cycle) of mitochondria, the cell's powerhouse which generates ATP (Adenosine triphosphate) through oxidative phosphorylation. This disruption of the mitochondria is brought on by ROS production which causes cellular aging in an older individual (Cui et al., 2012). Another major source of ROS is NADPH oxidase, which generates O_2^- for immune responses, while excessive activation of which can lead to OS and inflammation. Additionally, peroxisomes produce H_2O_2 during lipid metabolism, and xanthine oxidase involved in purine metabolism generates O_2^- and H_2O_2, with its elevated activities linked to conditions like gout and CVD. Enzymes involved in arachidonic acid metabolism also produce ROS as a byproduct during inflammatory responses, while nitric oxide (NO), produced by nitric oxide synthase (NOS), reacts with O_2^- to form peroxynitrite ($ONOO^-$), a potent oxidant involved in various diseases (Knight, 1998; Hekimi et al., 2011).

Besides internal sources, external environmental exposures can also elevate ROS. For instance, pollutants such as heavy metals, particulate matter, and volatile organic compounds generate free radicals or deplete antioxidant defenses, thus exacerbating OS. Ionizing radiations such as ultraviolet (UV) light and X-rays directly produce ROS in biological tissues, contributing to skin cancer risk. Additionally, cigarette smoke, which contains free radicals and oxidants, raises ROS levels in the lungs and systemic circulation, leading to respiratory diseases. Excessive alcohol consumption increases ROS through metabolic pathways in the liver, potentially resulting in alcoholic liver disease. Moreover, dietary factors can either exacerbate or alleviate OS; high-fat diets increase OS from lipid peroxidation, whereas antioxidant-rich diets such as fruits and vegetables can mitigate ROS levels (Yang & Omaye, 2009; Daiber et al., 2020; Priyadarshanee et al., 2022). In addition to diet, exercise also plays a dual role, while moderate exercise benefits health, excessive or intense physical activity can elevate ROS production. This is particularly true in endurance athletes, where prolonged exercise induces OS and muscle damage (Finaud et al., 2006; Patil et al., 2012).

Figure 1. Factors contributing to oxidative stress and aging.

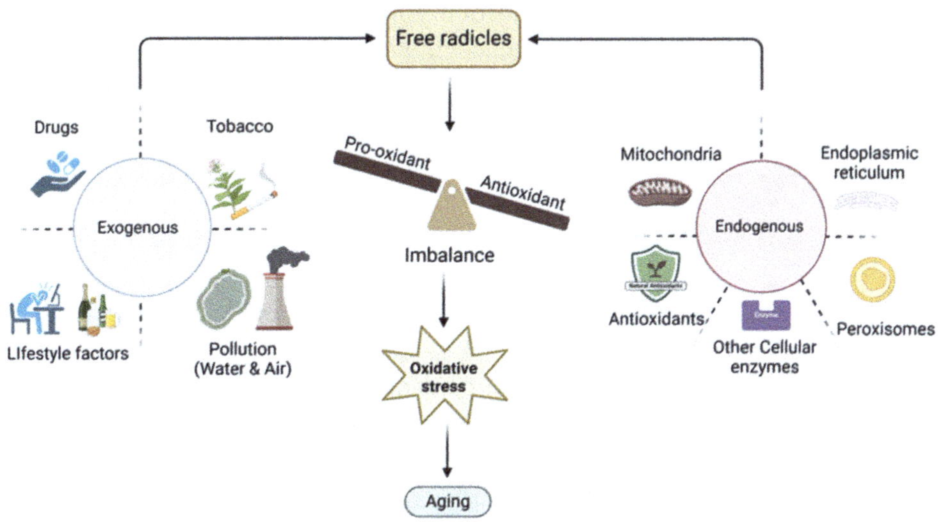

Health Implications of Oxidative Stress in Aging

Oxidative stress is a significant factor in the aging process, contributing to various health issues and age-related diseases. It occurs when there is an imbalance between the production of reactive oxygen species (ROS) and the body's ability to neutralize them through antioxidant defenses, leading to cellular damage. The health implications of oxidative stress are widespread, impacting multiple organ systems and accelerating aging-related various diseases including degenerative changes.

Cardiovascular Diseases (CVD)

Cardiovascular diseases are among the leading causes of morbidity and mortality in elderly population. Elevated ROS levels lead to endothelial dysfunction, characterized by reduced nitric oxide availability, which is essential for vascular relaxation (Alique et al., 2015; Jung et al., 2015). Additionally, the oxidation of low-density lipoprotein (LDL) cholesterol to oxidized LDL (oxLDL) is a critical process which promotes atherosclerosis (Schleicher & Friess, 2007). Oxidative damage can further lead to hypertension, heart failure and an increased risk of myocardial infarction. As an individual age the levels of antioxidants enzymes like SOD and glutathione peroxidase (GSH-px) decline resulting in exacerbation of oxidative damage in cardiovascular tissues (Alique et al., 2015; Jung et al., 2015).

Neurodegenerative Diseases (NDD)

Oxidative stress is closely related to the onset and progression of NDD, such as Parkinson's disease (PD) and Alzheimer's disease (AD). Increased ROS production leads to neuronal damage, inflammation, and the formation of neurotoxic aggregates, such as amyloid-beta plaques in AD and alpha-synuclein in PD (Brand et al., 2022; Sehar et al., 2022). Mitochondrial dysfunction, a hallmark of neurodegeneration, further exacerbates OS by impairing energy production while increasing ROS production. The oxidative damage resulting in neuronal injury contributes to cognitive decline, memory loss, and motor dysfunction. Studies have shown a correlation between elevated OS biomarkers and cognitive impairment in older adults, suggesting that OS may serve as an early predictor of NDDs (Barnham et al., 2004; Chen et al., 2012).

Sarcopenia

Sarcopenia, the age-related loss of muscle mass and strength, is closely linked to OS. Increased ROS levels can lead to protein carbonylation and other post-translational modifications that impair muscle protein synthesis and increase proteolysis contributing to muscle degeneration (Meng & Yu, 2010). Additionally, OS can interfere with neuromuscular junctions, reducing acetylcholine release and impairing muscle contraction. Sarcopenia is associated with frailty, decreased physical function, and increased risk of falls and fractures in older adults. The loss of muscle mass and strength can significantly impact the quality of life and independence of older adults, making it a critical area of concern in geriatric health (Brioche & Lemoine-Morel, 2016).

Chronic Inflammation (Inflammaging)

Chronic inflammation, a hallmark of aging is exacerbated by OS. Increased ROS levels can activate inflammatory pathways, leading to the production of pro-inflammatory cytokines such as IL-6 and TNF-α. This chronic inflammatory state promotes OS and accelerates aging and age-related diseases such as CVD conditions, diabetes and NDD (Zuo et al., 2019; Cannizzo et al., 2011). The persistent inflammatory state can lead to tissue damage and dysfunction, further increasing the risk of morbidity and mortality in older adults (Zuo et al., 2019).

Cancer

Oxidative stress is a significant contributor to the initiation and progression of cancer. ROS can cause DNA damage, leading to mutations that drive tumorigenesis. Additionally, the inflammatory environment created by OS can promote cancer cell proliferation and metastasis (Li et al., 2024). The link between OS and cancer underscores the importance of monitoring oxidative damage in aging populations. Increased oxidative stress biomarkers have been linked with a higher incidence of various cancers, reinforcing the need for preventive strategies targeting OS (Di Carlo & Sorrentino, 2024).

Chronic Kidney Disease (CDK)

Oxidative stress is a significant contributor to the pathogenesis of CDK, elevation in ROS levels can lead to renal inflammation and fibrosis and the progressive loss of kidney function (Liguori et al., 2018). The decline in renal function with age is often accompanied by increased oxidative damage to renal tissues, exacerbating CKD progression and is associated with increased frailty and morbidity in the elderly. The interplay between OS and kidney function highlights the need for targeted interventions to manage oxidative damage and slow CDK progression in aging populations (Dounousi et al., 2006; Ebert et al., 2021).

Oxidative stress has profound health implications in aging, affecting multiple organ systems and contributing to various age-related diseases. The underlying mechanisms involve increased ROS production, mitochondrial dysfunction, chronic inflammation, and damage to macromolecules. A better understanding of these mechanisms is crucial for developing effective interventions to mitigate oxidative stress and promote healthy aging. Future research should focus on exploring antioxidant therapies and lifestyle modifications, such as diet and exercise, that can enhance the body's resilience against oxidative damage, ultimately improving health outcomes and quality of life in older adults (Yang et al., 2024).

Figure 2. Key contributors of aging

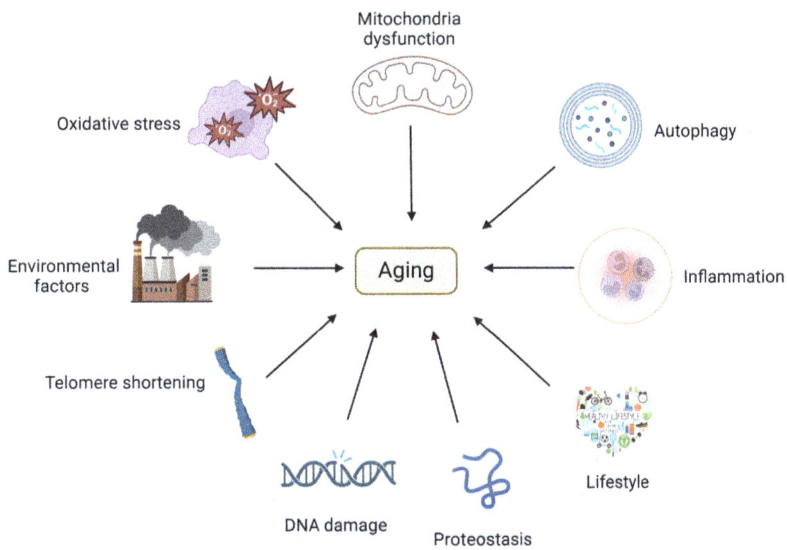

Natural Antioxidants a Key to Combating Oxidative Stress and Promoting Health

Natural antioxidants are essential for good health and averting conditions linked to OS because exogenous antioxidants cannot be produced by the body. Natural antioxidants are found in plants as their secondary metabolites and other products such as carotenoids, polyphenols, vitamins E and C. Each antioxidant has unique properties and health benefits, making it essential to consume a variety of fruits, vegetables, nuts, and whole grains. Since polyphenols are thought to be the most powerful antioxidants due to their ability to influence several signalling pathways and interact synergistically with other substances, such as vitamin C, a significant number of studies have been conducted on them. Numerous plants including *Murraya koenigii*, *Aronia melanocarpa*, *Ocimum sanctum*, *Ginkgo biloba*, *Nigella sativa* and others, have been researched for their high polyphenolic and other secondary metabolites content to quench OS and enhance longevity (Alambayan & Garg, 2020; Patel et al., 2020; Saliya & Usha, 2020). While supplements offer convenience, obtaining antioxidants from whole foods is generally recommended for the best possible health and well-being.

Polyphenols

Polyphenols are the most abundant antioxidants in the diet. They are secondary plant metabolites that represent a broad group of compounds with aromatic ring characterized by the presence of one or more hydroxyl groups with different structural complexities. Polyphenols include phenols and flavonoids and possess potent antioxidant, anti-inflammatory, anti-diabetic, neuroprotective and anti-aging properties (Dhalaria et al., 2020). Dietary sources include a diverse group of phytonutrients including berries (blueberries, strawberries), tea (green and black), dark chocolate, apples, onions, fruits, vegetables, cereals, dry legumes, fruit juices, and red wine. It also includes compounds like hydrolyzable tannins, condensed tannins, and different types of flavonoids like flavonols, flavones, isoflavones, anthocyanidins, and others. Polyphenols, with their antioxidative qualities and ability to activate a variety of cell receptors and signalling pathways, can support pro-apoptotic and cell survival mechanisms. By reducing oxidative stress, polyphenols may help prevent diseases like cancer, osteoporosis, cardiovascular disorders, neurological diseases, enhance cognitive function and reduce the risk of chronic diseases, according to epidemiological research (Crozier et al., 2006, Dhalaria et al., 2020). Moreover, studies including findings by Di Pietro et al. (2020), indicate that regular intake of polyphenol-rich foods helps lower blood pressure and improve endothelial function.

Vitamin C

Vitamin C (Vit C) is a highly effective antioxidant found in a variety of fruits and vegetables such as citrus fruits (oranges, lemons, grapefruits), berries (strawberries, blueberries, raspberries), kiwi, bell peppers, broccoli, and brussels sprouts. In addition to its antioxidant functions, Vit C aids in improving immune function, iron absorption and promotes collagen synthesis, which is vital for skin health and wound healing (Carr & Maggini, 2017; Pillar et al., 2017). Some research suggests that by reducing OS in brain cells, its antioxidant qualities may diminish the incidence of neurodegenerative illnesses like AD, PD, suggesting the link between Vit C and cognitive functions. Vit C also possesses anti-aging properties and is more popular in skin care to reduce wrinkles, enhance skin texture and prevent sun damage (Al-Niaimi & Chiang, 2017; Monacelli et al., 2017). Antioxidants neutralize free radicals by donating electrons to stabilise them and prevent cellular damage (Rakesh et al., 2021). For instance, Vit C is a potent water-soluble antioxidant that acts as a first line of defense against free radicals in the blood and plasma. It can neutralize various reactive oxygen species (ROS), including superoxide radicals and hydroxyl radicals, by donating an electron, Vit C transforms into a less reactive molecule, thereby reducing oxidative stress (Fang et al., 2002; Kim & Lee, 2004).

Vitamin E

Vitamin E (Vit E) or α-tocopherol is a lipid-soluble antioxidant found in cell membrane, wide range of foods, including spinach, broccoli, almonds, hazelnuts, and vegetable oils like sunflower oil and olive oil contain Vit E. It is believed Vit E has a role in the prevention of atherosclerosis through the inhibition of oxidative modifications of LDLs (Dutta & Dutta, 2003). Vit E can regenerate itself by interacting with other antioxidants, such as Vit C, which helps maintain its antioxidant capacity. The interaction between Vit C and Vit E is particularly important in lipid-rich environments, such as cell membranes, where Vit E protects lipids from oxidation (Wagner et al., 1996; Wolf et al., 1998). Several research have recently revealed that Vit E has a biological role, it protects against lipid peroxidation by reacting with lipid radicals, thus preventing the propagation of OS in cellular mechanisms and protecting the cell membrane. It also regulates signal transduction and gene expressions and also modulates the specific cell functions. Regular dietary intake of Vit E has been associated with the prevention of age-related macular degeneration and enhancements in immune function and skin health (Sarisözen et al., 2002; Christen et al., 2015)

Coenzyme Q10 (CoQ10)

Coenzyme Q10 is a naturally occurring cofactor (coenzyme) essential for cellular energy production and possesses powerful antioxidant and anti-aging properties. Natural sources of coenzyme Q10 include whole grains, spinach, broccoli, organ meats (liver, heart), and fatty fish (mackerel, salmon) (Arenas-jal et al., 2020; Lain et al., 2024). CoQ10 is essential in the mitochondria ETC cycle to generate ATP for various body functions. Naturally, the levels of CoQ10 decline as an individual ages, resulting in decreased production of ATP and an increase in the production of OS contributing to aging (Ayunin et al., 2022; Yang et al., 2022; Emeksiz, 2023). As a potent antioxidant, CoQ10 quenches free radicals, which can harm cells and hasten ageing process. It aids in regeneration of other antioxidants, including vitamins C and E, and shields cellular membranes from lipid peroxidation (Hernández-Camacho et al., 2018). CoQ10 also improves cellular metabolism, lowers oxidative damage, restores its levels in the skin, reduces wrinkles, stabilizes mitochondrial function and decreases ROS levels. Dietary supplementation alleviates heart failure symptoms and lowers the risk of CVD illness (Rabanal-Ruiz et al., 2021; Gutierrez et al., 2024). Hence CoQ10 is a major component in anti-aging therapies.

N-acetylcysteine (NAC)

N-acetylcysteine (NAC), an amino acid derivative has attracted interest for its possible anti-aging properties due to its antioxidants, anti-inflammatory capabilities. Studies have shown that NAC has the ability to quench OS and inflammation, which is the major cause of aging making it a candidate for promoting overall health and longevity. One of the antioxidants, GSH is largely produced by NAC as a precursor, by restoring GSH levels in the body, NAC can combat the harmful effects of OS on cellular integrity by preventing cellular damage of proteins, DNA and lipids (Shaposhnikov et al., 2018; Sohouli et al., 2023). NAC also exhibits direct antioxidant activity effects by scavenging the free radicals and lowering the proinflammatory cytokines, such as tumour necrosis factor- alpha (TNF- α) and interleukins, mitigating various age-related diseases and chronic conditions associated with aging. Various research indicates the importance of NAC in OS, particularly in mitochondrial dysfunction. By enhancing mitochondrial functions, NAC can shield the mitochondria by promoting the production of ATP and reduce fatigue in older individuals (Šalamon et al., 2019; Harmita et al., 2020; Bayoumi et al., 2021). NAC supplementation has shown to reduce oxidative stress indicating a potential role in enhancing healthy aging, it also prevents UV-induced damage and promotes skin elasticity. Overall, there is evidence that NAC promotes cognitive health and enhances aging by reducing OS in the brain (Ikonne et al., 2019)

Alpha-Lipoic Acid (ALP)

Alpha-lipoic acid (ALA) is a naturally occurring antioxidant with potential anti-aging properties. ALA functions in both aqueous and lipid environments, making it effective throughout the body. ALA is known for its ability to scavenge free radicals, which are unstable molecules that contribute to oxidative stress and cellular damage (Molz & Schröder, 2017; Superti & Russo, 2024). By neutralizing these free radicals, ALA shields the cells from oxidative damage, a key factor in aging. ALA regenerates other antioxidants such as Vit C and E and has shown to reduce inflammatory markers in the body, mitigating the effects of aging on various systems particularly in neurodegenerative diseases and metabolic disorders. Studies have shown that ALA plays an important role in improving mitochondrial health. As the mitochondrial efficiency declines with age, ALA enhance ATP production and supports overall health. Studies suggest that ALA may slow down the cognitive decline associated with aging by reducing OS in the brain and improving mitochondrial function. Some research indicates that combining ALA with other compounds may enhance its protective effects against NDD (Baeeri et al., 2019; Du et al., 2020).

Resveratrol

Resveratrol (3,5,4′-trihydroxystilbene) is a polyphenolic compound found in various foods, particularly red wine, grapes, peanuts, and berries. Resveratrol has strong antioxidant potential that combat OS, by reducing the markers of oxidative damage such as malondialdehyde (MDA) and protects cellular components against age related disease (Bhullar & Hubbard, 2015; Zhang et al., 2021). Resveratrol has been demonstrated to lessen age-related inflammation by modifying inflammatory pathways and blocking important mediators like nuclear factor kappa B (NF-κB). Resveratrol promotes autophagy and can boost mitochondrial biogenesis, activate key longevity proteins (AMPK and SIRT) and enhance longevity (Maroon, 2008). Research indicates that resveratrol can extend lifespan in various model organisms, including yeast, nematodes, fruit flies, and mice. Additionally, resveratrol has neuroprotective effects, improving cognitive function and memory by promoting neuronal survival, reducing neuroinflammation, and enhancing synaptic plasticity, making it a promising compound for countering age-related diseases and improving overall longevity (Kim et al., 2011; Marchal et al., 2013; Lee & Min, 2017).

ENZYMATIC ANTIOXIDANTS AND THEIR IMPACT ON AGING AND DISEASE

To combat oxidative stress, the body relies on a sophisticated network of antioxidants, molecules that can donate electrons to free radicals without becoming destabilized themselves. These can be categorized into enzymatic and non-enzymatic antioxidants. Antioxidants such as superoxide dismutase (SOD) is a crucial enzyme that catalyses the dismutation of superoxide radicals into H_2O_2 and oxygen. SOD exits in three main forms, cytosolic (Cy-SOD), mitochondrial (Mn-SOD), and extracellular (EC-SOD), each localized in different cellular compartments to efficiently detoxify superoxide in various environments. SOD is vital for protecting cells from oxidative damage, but its activity often declines with aging and age-related diseases. Catalase works alongside SOD to neutralize H_2O_2 by converting it into water and oxygen, predominantly within peroxisomes, where it detoxifies H_2O_2 generated during fatty acid oxidation. Thus, a decline in catalyse activity contributes to increased OS in aging. Glutathione peroxidase (GSH-Px) is another critical enzyme that reduces H_2O_2 and lipid peroxides using glutathione (GSH) as a cofactor. The activity of GSH-Px is a key marker of OS, and a decline in glutathione reductase activity regenerates reduced glutathione (GSH), which can lead to oxidative damage (Pajović et al., 2006; Rakesh et al., 2021).

In addition to enzymatic antioxidants, non-enzymatic antioxidants like Glutathione, an intracellular antioxidant composed of cysteine, glutamate, and glycine play a crucial role in detoxification and cellular protection (Pompella & Costantino, 2023). It is one of the most abundant non-enzymatic antioxidants in the body. It is reduced form of GSH that serves as the active antioxidant that detoxifies ROS and maintains redox balance, while also regenerating other antioxidants like vitamins C and E. Vit C (ascorbic acid) is a water-soluble antioxidant, scavenges free radicals and supports the regenerating of other antioxidants, particularly in the aqueous environment of cells. Vit E (tocopherol), a fat-soluble antioxidant, protects cell membranes from lipid peroxidation by donating electrons to lipid radicals. Together, these vitamins are essential for maintaining the body's overall antioxidant capacity.

Additionally, antioxidants such as polyphenols and flavonoids are a diverse group of compounds in plant-based foods that exhibit antioxidant effects by scavenging free radicals, chelating metal ions, and modulating oxidative stress-related signalling pathways (Kasprzak et al., 2015; Rakesh & Mahaboob, 2022). Polyphenols, for instance, have been shown to upregulate the expression of SOD and catalase, enhancing the body's defenses against oxidative damage (Zhang & Tsao, 2016). Consumption of polyphenols rich foods, such as fruits, vegetables, tea and red wine, is linked to various health benefits such as reduced inflammations and improved cardiovascular health (Polidori et al., 2001; Mirończuk-Chodakowska et al., 2018).

The body's antioxidant defense mechanisms are crucial for maintaining cellular homeostasis and preventing oxidative stress. Both enzymatic and non-enzymatic antioxidants work synergistically to neutralize ROS and protect cells from damage. Understanding these mechanisms can provide insights into potential therapeutic strategies for managing OS and promoting healthy aging. Through dietary interventions, lifestyle changes, and the enhancement of antioxidant defense, it may be possible to mitigate the effects of oxidative stress thereby improving quality of life.

Interplay of Antioxidants and Inflammation in Aging

Inflammation and oxidative stress are closely related and contribute to the development of various chronic diseases and decline in longevity. To combat these harmful effects many antioxidants are available in nature which possess a wide range of beneficial effects like antioxidant, anti-inflammatory, anti-diabetic, neuroprotective properties. Antioxidants help to reduce oxidative stress by neutralizing free radicals; by doing so, they can play a crucial role in preventing or managing chronic diseases. In addition to their direct effects on OS, some antioxidants also modulate immune function and cellular signaling pathways, further contributing to their therapeutic potential. Regular consumption of antioxidant-rich foods, such as fruits, vegetables, and herbs, can help maintain a balance between oxidative stress and inflammation, supporting overall health and well-being. For instance, curcumin an active compound in turmeric, has been shown to exhibit both antioxidant and anti-inflammatory effects. It can inhibit the activation of nuclear factor kappa B (NF-κB), a transcription factor that regulates the expression of pro-inflammatory cytokines. Curcumin helps protect against ailments such as arthritis and cardiovascular disease (Menon & Sudheer, 2007; Roy et al.,2022).

ROLE OF NATURAL PRODUCTS AND PLANT EXTRACTS IN PROMOTING LONGEVITY

Several plant extracts and other natural products have shown potential in promoting longevity by influencing cellular repair, metabolism, and inflammation. *Curcuma longa* (turmeric) and its active compound curcumin exhibits both antioxidant and anti-inflammatory properties by reducing oxidative stress and mitigating inflammation and accelerates aging (Menon & Sudheer, 2007). Other substances like *Astragalus membranaceus* have gained attention for their potential to extend lifespan by modulating the immune system and promoting cellular repair. *Astragalus* activates the telomerase enzyme, which maintains telomere length and supports chromosomal stability and cellular longevity (Wang et al., 2013). Plant compounds like Epigallocatechin gallate (EGCG) from green tea activate the AMPK pathway, enhancing mitochondrial function, increasing energy production, promoting cellular repair, and improving metabolic health. Additionally, Berberine, found in several plants, activates AMPK, which improves glucose metabolism, reduces oxidative stress, and combats age-related diseases. Together, these compounds not only boost antioxidant defenses but also regulate metabolism, reduce inflammation, and promote cellular repair, contributing to a longer and healthier life (Barzilai et al., 2018). Additionally, spices like *Nigella sativa* seeds and its active compound thymoquinone, mitigate oxidative damage by supporting the overall health, contributing to an extended life span in the *Drosophila* model. The mechanisms of action of antioxidants are multifaceted and involve direct scavenging of free radicals, repair of oxidized molecules, chelation of metal ions, regeneration of other antioxidants, modulation of antioxidant enzyme activity, and anti-inflammatory effects (Bawani & Anandhi, 2021; Kumar et al., 2024).

Natural vs. Synthetic Antioxidants: A Comparative Analysis

There is always an ongoing debate about whether natural or synthetic antioxidants are superior, a topic that continues to be of interest in nutritional science. Many natural antioxidants (from fruits, vegetables, or herbs) are more effective due to their molecular complexity and interaction with other molecules in diet (Walter et al., 2001; Tsao, 2015). On the other hand, synthetic antioxidants include compounds like butylated hydroxytoluene (BHT) and butylated hydroxyanisole (BHA), which have been functionally used in the food industry to prevent lipid oxidation and for their economic advantages (Uzombah, 2022). However, their long-term safety (especially their pro-oxidant effects at high concentrations) has led to growing research in natural alternatives.

Synergistic Effects of Natural Dietary Antioxidants and Endogenous Antioxidants

The intricate interplay between a natural dietary antioxidant-rich diet and endogenous antioxidant systems plays an important role in maintaining oxidative balance, thereby reducing the risk of chronic diseases. Natural antioxidants (such as polyphenols, carotenoids, flavonoids, vitamins C and E) exert their protective effects by scavenging free radicals and improving the action of cellular defense mechanisms. These compounds display synergistic effects on bioactivity when consumed collaboratively in an antioxidant rich diet (Walter et al., 2001; Tsao, 2015), potentially providing greater bioactivity than isolated antioxidant compounds. Additionally, the endogenous antioxidant defense system, which includes glutathione peroxidase (GPx), catalase, and superoxide dismutase (SOD), functions in tandem with dietary antioxidants to counteract oxidative stress and lower the risk of chronic diseases like cancer, neurodegeneration, and cardiovascular disease (Aguilar et al., 2016).

Practical Implications of Antioxidants

Antioxidants have extensive practical uses in medicine, nutrition, dermatology, and industry due to their ability to defend against oxidative stress.

1. In medicine they protect the neurons against OS mediated injuries and mitigate the risk of various NDD conditions and other diseases like cardiovascular disease, and prevent cancer by reducing DNA damage.
2. In nutrition antioxidants like vitamins (Vit E and C, beta-carotene) are used in dietary supplements to enhance the immune system and overall health. Natural sources such as berries, dark chocolate and green tea also provide various health benefits.
3. In dermatology antioxidants such as vitamin C, retinol, and niacinamide are used in anti-aging treatments to reduce wrinkles and skin damage. They also protect the skin from UV rays and reduce oxidative stress.
4. In industries, antioxidants stabilize drugs and extend the shelf life of food and beverages ensuring the quality of the products by inhibiting the oxidation.

Future Direction: Investigating nanotechnology-based delivery of antioxidants for enhanced bioavailability, and comparisons between natural and synthetic antioxidants are required. Furthermore, personalized antioxidant therapy, based on individual OS levels, is also being developed as a potential method in precision medicine.

Figure 3. Natural antioxidants and their beneficial role in aging related conditions

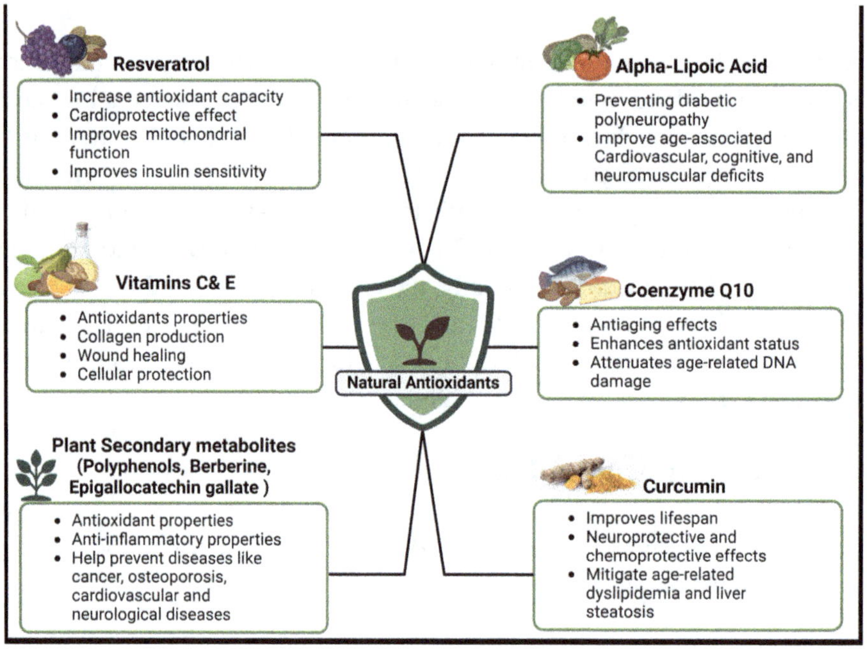

Table 1. Natural antioxidants and their health benefits

Natural Antioxidant	Source	Compounds	Mechanism of Action	Benefits	References
β-Carotene	Carrots, Sweet potatoes	Carotenoids	Enhance antioxidant enzyme activity by reducing ROS levels	Reduction in tissue fibrosis, improvement in cognitive function and enhances aging	Paiva & Russell, 1999; Boccardi et al., 2020; Abrego-Guandique et al., 2023
Lycopene	Tomatoes	Carotenoids	Protection of cells against oxidative damage	Supports liver, kidney and brain health	Abir et al., 2023; Kulawik et al., 2023
Niacinamide	Meat, fish, nuts	Niacinamide	Protection against UV damage	Improves skin health and reduces signs of aging	Chiu et al., 2007; Zhen et al., 2019; Boo, 2021
Vitamin E	Nuts, Seeds, Spinach	Tocopherols	Protects against lipid peroxidation	Reduces the risk of heart disease	Kunert & Ederer, 1985; Devi & Kiran,2004
Vitamin C	Citrus fruits and Strawberries	Ascorbic acid	Mitigates ROS, regenerates other antioxidants	Boost immune function and promote skin health	Padayatty et al., 2003; Harrison, 2012; Monacelli et al., 2017
Flavonoids	Berries, tea, apples	Quercetin (Various compounds)	Scavenge free radicals, inhibit inflammation	Improve cardiovascular health	Pietta,2000; Mondal & Rahaman, 2020
Phenolic compounds	Apples, Berries	Flavonoids	Inhibits OS by scavenging free radicals	Anti-inflammatory reduces risk of cancer	Obrenovich et al., 2010; Wang et al., 2022
Selenium	Brazil nuts, Mushrooms	Selenoproteins	Cofactor for glutathione peroxidase, antioxidant enzymes	Protects immune function and reduces risk of cancer	Hartman et al., 1998; Yang et al., 2019
Ferulic Acid	Whole grains	Phenolic acid	Mitigates free radicals	Linked to lower risk of chronic diseases	Mancuso & Santangelo, 2014; Wagle et al., 2021
Thymoquinone	*Nigella sativa* (Black seeds)	Thymoquinone	Scavenge free radicals, inhibit lipid peroxidation	Anti-inflammatory and antioxidant properties	Harphoush et al., 2019; Forouzanfar & Hosseinzadeh, 2020
Rosmarinic Acid	Rosemary, mint	Roamarinic acid	Antioxidant and anti-inflammatory properties	Improve cognitive function and reduces inflammation	Zhang et al., 2015; Nadeem et al., 2019
Anthocyanins	Berries (Blueberriers, black berries)	Anthocyanins	Scavenge free radicals and protects cell membrane	Improve cognitive function and improve cardiovascular health	Martín et al., 2017; Chen et al., 2022
Gingerol	Ginger (*Zingiber officinale*)	Gingerol	Inhibits lipid peroxidation and scavenges free radicals	Anti-inflammatory, promotes longevity	Lee et al., 2018; Xu et al.,2022
Goji Berries	Goji Berries	Various antioxidants	Scavenges free radicals	Improves immune function and skin health	de Freitas Rodrigues et al., 2021; Vidović et al.,2022

continued on following page

Table 1. Continued

Natural Antioxidant	Source	Compounds	Mechanism of Action	Benefits	References
Resveratrol	Grapes, peanuts, blueberries, red wine	Resveratrol	Activates SIRT1, enhances mitochondrial biogenesis.	Aid in management of illnesses associated with age like obesity, cancer, heart disease, neurodegenerative diseases, suppress oxidative stress, regulate apoptosis	Valenzano & Cellerino, 2006; Markus & Morris, 2008; Santos et al.,2023
Quercetin	Grapes, peaches, onions, garlic	Quercetin	Reduces oxidative damage, Regulates levels of MDA, TNF-a and increases SOD, CAT and GSH-PX,	Neuroprotective effect via antioxidant, anti-inflammatory, Protects against diabetes, cardiovascular diseases	Pozos-Nonato et al.,2023; Raina et al., 2023
N-acetylcysteine (NAC)	Supplement derived from cysteine	N-acetylcysteine (NAC)	Restores GSH levels, scavenges free radicals	Improve central nervous system, neuropsychiatric diseases, cardiovascular disease, protect cellular damage	Niraula & Kim, 2019; Šalamon et al.,2019
Alpha-Lipoic Acid	Broccoli, spinach, potatoes, yeast, tomatoes	Alpha-Lipoic Acid	Regenerates other antioxidants, chelates metals, reduces ROS	Improves mitochondrial function, slows cognitive decline. Improve age-associated cardiovascular, cognitive, and neuromuscular deficits	Shay et al., 2009; Shanaida et al., 2025

Ongoing Debates: Natural Antioxidants vs Synthetic Antioxidant Drugs

Antioxidants derived from natural sources or laboratory synthesized play an essential role in countering oxidative damage. Nonetheless, there are still debates over the long-term advantages, bioavailability and absorption, safety and effectiveness of natural antioxidants vs synthetic antioxidant medications. Synthetic antioxidants offer concentrated and powerful effects but may raise safety issues. Whereas, natural antioxidants are frequently commended for their comprehensive health advantages and decreased likelihood of negative side effects.

Efficacy of Dietary Antioxidants vs Synthetic Antioxidant Drugs

Dietary antioxidants and synthetic antioxidant drugs are still subject to high controversy regarding their efficacy. Dietary antioxidants, derived from fruits, vegetables, and whole foods provide broad-spectrum defense against oxidative stress by supplying a variety of bioactive substances. Antioxidants naturally present in food, including Vit C, Vit E and polyphenols, act in synergy to enhance cellular protective mechanisms (Tsao, 2015).

Conversely, synthetic antioxidant drugs have been designed specifically to administer precise doses of antioxidant compounds for controllable and measurable effects. Synthetic antioxidant drugs, such as butylated hydroxyanisole and edaravone, are designed to target specific oxidative pathways, providing fast and effective intervention in oxidative stress-related conditions (Goossens et al., 1995; Firuzi et al., 2011; Mizobuchi et al., 2022). While antioxidants demonstrate efficacy in acute conditions, long-term use raises concerns regarding toxicity and the potential for paradoxical pro-oxidant effects (Sotler et al., 2019).

Bioavailability and Absorption

The effectiveness of an antioxidant in-vivo is highly dependent on its bioavailability, which is determined by solubility, metabolic stability, and absorption. Since these factors determine its uptake and utilization, the therapeutic efficacy of antioxidants can be highly variable. For example, some polyphenols are subject to extensive metabolism in the liver and gut, which can result in variabilities in their bioavailability and biological activity (Marín et al., 2015). Moreover, Variable absorption is observed in natural antioxidants, whereas synthetic antioxidants offer consistent and measurable impact (Pokorný, 2007).

Regulatory and Safety Concerns

The regulatory landscape for antioxidant-based drugs and supplements is complex. Dietary antioxidants as part of diet are commonly taken as supplements, and they are not adequately regulated. In contrast, regulatory agencies (such as the FDA, EMA etc.) test synthetic antioxidant drugs thoroughly before marketing. In light of this, safety concerns surrounding high-dose antioxidant supplementation have also been on the rise, as excessive concentrations may elicit pro-oxidant effect (Liu, 2014). Furthermore, regulatory authorities emphasize the need for large-scale and rigorously controlled studies to better understand the scientific substantiation of health claims of antioxidant supplements (Santini et al., 2018). Natural antioxidants are known to boost health and longevity, whereas synthetic antioxidants allow a more targeted approach to combat age-related diseases. Additional studies would be warranted to examine personalized interventions combining natural and pharmacological strategies to achieve the best possible aging outcomes.

Gender Differences in Antioxidant Effects

Emerging studies indicate that sex may be an imperative modifying factor that impacts the metabolism and activity of antioxidant molecules (Tiberi et al., 2023). For instance, Estrogen is a recognized antioxidant that underscores the improved oxidative stress tolerance in women via MAPK activation, which in turn activates the NFkB signalling pathway, resulting in the up-regulation of the expression of longevity-related genes that may be implicated in gender differences on age-associated diseases like cardiovascular diseases (Vina et al., 2011). Studies have shown that men need more dietary antioxidants in their diet to counteract lower endogenous protective mechanisms (Tiberi et al., 2023). These distinctions call for specific dietary guidelines on a gender-based basis for individual-based antioxidant metabolism.

Age-Specific Antioxidant Effects

Endogenous antioxidant defense mechanisms decline with age, increasing susceptibility to oxidative stress related diseases. Dietary antioxidants are not equally effective at mitigating age-related oxidative damage at all life stages. In young people, antioxidants mainly act preventively against oxidative stress, whereas in older subjects, they have a reparative function, limiting accumulated oxidative damage (Tan et al., 2018). Specific antioxidants like resveratrol and curcumin have demonstrated anti-aging characteristics by modulating mitochondrial role and impacting inflammation (Ungvari et al., 2011; Trujillo et al., 2014). Furthermore, evidence indicates that higher consumption of antioxidants such as Vit C (Scarmeas et al., 2003) and Vit E (Morris et al., 2002) are linked with reduction in cognitive decline and greater neuroprotection among older individuals. Therefore, age-specific dietary recommendations should consider the progressive deterioration of endogenous antioxidant defenses.

Interactions Between Antioxidants and Medications

Interactions in the concurrent usage of dietary antioxidants with pharmaceutical agents may be beneficial or adverse. For instance, certain flavonoids such as quercetin and catechins have been shown to modulate the activity of cytochrome P450 enzymes and thereby affect drug metabolism (Misaka et al., 2013; Rastogi & Jana, 2014). Antioxidants may also protect healthy cells from oxidative impairment that is meant to damage them during chemotherapy and radiotherapy (Simone et al., 2007). Besides, there is evidence that high-dose vitamin C supplementation might impair the efficacy of certain chemotherapeutic drugs (Heaney et al., 2008). Since the effects of antioxidant-drug interactions in the clinic may have a double-edged nature, careful design might help maximize the therapeutic effects of antioxidants without interfering with the action of the drugs used.

Drawbacks of Antioxidant Supplements

The potential benefits of antioxidants have gained enormous popularity in recent years owing to their immense benefits in preventing aging related ailments and chronic diseases including cardiovascular disease, cancer, and neurodegenerative disorders. However, the scientific community remains divided over the safety and effectiveness of antioxidant supplements. Meta-analysis studies, like that of Vivekananthan et al., 2003, suggest higher dietary intake of antioxidants like Vit C and Vit E supplements to be associated with lowering the risk of cardiovascular diseases. Besides, Vit C is also known to play a role in stimulating the production of white blood cells and antibodies, thereby enhancing immune function (Jafari et al., 2019). Moreover, studies exploring the potential protective effects of selenium and beta-carotene have reported to reduce the incidence of prostate cancer in men with a low baseline level of selenium (Hartman et al., 1998).

Despite the promising benefits of dietary antioxidant supplements, the efficacy of their role in alleviating age-related ailments remains inconclusive. For instance, A randomized control study on over 35000 women investigated the efficacy of Vit E supplementation on cancer and major cardiovascular events and reported no substantial beneficial effects of Vit E supplementation (Moyad, 2002). Likewise, other trials have also reported antioxidant supplementation to have no significant reduction in the incidence of cancer or overall mortality (Peters et al., 2008).

Moreover, higher doses of antioxidant supplements have reported to cause adverse effects and even increase the risk of certain health conditions. Vit E, for instance, at higher dosages has been reported to increase the risk of haemorrhagic stroke and has also been found to interfere with anticoagulating medications (Maggio et al., 2024). Likewise, reports suggest antioxidants act as pro-oxidants under certain conditions, thereby potentially aggravating oxidative stress rather than alleviating it, as found in the case of high dosages of beta-carotene supplements, where it was reported to be associated with an increased risk of lung cancer in smokers. (Tanvetyanon & Bepler, 2008). Besides, antioxidant supplements may also interact adversely with various medications thereby altering the effectiveness of the medication and increasing the risk of developing adverse side effects. For example, Vit E can enhance the effects of blood-thinning medications, leading to an increased risk of bleeding (Meganathan et al., 2008). Therefore, it is recommended to consult healthcare professionals for the usage of dietary supplementations to avoid possible and unintended side effects. Besides, excessive focus on supplements could lead people to overlook the value of a balanced, healthy diet consisting of whole foods. The effectiveness of supplementation varies significantly among individuals due to various factors like genetic variations, environmental influence, higher baseline antioxidant status and lifestyle factors. Hence there may exist a "therapeutic window" during which the supplementation could be most beneficial (Hirsh et al., 1998). Besides, excessive focus on supplements may result in individuals neglecting the importance of a balanced diet rich in whole foods. Therefore, it is recommended to consult a healthcare professional to prevent potential and unforeseen adverse effects. Moreover, as the long-term effects of high-dose antioxidant supplements remain ambiguous, organizations like The American Heart Association recommend a balanced diet with antioxidant-rich foods rather than relying on supplementation, citing the need for more studies to establish clear guidelines for antioxidant supplementation (Lichtenstein et al., 2006).

Current Research and Controversies

Research on antioxidant supplements continues to evolve, with ongoing studies investigating their potential benefits and mechanisms of action. To determine whether targeted supplementation can yield a more favorable and positive outcome, recent studies have focused on specific populations, such as individuals with low antioxidant status or those at high risk for chronic diseases. For instance, in populations that are prone to higher levels of oxidative stress such as individuals with smoking habits or with chronic inflammatory conditions. Further studies are required to clarify if the antioxidant supplementation can provide protective benefits (Sharifi-Rad et al., 2020). The lack of consensus on the efficacy of antioxidant supplements has led to controversies surrounding supplementation guidelines. Although some studies have reported the association of antioxidants to lower the risk of age-related diseases, other investigations contradict these findings, demonstrating no significant benefits of such supplementation. Given the multifactorial nature of aging related diseases and the complexity of the aging process, drawing a definitive conclusion on the efficacy of antioxidant supplementation in aging is a challenging endeavour. Hence, future research could perhaps proceed to venture towards tailoring antioxidant supplementation towards targeted populations based on genetic, lifestyle, and health factors.

An emerging field of Nutrigenomics may offer one such avenue as it deals with the studies of the interaction between nutrition and genes, focusing on how dietary components influence gene expression and how genetic variations affect individual responses to nutrients. Nutrients are known to modulate gene expression through various mechanisms including epigenetic modifications, transcription factor activation, and signalling pathways. Hence, the field of nutrigenomics has gained significant attention in recent times. Certain phytochemicals found in fruits and vegetables are known to activate transcription factors that promote antioxidant defense mechanisms (Virgili et al., 2008). Likewise, Vit C and E with their antioxidant properties can modify oxidative stress response by modulating the expression of genes involved (Bonucci et al., 2018). Similarly, certain variations in genes encoding antioxidant enzymes, including that of superoxide dismutase (SOD) and glutathione peroxidase (GPx) may also give rise to differences in the antioxidant capacity among individuals (Bentley et al., 2008).

Furthermore, genetic variations in genes of antioxidant enzymes have shown to influence the efficacy of dietary antioxidants. Individuals with certain polymorphisms in GPx genes, for example, may reduce the enzyme activity, thereby affecting their antioxidant properties (Voetsch et al., 2007). Individuals with a genetic predisposition to oxidative stress, for instance, may benefit from an increased intake of antioxidant rich food such as leafy vegetables, berries and nuts (Tan et al., 2018). Therefore, by understanding the genetic profile of an individual or specific populations, nutrigenomics can help guide dietary interventions including antioxidation supplementation alongside antioxidant-rich whole food.

The approach of personalizing nutrition in nutrigenomics can significantly enhance the effectiveness of dietary interventions. This will better guide healthcare providers to tailor dietary recommendations to optimize antioxidant supplementation intake, therefore minimising any adverse side effects that may arise due to dietary supplementation while maximising the overall benefit of health outcomes.

Recent Advancements in Antioxidant Research

Recent developments in antioxidant research have focused on new delivery systems, such as gut microbiota-mediated metabolism and the discovery of bioactive molecules. The use of nanotechnology leads to the improvement of stability, bioavailability, and targeted delivery of antioxidants by nano-based formulations, including liposomes and polymeric nanoparticles. These carriers safeguard active molecules from early degradation and enable targeted release at particular locations, thus enhancing therapeutic effect (Khalil et al., 2019). Gut microbiota plays a vital role in the biotransformation and absorption of polyphenols, which in turn activates or inhibits polyphenol's potential health benefits. Only a small quantity of dietary polyphenols is absorbed in small intestine; the rest passes on to the colon, where gut bacteria metabolize them into bioactive compounds. Such metabolism by microbes can improve the bioavailability and activity of polyphenols and may lead to health benefits (Wang & Zheng., 2022).

The interaction of dietary antioxidants, endogenous defense mechanisms, and lifestyle variables determines their overall effectiveness. Optimizing antioxidant therapy requires knowledge of bioavailability, age and gender-specific requirements, and drug interactions. Future studies may focus on personalized nutrition techniques to optimize their benefits.

FUTURE DIRECTIONS AND CHALLENGES

Nutrigenomics, even though shown to have a promising potential, various challenges still prevail. Amongst the challenges is the need to establish a clear link between specific genetic variations and dietary responses. As well as to identify specific genetic and environmental factors that can influence metabolic efficiency and develop personalized dietary interventions that consider individual metabolic profiles. Along with conducting clinical trials to evaluate the effectiveness of the customized dietary approaches in improving the antioxidant status. Moreover, large scale studies are required to validate the findings, develop user friendly genetic testing methods for dietary planning and educate healthcare professionals on the implications of nutrigenomics in their clinical practice.

Customized dietary planning based on genetic testing may raise ethical considerations as well, including concerns over potential genetic discrimination and privacy concerns. Hence, it is essential to have well established guidelines and protocols to protect the genetic information of the individual. Furthermore, there is a need to make genetic testing more accessible and affordable for the general population. Creating awareness among the general population about the benefits as well as the limitations of genetic testing-based dietary planning is highly important for its smooth implementation.

Antioxidant-Based Drugs in Development and Clinical Challenges

Many pharmaceutical and biotech establishments are now pursuing oxidative stress target therapy. For instance, the use of bardoxolone methyl for kidney disease (Pergola et al., 2011) and edaravone for neurodegenerative diseases (Jiao et al., 2015). Furthermore, mitochondrial-targeted antioxidants like MitoQ (Rossman et al., 2018), SkQ1 (Demyanenko et al., 2015) are being explored for their clinical applications in anti-aging treatments for the management of age-related clinical conditions. Translating promising preclinical results into effective clinical therapies has proven challenging for antioxidant-based drugs. One big problem is the lack of consistency in clinical study results, as many antioxidant substances have demonstrated benefits in (animal) models but do not exhibit significant effectiveness in human studies. These differences are mainly due to differences in metabolism, bioavailability, and complex pathways of oxidative stress in humans.

Challenges Implementations

Unlike pharmaceutical drugs, dietary supplements are not subjected to the rigorous process of testing and approval. Hence, regulating dietary supplements presents a significant challenge for clinical usage, which may result in variability in the efficacy and quality of the product. The variability arising from the lack of standardization in the production of dietary supplements can effectively complicate clinical studies, making it difficult to establish clear guidelines for its clinical applications, leading to concerns over its safety and efficacy. Therefore, establishing clear guidelines for the testing and marketing dietary antioxidant supplements is essential for ensuring consumer safety. Besides, such research probing the effectiveness of natural antioxidants and their clinical applications may often face funding challenges that further hinder the advancement of knowledge in this area in terms of large-scale controlled clinical trials compared to pharmaceutical research.

CONCLUSIONS

Aging is a multifaceted process shaped by the intricate interplay of biological mechanisms, environmental exposures, and genetic predispositions. Additionally, lifestyle factors such as physical activity, nutrition, and sleep quality along with environmental stressors like pollution and socioeconomic disparities exacerbate age-related vulnerabilities significantly influence health span. The biological hallmarks of aging namely genomic instability, mitochondrial dysfunction, telomere shortening and cellular senescence, underscore the progressive decline in physiological resilience. Furthermore, genetic variations modulate individual susceptibility to aging and disease, with emerging insights into epigenetic regulation offering promising avenues for intervention.

Oxidative stress emerges as a central driver of aging, contributing to the manifestation of various conditions such as cardiovascular, neurodegenerative, metabolic, and immune disorders. While antioxidants from natural sources play a critical role in mitigating oxidative damage, the efficacy of supplemental antioxidants remains contentious, with risks of adverse effects at high doses. This highlights the importance of prioritizing whole-food, nutrient-dense diets over unregulated supplementation.

Current trends in research are directed towards personalized approaches, such as nutrigenomics, to tailor interventions based on genetic and metabolic profiles. However, challenges persist, including the need for rigorous clinical trials, standardization of supplements, and ethical considerations in genetic testing. Furthermore, efforts could be made to address these gaps through an interdisciplinary approach, large-scale studies, and public health strategies that integrate lifestyle, environmental, and genetic factors.

The understanding of the role of antioxidants in aging is still evolving. While numerous studies have demonstrated the potential benefits of various natural products and dietary supplements, significant gaps remain in our knowledge. Most existing research is based on laboratory-adapted species, which may not accurately reflect the effects in diverse human populations. Further studies are required for deeper insights into the specific mechanisms by which antioxidants influence the aging processes. Current studies often lack comprehensive analyses of how these compounds interact with cellular pathways involved in aging. Moreover, many natural products suffer from low bioavailability, which limits their effectiveness. Studies must also focus on improving the absorption and utilization of these compounds in the human body.

Existing clinical trials often yield inconsistent results, primarily due to small sample sizes and a lack of rigorous methodologies. Future studies should aim for larger, well-controlled trials to provide more precise insights into the efficacy of antioxidants. Most studies do not account for the genetic and environmental diversity of human populations. Further research could include a broader range of subjects to understand how different demographics respond to antioxidant interventions.

Ultimately, promoting healthy aging requires a holistic strategy combining preventive healthcare, equitable access to resources, and advances in personalized medicine to enhance the quality of life and longevity in an increasingly aging global population.

ACKNOWLEDGEMENT

We would like to express our heartfelt gratitude to **Bangalore University** for providing the academic environment and resources that made this work possible. Special thanks to **Prof. D. Usha Anandhi, Prof. P Mahaboob Basha,** and **Prof. B. P. Harini** for their invaluable guidance, insightful feedback, and unwavering support throughout the process of writing this book chapter. Their expertise and encouragement have been instrumental in shaping this work. We are deeply appreciative of their contributions and commitment to fostering academic excellence.

REFERENCES

Abdul, Q. A., Yu, B. P., Chung, H. Y., Jung, H. A., & Choi, J. S. (2017). Epigenetic modifications of gene expression by lifestyle and environment. *Archives of Pharmacal Research, 40*(11), 1219–1237. DOI: 10.1007/s12272-017-0973-3 PMID: 29043603

Abir, M. H., Mahamud, A. S. U., Tonny, S. H., Anu, M. S., Hossain, K. S., Protic, I. A., & Uddin, M. J. (2023). Pharmacological potentials of lycopene against aging and aging-related disorders: A review. *Food Science & Nutrition, 11*(10), 5701–5735. DOI: 10.1002/fsn3.3523 PMID: 37823149

Abrego-Guandique, D. M., Bonet, M. L., Caroleo, M. C., Cannataro, R., Tucci, P., Ribot, J., & Cione, E. (2023). The effect of beta-carotene on cognitive function: A systematic review. *Brain Sciences, 13*(10), 1468. DOI: 10.3390/brainsci13101468 PMID: 37891835

Addo, K. M., & Khan, H. (2024). Factors affecting healthy aging and its interconnected pathways. *Turkish Journal of Healthy Aging Medicine*, (1), 9–24.

Aguilar, T. A. F., Navarro, B. C. H., & Pérez, J. A. M. (2016). *Endogenous antioxidants: a review of their role in oxidative stress*. IntechOpen.

Al-Niaimi, F., & Chiang, N. Y. Z. (2017). Topical vitamin C and the skin: Mechanisms of action and clinical applications. *The Journal of Clinical and Aesthetic Dermatology, 10*(7), 14. PMID: 29104718

Alambayan, J., & Garg, V. (2020). Overview on Phyto-based Treatment for Anxiety. *Current Psychopharmacology, 9*(3), 185–210. DOI: 10.2174/2211556009999200723122833

Alique, M., Luna, C., Carracedo, J., & Ramírez, R. (2015). LDL biochemical modifications: A link between atherosclerosis and aging. *Food & Nutrition Research, 59*(1), 29240. DOI: 10.3402/fnr.v59.29240 PMID: 26637360

Almohaisen, N., Gittins, M., Todd, C., Sremanakova, J., Sowerbutts, A. M., Aldossari, A., & Burden, S. (2022). Prevalence of undernutrition, frailty and sarcopenia in community-dwelling people aged 50 years and above: Systematic review and meta-analysis. *Nutrients, 14*(8), 1537. DOI: 10.3390/nu14081537 PMID: 35458101

Anton, S. D., Cruz-Almeida, Y., Singh, A., Alpert, J., Bensadon, B., Cabrera, M., & Pahor, M. (2020). Innovations in Geroscience to enhance mobility in older adults. *Experimental Gerontology, 142*, 111123. DOI: 10.1016/j.exger.2020.111123 PMID: 33191210

Arenas-Jal, M., Suñé-Negre, J. M., & García-Montoya, E. (2020). Coenzyme Q10 supplementation: Efficacy, safety, and formulation challenges. *Comprehensive Reviews in Food Science and Food Safety, 19*(2), 574–594. DOI: 10.1111/1541-4337.12539 PMID: 33325173

Ayunin, Q., Miatmoko, A., Soeratri, W., Erawati, T., Susanto, J., & Legowo, D. (2022). Improving the anti-ageing activity of coenzyme Q10 through protransfersome-loaded emulgel. *Scientific Reports, 12*(1), 906. DOI: 10.1038/s41598-021-04708-4 PMID: 35042910

Baeeri, M., Bahadar, H., Rahimifard, M., Navaei-Nigjeh, M., Khorasani, R., Rezvanfar, M. A., & Abdollahi, M. (2019). α-Lipoic acid prevents senescence, cell cycle arrest, and inflammatory cues in fibroblasts by inhibiting oxidative stress. *Pharmacological Research, 141*, 214–223. DOI: 10.1016/j.phrs.2019.01.003 PMID: 30611855

Barinova, G. M., Gaeva, D. V., & Krasnov, E. V. (2020). Hazardous chemicals and air, water, and soil pollution and contamination. *Good Health and Well-Being*, 255-266.

Barnham, K. J., Masters, C. L., & Bush, A. I. (2004). Neurodegenerative diseases and oxidative stress. *Nature Reviews. Drug Discovery, 3*(3), 205–214. DOI: 10.1038/nrd1330 PMID: 15031734

Barzilai, N., Cuervo, A. M., & Austad, S. (2018). Aging as a biological target for prevention and therapy. *Journal of the American Medical Association, 320*(13), 1321–1322. DOI: 10.1001/jama.2018.9562 PMID: 30242337

Basha, P. M., Rakesh, H., & Mani, S. S. (2021). Correlates of sperm quality parameters and oxidative stress indices in diabetic rats exposed to cold stress: Role of Moringa oleifera leaf extract. *Journal of Applied Biology and Biotechnology, 9*(05), 70–77.

Bawani, S. S., & Anandhi, D. U. (2021). GC-MS analysis of nigella sativa seed extract and its ameliorative effects on transgenic drosophila model of Parkinson disease. *International Journal of Innovative Science and Research Technology, 4*, 16–22.

Bayoumi, M., Arafa, M. G., Nasr, M., & Sammour, O. A. (2021). Nobiletin-loaded composite penetration enhancer vesicles restore the normal miRNA expression and the chief defence antioxidant levels in skin cancer. *Scientific Reports, 11*(1), 20197. DOI: 10.1038/s41598-021-99756-1 PMID: 34642396

Bentley, A. R., Emrani, P., & Cassano, P. A. (2008). Genetic variation and gene expression in antioxidant related enzymes and risk of COPD: A systematic review. *Thorax, 63*(11), 956–961. DOI: 10.1136/thx.2007.086199 PMID: 18566111

Bhullar, K. S., & Hubbard, B. P. (2015). Lifespan and healthspan extension by resveratrol. Biochimica et Biophysica Acta (BBA)-. *Biochimica et Biophysica Acta. Molecular Basis of Disease, 1852*(6), 1209–1218. DOI: 10.1016/j.bbadis.2015.01.012

Blackburn, E. H., Epel, E. S., & Lin, J. (2015). Human telomere biology: A contributory and interactive factor in aging, disease risks, and protection. *Science, 350*(6265), 1193–1198. DOI: 10.1126/science.aab3389 PMID: 26785477

Bloom, I., Edwards, M., Jameson, K. A., Syddall, H. E., Dennison, E., Gale, C. R., & Robinson, S. (2017). Influences on diet quality in older age: The importance of social factors. *Age and Ageing*, *46*(2), 277–283. PMID: 27744301

Boccardi, V., Arosio, B., Cari, L., Bastiani, P., Scamosci, M., Casati, M., & Mecocci, P. (2020). Beta-carotene, telomerase activity and Alzheimer's disease in old age subjects. *European Journal of Nutrition*, *59*(1), 119–126. DOI: 10.1007/s00394-019-01892-y PMID: 30649596

Bonucci, J., Gragnani, A., Trincado, M. M., Vincentin, V., Correa, S. A. A., & Ferreira, L. M. (2018). The role of vitamin C in the gene expression of oxidative stress markers in fibroblasts from burn patients. *Acta Cirurgica Brasileira*, *33*(08), 703–712. DOI: 10.1590/s0102-865020180080000006 PMID: 30208132

Boo, Y. C. (2021). Mechanistic basis and clinical evidence for the applications of nicotinamide (niacinamide) to control skin aging and pigmentation. *Antioxidants*, *10*(8), 1315. DOI: 10.3390/antiox10081315 PMID: 34439563

Brand, A. L., Lawler, P. E., Bollinger, J. G., Li, Y., Schindler, S. E., Li, M., & Bateman, R. J. (2022). The performance of plasma amyloid beta measurements in identifying amyloid plaques in Alzheimer's disease: A literature review. *Alzheimer's Research & Therapy*, *14*(1), 195. DOI: 10.1186/s13195-022-01117-1 PMID: 36575454

Brioche, T., & Lemoine-Morel, S. (2016). Oxidative stress, sarcopenia, antioxidant strategies and exercise: Molecular aspects. *Current Pharmaceutical Design*, *22*(18), 2664–2678. DOI: 10.2174/1381612822666160219120531 PMID: 26891808

Campisi, J., & Robert, L. (2014). Cell senescence: Role in aging and age-related diseases. *Aging (Albany NY)*, *39*, 45–61. PMID: 24862014

Cannizzo, E. S., Clement, C. C., Sahu, R., Follo, C., & Santambrogio, L. (2011). Oxidative stress, inflamm-aging and immunosenescence. *Journal of Proteomics*, *74*(11), 2313–2323. DOI: 10.1016/j.jprot.2011.06.005 PMID: 21718814

Carr, A. C., & Maggini, S. (2017). Vitamin C and immune function. *Nutrients*, *9*(11), 1211. DOI: 10.3390/nu9111211 PMID: 29099763

Chen, X., Guo, C., & Kong, J. (2012). Oxidative stress in neurodegenerative diseases☆. *Neural Regeneration Research*, *7*(5), 376–385. PMID: 25774178

Chiu, P. C., Chan, C. C., Lin, H. M., & Chiu, H. C. (2007). The clinical anti-aging effects of topical kinetin and niacinamide in Asians: A randomized, double-blind, placebo-controlled, split-face comparative trial. *Journal of Cosmetic Dermatology*, *6*(4), 243–249. DOI: 10.1111/j.1473-2165.2007.00342.x PMID: 18047609

Christen, W. G., Glynn, R. J., Gaziano, J. M., Darke, A. K., Crowley, J. J., Goodman, P. J., & Klein, E. A. (2015). Age-related cataract in men in the selenium and vitamin e cancer prevention trial eye endpoints study: A randomized clinical trial. *JAMA Ophthalmology*, *133*(1), 17–24. DOI: 10.1001/jamaophthalmol.2014.3478 PMID: 25232809

Clarke, T. L., & Mostoslavsky, R. (2022). DNA repair as a shared hallmark in cancer and ageing. *Molecular Oncology*, *16*(18), 3352–3379. DOI: 10.1002/1878-0261.13285 PMID: 35834102

Crowley, K. (2011). Sleep and sleep disorders in older adults. *Neuropsychology Review*, *21*(1), 41–53. DOI: 10.1007/s11065-010-9154-6 PMID: 21225347

Crozier, A., Yokota, T., Jaganath, I. B., Marks, S., Saltmarsh, M., & Clifford, M. N. (2006). Secondary metabolites in fruits, vegetables, beverages and other plant based dietary components. *Plant secondary metabolites: Occurrence, structure and role in the human diet*, 208-302.

Cui, H., Kong, Y., & Zhang, H. (2012). Oxidative stress, mitochondrial dysfunction, and aging. *Journal of Signal Transduction*, *2012*(1), 646354. PMID: 21977319

Daiber, A., Kuntic, M., Hahad, O., Delogu, L. G., Rohrbach, S., Di Lisa, F., & Münzel, T. (2020). Effects of air pollution particles (ultrafine and fine particulate matter) on mitochondrial function and oxidative stress–Implications for cardiovascular and neurodegenerative diseases. *Archives of Biochemistry and Biophysics*, *696*, 108662. DOI: 10.1016/j.abb.2020.108662 PMID: 33159890

de Freitas Rodrigues, C., Boldori, J. R., Soares, M. V., Somacal, S., Emanuelli, T., Izaguirry, A., & Denardin, C. C. (2021). Goji berry (Lycium barbarum L.) juice reduces lifespan and premature aging of Caenorhabditis elegans: Is it safe to consume it? *Food Research International*, *144*, 110297. DOI: 10.1016/j.foodres.2021.110297 PMID: 34053563

Demyanenko, I. A., Popova, E. N., Zakharova, V. V., Ilyinskaya, O. P., Vasilieva, T. V., Romashchenko, V. P., & Chernyak, B. V. (2015). Mitochondria-targeted antioxidant SkQ1 improves impaired dermal wound healing in old mice. *Aging (Albany NY)*, *7*(7), 475–485. DOI: 10.18632/aging.100772 PMID: 26187706

Devi, S. A., & Kiran, T. R. (2004). Regional responses in antioxidant system to exercise training and dietary vitamin E in aging rat brain. *Neurobiology of Aging*, *25*(4), 501–508. DOI: 10.1016/S0197-4580(03)00112-X PMID: 15013571

Dhalaria, R., Verma, R., Kumar, D., Puri, S., Tapwal, A., Kumar, V., & Kuca, K. (2020). Bioactive compounds of edible fruits with their anti-aging properties: A comprehensive review to prolong human life. *Antioxidants*, *9*(11), 1123. DOI: 10.3390/antiox9111123 PMID: 33202871

Di Bona, D., Accardi, G., Virruso, C., Candore, G., & Caruso, C. (2014). Association between genetic variations in the insulin/insulin-like growth factor (Igf-1) signaling pathway and longevity: A systematic review and meta-analysis. *Current Vascular Pharmacology*, *12*(5), 674–681. DOI: 10.2174/15701611 11666131218152807 PMID: 24350933

Di Carlo, E., & Sorrentino, C. (2024). Oxidative stress and age-related tumors. *Antioxidants*, *13*(9), 1109. DOI: 10.3390/antiox13091109 PMID: 39334768

Dounousi, E., Papavasiliou, E., Makedou, A., Ioannou, K., Katopodis, K. P., Tselepis, A., & Tsakiris, D. (2006). Oxidative stress is progressively enhanced with advancing stages of CKD. *American Journal of Kidney Diseases*, *48*(5), 752–760. DOI: 10.1053/j.ajkd.2006.08.015 PMID: 17059994

Du, G., Qiao, Y., Zhuo, Z., Zhou, J., Li, X., Liu, Z., & Chen, H. (2020). Lipoic acid rejuvenates aged intestinal stem cells by preventing age-associated endosome reduction. *EMBO Reports*, *21*(8), e49583. DOI: 10.15252/embr.201949583 PMID: 32648369

Duan, R. R., Hao, K., & Yang, T. (2020). Air pollution and chronic obstructive pulmonary disease. *Chronic Diseases and Translational Medicine*, *6*(04), 260–269. DOI: 10.1016/j.cdtm.2020.05.004 PMID: 33336171

Dutta, A., & Dutta, S. K. (2003). Vitamin E and its role in the prevention of atherosclerosis and carcinogenesis: A review. *Journal of the American College of Nutrition*, *22*(4), 258–268. DOI: 10.1080/07315724.2003.10719302 PMID: 12897039

Ebert, T., Neytchev, O., Witasp, A., Kublickiene, K., Stenvinkel, P., & Shiels, P. G. (2021). Inflammation and oxidative stress in chronic kidney disease and dialysis patients. *Antioxidants & Redox Signaling*, *35*(17), 1426–1448. DOI: 10.1089/ars.2020.8184 PMID: 34006115

Emeksiz, M. A. C. (2023). Biotin, Folic acid, and Coenzyme Q for Skin Health. Supplements in Dermatology, 112.

Epel, E. S., Lin, J., Wilhelm, F. H., Wolkowitz, O. M., Cawthon, R., Adler, N. E., & Blackburn, E. H. (2006). Cell aging in relation to stress arousal and cardiovascular disease risk factors. *Psychoneuroendocrinology*, *31*(3), 277–287. DOI: 10.1016/j.psyneuen.2005.08.011 PMID: 16298085

Esposito, R., Fiorini, L., Limosani, R., Bonaccorsi, M., Manzi, A., Cavallo, F., & Dario, P. (2016). Supporting active and healthy aging with advanced robotics integrated in smart environment. In *Optimizing assistive technologies for aging populations* (pp. 46–77). IGI Global. DOI: 10.4018/978-1-4666-9530-6.ch003

Finaud, J., Lac, G., & Filaire, E. (2006). Oxidative stress: Relationship with exercise and training. *Sports Medicine (Auckland, N.Z.)*, *36*(4), 327–358. DOI: 10.2165/00007256-200636040-00004 PMID: 16573358

Firuzi, O., Miri, R., Tavakkoli, M., & Saso, L. (2011). Antioxidant therapy: Current status and future prospects. *Current Medicinal Chemistry*, *18*(25), 3871–3888. DOI: 10.2174/092986711803414368 PMID: 21824100

Fisher, J. E., Loft, S., Ulrik, C. S., Raaschou-Nielsen, O., Hertel, O., Tjønneland, A., & Andersen, Z. J. (2016). Physical activity, air pollution, and the risk of asthma and chronic obstructive pulmonary disease. *American Journal of Respiratory and Critical Care Medicine*, *194*(7), 855–865. DOI: 10.1164/rccm.201510-2036OC PMID: 27653737

Forouzanfar, F., & Hosseinzadeh, H. (2020). Protective role of Nigella sativa and thymoquinone in oxidative stress: a review. Nuts and seeds in health and disease prevention, 127-146.

Gasek, N. S., Kuchel, G. A., Kirkland, J. L., & Xu, M. (2021). Strategies for targeting senescent cells in human disease. *Nature Aging*, *1*(10), 870–879. DOI: 10.1038/s43587-021-00121-8 PMID: 34841261

Gentilini, D., Mari, D., Castaldi, D., Remondini, D., Ogliari, G., Ostan, R., & Vitale, G. (2013). Role of epigenetics in human aging and longevity: Genome-wide DNA methylation profile in centenarians and centenarians' offspring. *Age (Dordrecht, Netherlands)*, *35*(5), 1961–1973. DOI: 10.1007/s11357-012-9463-1 PMID: 22923132

Goossens, V., Grooten, J., De Vos, K., & Fiers, W. (1995). Direct evidence for tumor necrosis factor-induced mitochondrial reactive oxygen intermediates and their involvement in cytotoxicity. *Proceedings of the National Academy of Sciences of the United States of America*, *92*(18), 8115–8119. DOI: 10.1073/pnas.92.18.8115 PMID: 7667254

Halliwell, B. (2006). Reactive species and antioxidants. Redox biology is a fundamental theme of aerobic life. *Plant Physiology*, *141*(2), 312–322. DOI: 10.1104/pp.106.077073 PMID: 16760481

Harmita, H., Iskandarsyah, I., & Afifah, S. F. (2020). Effect of transfersome formulation on the stability and antioxidant activity of N-acetylcysteine in anti-aging cream. *International Journal of Applied Pharmaceutics*, *12*(1), 156–162. DOI: 10.22159/ijap.2020.v12s1.FF034

Harrison, F. E. (2012). A critical review of vitamin C for the prevention of age-related cognitive decline and Alzheimer's disease. *Journal of Alzheimer's Disease*, *29*(4), 711–726. DOI: 10.3233/JAD-2012-111853 PMID: 22366772

Hartman, T. J., Albanes, D., Rautalahti, M., Tangrea, J. A., Virtamo, J., Stolzenberg, R., & Taylor, P. R. (1998). Physical activity and prostate cancer in the alpha-tocopherol, beta-carotene (ATBC) cancer prevention study (Finland). *Cancer Causes & Control*, *9*(1), 11–18. DOI: 10.1023/A:1008889001519 PMID: 9486459

Heaney, M. L., Gardner, J. R., Karasavvas, N., Golde, D. W., Scheinberg, D. A., Smith, E. A., & O'Connor, O. A. (2008). Vitamin C antagonizes the cytotoxic effects of antineoplastic drugs. *Cancer Research*, *68*(19), 8031–8038. DOI: 10.1158/0008-5472.CAN-08-1490 PMID: 18829561

Hekimi, S., Lapointe, J., & Wen, Y. (2011). Taking a "good" look at free radicals in the aging process. *Trends in Cell Biology*, *21*(10), 569–576. DOI: 10.1016/j.tcb.2011.06.008 PMID: 21824781

Hernández-Camacho, J. D., Bernier, M., López-Lluch, G., & Navas, P. (2018). Coenzyme Q10 supplementation in aging and disease. *Frontiers in Physiology*, *9*, 44. DOI: 10.3389/fphys.2018.00044 PMID: 29459830

Hill, W. G., & Mulder, H. A. (2010). Genetic analysis of environmental variation. *Genetical Research*, *92*(5-6), 381–395. DOI: 10.1017/S0016672310000546 PMID: 21429270

Hirsh, J., Dalen, J. E., Anderson, D. R., Poller, L., Bussey, H., Ansell, J., Deykin, D., & Brandt, J. T. (1998). Oral anticoagulants: Mechanism of action, clinical effectiveness, and optimal therapeutic range. *Chest*, *114*(5), S445. DOI: 10.1378/chest.114.5_Supplement.445S PMID: 9822057

Hoeijmakers, J. H. (2009). DNA damage, aging, and cancer. *The New England Journal of Medicine*, *361*(15), 1475–1485. DOI: 10.1056/NEJMra0804615 PMID: 19812404

Huang, W., Hickson, L. J., Eirin, A., Kirkland, J. L., & Lerman, L. O. (2022). Cellular senescence: The good, the bad and the unknown. *Nature Reviews. Nephrology*, *18*(10), 611–627. DOI: 10.1038/s41581-022-00601-z PMID: 35922662

Huxhold, O., Miche, M., & Schüz, B. (2014). Benefits of having friends in older ages: Differential effects of informal social activities on well-being in middle-aged and older adults. *The Journals of Gerontology. Series B, Psychological Sciences and Social Sciences*, *69*(3), 366–375. DOI: 10.1093/geronb/gbt029 PMID: 23682165

Ikonne, U. S., Vann, P. H., Wong, J. M., Forster, M. J., & Sumien, N. (2019). Supplementation with N-acetyl cysteine affects motor and cognitive function in young but not old mice. *The Journal of Nutrition*, *149*(3), 463–470. DOI: 10.1093/jn/nxy287 PMID: 30770531

Jafari, D., Esmaeilzadeh, A., Mohammadi-Kordkhayli, M., & Rezaei, N. (2019). Vitamin C and the immune system. *Nutrition and immunity*, 81-102.

Jiao, S. S., Yao, X. Q., Liu, Y. H., Wang, Q. H., Zeng, F., Lu, J. J., & Wang, Y. J. (2015). Edaravone alleviates Alzheimer's disease-type pathologies and cognitive deficits. *Proceedings of the National Academy of Sciences of the United States of America*, *112*(16), 5225–5230. DOI: 10.1073/pnas.1422998112 PMID: 25847999

Johnson, A. A., Akman, K., Calimport, S. R., Wuttke, D., Stolzing, A., & De Magalhaes, J. P. (2012). The role of DNA methylation in aging, rejuvenation, and age-related disease. *Rejuvenation Research*, *15*(5), 483–494. DOI: 10.1089/rej.2012.1324 PMID: 23098078

Jung, S., Kim, M., Ryu, H. J., Chae, J. S., Lee, S. H., & Lee, J. H. (2015). Age-related increase in LDL-cholesterol is associated with enhanced oxidative stress and disturbed sphingolipid metabolism. *Metabolomics*, *11*(1), 40–49. DOI: 10.1007/s11306-014-0669-3

Kasprzak, M. M., Erxleben, A., & Ochocki, J. (2015). Properties and applications of flavonoid metal complexes. *RSC Advances*, *5*(57), 45853–45877. DOI: 10.1039/C5RA05069C

Khalil, I., Yehye, W. A., Etxeberria, A. E., Alhadi, A. A., Dezfooli, S. M., Julkapli, N. B. M., & Seyfoddin, A. (2019). Nanoantioxidants: Recent trends in antioxidant delivery applications. *Antioxidants*, *9*(1), 24. DOI: 10.3390/antiox9010024 PMID: 31888023

Kim, S. I., Jung, J. W., Ahn, Y. J., Restifo, L. L., & Kwon, H. W. (2011). Drosophila as a model system for studying lifespan and neuroprotective activities of plant-derived compounds. *Journal of Asia-Pacific Entomology*, *14*(4), 509–517. DOI: 10.1016/j.aspen.2011.07.001

Knight, J. A. (1998). Free radicals: Their history and current status in aging and disease. *Annals of Clinical and Laboratory Science*, *28*(6), 331–346. PMID: 9846200

Koppenol, W., Moreno, J., Pryor, W. A., Ischiropoulos, H., & Beckman, J. (1992). Peroxynitrite, a cloaked oxidant formed by nitric oxide and superoxide. *Chemical Research in Toxicology*, *5*(6), 834–842. DOI: 10.1021/tx00030a017 PMID: 1336991

Kulawik, A., Cielecka-Piontek, J., & Zalewski, P. (2023). The importance of antioxidant activity for the health-promoting effect of lycopene. *Nutrients*, *15*(17), 3821. DOI: 10.3390/nu15173821 PMID: 37686853

Kumar, P. P., Bawani, S. S., Anandhi, D. U., & Prashanth, K. H. (2024). Dietary supplementation with thymoquinone inhibits rotenone induced developmental toxicity in Drosophila melanogaster: Focus on ovary and larval development. *Food Bioscience*, *62*, 105233. DOI: 10.1016/j.fbio.2024.105233

Kunert, K. J., & Ederer, M. (1985). Leaf aging and lipid peroxidation: The role of the antioxidants vitamin C and E. *Physiologia Plantarum*, *65*(1), 85–88. DOI: 10.1111/j.1399-3054.1985.tb02364.x

Lee, E. B., Kim, J. H., An, C. W., Kim, Y. J., Noh, Y. J., Kim, S. J., Kim, D. K., Shrestha, A. C., Ham, H.-N., Leem, J.-Y., Jo, H.-K., Kim, D.-S., Moon, K. H., Lee, J. H., Jeong, K. O., & Kim, D. K. (2018). Longevity and stress resistant property of 6-gingerol from Zingiber officinale Roscoe in Caenorhabditis elegans. *Biomolecules & Therapeutics*, *26*(6), 568–575. DOI: 10.4062/biomolther.2017.215 PMID: 29534560

Lee, S. H., & Min, K. J. (2017). Lifespan-Extending Effect of Resveratrol and Other Phytochemicals.

Li, K., Deng, Z., Lei, C., Ding, X., Li, J., & Wang, C. (2024). The Role of Oxidative Stress in Tumorigenesis and Progression. *Cells*, *13*(5), 441. DOI: 10.3390/cells13050441 PMID: 38474405

Lichtenstein, A. H., Appel, L. J., Brands, M., Carnethon, M., Daniels, S., Franch, H. A., & Wylie-Rosett, J. (2006). Diet and lifestyle recommendations revision 2006: A scientific statement from the American Heart Association Nutrition Committee. *Circulation*, *114*(1), 82–96. DOI: 10.1161/CIRCULATIONAHA.106.176158 PMID: 16785338

Liguori, I., Russo, G., Curcio, F., Bulli, G., Aran, L., Della-Morte, D., & Abete, P. (2018). Oxidative stress, aging, and diseases. *Clinical Interventions in Aging*, *13*, 757–772. DOI: 10.2147/CIA.S158513 PMID: 29731617

Liu, Z. Q. (2014). Antioxidants may not always be beneficial to health. *Nutrition (Burbank, Los Angeles County, Calif.)*, *30*(2), 131–133. DOI: 10.1016/j.nut.2013.04.006 PMID: 23993796

Lombard, D. B., Chua, K. F., Mostoslavsky, R., Franco, S., Gostissa, M., & Alt, F. W. (2005). DNA repair, genome stability, and aging. *Cell*, *120*(4), 497–512. DOI: 10.1016/j.cell.2005.01.028 PMID: 15734682

López-Otín, C., Blasco, M. A., Partridge, L., Serrano, M., & Kroemer, G. (2013). The hallmarks of aging. *Cell*, *153*(6), 1194–1217. DOI: 10.1016/j.cell.2013.05.039 PMID: 23746838

Maggio, E., Bocchini, V. P., Carnevale, R., Pignatelli, P., Violi, F., & Loffredo, L. (2024). Vitamin E supplementation (alone or with other antioxidants) and stroke: A meta-analysis. *Nutrition Reviews*, *82*(8), 1069–1078. DOI: 10.1093/nutrit/nuad114 PMID: 37698992

Mancuso, C., & Santangelo, R. (2014). Ferulic acid: Pharmacological and toxicological aspects. *Food and Chemical Toxicology*, *65*, 185–195. DOI: 10.1016/j.fct.2013.12.024 PMID: 24373826

Marchal, J., Pifferi, F., & Aujard, F. (2013). Resveratrol in mammals: Effects on aging biomarkers, age-related diseases, and life span. *Annals of the New York Academy of Sciences*, *1290*(1), 67–73. DOI: 10.1111/nyas.12214 PMID: 23855467

Marín, L., Miguélez, E. M., Villar, C. J., & Lombó, F. (2015). Bioavailability of dietary polyphenols and gut microbiota metabolism: Antimicrobial properties. *BioMed Research International*, *2015*(1), 905215. DOI: 10.1155/2015/905215 PMID: 25802870

Markus, M. A., & Morris, B. J. (2008). Resveratrol in prevention and treatment of common clinical conditions of aging. *Clinical Interventions in Aging*, *3*(2), 331–339. PMID: 18686754

Maroon, J. (2008). *The longevity factor: how resveratrol and red wine activate genes for a longer and healthier life*. Simon and Schuster.

Martín, J., Kuskoski, E. M., Navas, M. J., & Asuero, A. G. (2017). Antioxidant capacity of anthocyanin pigments. Flavonoids-from biosynthesis to human health, 3, 205-255.

Mates, J. M. (2000). Effects of antioxidant enzymes in the molecular control of reactive oxygen species toxicology. *Toxicology*, *153*(1-3), 83–104. DOI: 10.1016/S0300-483X(00)00306-1 PMID: 11090949

McMaughan, D. J., Oloruntoba, O., & Smith, M. L. (2020). Socioeconomic status and access to healthcare: Interrelated drivers for healthy aging. *Frontiers in Public Health*, *8*, 231. DOI: 10.3389/fpubh.2020.00231 PMID: 32626678

Meganathan, P., Selvaduray, K. R., & Nesaretnam, K. (2008). Blood Thinning Effects and Phytonutrients. *Malays. Oil J.*, *23*(2), 8–12.

Meng, S. J., & Yu, L. J. (2010). Oxidative stress, molecular inflammation and sarcopenia. *International Journal of Molecular Sciences*, *11*(4), 1509–1526. DOI: 10.3390/ijms11041509 PMID: 20480032

Menon, V. P., & Sudheer, A. R. (2007). Antioxidant and anti-inflammatory properties of curcumin. *The molecular targets and therapeutic uses of curcumin in health and disease*, 105-125.

Mirończuk-Chodakowska, I., Witkowska, A. M., & Zujko, M. E. (2018). Endogenous non-enzymatic antioxidants in the human body. *Advances in Medical Sciences*, *63*(1), 68–78. DOI: 10.1016/j.advms.2017.05.005 PMID: 28822266

Misaka, S., Kawabe, K., Onoue, S., Werba, J. P., Giroli, M., Tamaki, S., & Yamada, S. (2013). Effects of green tea catechins on cytochrome P450 2B6, 2C8, 2C19, 2D6 and 3A activities in human liver and intestinal microsomes. *Drug Metabolism and Pharmacokinetics*, *28*(3), 244–249. DOI: 10.2133/dmpk.DMPK-12-RG-101 PMID: 23268924

Mizobuchi, M., Ishidoh, K., & Kamemura, N. (2022). A comparison of cell death mechanisms of antioxidants, butylated hydroxyanisole and butylated hydroxytoluene. *Drug and Chemical Toxicology*, *45*(4), 1899–1906. DOI: 10.1080/01480545.2021.1894701 PMID: 34013795

Molz, P., & Schröder, N. (2017). Potential therapeutic effects of lipoic acid on memory deficits related to aging and neurodegeneration. *Frontiers in Pharmacology*, *8*, 849. DOI: 10.3389/fphar.2017.00849 PMID: 29311912

Monacelli, F., Acquarone, E., Giannotti, C., Borghi, R., & Nencioni, A. (2017). Vitamin C, aging and Alzheimer's disease. *Nutrients*, *9*(7), 670. DOI: 10.3390/nu9070670 PMID: 28654021

Mondal, S., & Rahaman, S. T. (2020). Flavonoids: A vital resource in healthcare and medicine. *Pharmacy & Pharmacology International Journal*, *8*(2), 91–104. DOI: 10.15406/ppij.2020.08.00285

Morris, M. C., Evans, D. A., Bienias, J. L., Tangney, C. C., & Wilson, R. S. (2002). Vitamin E and cognitive decline in older persons. *Archives of Neurology, 59*(7), 1125–1132. DOI: 10.1001/archneur.59.7.1125 PMID: 12117360

Moyad, M. A. (2002). Selenium and vitamin E supplements for prostate cancer: Evidence or embellishment? *Urology, 59*(4), 9–19. DOI: 10.1016/S0090-4295(01)01190-6 PMID: 11937432

Nadeem, M., Imran, M., Aslam Gondal, T., Imran, A., Shahbaz, M., Muhammad Amir, R., & Martins, N. (2019). Therapeutic potential of rosmarinic acid: A comprehensive review. *Applied Sciences (Basel, Switzerland), 9*(15), 3139. DOI: 10.3390/app9153139

Obrenovich, M. E., Nair, N. G., Beyaz, A., Aliev, G., & Reddy, V. P. (2010). The role of polyphenolic antioxidants in health, disease, and aging. *Rejuvenation Research, 13*(6), 631–643. DOI: 10.1089/rej.2010.1043 PMID: 20818981

Ortolá, R., García-Esquinas, E., García-Varela, G., Struijk, E. A., Rodríguez-Artalejo, F., & López-García, E. (2019). Influence of changes in diet quality on unhealthy aging: The seniors-ENRICA cohort. *The American Journal of Medicine, 132*(9), 1091–1102. DOI: 10.1016/j.amjmed.2019.03.023 PMID: 30981558

Padayatty, S. J., Katz, A., Wang, Y., Eck, P., Kwon, O., Lee, J. H., & Levine, M. (2003). Vitamin C as an antioxidant: Evaluation of its role in disease prevention. *Journal of the American College of Nutrition, 22*(1), 18–35. DOI: 10.1080/07315724.2003.10719272 PMID: 12569111

Paiva, S. A., & Russell, R. M. (1999). β-carotene and other carotenoids as antioxidants. *Journal of the American College of Nutrition, 18*(5), 426–433. DOI: 10.1080/07315724.1999.10718880 PMID: 10511324

Pajović, S. B., Saičić, Z. S., Pejić, S., Kasapović, J., Stojiljković, V., & Kanazir, D. T. (2006). Antioxidative biomarkers and cancerogenesis. *Jugoslovenska medicinska biohemija, 25*(4), 397-402.

Palmer, A. K., & Jensen, M. D. (2022). Metabolic changes in aging humans: Current evidence and therapeutic strategies. *The Journal of Clinical Investigation, 132*(16), e158451. DOI: 10.1172/JCI158451 PMID: 35968789

Patel, A., Tiwari, S., Pandey, N., Gupta, D., & Prasad, S. M. (2020). Role of spices beyond a flavouring agent: The antioxidant and medicinal properties. In *Ethnopharmacological Investigation of Indian Spices* (pp. 5–35). IGI Global Scientific Publishing. DOI: 10.4018/978-1-7998-2524-1.ch002

Patil, H. R., O'Keefe, J. H., Lavie, C. J., Magalski, A., Vogel, R. A., & McCullough, P. A. (2012). Cardiovascular damage resulting from chronic excessive endurance exercise. *Missouri Medicine, 109*(4), 312. PMID: 22953596

Pearson, P., Lewis, S. A., Britton, J., Young, I. S., & Fogarty, A. (2006). The pro-oxidant activity of high-dose vitamin E supplements in vivo. *BioDrugs, 20*(5), 271–273. DOI: 10.2165/00063030-200620050-00002 PMID: 17025373

Pergola, P. E., Raskin, P., Toto, R. D., Meyer, C. J., Huff, J. W., Grossman, E. B., & Warnock, D. G. (2011). Bardoxolone methyl and kidney function in CKD with type 2 diabetes. *The New England Journal of Medicine, 365*(4), 327–336. DOI: 10.1056/NEJMoa1105351 PMID: 21699484

Peters, D. H., Garg, A., Bloom, G., Walker, D. G., Brieger, W. R., & Hafizur Rahman, M. (2008). Poverty and access to health care in developing countries. *Annals of the New York Academy of Sciences*, *1136*(1), 161–171. DOI: 10.1196/annals.1425.011 PMID: 17954679

Pickering, C., & Kiely, J. (2017). ACTN3: More than just a gene for speed. *Frontiers in Physiology*, *8*, 1080. DOI: 10.3389/fphys.2017.01080 PMID: 29326606

Pietta, P. G. (2000). Flavonoids as antioxidants. *Journal of Natural Products*, *63*(7), 1035–1042. DOI: 10.1021/np9904509 PMID: 10924197

Pokorný, J. (2007). Are natural antioxidants better–and safer–than synthetic antioxidants? *European Journal of Lipid Science and Technology*, *109*(6), 629–642. DOI: 10.1002/ejlt.200700064

Polidori, M. C., Cherubini, A., Senin, U., & Mecocci, P. (2001). Peripheral non-enzymatic antioxidant changes with human aging: A selective status report. *Biogerontology*, *2*(2), 99–104. DOI: 10.1023/A:1011593319127 PMID: 11708381

Polidori, M. C., Mecocci, P., Cherubini, A., & Senin, U. (2000). Physical activity and oxidative stress during aging. *International Journal of Sports Medicine*, *21*(03), 154–157. DOI: 10.1055/s-2000-8881 PMID: 10834344

Pompella, M., & Costantino, L. (2023). ESG disclosure and sustainability transition: A new metric and emerging trends in responsible investments. *TalTech Journal of European Studies*, *13*(1), 8–39. DOI: 10.2478/bjes-2023-0002

Pozos-Nonato, S., Domínguez-Delgado, C. L., Campos-Santander, K. A., Benavides, A. A., Pacheco-Ortin, S. M., Higuera-Piedrahita, R. I., & Molina-Trinidad, E. M. (2023). Novel nanotechnological strategies for skin anti-aging. *Current Pharmaceutical Biotechnology*, *24*(11), 1397–1419. DOI: 10.2174/1389201024666221223095315 PMID: 36567280

Priyadarshanee, M., Mahto, U., & Das, S. (2022). Mechanism of toxicity and adverse health effects of environmental pollutants. In *Microbial biodegradation and bioremediation* (pp. 33–53). Elsevier.

Raina, K., Kumari, R., Thakur, P., Sharma, R., Singh, R., Thakur, A., & Chaudhary, A. (2023). Mechanistic role and potential of Ayurvedic herbs as anti-aging therapies. *Drug Metabolism and Personalized Therapy*. Advance online publication. DOI: 10.1515/dmdi-2023-0024

Rakesh, H., & Basha, P. M. (2022). Total Phenolic, Total Flavonoid and Free Radical Scavenging Potential of Moringa Oleifera Leaf and Tribulus Terrestris Fruit Extracts. *International Journal of Science and Research, Vol*, *11*(11), 1363–1373.

Rakesh, H., Mani, S. S., & Basha, P. M. (2021). Chronic cold exposure aggravates oxidative stress in reproductive organs of STZ-induced diabetic rats: Protective role of Moringa oleifera. *Journal of Applied Biology and Biotechnology*, *9*(03), 114–120.

Ramos, A. F., Fonseca, C., & Henriques, A. (2020). Developing and managing health systems and organizations for an aging society. In *Handbook of Research on Health Systems and Organizations for an Aging Society* (pp. 62–68). IGI Global. DOI: 10.4018/978-1-5225-9818-3.ch005

Rasinaho, M., Hirvensalo, M., Leinonen, R., Lintunen, T., & Rantanen, T. (2007). Motives for and barriers to physical activity among older adults with mobility limitations. *Journal of Aging and Physical Activity*, *15*(1), 90–102. DOI: 10.1123/japa.15.1.90 PMID: 17387231

Rastogi, H., & Jana, S. (2014). Evaluation of inhibitory effects of caffeic acid and quercetin on human liver cytochrome p450 activities. *Phytotherapy Research*, *28*(12), 1873–1878. DOI: 10.1002/ptr.5220 PMID: 25196644

Rogeri, P. S., Zanella, R.Jr, Martins, G. L., Garcia, M. D., Leite, G., Lugaresi, R., & Lancha, A. H.Jr. (2021). Strategies to prevent sarcopenia in the aging process: Role of protein intake and exercise. *Nutrients*, *14*(1), 52. DOI: 10.3390/nu14010052 PMID: 35010928

Rossman, M. J., Santos-Parker, J. R., Steward, C. A., Bispham, N. Z., Cuevas, L. M., Rosenberg, H. L., & Seals, D. R. (2018). Chronic supplementation with a mitochondrial antioxidant (MitoQ) improves vascular function in healthy older adults. *Hypertension*, *71*(6), 1056–1063. DOI: 10.1161/HYPERTENSIONAHA.117.10787 PMID: 29661838

Roy, A., Das, S., Chatterjee, I., Roy, S., & Chakraborty, R. (2022). Anti-inflammatory effects of different dietary antioxidants. In *Plant Antioxidants and Health* (pp. 1–25). Springer International Publishing.

Rufini, A., Tucci, P., Celardo, I., & Melino, G. (2013). Senescence and aging: The critical roles of p53. *Oncogene*, *32*(43), 5129–5143. DOI: 10.1038/onc.2012.640 PMID: 23416979

Salameh, Y., Bejaoui, Y., & El Hajj, N. (2020). DNA methylation biomarkers in aging and age-related diseases. *Frontiers in Genetics*, *11*, 480672. DOI: 10.3389/fgene.2020.00171 PMID: 32211026

Šalamon, Š., Kramar, B., Marolt, T. P., Poljšak, B., & Milisav, I. (2019). Medical and dietary uses of N-acetylcysteine. *Antioxidants*, *8*(5), 111. DOI: 10.3390/antiox8050111 PMID: 31035402

Saliya, S. B., & Usha, D. A. (2020). Evaluation of Phytochemical Antioxidant Properties and Quantification of Thymoquinone in Nigella sativa L. Seed Extract, *International Journal of Science and Research (IJSR), Vol* (9)9, 228-234.

Santini, A., Cammarata, S. M., Capone, G., Ianaro, A., Tenore, G. C., Pani, L., & Novellino, E. (2018). Nutraceuticals: Opening the debate for a regulatory framework. *British Journal of Clinical Pharmacology*, *84*(4), 659–672. DOI: 10.1111/bcp.13496 PMID: 29433155

Santos, M. A., Franco, F. N., Caldeira, C. A., de Araújo, G. R., Vieira, A., & Chaves, M. M. (2023). Resveratrol has its antioxidant and anti-inflammatory protective mechanisms decreased in aging. *Archives of Gerontology and Geriatrics*, *107*, 104895. DOI: 10.1016/j.archger.2022.104895 PMID: 36525827

Sarisözen, B., Durak, K. E. M. A. L., Dincer, G., & Bilgen, O. F. (2002). The effects of vitamins E and C on fracture healing in rats. *The Journal of International Medical Research*, *30*(3), 309–313. DOI: 10.1177/147323000203000312 PMID: 12166348

Schleicher, E., & Friess, U. (2007). Oxidative stress, AGE, and atherosclerosis. *Kidney International*, *72*, S17–S26. DOI: 10.1038/sj.ki.5002382 PMID: 17653206

Sehar, U., Rawat, P., Reddy, A. P., Kopel, J., & Reddy, P. H. (2022). Amyloid beta in aging and Alzheimer's disease. *International Journal of Molecular Sciences*, *23*(21), 12924. DOI: 10.3390/ijms232112924 PMID: 36361714

Shanaida, M., Lysiuk, R., Mykhailenko, O., Hudz, N., Abdulsalam, A., Gontova, T., & Bjørklund, G. (2025). Alpha-lipoic acid: An antioxidant with anti-aging properties for disease therapy. *Current Medicinal Chemistry*, *32*(1), 23–54. DOI: 10.2174/0109298673300496240416114827 PMID: 38644711

Shaposhnikov, M. V., Zemskaya, N. V., Koval, L. A., Schegoleva, E. V., Zhavoronkov, A., & Moskalev, A. A. (2018). Effects of N-acetyl-L-cysteine on lifespan, locomotor activity and stress-resistance of 3 Drosophila species with different lifespans. *Aging (Albany NY)*, *10*(9), 2428–2458. DOI: 10.18632/aging.101561 PMID: 30243020

Sharief, R., & Mahaboob, A. (2020). Consequential exposure to hypothermia in gestational diabetic rats induces oxidative changes in the brain of offspring.

Shay, K. P., Moreau, R. F., Smith, E. J., Smith, A. R., & Hagen, T. M. (2009). Alpha-lipoic acid as a dietary supplement: Molecular mechanisms and therapeutic potential. Biochimica et Biophysica Acta (BBA)-. *Biochimica et Biophysica Acta. G, General Subjects*, *1790*(10), 1149–1160. DOI: 10.1016/j.bbagen.2009.07.026 PMID: 19664690

Shinohara, M., Kanekiyo, T., Tachibana, M., Kurti, A., Shinohara, M., Fu, Y., & Bu, G. (2020). APOE2 is associated with longevity independent of Alzheimer's disease. *eLife*, *9*, e62199. DOI: 10.7554/eLife.62199 PMID: 33074098

Sies, H., Stahl, W., & Sundquist, A. R. (1992). Antioxidant functions of vitamins. Vitamins E and C, beta-carotene, and other carotenoids. *Annals of the New York Academy of Sciences*, *669*(1), 7–20. DOI: 10.1111/j.1749-6632.1992.tb17085.x PMID: 1444060

Simone, C. B.II, Simone, N. L., Simone, V., & Simone, C. B. (2007). Antioxidants and other nutrients do not interfere with chemotherapy or radiation therapy and can increase kill and increase survival, Part 2. *Alternative Therapies in Health and Medicine*, *13*(2), 40–47. PMID: 17405678

Sohouli, M. H., Eslamian, G., Malekpour Alamdari, N., Abbasi, M., Fazeli Taherian, S., Behtaj, D., & Zand, H. (2023). Effects of N-acetylcysteine on aging cell and obesity complications in obese adults: A randomized, double-blind clinical trial. *Frontiers in Nutrition*, *10*, 1237869. DOI: 10.3389/fnut.2023.1237869 PMID: 37794966

Sotler, R., Poljšak, B., Dahmane, R., Jukić, T., Pavan Jukić, D., Rotim, C., & Starc, A. (2019). Prooxidant activities of antioxidants and their impact on health. *Acta Clinica Croatica, 58*(4.), 726-736.

Spulber, D. (2015). Socio-psychological aspects" happy old age" and opportunities of social services in its provision. *Историческая и социально-образовательная мысль [Historical and socio-educational thought], 7*(7 (eng)), 67-75.

Srivastava, I., Thukral, N., & Hasija, Y. (2015). Genetics of human age related disorders. *Uspekhi Gerontologii*, *28*(2), 228–247. PMID: 26856084

Steptoe, A., & Zaninotto, P. (2020). Lower socioeconomic status and the acceleration of aging: An outcome-wide analysis. *Proceedings of the National Academy of Sciences of the United States of America, 117*(26), 14911–14917. DOI: 10.1073/pnas.1915741117 PMID: 32541023

Superti, F., & Russo, R. (2024). Alpha-Lipoic Acid: Biological Mechanisms and Health Benefits. *Antioxidants, 13*(10), 1228. DOI: 10.3390/antiox13101228 PMID: 39456481

Tan, B. L., Norhaizan, M. E., & Liew, W. P. P. (2018). Nutrients and oxidative stress: Friend or foe? *Oxidative Medicine and Cellular Longevity, 2018*(1), 9719584. DOI: 10.1155/2018/9719584 PMID: 29643982

Tan, B. L., Norhaizan, M. E., Liew, W. P. P., & Sulaiman Rahman, H. (2018). Antioxidant and oxidative stress: A mutual interplay in age-related diseases. *Frontiers in Pharmacology, 9*, 1162. DOI: 10.3389/fphar.2018.01162 PMID: 30405405

Tanvetyanon, T., Eikman, E. A., Sommers, E., Robinson, L., Boulware, D., & Bepler, G. (2008). Computed tomography response, but not positron emission tomography scan response, predicts survival after neoadjuvant chemotherapy for resectable non–small-cell lung cancer. *Journal of Clinical Oncology, 26*(28), 4610–4616. DOI: 10.1200/JCO.2008.16.9383 PMID: 18824709

Tiberi, J., Cesarini, V., Stefanelli, R., Canterini, S., Fiorenza, M. T., & La Rosa, P. (2023). Sex differences in antioxidant defence and the regulation of redox homeostasis in physiology and pathology. *Mechanisms of Ageing and Development, 211*, 111802. DOI: 10.1016/j.mad.2023.111802 PMID: 36958540

To, T., Zhu, J., Larsen, K., Simatovic, J., Feldman, L., Ryckman, K., & Carlsten, C. (2016). Progression from asthma to chronic obstructive pulmonary disease. Is air pollution a risk factor? *American Journal of Respiratory and Critical Care Medicine, 194*(4), 429–438. DOI: 10.1164/rccm.201510-1932OC PMID: 26950751

Tremblay, M. S., Colley, R. C., Saunders, T. J., Healy, G. N., & Owen, N. (2010). Physiological and health implications of a sedentary lifestyle. *Applied Physiology, Nutrition, and Metabolism, 35*(6), 725–740. DOI: 10.1139/H10-079 PMID: 21164543

Trichopoulou, A. (2004). Traditional Mediterranean diet and longevity in the elderly: A review. *Public Health Nutrition, 7*(7), 943–947. DOI: 10.1079/PHN2004558 PMID: 15482622

Trovato, G. M. (2012). Behavior, nutrition and lifestyle in a comprehensive health and disease paradigm: Skills and knowledge for a predictive, preventive and personalized medicine. *The EPMA Journal, 3*(1), 1–15. DOI: 10.1007/s13167-012-0141-2 PMID: 22738244

Trujillo, J., Granados-Castro, L. F., Zazueta, C., Andérica-Romero, A. C., Chirino, Y. I., & Pedraza-Chaverrí, J. (2014). Mitochondria as a target in the therapeutic properties of curcumin. *Archiv der Pharmazie, 347*(12), 873–884. DOI: 10.1002/ardp.201400266 PMID: 25243820

Tsao, R. (2015). Synergistic interactions between antioxidants used in food preservation. In *Handbook of antioxidants for food preservation* (pp. 335–347). Woodhead Publishing. DOI: 10.1016/B978-1-78242-089-7.00013-0

Ungvari, Z., Sonntag, W. E., de Cabo, R., Baur, J. A., & Csiszar, A. (2011). Mitochondrial protection by resveratrol. *Exercise and Sport Sciences Reviews*, *39*(3), 128–132. DOI: 10.1097/JES.0b013e3182141f80 PMID: 21383627

Uzombah, T. A. (2022). The implications of replacing synthetic antioxidants with natural ones in the food systems. In *Natural food additives*. IntechOpen. DOI: 10.5772/intechopen.103810

Valenzano, D. R., & Cellerino, A. (2006). Resveratrol and the pharmacology of aging: A new vertebrate model to validate an old molecule. *Cell Cycle (Georgetown, Tex.)*, *5*(10), 1027–1032. DOI: 10.4161/cc.5.10.2739 PMID: 16687936

Vidović, B. B., Milinčić, D. D., Marčetić, M. D., Djuriš, J. D., Ilić, T. D., Kostić, A. Ž., & Pešić, M. B. (2022). Health benefits and applications of goji berries in functional food products development: A review. *Antioxidants*, *11*(2), 248. DOI: 10.3390/antiox11020248 PMID: 35204130

Vina, J., Gambini, J., Lopez-Grueso, R. M., Abdelaziz, K., Jove, M., & Borras, C. (2011). Females live longer than males: Role of oxidative stress. *Current Pharmaceutical Design*, *17*(36), 3959–3965. DOI: 10.2174/138161211798764942 PMID: 22188448

Virgili, F., & Marino, M. (2008). Regulation of cellular signals from nutritional molecules: A specific role for phytochemicals, beyond antioxidant activity. *Free Radical Biology & Medicine*, *45*(9), 1205–1216. DOI: 10.1016/j.freeradbiomed.2008.08.001 PMID: 18762244

Vivekananthan, D. P., Penn, M. S., Sapp, S. K., Hsu, A., & Topol, E. J. (2003). Use of antioxidant vitamins for the prevention of cardiovascular disease: Meta-analysis of randomised trials. *Lancet*, *361*(9374), 2017–2023. DOI: 10.1016/S0140-6736(03)13637-9 PMID: 12814711

Voetsch, B., Jin, R. C., Bierl, C., Benke, K. S., Kenet, G., Simioni, P., & Loscalzo, J. (2007). Promoter polymorphisms in the plasma glutathione peroxidase (GPx-3) gene. *Stroke*.

Wagle, S., Sim, H. J., Bhattarai, G., Choi, K. C., Kook, S. H., Lee, J. C., & Jeon, Y. M. (2021). Supplemental ferulic acid inhibits total body irradiation-mediated bone marrow damage, bone mass loss, stem cell senescence, and hematopoietic defect in mice by enhancing antioxidant defense systems. *Antioxidants*, *10*(8), 1209. DOI: 10.3390/antiox10081209 PMID: 34439457

Walter, P., Hornig, D., & Moser, U. (2001). Synergistic effects of antioxidant vitamins. In *Functions of Vitamins Beyond Recommended Dietary Allowances: European Academy of Nutritional Sciences Workshop, Nice, October 1997: Proceedings* (No. 55, p. 68). Karger Medical and Scientific Publishers.

Wang, C., Wang, C., Tang, K., Rao, Z., & Chen, J. (2022). Effects of different aging methods on the phenolic compounds and antioxidant activity of red wine. *Fermentation (Basel, Switzerland)*, *8*(11), 592. DOI: 10.3390/fermentation8110592

Wang, X., Qi, Y., & Zheng, H. (2022). Dietary polyphenol, gut microbiota, and health benefits. *Antioxidants*, *11*(6), 1212. DOI: 10.3390/antiox11061212 PMID: 35740109

Wang, Y., Zhang, Z., Chi, Y., Zhang, Q., Xu, F., Yang, Z., & Han, Z. C. (2013). Long-term cultured mesenchymal stem cells frequently develop genomic mutations but do not undergo malignant transformation. *Cell Death & Disease*, *4*(12), e950–e950. DOI: 10.1038/cddis.2013.480 PMID: 24309937

Willcox, D. C., Willcox, B. J., Hsueh, W. C., & Suzuki, M. (2006). Genetic determinants of exceptional human longevity: Insights from the Okinawa Centenarian Study. *Age (Dordrecht, Netherlands)*, *28*(4), 313–332. DOI: 10.1007/s11357-006-9020-x PMID: 22253498

Willie-Tyndale, D., Holder-Nevins, D., Mitchell-Fearon, K., James, K., Laws, H., Waldron, N. K., & Eldemire-Shearer, D. (2016). Participation in social activities and the association with socio-demographic and health-related factors among community-dwelling older adults in Jamaica. *Journal of Cross-Cultural Gerontology*, *31*(4), 427–447. DOI: 10.1007/s10823-016-9297-x PMID: 27475790

Xu, T., Tao, M., Li, R., Xu, X., Pan, S., & Wu, T. (2022). Longevity-promoting properties of ginger extract in Caenorhabditis elegans via the insulin/IGF-1 signaling pathway. *Food & Function*, *13*(19), 9893–9903. DOI: 10.1039/D2FO01602H PMID: 36052763

Yang, H., Qazi, I. H., Pan, B., Angel, C., Guo, S., Yang, J., & Zhou, G. (2019). Dietary selenium supplementation ameliorates female reproductive efficiency in aging mice. *Antioxidants*, *8*(12), 634. DOI: 10.3390/antiox8120634 PMID: 31835711

Yang, J., Luo, J., Tian, X., Zhao, Y., Li, Y., & Wu, X. (2024). Progress in understanding oxidative stress, aging, and aging-related diseases. *Antioxidants*, *13*(4), 394. DOI: 10.3390/antiox13040394 PMID: 38671842

Yang, W., & Omaye, S. T. (2009). Air pollutants, oxidative stress and human health. *Mutation Research/Genetic Toxicology and Environmental Mutagenesis*, *674*(1-2), 45–54. DOI: 10.1016/j.mrgentox.2008.10.005 PMID: 19013537

Yang, Z., Zhang, Y., Yang, S., Ding, Y., & Qu, Y. (2022). Low-dose resveratrol inhibits RIPK3-mediated necroptosis and delays the onset of age-related hearing loss. *Frontiers in Pharmacology*, *13*, 910308. DOI: 10.3389/fphar.2022.910308 PMID: 35846996

Zhang, H., & Tsao, R. (2016). Dietary polyphenols, oxidative stress and antioxidant and anti-inflammatory effects. *Current Opinion in Food Science*, *8*, 33–42. DOI: 10.1016/j.cofs.2016.02.002

Zhang, Y., Chen, X., Yang, L., Zu, Y., & Lu, Q. (2015). Effects of rosmarinic acid on liver and kidney antioxidant enzymes, lipid peroxidation and tissue ultrastructure in aging mice. *Food & Function*, *6*(3), 927–931. DOI: 10.1039/C4FO01051E PMID: 25635678

Zhen, A. X., Piao, M. J., Kang, K. A., Fernando, P. D. S. M., Kang, H. K., Koh, Y. S., & Hyun, J. W. (2019). Niacinamide protects skin cells from oxidative stress induced by particulate matter. *Biomolecules & Therapeutics*, *27*(6), 562–569. DOI: 10.4062/biomolther.2019.061 PMID: 31272139

Ziv, E., & Hu, D. (2011). Genetic variation in insulin/IGF-1 signaling pathways and longevity. *Ageing Research Reviews*, *10*(2), 201–204. DOI: 10.1016/j.arr.2010.09.002 PMID: 20868776

Zuo, L., Prather, E. R., Stetskiv, M., Garrison, D. E., Meade, J. R., Peace, T. I., & Zhou, T. (2019). Inflammaging and oxidative stress in human diseases: From molecular mechanisms to novel treatments. *International Journal of Molecular Sciences*, *20*(18), 4472. DOI: 10.3390/ijms20184472 PMID: 31510091

Chapter 9
Herbal Solutions for Longevity:
Anti-Ageing Compounds From Traditional Medicine

Tiago Manuel Horta Reis da Silva
https://orcid.org/0000-0001-5220-1718
King's College London, UK

ABSTRACT

This chapter delves into the realm of traditional medicine to uncover natural compounds with potential anti-ageing properties. It examines the historical context and foundational principles of traditional medical systems, emphasising their holistic approaches to health and longevity. The chapter identifies key herbal compounds renowned for their anti-ageing effects, exploring their mechanisms of action, including antioxidant activity, anti-inflammatory properties, and modulation of cellular pathways. Furthermore, it evaluates the scientific evidence supporting these claims, discusses the integration of these herbal solutions into modern healthcare, and addresses safety considerations. The chapter concludes by highlighting future research directions and the importance of a balanced approach to incorporating traditional herbal remedies into contemporary anti-ageing strategies.

1. INTRODUCTION

The phenomenon of ageing has garnered significant attention in contemporary research, particularly as it relates to the quest for longevity. Ageing is not merely a biological process but a multifaceted phenomenon influenced by genetic, environmental, and lifestyle factors (Reis da Silva, 2024a; Reis da Silva, 2025a). The complexities of ageing are underscored by its association with various chronic diseases, including cardiovascular diseases, diabetes, and neurodegenerative disorders, which collectively contribute to a decline in healthspan — the period of life spent in good health (Fischer et al., 2022; Raymond, 2024; Reis da Silva, 2024b). As the global population ages, understanding the mechanisms underlying ageing and identifying strategies to enhance longevity and healthspan have become paramount (Reis da

DOI: 10.4018/979-8-3693-9730-5.ch009

Silva, 2023; Lyu, 2024; Reis da Silva, 2024c). This chapter aims to provide a comprehensive overview of ageing, the quest for longevity, and the role of traditional medicine in promoting healthspan.

Traditional medicine has long been a cornerstone of health practices across various cultures, offering insights into holistic approaches to health and longevity (Reis da Silva, 2025b). Many traditional medicinal systems emphasise the importance of maintaining balance within the body, often through the use of natural compounds derived from plants and herbs (Reis da Silva, 2025b). Recent studies have highlighted the potential of these natural compounds, such as resveratrol and metformin, in promoting longevity and mitigating age-related decline (Todorova, 2024). Moreover, the integration of traditional medicine with modern scientific research has opened new avenues for understanding the biochemical pathways involved in aging and longevity (Pasupuleti, 2024). This chapter will explore how traditional medicine contributes to the broader discourse on healthspan and longevity, providing a synthesis of historical practices and contemporary scientific findings.

The purpose of this chapter is to elucidate the intricate relationship between ageing, longevity, and traditional medicine. By examining the historical context and current scientific advancements, the aim is to highlight the potential of traditional medicinal practices in enhancing healthspan and promoting longevity. The scope of this chapter encompasses a review of ageing mechanisms, the role of traditional medicine in health promotion, and an exploration of emerging research that bridges these domains. Through this comprehensive analysis, we seek to contribute to the ongoing dialogue surrounding aging and longevity, emphasising the importance of an integrative approach that respects both traditional knowledge and modern scientific inquiry.

2. FOUNDATIONS OF TRADITIONAL MEDICINE

The exploration of traditional medicine offers a rich tapestry of historical perspectives on ageing, health, and longevity. Various traditional medical systems have developed unique frameworks that reflect their cultural, spiritual, and philosophical underpinnings (Reis da Silva, 2025b). For instance, African traditional medicine encompasses a holistic health care system that integrates divination, spiritualism, and herbalism, emphasising the interconnectedness of mind, body, and spirit in the healing process (Ozioma & NwamakaChinwe, 2019). Similarly, Ayurveda, one of the oldest medical systems in the world, provides insights into healthy living and longevity through its principles of balance and harmony within the body (Yao et al., 2023). These historical perspectives reveal that ageing is not merely a biological phenomenon but is deeply influenced by cultural beliefs and practices that have evolved over centuries.

The core principles guiding these traditional approaches to ageing often revolve around the concepts of balance, harmony, and the interconnectedness of body, mind, and spirit. Traditional medical systems emphasise preventive care and the maintenance of health rather than merely treating diseases as they arise. This preventive focus is evident in practices such as regular detoxification in Ayurveda and the seasonal adjustments in diet and lifestyle recommended in TCM (Yadav, 2024; Wang, 2024). The historical emphasis on prevention and holistic care reflects a deep understanding of the ageing process and its implications for overall health.

A comparative analysis of different traditional medical practices reveals both commonalities and distinctions in their approaches to ageing. While Ayurveda and TCM share a holistic perspective, their methodologies and specific practices differ significantly. Ayurveda employs a personalised approach based on individual constitution (Prakriti), whereas TCM focuses on the balance of energy and the flow of Qi (Yadav, 2024; Wang, 2024). Additionally, indigenous healing practices often incorporate spiritual elements that may not be as pronounced in Ayurveda or TCM, highlighting the diverse ways in which cultures understand and address aging (Baez, 2024; Abdullah, 2023).

2.1 Historical Perspectives on Ageing in Traditional Medical Systems

The historical perspectives on ageing in traditional medical systems provide a rich context for understanding how various cultures have approached the complexities of ageing and health. Traditional medical systems, such as Ayurveda, Traditional Chinese Medicine (TCM), and indigenous healing practices, have long recognised ageing as a multifaceted process influenced by physical, emotional, and spiritual factors. These systems have developed unique frameworks that not only address the biological aspects of ageing but also emphasise the importance of maintaining balance and harmony within the individual (Elendu, 2024).

In Ayurveda, for instance, the concept of "Rasayana," which translates to rejuvenation, plays a pivotal role in promoting longevity and vitality. This ancient Indian system of medicine emphasises the use of specific herbs, dietary practices, and lifestyle modifications to enhance overall health and mitigate the effects of ageing (Yadav, 2024; Baliga et al., 2015). The historical texts of Ayurveda detail various regenerative therapies that have been practiced for centuries, showcasing a holistic understanding of health that integrates physical, mental, and spiritual well-being (Yadav, 2024). Similarly, TCM has a profound historical perspective on ageing, where concepts such as Qi (vital energy) and the balance of Yin and Yang are central to maintaining health throughout the ageing process. TCM practitioners utilise herbal remedies, acupuncture, and dietary recommendations to support the body's natural resilience against age-related decline (Wang, 2024).

Moreover, indigenous healing systems across the globe have their own historical narratives regarding ageing. For example, many Native American tribes view ageing as a natural progression that is honoured and respected within their communities. Elders are often seen as repositories of wisdom and knowledge, and traditional practices are employed to ensure their health and well-being (Baez, 2024; Abdullah, 2023). These cultural perspectives highlight the importance of community and social support in the ageing process, contrasting with more individualistic approaches often found in Western medicine.

2.2 Core Principles Guiding Traditional Approaches to Health and Longevity

Core principles guiding traditional approaches to health and longevity often revolve around the concepts of balance, harmony, and the integration of physical, mental, and spiritual health. In Traditional Chinese Medicine, for example, the philosophy of yin and yang illustrates the importance of balance in maintaining health and preventing disease. While the reference provided Liu et al. (2023) discusses the role of TCM in self-care practices, it does not specifically address the philosophy of yin and yang or its implications for ageing. Therefore, this claim will be stated without citation. Furthermore, traditional practices often emphasise the use of natural remedies, such as herbal medicines, which have been utilized for centuries to support health and mitigate the effects of ageing (Jütte et al., 2017). The holistic nature of these approaches underscores the significance of lifestyle factors, including diet, exercise, and mental well-being, in promoting a longer, healthier life.

2.3 Comparative Analysis of Different Traditional Medical Practices

A comparative analysis of different traditional medical practices reveals both unique methodologies and shared philosophies across cultures. For instance, while African traditional medicine focuses on spiritual and communal aspects of healing, Ayurveda emphasises dietary practices and herbal formulations tailored to individual constitutions (Ozioma & NwamakaChinwe, 2019; Yao et al., 2023). In contrast, TCM employs a systematic approach that includes acupuncture, herbal medicine, and dietary therapy, all aimed at restoring balance and harmony within the body. Despite these differences, a common thread among these systems is the recognition of the individual's role in their health and the importance of preventive measures in managing ageing and promoting longevity. This comparative perspective not only highlights the diversity of traditional medical practices but also emphasises the potential for integrating these approaches into contemporary health care systems to enhance overall well-being.

3. KEY HERBAL COMPOUNDS WITH ANTI-AGEING POTENTIAL

The identification of prominent herbs used in traditional medicine for longevity reveals a wealth of knowledge accumulated over centuries. Various cultures have harnessed the therapeutic potential of specific plants to promote health and mitigate the effects of ageing. For instance, in TCM, herbs such as Ginseng (Panax ginseng) and Goji berries (Lycium barbarum) are renowned for their adaptogenic and antioxidant properties, respectively, which are believed to enhance vitality and longevity (Cho et al., 2023). Similarly, Ayurvedic practices highlight the use of Ashwagandha (Withania somnifera) and Turmeric (Curcuma longa) for their rejuvenating effects and ability to combat oxidative stress (Kim, 2023; Luo et al., 2019). These herbs not only reflect the traditional wisdom of their respective cultures but also serve as a foundation for contemporary research into their anti-ageing potential.

The phytochemical constituents relevant to anti-ageing found in these herbs include a variety of bioactive compounds known for their antioxidant, anti-inflammatory, and neuroprotective properties. For example, curcumin, the active component of turmeric, has been shown to possess potent antioxidant activities, which help in neutralising free radicals and reducing oxidative stress associated with ageing (Sharifi-Rad et al., 2020). Similarly, flavonoids such as quercetin and resveratrol, found in various plants, exhibit significant anti-inflammatory effects and have been linked to improved cardiovascular health and longevity (Chaiyana et al., 2021; Sharifi-Rad et al., 2020). These phytochemicals not only contribute to the therapeutic effects of traditional herbs but also provide a scientific basis for their use in promoting healthspan and longevity.

Traditional uses of these herbs often encompass a holistic approach to health, integrating physical, mental, and spiritual well-being. For instance, Ginseng has been traditionally used to enhance energy levels and improve mental clarity, while Goji berries are consumed for their purported benefits in promoting eye health and boosting the immune system (Sangkaew, 2024). Contemporary applications of these herbs have expanded to include dietary supplements, functional foods, and topical formulations aimed at addressing age-related concerns such as skin ageing and cognitive decline. Recent studies have demonstrated the efficacy of herbal extracts in clinical settings, highlighting their potential as complementary therapies in modern medicine (Karapetyan & Barseghyan, 2022; Sharifi-Rad et al., 2020).

Moreover, the integration of traditional herbal medicine with modern scientific methodologies has led to the discovery of novel formulations and delivery systems that enhance the bioavailability and efficacy of these compounds. For example, the development of herbal nanocosmetics has shown promise in improving skin hydration and elasticity, thereby addressing signs of ageing (Sharifi-Rad et al., 2020). Additionally, research into the synergistic effects of herbal combinations has revealed enhanced therapeutic outcomes, further validating the traditional practices of using multiple herbs in conjunction (Chang et al., 2021).

3.1 Prominent Herbs Used in Traditional Medicine for Longevity

Traditional medicine systems across the globe have long recognised the importance of specific herbs in promoting longevity and mitigating the effects of ageing. For instance, **Ginseng** (Panax ginseng) is a cornerstone of Traditional Chinese Medicine (TCM), celebrated for its adaptogenic properties that enhance vitality and resilience against stress (Xia et al., 2022). Similarly, **Ashwagandha** (Withania somnifera), a prominent herb in Ayurveda, is revered for its ability to rejuvenate the body and mind, thereby supporting overall health and longevity (Hussain et al., 2023). Other notable herbs include **Goji berries** (Lycium barbarum), known for their antioxidant properties, and **Turmeric** (Curcuma longa), which contains curcumin, a compound recognised for its anti-inflammatory and neuroprotective effects (Jazani et al., 2019).

In addition to these well-known herbs, lesser-known plants such as **Dendrobium** species have also been utilized in traditional practices for their tonic and anti-ageing properties (Čáková et al., 2017). The historical use of these herbs is often documented in ancient texts, which detail their applications in enhancing health and prolonging life. For example, the **Donguibogam**, a classic Korean medical text, lists numerous herbs with anti-ageing effects, emphasising the holistic approach of traditional medicine in addressing the aging process (Čáková et al., 2017).

3.2 Phytochemical Constituents Relevant to Anti-Aging

The efficacy of these herbs in promoting longevity can be attributed to their rich phytochemical profiles. Many of these plants contain a variety of bioactive compounds that exhibit antioxidant, anti-inflammatory, and neuroprotective properties. For instance, Ginseng is rich in ginsenosides, which have been shown to enhance cognitive function and reduce oxidative stress (Xia et al., 2022). Similarly, Ashwagandha contains withanolides, which are known for their ability to combat oxidative stress and inflammation, thereby contributing to its anti-ageing effects (Kumar et al., 2015).

Curcumin, the active ingredient in turmeric, is another potent phytochemical that has garnered attention for its ability to modulate multiple signaling pathways involved in ageing and age-related diseases (Jazani et al., 2019). Studies have demonstrated that curcumin can inhibit the NF-κB pathway, which plays a crucial role in inflammation and aging (Park, 2024). Additionally, Goji berries are rich in carotenoids and polysaccharides, compounds that contribute to their antioxidant capacity and potential to enhance immune function (Jazani et al., 2019).

Moreover, the synergistic effects of these phytochemicals are significant. For example, the combination of ginsenosides from Ginseng and curcumin from turmeric has been shown to enhance neuroprotective effects, suggesting that multi-herb formulations may offer greater benefits than single-herb extracts (Eng et al., 2019). This highlights the importance of understanding the complex interactions between various phytochemicals in traditional herbal medicine.

3.3 Traditional Uses and Contemporary Applications

Historically, these herbs have been employed in various forms, including teas, tinctures, and powders, to promote health and longevity. In Ayurveda, Ashwagandha is often used as a rejuvenating tonic, particularly for the elderly, to enhance vitality and reduce the effects of stress (Hussain et al., 2023). Similarly, Ginseng has been traditionally consumed to improve energy levels and cognitive function, making it a popular choice among older adults seeking to maintain their mental acuity (Xia et al., 2022). In contemporary applications, the use of these herbs has expanded significantly. The rise of the wellness industry has led to the incorporation of traditional herbs into dietary supplements, functional foods, and skincare products. For instance, Turmeric is now widely available as a dietary supplement due to its anti-inflammatory properties, while Ginseng is commonly found in energy drinks and health supplements aimed at enhancing physical and mental performance (Jazani et al., 2019).

Furthermore, modern research has validated many of the traditional uses of these herbs. Clinical studies have demonstrated the efficacy of Goji berries in improving immune function and reducing oxidative stress, aligning with their historical applications in traditional medicine (Jazani et al., 2019). Similarly, the neuroprotective effects of Ginseng and Ashwagandha have been substantiated through various scientific investigations, reinforcing their roles in contemporary health practices (Xia et al., 2022; Kumar et al., 2015). The integration of traditional herbal medicine with modern scientific methodologies has also led to the development of novel formulations that enhance the bioavailability and efficacy of these compounds. For example, the use of nanotechnology in delivering herbal extracts has shown promise in improving their therapeutic effects, particularly in skincare applications (Kanlayavattanakul, 2024). This innovative approach not only preserves the traditional knowledge surrounding these herbs but also adapts it to meet the demands of modern consumers.

4. MECHANISMS OF ACTION

The mechanisms through which herbal compounds exert their anti-ageing effects are multifaceted, encompassing antioxidant activities, anti-inflammatory effects, modulation of cellular senescence and apoptosis, and influences on metabolic and hormonal regulation. Understanding these mechanisms is crucial for harnessing the therapeutic potential of herbal medicine in promoting longevity and mitigating age-related diseases.

4.1 Antioxidant Activities

Oxidative stress, characterised by an imbalance between reactive oxygen species (ROS) production and antioxidant defenses, is a significant contributor to ageing and age-related diseases. Herbal compounds exhibit potent antioxidant activities that help neutralise ROS, thereby reducing oxidative damage to cellular components such as lipids, proteins, and DNA (Sharma et al., 2019; Park et al., 2021). For instance, ***Curcuma longa*** (turmeric) contains curcumin, a well-known antioxidant that has been shown to scavenge free radicals and enhance the body's endogenous antioxidant defenses (Cai et al., 2021).

Similarly, ***Zingiber officinale*** (ginger) has been reported to possess strong antioxidant properties, which contribute to its protective effects against oxidative stress-related conditions (Park et al., 2021).

The antioxidant mechanisms of these herbs often involve the upregulation of antioxidant enzymes such as superoxide dismutase (SOD), catalase, and glutathione peroxidase (Shivlingesh et al., 2024). For example, studies have demonstrated that extracts from ***Cinnamomum verum*** (cinnamon) can enhance the activity of these enzymes, thereby providing a protective effect against oxidative stress (Hamidpour et al., 2015). Moreover, the polyphenolic compounds found in various herbs, such as flavonoids and phenolic acids, play a crucial role in their antioxidant activities by donating electrons to neutralize free radicals (Adha, 2025). This electron donation not only mitigates oxidative stress but also prevents the initiation of lipid peroxidation, a process that can lead to cellular damage and aging (Hamidpour et al., 2015).

4.2 Anti-Inflammatory Effects and Modulation of Inflammatory Pathways

Chronic inflammation is another critical factor in the ageing process, contributing to the development of various age-related diseases, including cardiovascular diseases, neurodegenerative disorders, and cancer (Reis da Silva, 2024b). Herbal medicines have been shown to possess significant anti-inflammatory properties, which can modulate inflammatory pathways and reduce the risk of these diseases (Wang, 2024; Chi et al., 2021). For instance, ***Boswellia serrata*** has been extensively studied for its ability to inhibit pro-inflammatory cytokines such as TNF-α and IL-6, thereby alleviating inflammation (Komariah et al., 2023).

The anti-inflammatory effects of herbal compounds often involve the inhibition of key signaling pathways, including the nuclear factor-kappa B (NF-κB) and mitogen-activated protein kinase (MAPK) pathways. By inhibiting these pathways, herbal extracts can reduce the expression of inflammatory mediators and cytokines, leading to decreased inflammation (Nurani et al., 2021; Rui, 2023). For example, ***Glycyrrhiza glabra*** (licorice) has been shown to inhibit the activation of NF-κB, thereby reducing the production of inflammatory cytokines (Iitsuka et al., 2018). Furthermore, the anti-inflammatory effects of herbs can also be attributed to their ability to modulate the immune response, promoting a balanced immune system that can effectively respond to pathogens while minimizing excessive inflammation (Thariwong et al., 2021).

4.3 Influence on Cellular Senescence and Apoptosis

Cellular senescence, characterised by a permanent state of cell cycle arrest, is a hallmark of ageing and contributes to tissue dysfunction and the aging process. Herbal compounds have been shown to influence cellular senescence and apoptosis, thereby promoting healthier ageing. For instance, ***Withania somnifera*** (ashwagandha) has been reported to induce apoptosis in cancer cells while protecting normal cells from oxidative stress-induced senescence (Ghahremanlo et al., 2018). This selective induction of apoptosis is crucial for eliminating damaged cells that could otherwise contribute to ageing and disease.

Moreover, certain herbal compounds can modulate the expression of genes associated with senescence and apoptosis. For example, **Curcumin** has been shown to downregulate the expression of p53, a key regulator of the cell cycle and apoptosis, thereby promoting cell survival under stress conditions (Qiang et al., 2023). Additionally, the activation of sirtuins, a family of proteins involved in cellular regulation and longevity, has been linked to the consumption of various herbal compounds, including resveratrol found in ***Vitis vinifera*** (grapes) (Ara et al., 2018). Sirtuins play a vital role in promoting cellular health by enhancing DNA repair mechanisms and regulating metabolic processes, ultimately influencing the aging process.

4.4 Impact on Metabolic and Hormonal Regulation

Herbal compounds also exert significant effects on metabolic and hormonal regulation, which are essential for maintaining overall health and longevity. For instance, **Cinnamon** has been shown to improve insulin sensitivity and regulate blood glucose levels, making it a valuable herb for managing metabolic disorders such as type 2 diabetes (Kusmardi et al., 2021). The active components in cinnamon, such as cinnamaldehyde, have been demonstrated to enhance insulin signalling pathways, thereby promoting better glucose metabolism (Ahn et al., 2022).

In addition to metabolic regulation, herbal medicines can also influence hormonal balance. For example, **Ashwagandha** has been reported to reduce cortisol levels, a hormone associated with stress, thereby promoting a balanced hormonal environment conducive to health and longevity (Suh et al., 2021). The adaptogenic properties of ashwagandha help the body cope with stress, which is crucial for maintaining hormonal balance and preventing the negative effects of chronic stress on health.

Furthermore, the modulation of metabolic pathways by herbal compounds can have far-reaching effects on overall health. For instance, ***Camellia sinensis*** (green tea) contains catechins, which have been shown to enhance lipid metabolism and promote weight loss (Cho, 2023). This effect is particularly important in the context of ageing, as maintaining a healthy weight is associated with a reduced risk of age-related diseases.

5. SCIENTIFIC EVIDENCE AND CLINICAL STUDIES

The quest for effective anti-ageing interventions has led to a growing body of research focused on the potential of herbal compounds. This section reviews the scientific evidence supporting the anti-ageing claims of various herbs, highlighting in vitro and in vivo studies, clinical trials evaluating efficacy and safety, and a critical appraisal of existing research to identify gaps.

5.1 Review of In Vitro and In Vivo Studies Supporting Anti-Ageing Claims

Numerous in vitro studies have demonstrated the anti-aging potential of various herbal compounds through mechanisms such as antioxidant activity, anti-inflammatory effects, and modulation of cellular senescence. For instance, **Quercetin**, a flavonoid found in many fruits and vegetables, has been shown to exhibit significant antioxidant and anti-inflammatory properties. In vitro studies indicate that quercetin can reduce oxidative stress and inflammation in human cells, which are critical factors in the aging process (Shen et al., 2021). Furthermore, quercetin has been reported to attenuate the effects of age-related diseases, such as rheumatoid arthritis and inflammatory bowel disease, in animal models (Shen et al., 2021).

Another notable example is ***Lycium barbarum*** (goji berries), which has been extensively studied for its antioxidant properties. Gao et al. (2017) reported that extracts from Lycium barbarum can enhance the body's endogenous antioxidant defenses, thereby reducing oxidative damage associated with ageing. In vivo studies have shown that these extracts can improve cognitive function and protect against neurodegenerative diseases in aged mice, supporting their traditional use in promoting longevity (Gao et al., 2017).

In addition to antioxidant effects, several herbs have demonstrated anti-inflammatory properties that contribute to their anti-ageing potential. For example, **Ginger** (*Zingiber officinale*) and **Turmeric** (*Curcuma longa*) have been shown to inhibit pro-inflammatory cytokines and pathways, such as NF-κB and MAPK, in various cell types (Zhou et al., 2022; Özkur et al., 2022). In vitro studies have indicated that these herbs can significantly reduce inflammation in human keratinocytes and fibroblasts, which are essential for skin health and ageing (Zhou et al., 2022). Moreover, in vivo studies have confirmed that ginger and turmeric can alleviate inflammation and oxidative stress in animal models, further supporting their role in healthy aging (Özkur et al., 2022).

5.2 Clinical Trials Evaluating Efficacy and Safety

Clinical trials investigating the efficacy and safety of herbal compounds for anti-ageing purposes have also emerged. For instance, a systematic review of clinical trials involving **Ginseng** (*Panax ginseng*) highlighted its potential benefits in improving cognitive function, reducing fatigue, and enhancing overall well-being in older adults (Szczuka et al., 2019). The review concluded that while ginseng is generally safe, further large-scale studies are needed to establish definitive efficacy and safety profiles.

Similarly, clinical trials evaluating the effects of **Ashwagandha** (*Withania somnifera*) on stress reduction and cognitive function in older adults have shown promising results. Participants reported significant improvements in stress levels and cognitive performance after supplementation with ashwagandha extract (Raguraman & Subramaniam, 2016). These findings align with the herb's traditional use in Ayurvedic medicine as a rejuvenating tonic.

Moreover, a meta-analysis examining the effects of Qigong, which incorporates traditional Chinese medicine principles, found that this practice could improve various health parameters associated with ageing, including balance, flexibility, and mental health (Yu et al., 2020). However, the authors noted that the quality of the included studies varied, and more rigorous trials are necessary to confirm these benefits.

Despite the promising results from clinical trials, there remains a need for further research to establish standardised dosages, long-term safety, and the mechanisms underlying the observed benefits. Many studies have small sample sizes and lack control groups, which limits the generalizability of their findings.

5.3 Critical Appraisal of Existing Research and Identification of Gaps

While the existing body of research provides valuable insights into the anti-ageing potential of herbal compounds, several gaps and limitations warrant attention. First, many studies focus on single herbs or compounds, neglecting the potential synergistic effects of multi-herb formulations commonly used in traditional medicine. For example, the combination of ginger and turmeric has been shown to enhance anti-inflammatory effects beyond those of each herb alone (Zhou et al., 2022). Future research should explore the efficacy of these combinations in both in vitro and clinical settings.

Second, the majority of studies rely on animal models or in vitro systems, which may not fully replicate human physiology. Although these models are essential for understanding mechanisms of action, clinical trials are crucial for confirming efficacy and safety in human populations. There is a pressing need for well-designed, large-scale clinical trials that assess the long-term effects of herbal interventions on ageing-related outcomes. Additionally, the variability in the quality and preparation of herbal products poses a challenge for research. Factors such as growing conditions, harvesting methods, and extraction processes can significantly influence the bioactive content of herbal preparations (Gao et al., 2017). Standardisation of herbal products is essential to ensure consistent dosing and efficacy across studies.

Furthermore, the mechanisms by which herbal compounds exert their anti-ageing effects remain poorly understood. While many studies have identified antioxidant and anti-inflammatory activities, the specific pathways and molecular targets involved in these processes require further elucidation. For instance, the role of non-coding RNAs in the regulation of ageing-related pathways is an emerging area of research that has yet to be explored in the context of herbal medicine (Dong et al., 2019).

Finally, there is a need for interdisciplinary approaches that integrate traditional knowledge with modern scientific methodologies. Collaborations between herbalists, pharmacologists, and clinical researchers can facilitate the development of evidence-based herbal interventions for ageing and age-related diseases.

6. INTEGRATION INTO MODERN HEALTHCARE

The integration of herbal solutions into modern healthcare presents both challenges and opportunities. As interest in complementary and alternative medicine continues to grow, there is an increasing recognition of the potential benefits of herbal remedies in promoting health and longevity. However, several barriers must be addressed to facilitate their incorporation into mainstream medical practice. This section explores the challenges and opportunities associated with integrating herbal solutions, regulatory considerations for standardization, and case studies of successful integrative approaches.

6.1 Challenges and Opportunities in Incorporating Herbal Solutions

One of the primary challenges in integrating herbal solutions into modern healthcare is the lack of standardised dosing and quality control. Unlike pharmaceutical drugs, which undergo rigorous testing and regulation, herbal products often vary significantly in their composition, potency, and purity. This variability can lead to inconsistent therapeutic outcomes and raises concerns about safety and efficacy (Zhang et al., 2020; Peltzer & Pengpid, 2019). For instance, a study conducted in Thailand found that many chronic disease patients used herbal medicines without proper guidance, leading to potential interactions with conventional medications (Peltzer & Pengpid, 2019). This underscores the need for healthcare providers to be well-informed about herbal remedies to ensure safe and effective use.

Another challenge is the prevailing scepticism among some healthcare professionals regarding the efficacy of herbal medicine. Despite a growing body of evidence supporting the benefits of various herbal compounds, many practitioners remain unconvinced due to a lack of high-quality clinical trials and standardised research methodologies (Jung, 2024). This scepticism can hinder the acceptance of herbal solutions as viable treatment options within conventional medical settings.

However, there are significant opportunities for integrating herbal solutions into modern healthcare. The increasing consumer demand for natural and holistic approaches to health has prompted many healthcare providers to explore complementary therapies, including herbal medicine. For example, the use of herbal supplements alongside conventional cancer treatments has gained traction, with studies indicating that certain herbal compounds can enhance the efficacy of chemotherapy while reducing side effects (Pandeya et al., 2021; Cho et al., 2023). This presents an opportunity for healthcare professionals to adopt a more integrative approach, combining the strengths of both conventional and herbal medicine.

Moreover, the growing interest in personalised medicine aligns well with herbal solutions, as many herbal remedies can be tailored to individual patient needs. By considering factors such as genetics, lifestyle, and health status, healthcare providers can develop personalised herbal treatment plans that complement conventional therapies (Hawash, 2024). This personalised approach not only enhances patient satisfaction but also improves treatment outcomes.

6.2 Regulatory Considerations and Standardization of Herbal Products

The regulatory landscape for herbal products varies significantly across countries, impacting their integration into modern healthcare. In some regions, herbal medicines are classified as dietary supplements, which may not require the same level of scrutiny as pharmaceutical drugs. This lack of regulation can lead to concerns about product quality, safety, and efficacy (Domfeh et al., 2023). For instance, a systematic review highlighted the prevalence of undeclared synthetic pharmaceuticals in herbal weight loss products, raising significant safety concerns (Adha, 2025).

To address these issues, there is a pressing need for standardised regulations governing the production, labelling, and marketing of herbal products. Regulatory bodies should establish clear guidelines for quality control, ensuring that herbal remedies meet specific safety and efficacy standards. This could involve implementing Good Manufacturing Practices (GMP) for herbal products, similar to those required for pharmaceutical manufacturing (Ahn et al., 2022). Such regulations would not only enhance consumer confidence in herbal remedies but also facilitate their acceptance within the medical community.

Standardisation of herbal products is also crucial for research purposes. Many studies have reported variations in the bioactive constituents of herbal preparations due to differences in growing conditions, harvesting methods, and extraction processes (Vasudev et al., 2021). Establishing standardised extraction methods

7. SAFETY AND ETHICAL CONSIDERATIONS

The integration of herbal medicine into modern healthcare systems raises significant safety and ethical considerations. While herbal remedies are often perceived as safe due to their natural origins, they can pose risks, including potential adverse effects and herb-drug interactions. Additionally, ethical issues related to sourcing and using traditional herbs must be addressed to ensure responsible practices. This section discusses these aspects in detail, providing guidelines for practitioners and consumers.

7.1 Potential Adverse Effects and Herb-Drug Interactions

Despite the common belief that herbal remedies are safer than conventional pharmaceuticals, they can cause adverse effects and interact with prescribed medications. A systematic review by Jayasinghe and Jayawardena (2019) highlighted that while herbal medicine is often perceived as safe, there are documented cases of toxicity associated with various herbal products. For instance, certain herbs can lead to gastrointestinal distress, allergic reactions, or even more severe complications such as liver damage (Amadi & Orisakwe, 2018).

Moreover, herb-drug interactions can significantly impact patient safety. Many patients using herbal remedies do not disclose this information to their healthcare providers, which can lead to unintended consequences. Alqathama et al. (2020) found that nearly half of the diabetic patients surveyed did not consult their doctors before starting herbal remedies, which raises concerns about potential interactions with diabetes medications. Such interactions can either enhance or diminish the effects of conventional drugs, leading to suboptimal therapeutic outcomes or increased toxicity.

For example, **St. John's Wort** (*Hypericum perforatum*) is known to induce cytochrome P450 enzymes, which can accelerate the metabolism of various medications, including antidepressants and anticoagulants, potentially reducing their effectiveness (Izzo et al., 2016). Similarly, **Ginger** and **Garlic** have been reported to interact with anticoagulant medications, increasing the risk of bleeding (Alhumaid, 2023). These examples underscore the importance of healthcare providers being aware of patients' herbal use to manage potential risks effectively.

7.2 Ethical Issues in Sourcing and Using Traditional Herbs

The ethical considerations surrounding the sourcing and use of traditional herbs are multifaceted. One major concern is the sustainability of herbal resources. Overharvesting of certain plants can lead to depletion of natural populations, threatening biodiversity and the livelihoods of communities that rely on these resources (Alanazi, 2023). Ethical sourcing practices are essential to ensure that herbal products are obtained sustainably and do not contribute to environmental degradation.

Additionally, there are ethical implications related to the commercialisation of traditional knowledge. Indigenous communities often possess extensive knowledge about the medicinal properties of local plants, which has been passed down through generations. However, the appropriation of this knowledge by commercial enterprises without proper compensation or acknowledgment raises ethical concerns (Alhur, 2024). It is crucial to establish fair trade practices and benefit-sharing agreements that respect the rights of indigenous peoples and ensure they receive recognition and compensation for their contributions to herbal medicine.

Furthermore, the lack of regulation surrounding herbal products can lead to issues of quality and safety. Many herbal remedies are marketed without adequate testing for efficacy or safety, putting consumers at risk. Ethical marketing practices should ensure that consumers are well-informed about the potential risks and benefits of herbal products, as well as any scientific evidence supporting their use (Yazıcı & Güney, 2023).

7.3 Guidelines for Practitioners and Consumers

To navigate the complexities of herbal medicine safely and ethically, several guidelines can be established for both practitioners and consumers:

1. **Education and Training:** Healthcare practitioners should receive training in herbal medicine to understand the potential benefits and risks associated with herbal remedies. This knowledge will enable them to provide informed recommendations and monitor for potential herb-drug interactions (Ali, 2024).

2. **Open Communication:** Patients should be encouraged to disclose their use of herbal remedies to their healthcare providers. Open communication can help identify potential interactions and ensure that all aspects of a patient's treatment plan are coordinated effectively (Sharifi-Rad et al., 2018).
3. **Quality Assurance:** Consumers should seek herbal products from reputable sources that adhere to quality control standards. Certifications from regulatory bodies can help ensure that herbal products are safe, effective, and free from contaminants (Elmaghraby, 2023).
4. **Informed Decision-Making:** Consumers should be educated about the potential risks and benefits of herbal remedies. This includes understanding that "natural" does not always equate to "safe" and that herbal products can have side effects and interactions similar to conventional medications (Heiran et al., 2021).
5. **Sustainable Practices**: Both practitioners and consumers should advocate for sustainable sourcing of herbal products. Supporting companies that prioritise ethical harvesting and fair trade practices can help protect biodiversity and support local communities (Chiarioni, 2023).
6. **Research and Evidence:** Ongoing research is essential to establish the safety and efficacy of herbal remedies. Consumers should look for products that have been studied in clinical trials and have evidence supporting their use for specific health conditions (Nunavath, 2024).
7. **Regulatory Compliance:** Regulatory bodies should implement and enforce guidelines for the production and marketing of herbal products. This includes establishing standards for labelling, quality control, and safety evaluations to protect consumers (Khdour et al., 2016).

8. FUTURE DIRECTIONS AND RESEARCH PRIORITIES

The field of herbal anti-ageing research is rapidly evolving, driven by emerging trends, technological advancements, and a growing interest in natural remedies. As the scientific community increasingly recognises the potential of herbal compounds in promoting longevity and mitigating age-related diseases, it is essential to identify future research priorities and collaborative opportunities. This section discusses emerging trends in herbal anti-ageing research, technological advancements in studying herbal compounds, and recommendations for future studies and collaborations.

8.1 Emerging Trends in Herbal Anti-Ageing Research

One of the most significant trends in herbal anti-ageing research is the increasing focus on the molecular mechanisms underlying the effects of herbal compounds. Recent studies have highlighted the ability of various herbal components to modulate cellular pathways associated with ageing, such as oxidative stress, inflammation, and apoptosis. For example, Liu et al. (2019) demonstrated that herbal medicine can activate telomerase, enhance antioxidant capacity, and regulate ageing-related pathways, providing new insights into the therapeutic potential of these natural products. This trend emphasises the need for further exploration of the biochemical pathways influenced by herbal compounds, which could lead to the development of targeted anti-ageing therapies.

Another emerging trend is the integration of traditional knowledge with modern scientific methodologies. As researchers seek to validate the efficacy of traditional herbal remedies, there is a growing emphasis on conducting rigorous clinical trials and systematic reviews. For instance, systematic reviews of in vivo studies have begun to consolidate evidence supporting the anti-ageing effects of various herbs, such as *Gastrodiae Rhizoma* and Lycium barbarum (Cho et al., 2023). This trend highlights the importance of bridging the gap between traditional herbal medicine and contemporary scientific research, fostering a more comprehensive understanding of herbal efficacy.

Additionally, there is a rising interest in the development of multi-herb formulations that leverage the synergistic effects of various herbal compounds. Research has shown that combining different herbs can enhance their therapeutic effects, leading to improved outcomes in managing age-related conditions (Peltzer & Pengpid, 2019). This trend encourages the exploration of traditional herbal combinations and their potential applications in modern healthcare.

8.2 Technological Advancements in Studying Herbal Compounds

Technological advancements are playing a crucial role in advancing herbal anti-ageing research. High-throughput screening techniques, for example, enable researchers to rapidly evaluate the biological activities of numerous herbal extracts and their constituents. This approach facilitates the identification of promising candidates for further study and accelerates the drug discovery process (Menghini et al., 2016). Furthermore, advancements in molecular biology techniques, such as CRISPR and RNA sequencing, allow for a deeper understanding of the genetic and epigenetic mechanisms influenced by herbal compounds (El-Dahiyat et al., 2020).

Nanotechnology is another area of innovation that holds promise for enhancing the delivery and efficacy of herbal remedies. Herbal nanoformulations, which use nanoparticles to encapsulate bioactive compounds, can improve the bioavailability and targeted delivery of these compounds to specific tissues (Park et al., 2021). For instance, studies have demonstrated that nanoemulsions of herbal extracts can enhance skin penetration and improve anti-ageing effects, making them valuable for cosmetic applications (Buhrmann et al., 2020). The integration of nanotechnology into herbal medicine research presents exciting opportunities for developing more effective and safer herbal products.

Moreover, the use of computational methods and systems biology approaches is gaining traction in herbal research. These methodologies allow researchers to model the complex interactions between herbal compounds and biological systems, providing insights into their mechanisms of action and potential therapeutic applications (Cho et al., 2023). By leveraging these technological advancements, researchers can better understand the multifaceted effects of herbal remedies on ageing and age-related diseases.

8.3 Recommendations for Future Studies and Collaborations

To maximise the potential of herbal anti-ageing research, several recommendations can be made for future studies and collaborations:

1. **Standardisation of Herbal Products:** Future research should prioritise the standardisation of herbal products to ensure consistent quality and potency. Establishing guidelines for the cultivation, harvesting, and processing of herbal materials will enhance the reliability of research findings and improve consumer safety (Kim, 2023).
2. **Interdisciplinary Collaborations:** Collaborative efforts between herbalists, pharmacologists, biochemists, and clinicians are essential for advancing herbal research. Interdisciplinary teams can facilitate the integration of traditional knowledge with modern scientific methodologies, leading to more comprehensive studies and innovative therapeutic approaches (Hawash, 2024).

3. **Longitudinal Clinical Trials:** Conducting well-designed, long-term clinical trials is crucial for evaluating the safety and efficacy of herbal remedies in ageing populations. These studies should focus on diverse demographic groups to assess the effects of herbal interventions across different populations (Sangkaew, 2024).
4. **Exploration of Synergistic Effects:** Future studies should investigate the synergistic effects of multi-herb formulations. Research into traditional combinations of herbs can provide valuable insights into their collective therapeutic potential and inform the development of more effective anti-ageing products (Tai et al., 2021).
5. **Focus on Mechanisms of Action:** Understanding the molecular mechanisms through which herbal compounds exert their effects is essential for developing targeted therapies. Future research should employ advanced techniques, such as proteomics and metabolomics, to elucidate the pathways influenced by herbal remedies (Karapetyan & Barseghyan, 2022).
6. **Public Awareness and Education:** Increasing public awareness of the benefits and risks associated with herbal medicine is vital. Educational programs should be developed to inform consumers about the safe use of herbal remedies and the importance of consulting healthcare professionals before starting any herbal treatment (Costa et al., 2022).
7. **Regulatory Frameworks:** Establishing clear regulatory frameworks for herbal products will enhance consumer safety and promote responsible practices within the herbal industry. Regulatory bodies should work to create guidelines that ensure the quality, safety, and efficacy of herbal remedies (Domfeh et al., 2023).

9. CONCLUSION

The exploration of herbal solutions for promoting longevity and mitigating the effects of ageing has garnered significant attention in recent years. This review has highlighted key findings from various studies, emphasising the potential of herbal compounds to contribute to anti-ageing strategies. As the body of evidence supporting the efficacy of herbal remedies continues to grow, it is essential to adopt a balanced and evidence-based approach to their integration into modern healthcare.

9.1 Summary of Key Findings

The research presented in this review underscores the multifaceted benefits of herbal compounds in promoting longevity. Numerous studies have demonstrated the antioxidant, anti-inflammatory, and immunomodulatory properties of various herbs, which play crucial roles in combating age-related diseases. For instance, compounds such as curcumin from turmeric and ginsenosides from ginseng have shown promise in enhancing cellular health and reducing oxidative stress (Luo et al., 2019). Furthermore, the potential of multi-herb formulations to synergistically enhance therapeutic effects presents exciting opportunities for developing more effective anti-ageing interventions (Suzana, 2024). Emerging trends in herbal anti-aging research indicate a shift towards understanding the molecular mechanisms underlying the effects of these compounds. This includes the exploration of pathways related to cellular senescence, apoptosis, and metabolic regulation (Suzana, 2024). Technological advancements, such as high-throughput screening and nanotechnology, are facilitating the discovery and development of novel herbal formulations with enhanced bioavailability and efficacy (Woodley et al., 2021).

While the potential benefits of herbal remedies are promising, it is crucial to approach their use with caution. The variability in the quality and composition of herbal products can lead to inconsistent therapeutic outcomes, which undermines the credibility of herbal medicine (Cai et al., 2021). Therefore, a balanced approach that combines traditional knowledge with rigorous scientific research is essential for ensuring the safety and efficacy of herbal interventions.

Healthcare practitioners must be well-informed about the potential risks and benefits of herbal remedies, including possible herb-drug interactions and adverse effects (Li & Zhang, 2020). Encouraging open communication between patients and healthcare providers regarding the use of herbal supplements is vital for optimizing treatment outcomes and minimizing risks. Furthermore, regulatory frameworks should be established to ensure the quality and safety of herbal products, thereby enhancing consumer confidence in their use (Salm, 2023).

9.2 Final Thoughts

In conclusion, traditional herbal solutions hold significant promise for promoting longevity and enhancing healthspan. As research continues to unveil the mechanisms through which these compounds exert their effects, it is essential to prioritise future studies that focus on standardisation, quality control, and the exploration of synergistic effects in multi-herb formulations. Collaborative efforts between researchers, healthcare practitioners, and regulatory bodies will be crucial in advancing the field of herbal medicine and integrating these solutions into modern healthcare practices.

The potential of herbal remedies to address age-related health challenges is vast, and with a commitment to evidence-based research and ethical practices, traditional herbal solutions can play a vital role in the quest for healthier ageing. As we move forward, embracing the wisdom of traditional medicine while leveraging modern scientific advancements will pave the way for innovative approaches to longevity and well-being.

REFERENCES

Abdullah, V., Wahidin, W., Wibowo, D. P., & Mariani, R. (2023). Cross-cultural analysis of the role of traditional medicine in health access in Indonesia. *West Science Interdisciplinary Studies, 1*(10), 940–947. DOI: 10.58812/wsis.v1i10.279

Adha, S., Afifah, N., Latarissa, I., Iftinan, G., Kusuma, A., Febriyanti, R., Barliana, M., & Lestari, K. (2025). Herbal medicines as complementary therapy for managing complications in covid-19 patients with diabetes mellitus. *Diabetes, Metabolic Syndrome and Obesity, 18*, 135–146. DOI: 10.2147/DMSO.S498774 PMID: 39840393

Ahn, H., Park, D., Shin, M., Nguyen, Q., Park, J., Kim, D., Kang, K. S., & Lee, H. (2022). The ameliorating effect of lizhong-tang on antibiotic-associated imbalance in the gut microbiota in mouse. *Applied Sciences (Basel, Switzerland), 12*(14), 6943. DOI: 10.3390/app12146943

Alanazi, A. (2023). Saudi people's knowledge and attitudes about herbals' side effects and their interactions with medications. *Journal of Pharmaceutical Research International, 35*(35), 41–53. DOI: 10.9734/jpri/2023/v35i357486

Alhumaid, M. (2023). *Pharmacists and herbal medications: identifying potential interactions with conventional drugs*. SFS., DOI: 10.53555/sfs.v10i5.2312

Alhur, A. (2024). Community insights on drug-herbal interactions: A study from hail, Saudi Arabia. *Cureus*. Advance online publication. DOI: 10.7759/cureus.72529 PMID: 39606543

Ali, H., Alharbi, S. F., Iskandar, R. A., Mira, G. B., Yanogue, A. S., & Albоualy, E. A. (2024). Perception and use of herbal medicine in general practice patients: A cross-sectional study in Saudi Arabia. *Cureus*. Advance online publication. DOI: 10.7759/cureus.56806 PMID: 38654786

Alqathama, A., Alluhiabi, G., Baghdadi, H., Aljahani, L., Khan, O., Jabal, S., Makkawi, S., & Alhomoud, F. (2020). Herbal medicine from the perspective of type ii diabetic patients and physicians: What is the relationship? *BMC Complementary Medicine and Therapies, 20*(1), 65. Advance online publication. DOI: 10.1186/s12906-020-2854-4 PMID: 32111222

Amadi, C., & Orisakwe, O. (2018). Herb-induced liver injuries in developing nations: An update. *Toxics, 6*(2), 24. DOI: 10.3390/toxics6020024 PMID: 29673137

Ara, T., Nakatani, S., Kobata, K., Sogawa, N., & Sogawa, C. (2018). The biological efficacy of natural products against acute and chronic inflammatory diseases in the oral region. *Medicines (Basel, Switzerland), 5*(4), 122. DOI: 10.3390/medicines5040122 PMID: 30428613

Baez, M. (2024). Traditional medicine in Latin America: A holistic approach to health. *Community and Interculturality in Dialogue, 4*, 120. DOI: 10.56294/cid2024120

Baliga, M., Meera, S., Shivashankara, A., Palatty, P., & Haniadka, R. (2015). The health benefits of Indian traditional ayurvedic Rasayana (anti-aging) drugs., 151-161. DOI: 10.1016/B978-0-12-418680-4.00016-6

Buhrmann, C., Honarvar, A., Setayeshmehr, M., Karbasi, S., Shakibaei, M., & Valiani, A. (2020). Herbal remedies as potential in cartilage tissue engineering: An overview of new therapeutic approaches and strategies. *Molecules (Basel, Switzerland)*, *25*(13), 3075. DOI: 10.3390/molecules25133075 PMID: 32640693

Cai, M., Ni, W., Han, L., Chen, W., & Peng, D. (2021). Research progress of therapeutic enzymes and their derivatives: Based on herbal medicinal products in rheumatoid arthritis. *Frontiers in Pharmacology*, *12*, 626342. Advance online publication. DOI: 10.3389/fphar.2021.626342 PMID: 33796022

Čáková, V., Bonté, F., & Lobstein, A. (2017). Dendrobium: Sources of active ingredients to treat age-related pathologies. *Aging and Disease*, *8*(6), 827. DOI: 10.14336/AD.2017.0214 PMID: 29344419

Chaiyana, W., Charoensup, W., Sriyab, S., Punyoyai, C., & Neimkhum, W. (2021). Herbal extracts as potential antioxidant, anti-aging, anti-inflammatory, and whitening cosmeceutical ingredients. *Chemistry & Biodiversity*, *18*(7), e2100245. Advance online publication. DOI: 10.1002/cbdv.202100245 PMID: 33989453

Chang, Y., Zhang, D., Yang, G., Zheng, Y., & Guo, L. (2021). Screening of anti-lipase components of artemisia argyi leaves based on spectrum-effect relationships and hplc-ms/ms. *Frontiers in Pharmacology*, *12*, 675396. Advance online publication. DOI: 10.3389/fphar.2021.675396 PMID: 34025435

Chi, J., Sun, L., Cai, L., Liu, F., Shao, C., Shang, L., & Zhao, Y. (2021). Chinese herb microneedle patch for wound healing. *Bioactive Materials*, *6*(10), 3507–3514. DOI: 10.1016/j.bioactmat.2021.03.023 PMID: 33817424

Chiarioni, G., Popa, S. L., Ismaiel, A., Pop, C., Dumitrascu, D. I., Brata, V. D., Duse, T. A., Incze, V., & Surdea-Blaga, T. (2023). Herbal remedies for constipation-predominant irritable bowel syndrome: A systematic review of randomized controlled trials. *Nutrients*, *15*(19), 4216. DOI: 10.3390/nu15194216 PMID: 37836500

Cho, M., Park, J.-W., Kim, J., & Ko, S.-J. (2023). The influence of herbal medicine on serum motilin and its effect on human and animal model: A systematic review. *Frontiers in Pharmacology*, *14*, 1286333. Advance online publication. DOI: 10.3389/fphar.2023.1286333 PMID: 38161695

Cho, S., Lee, H., Kwon, S., Park, S., Jung, W., Moon, S., Park, J.-M., & Ko, C. (2023). A systematic review of in vivo studies of the efficacy of herbal medicines for anti-aging in the last five years. *Pharmaceuticals (Basel, Switzerland)*, *16*(3), 448. DOI: 10.3390/ph16030448 PMID: 36986547

Costa, E., Magalhães, W., & Stasi, L. (2022). Recent advances in herbal-derived products with skin anti-aging properties and cosmetic applications. *Molecules (Basel, Switzerland)*, *27*(21), 7518. DOI: 10.3390/molecules27217518 PMID: 36364354

Domfeh, S., Kyeremeh, G., & Belifini, M. (2023). Evaluation of anti-candida albicans activities of herbal preparations sold at the Kumasi central market in the Ashanti region of Ghana. Evidence-Based Complementary and Alternative Medicine, 2023(1). DOI: 10.1155/2023/6162532

Dong, Y., Chen, H., Gao, J., Liu, Y., Li, J., & Wang, J. (2019). Bioactive ingredients in chinese herbal medicines that target non-coding rnas: Promising new choices for disease treatment. *Frontiers in Pharmacology*, *10*, 515. Advance online publication. DOI: 10.3389/fphar.2019.00515 PMID: 31178721

El-Dahiyat, F., Rashrash, M., Abuhamdah, S., Farha, R., & Babar, Z. (2020). Herbal medicines: A cross-sectional study to evaluate the prevalence and predictors of use among Jordanian adults. *Journal of Pharmaceutical Policy and Practice*, *13*(1), 2. Advance online publication. DOI: 10.1186/s40545-019-0200-3 PMID: 31988754

Elendu, C. (2024). The evolution of ancient healing practices: from shamanism to Hippocratic medicine: a review. *Medicine*, *103*(28), e39005. DOI: 10.1097/MD.0000000000039005 PMID: 38996102

Elmaghraby, D., Alsalman, G. A., Alawadh, L. H., Al-Abdulqader, S. A., Alaithan, M. M., & Alnuwaysir, B. I. (2023). Integrated traditional herbal medicine in the treatment of gastrointestinal disorder: The pattern of use and the knowledge of safety among the eastern region Saudi population. *BMC Complementary Medicine and Therapies*, *23*(1), 373. Advance online publication. DOI: 10.1186/s12906-023-04197-0 PMID: 37872543

Eng, Y., Lee, C., Lee, W., Huang, C., & Chang, J. (2019). Unraveling the molecular mechanism of traditional Chinese medicine: Formulas against acute airway viral infections as examples. *Molecules (Basel, Switzerland)*, *24*(19), 3505. DOI: 10.3390/molecules24193505 PMID: 31569633

Fischer, F., Grigolon, G., Benner, C., & Ristow, M. (2022). Evolutionarily conserved transcription factors as regulators of longevity and targets for geroprotection. *Physiological Reviews*, *102*(3), 1449–1494. DOI: 10.1152/physrev.00017.2021 PMID: 35343830

Gao, Y., Wei, Y., Wang, Y., Gao, F., & Chen, Z. (2017). Lycium barbarum: A traditional Chinese herb and a promising anti-aging agent. *Aging and Disease*, *8*(6), 778. DOI: 10.14336/AD.2017.0725 PMID: 29344416

Ghahremanlo, A., Boroumand, N., Ghazvini, K., & Hashemy, S. (2018). Herbal medicine in oral lichen planus. *Phytotherapy Research*, *33*(2), 288–293. DOI: 10.1002/ptr.6236 PMID: 30421555

Hamidpour, R., Hamidpour, M., Hamidpour, S., & Shahlari, M. (2015). Cinnamon from the selection of traditional applications to its novel effects on the inhibition of angiogenesis in cancer cells and prevention of Alzheimer's disease, and a series of functions such as antioxidant, anticholesterol, antidiabetes, antibacterial, antifungal, nematicidal, acaracidal, and repellent activities. *Journal of Traditional and Complementary Medicine*, *5*(2), 66–70. DOI: 10.1016/j.jtcme.2014.11.008 PMID: 26151013

Hawash, M., Jaradat, N., Salhi, N. A., Shatreet, B., Asbah, A. A., & Hawash, Y. H. (2024). Assessing the therapeutic potential and safety of traditional anti-obesity herbal blends in Palestine. *Scientific Reports*, *14*(1), 1919. Advance online publication. DOI: 10.1038/s41598-024-52172-7 PMID: 38253703

Heiran, A., Lankarani, K., Bradley, R., Simab, A., & Pasalar, M. (2021). Efficacy of herbal treatments for functional dyspepsia: A systematic review and meta-analysis of randomized clinical trials. *Phytotherapy Research*, *36*(2), 686–704. DOI: 10.1002/ptr.7333 PMID: 34851546

Hussain, M., Al-Qahtani, S., Ahmad, S., & Iqbal, M. (2023). A comprehensive scientific claims on ethnobotany, phytochemical pharmacological and toxicology of withania somnifera (l.) dunal. *Journal of Drug Delivery and Therapeutics*, *13*(3), 194–207. DOI: 10.22270/jddt.v13i3.6003

Iitsuka, H., Koizumi, K., Inujima, A., Suzaki, M., Mizuno, Y., Takeshita, Y., Eto, T., Otsuka, Y., Shimada, R., Liu, M., Ikeda, K., Nakano, M., Suzuki, R., Maruyama, K., Zhou, Y., Sakurai, H., & Shibahara, N. (2018). Discovery of a sugar-based nanoparticle universally existing in boiling herbal water extracts and their immunostimulant effect. *Biochemistry and Biophysics Reports*, *16*, 62–68. DOI: 10.1016/j.bbrep.2018.08.004 PMID: 30338298

Izzo, A., Hoon-Kim, S., Radhakrishnan, R., & Williamson, E. (2016). A critical approach to evaluating clinical efficacy, adverse events and drug interactions of herbal remedies. *Phytotherapy Research*, *30*(5), 691–700. DOI: 10.1002/ptr.5591 PMID: 26887532

Jayasinghe, C., & Jayawardena, U. (2019). Toxicity assessment of herbal medicine using zebrafish embryos: A systematic review. *Evidence-Based Complementary and Alternative Medicine : eCAM*, *2019*, 1–17. DOI: 10.1155/2019/7272808 PMID: 31781278

Jazani, A., Azgomi, H., Azgomi, A., & Azgomi, R. (2019). A comprehensive review of clinical studies with herbal medicine on polycystic ovary syndrome (PCOS). *Daru : Journal of Faculty of Pharmacy, Tehran University of Medical Sciences*, *27*(2), 863–877. DOI: 10.1007/s40199-019-00312-0 PMID: 31741280

Jung, T., & Cheon, C. (2024). Synergistic and additive effects of herbal medicines in combination with chemotherapeutics: A scoping review. *Integrative Cancer Therapies*, *23*, 15347354241259416. Advance online publication. DOI: 10.1177/15347354241259416 PMID: 38867515

Jütte, R., Heinrich, M., Helmstädter, A., Langhorst, J., Meng, G., Niebling, W., Pommerening, T., & Trampisch, H. (2017). Herbal medicinal products – evidence and tradition from a historical perspective. *Journal of Ethnopharmacology*, *207*, 220–225. DOI: 10.1016/j.jep.2017.06.047 PMID: 28668645

Kanlayavattanakul, M., Khongkow, M., & Lourith, N. (2024). Wound healing and photoprotection properties of acanthus ebracteatus vahl. extracts standardized in verbascoside. *Scientific Reports*, *14*(1), 1904. Advance online publication. DOI: 10.1038/s41598-024-52511-8 PMID: 38253627

Karapetyan, H., & Barseghyan, E. (2022). Effect of hypericum alpestre and rumexob tusifolius l. extractson the alterations of proline quantity in various rat organs. *Biological Journal of Armenia*, ●●●, 38–43. DOI: 10.54503/0366-5119-2022.74.3-38

Khdour, M., Kurdi, M., Hallak, H., Jarab, A., Dweib, M., & Al-Shahed, Q. (2016). Pharmacists' knowledge, attitudes and practices towards herbal remedies in west bank, Palestine. *International Archives of Medicine*. Advance online publication. DOI: 10.3823/1974

Kim, H., Kim, S.-Y., Bae, H. J., Choi, Y.-Y., An, J.-Y., Cho, Y. E., Cho, S.-Y., Lee, S.-J., Lee, S., Sin, M. S., Yun, Y. M., Lee, J. R., & Park, S. J. (2023). Anti-inflammatory effects of the lk5 herbal complex on lps- and il-4/il-13-stimulated hacat cells and a dncb-induced animal model of atopic dermatitis in balb/c mice. *Pharmaceutics*, *16*(1), 40. DOI: 10.3390/pharmaceutics16010040 PMID: 38258052

Komariah, M., Amirah, S., Maulana, S., Abdurrahman, M., Ibrahim, K., Platini, H., Lele, J. A. J. M. N., Kohar, K., Rahayuwati, L., & Firdaus, M. (2023). The efficacy of herbs as complementary and alternative therapy in recovery and clinical outcome among people with covid-19: A systematic review, meta-analysis, and meta-regression. *Therapeutics and Clinical Risk Management, 19*, 611–627. DOI: 10.2147/TCRM.S405507 PMID: 37484695

Kumar, V., Dey, A., Hadimani, M., Marcovic, T., & Emerald, M. (2015). Chemistry and pharmacology of withania somnifera: an update. Tang [Humanitas Medicine], 5(1), 1.1-1.13. DOI: 10.5667/tang.2014.0030

Kusmardi, K., Wiyarta, E., Estuningtyas, A., Sahar, N., Midoen, Y., & Tedjo, A. (2021). Potential of phaleria macrocarpa leaves ethanol extract to upregulate the expression of caspase-3 in mouse distal colon after dextran sodium sulphate induction. *Pharmacognosy Journal, 13*(1), 23–29. DOI: 10.5530/pj.2021.13.4

Li, X., & Zhang, S. (2020). Recent advance in treatment of osteoarthritis by bioactive components from herbal medicine. *Chinese Medicine, 15*(1), 80. Advance online publication. DOI: 10.1186/s13020-020-00363-5 PMID: 32765641

Liu, Y., Wei-liang, W., Gao, R., & Liu, Y. (2019). New insights for cellular and molecular mechanisms of aging and aging-related diseases: Herbal medicine as potential therapeutic approach. *Oxidative Medicine and Cellular Longevity, 2019*, 1–25. DOI: 10.1155/2019/4598167 PMID: 31915506

Liu, Y., Zheng, Z., Wang, X., Xia, J., Zhu, X., Cheng, F., & Li, Y. (2023). Factors associated with the incidence and the expenditure of self-medication among middle-aged and older adults in China: A cross-sectional study. *Frontiers in Public Health, 11*, 1120101. Advance online publication. DOI: 10.3389/fpubh.2023.1120101 PMID: 37124784

Luo, H., Vong, C., Chen, H., Gao, Y., Lyu, P., Qiu, L., Zhao, M., Liu, Q., Cheng, Z., Zou, J., Yao, P., Gao, C., Wei, J., Ung, C. O. L., Wang, S., Zhong, Z., & Wang, Y. (2019). Naturally occurring anti-cancer compounds: Shining from Chinese herbal medicine. *Chinese Medicine, 14*(1), 48. Advance online publication. DOI: 10.1186/s13020-019-0270-9 PMID: 31719837

Lyu, Y., Fu, Q., Wilczok, D., Ying, K., King, A., Antebi, A., Vojta, A., Stolzing, A., Moskalev, A., Georgievskaya, A., Maier, A. B., Olsen, A., Groth, A., Simon, A. K., Brunet, A., Jamil, A., Kulaga, A., Bhatti, A., Yaden, B., & Bakula, D. (2024). Longevity biotechnology: Bridging ai, biomarkers, geroscience and clinical applications for healthy longevity. *Aging (Albany NY)*. Advance online publication. DOI: 10.18632/aging.206135 PMID: 39418098

Menghini, L., Ferrante, C., Leporini, L., Recinella, L., Chiavaroli, A., Leone, S., Pintore, G., Vacca, M., Orlando, G., & Brunetti, L. (2016). An hydroalcoholic chamomile extract modulates inflammatory and immune response in ht29 cells and isolated rat colon. *Phytotherapy Research, 30*(9), 1513–1518. DOI: 10.1002/ptr.5655 PMID: 27237110

Nunavath, R., & Nagappan, K. (2024). Identification of synthetic impurities and their significance in natural products quality control. *Natural Product Communications, 19*(5), 1934578X241252727. Advance online publication. DOI: 10.1177/1934578X241252727

Nurani, L., Rohman, A., Windarsih, A., Guntarti, A., Riswanto, F., Lukitaningsih, E., Fadzillah, N. A., & Rafi, M. (2021). Metabolite fingerprinting using 1h-nmr spectroscopy and chemometrics for classification of three curcuma species from different origins. *Molecules (Basel, Switzerland)*, *26*(24), 7626. DOI: 10.3390/molecules26247626 PMID: 34946709

Ozioma, E. and NwamakaChinwe, O. (2019). Herbal medicines in African traditional medicine.. DOI: 10.5772/intechopen.80348

Özkur, M., Benlier, N., Takan, I., Vasileiou, C., Georgakilas, A., Pavlopoulou, A., Cetin, Z., & Saygılı, E. (2022). Ginger for healthy ageing: A systematic review on current evidence of its antioxidant, anti-inflammatory, and anticancer properties. *Oxidative Medicine and Cellular Longevity*, *2022*, 1–16. DOI: 10.1155/2022/4748447 PMID: 35585878

Pandeya, P., Lamichhane, R., Lamichhane, G., Lee, K., Lee, H., Rhee, S., & Jung, H. (2021). 18kht01, a potent anti-obesity polyherbal formulation. *Frontiers in Pharmacology*, *12*, 807081. Advance online publication. DOI: 10.3389/fphar.2021.807081 PMID: 34975503

Park, J., Jeong, D., Song, M., & Kim, B. (2021). Recent advances in anti-metastatic approaches of herbal medicines in 5 major cancers: From traditional medicine to modern drug discovery. *Antioxidants*, *10*(4), 527. DOI: 10.3390/antiox10040527 PMID: 33801741

Park, S., Lee, Y. Y., Kim, M. H., & Kim, C.-E. (2024). Deciphering the systemic impact of herbal medicines on allergic rhinitis: A network pharmacological approach. *Life (Chicago, Ill.)*, *14*(5), 553. DOI: 10.3390/life14050553 PMID: 38792575

Pasupuleti, M. (2024). Ai and biotechnology for longevity: pioneering advances in human lifespan extension., 251-277. DOI: 10.62311/nesx/92465

Peltzer, K., & Pengpid, S. (2019). the use of herbal medicines among chronic disease patients in Thailand: A cross-sectional survey. *Journal of Multidisciplinary Healthcare*, *12*, 573–582. DOI: 10.2147/JMDH.S212953 PMID: 31413584

Qiang, R., Huang, H., Chen, J., Shi, X., Fan, Z., Xu, G., & Qiu, H. (2023). Carbon quantum dots derived from herbal medicine as therapeutic nanoagents for rheumatoid arthritis with ultrahigh lubrication and anti-inflammation. *ACS Applied Materials & Interfaces*, *15*(32), 38653–38664. DOI: 10.1021/acsami.3c06188 PMID: 37535012

Raguraman, V., & Subramaniam, J. (2016). withania somnifera root extract enhances telomerase activity in the human hela cell line. *Advances in Bioscience and Biotechnology*, *07*(04), 199–204. DOI: 10.4236/abb.2016.74018

Raymond, R. (2024). Biomedicines in longevity and aging the quest to resist biological decline. *Biomedicine (Taipei)*, *14*(1). Advance online publication. DOI: 10.37796/2211-8039.1433 PMID: 38533302

Reis da Silva, T. (2024a). The Evolution of Nursing for Older Adult: A Historical Perspective. Associative J Health Sci. 3(3). AJHS. 000561. 2024. DOI: . Link: https://crimsonpublishers.com/ajhs/pdf/AJHS.000561.pdfDOI: 10.31031/AJHS.2024.03.000561

Reis da Silva, T. H. (2023). Falls assessment and prevention in the nursing home and community. *British Journal of Community Nursing*, *28*(2), 68–72. DOI: 10.12968/bjcn.2023.28.2.68 PMID: 36735363

Reis da Silva, T. H (2024b). Oncology and Cancer Medicine: Understanding the complexities in Older Patients. Biomed J Sci & Tech Res 55(3)-2024. DOI: https://doi.org/DOI: 10.26717/BJSTR.2024.55.008720

Reis da Silva, T. H. (2024c). Falls prevention in older people and the role of nursing. *British Journal of Community Nursing*, *29*(7), 335–339. DOI: 10.12968/bjcn.2024.0005 PMID: 38963269

Reis da Silva, T. H. (2025b). Chapter 12 – Emotional Intelligence in Integrative Medicine: Enhancing Patient-Centred Care Through Humanised Technology. In Tikadar, S.; Liu, H.; Bhattacharya, P.; Bhattacharya, S. *Humanizing Technology With Emotional Intelligence*. Pp. 263-280. IGI Global Scientific Publishing. https://doi.org/DOI: 10.4018/979-8-3693-7011-7.ch012

Reis da Silva, T. M. (2025a). Integrative Approaches to Geriatric Care: Enhancing Physical and Mental Health Through AI-Driven Insights. In Jermsittiparsert, K., & Marzo, R. (Eds.), *Physical Health, Mental Health, and Human Well-Being in the Age of AI* (pp. 113–136). IGI Global Scientific Publishing., DOI: 10.4018/979-8-3693-6190-0.ch007

Rui, G., Qin, Z.-Y., Chang, Y.-Q., Zheng, Y.-G., Zhang, D., Yao, L.-M., & Guo, L. (2023). Chemical comparison and identification of xanthine oxidase inhibitors of dioscoreae hypoglaucae rhizoma and dioscoreae spongiosae rhizoma by chemometric analysis and spectrum–effect relationship. *Molecules (Basel, Switzerland)*, *28*(24), 8116. DOI: 10.3390/molecules28248116 PMID: 38138603

Salm, S., Rutz, J., van den Akker, M., Blaheta, R. A., & Bachmeier, B. E. (2023). Current state of research on the clinical benefits of herbal medicines for non-life-threatening ailments. *Frontiers in Pharmacology*, *14*, 1234701. Advance online publication. DOI: 10.3389/fphar.2023.1234701 PMID: 37841934

Sangkaew, W., Sianglum, W., Wunnoo, S., Voravuthikunchai, S. P., & Joycharat, N. (2024). Bioactive substance contents and therapeutic potential for skin inflammation of an herbal gel containing derris reticulata and glycyrrhiza glabra. *Pharmaceutical Biology*, *62*(1), 648–658. DOI: 10.1080/13880209.2024.2385456 PMID: 39150231

Sharifi-Rad, M., Lankatillake, C., Dias, D., Docea, A., Mahomoodally, M., Lobine, D., Chazot, P. L., Kurt, B., Boyunegmez Tumer, T., Catarina Moreira, A., Sharopov, F., Martorell, M., Martins, N., Cho, W. C., Calina, D., & Sharifi-Rad, J. (2020). Impact of natural compounds on neurodegenerative disorders: From preclinical to pharmacotherapeutics. *Journal of Clinical Medicine*, *9*(4), 1061. DOI: 10.3390/jcm9041061 PMID: 32276438

Sharma, P., Dwivedee, B., Bisht, D., Dash, A., & Kumar, D. (2019). The chemical constituents and diverse pharmacological importance of tinospora cordifolia. *Heliyon*, *5*(9), e02437. DOI: 10.1016/j.heliyon.2019.e02437 PMID: 31701036

Shen, P., Lin, W., Deng, X., Ba, X., Liang, H., Chen, Z., & Tu, S. (2021). Potential implications of quercetin in autoimmune diseases. *Frontiers in Immunology*, *12*, 689044. Advance online publication. DOI: 10.3389/fimmu.2021.689044 PMID: 34248976

Shivlingesh, K. K., Gangwar, C., Sharma, S., Kalsi, R., Asthana, G., & Gupta, V. (2024). Comparative Evaluation of Herbal Versus Non-herbal Dentifrice in Maintaining Oral Health of Young Adults. *Cureus*, *16*(7), e65331. DOI: 10.7759/cureus.65331 PMID: 39184597

Suh, W., Seo, Y., Jin, C., Cho, S., Park, S., Jung, W., Moon, S.-K., Park, J.-M., Ko, C.-N., Kwon, S., & Cho, K. (2021). Traditional east Asian herbal medicine for amyotrophic lateral sclerosis: A scoping review. *Evidence-Based Complementary and Alternative Medicine : eCAM*, *2021*, 1–22. DOI: 10.1155/2021/5674142 PMID: 34912464

Suzana, D., Kintoko, , Ilham, L. M., Bahri, M. S., & Sandy, T. A. (2024). Bibliometric analysis of herbal treatments for male infertility: Trends, efficacy, and future directions. *South Eastern European Journal of Public Health*, •••, 986–995. DOI: 10.70135/seejph.vi.2235

Szczuka, D., Nowak, A., Zakłos-Szyda, M., Kochan, E., Szymańska, G., Motyl, I., & Błasiak, J. (2019). American ginseng (panax quinquefolium l.) as a source of bioactive phytochemicals with pro-health properties. *Nutrients*, *11*(5), 1041. DOI: 10.3390/nu11051041 PMID: 31075951

Tai, C., El-Shazly, M., Tsai, Y., Csupor, D., Hohmann, J., Wu, Y., Tseng, T.-G., Chang, F.-R., & Wang, H. (2021). Uncovering modern clinical applications of fuzi and fuzi-based formulas: A nationwide descriptive study with market basket analysis. *Frontiers in Pharmacology*, *12*, 641530. Advance online publication. DOI: 10.3389/fphar.2021.641530 PMID: 33986674

Thariwong, S., Intharuksa, A., Sirisa-ard, P., Charoensup, W., & Chansakaow, S. (2021). Specification and dna barcoding of Thai traditional remedy for chronic kidney disease: Pikad tri-phol-sa-mut-than. *Plants*, *10*(10), 2023. DOI: 10.3390/plants10102023 PMID: 34685831

Todorova, M., Savova, M. S., Mihaylova, L. V., & Georgiev, M. I. (2024). Nurturing longevity through natural compounds: Where do we stand, and where do we go? *Food Frontiers*, *5*(2), 267–310. DOI: 10.1002/fft2.350

Vasudev, S., More, V., Ananthraju, K., & More, S. (2021). Potential of herbal cocktail of medicinal plant extracts against 'big four' snake venoms from India. *Journal of Ayurveda and Integrative Medicine*, *12*(3), 458–464. DOI: 10.1016/j.jaim.2021.04.006 PMID: 34334287

Wang, S., Fang, R., Huang, L., Zhou, L., Liu, H., Cai, M., Sha'aban, A., Yu, C., & Akkaif, M. (2024). Acupuncture in traditional Chinese medicine: A complementary approach for cardiovascular health. *Journal of Multidisciplinary Healthcare*, *17*, 3459–3473. DOI: 10.2147/JMDH.S476319 PMID: 39050695

Wang, X., Kong, Y., & Li, Z. (2024). Advantages of Chinese herbal medicine in treating rheumatoid arthritis: A focus on its anti-inflammatory and anti-oxidative effects. *Frontiers in Medicine*, *11*, 1371461. Advance online publication. DOI: 10.3389/fmed.2024.1371461 PMID: 38515982

Woodley, S., Mould, R., Sahuri-Arisoylu, M., Kalampouka, I., Booker, A., & Bell, J. (2021). Mitochondrial function as a potential tool for assessing function, quality and adulteration in medicinal herbal teas. *Frontiers in Pharmacology*, *12*, 660938. Advance online publication. DOI: 10.3389/fphar.2021.660938 PMID: 33981240

Xia, Z., Sun, B., Wen, J., Ma, R., Wang, F., Wang, Y., Li, Z., Jia, P., & Zheng, X. (2022). Research progress on metabolomics in the quality evaluation and clinical study of panax ginseng. *Biomedical Chromatography*, *37*(7), e5546. Advance online publication. DOI: 10.1002/bmc.5546 PMID: 36342761

Yadav, M. (2024). Integrating ayurvedic rasayana in geriatric care: A holistic approach to healthy aging. *IJAR*, *71-73*. Advance online publication. DOI: 10.36106/ijar/4505489

Yao, R., Heinrich, M., Zhang, B., Wei, X., Qi, Y., & Gao, W. (2023). Single botanical drugs in the ayurvedic pharmacopoeia of India—A quantitative ethnobotanical analysis. *Frontiers in Pharmacology*, *14*, 1136446. Advance online publication. DOI: 10.3389/fphar.2023.1136446 PMID: 37251315

Yazıcı, R., & Güney, İ. (2023). Serious multiorgan toxicity caused by mixed herbal tea ingestion: A case report. *Cureus*. Advance online publication. DOI: 10.7759/cureus.34000 PMID: 36811058

Yu, P., Li, W., Han, L., Ouyang, S., Cai, H., Wu, J., & Huang, Q. (2020). The efficacy and safety of health qigong for anti-aging. *Medicine*, *99*(49), e22877. DOI: 10.1097/MD.0000000000022877 PMID: 33285677

Zhang, D., Wu, K., Zhang, X., Deng, S., & Peng, B. (2020). In silico screening of Chinese herbal medicines with the potential to directly inhibit 2019 novel coronavirus. *Journal of Integrative Medicine*, *18*(2), 152–158. DOI: 10.1016/j.joim.2020.02.005 PMID: 32113846

Zhou, X., Afzal, S., Wohlmuth, H., Münch, G., Leach, D., Low, M., & Li, C. (2022). Synergistic anti-inflammatory activity of ginger and turmeric extracts in inhibiting lipopolysaccharide and interferon-γ-induced proinflammatory mediators. *Molecules (Basel, Switzerland)*, *27*(12), 3877. DOI: 10.3390/molecules27123877 PMID: 35745000

Chapter 10
Lifespan-Extending Natural Compounds

Odangowei Inetiminebi Ogidi
https://orcid.org/0000-0002-9961-893X
Bayelsa Medical University, Yenagoa, Nigeria

Christopher Unyime Ebong
Transition Minerals International Limited, Abuja, Nigeria

Charles German Ikimi
https://orcid.org/0000-0002-3729-8870
Federal University, Otuoke, Nigeria

ABSTRACT

Over the last decade, the revolution in ageing science has propelled advancements in therapies aimed at extending lifespan. The analysis of the traditional indicators of ageing has yielded reliable evidence to establish the existence of at least three new indicators, therefore creating opportunities for the advancement of innovative methods aimed at promoting lifespan. The pursuit of geroprotectors is highly intriguing, as it aims to identify the alchemical substance that promotes successful ageing and extends lifespan. Natural origin geroprotectors, including metformin, resveratrol, aspirin, and spermidine, are widely acknowledged as valuable agents that enhance longevity. Ongoing research is predominantly investigating the potential of plant secondary metabolites as pharmacological modulators of healthspan and lifespan. Therefore, this chapter rigorously evaluate the existing activities and significant findings in the area of longevity research.

INTRODUCTION

Ageing is a natural biological process characterised by a progressive decline in physiological functions and the emergence of age-related diseases, including cardiovascular disease, cancer, diabetes, and neurodegenerative disorders. These conditions diminish quality of life and present considerable economic and social challenges worldwide. The increasing ageing population has made research into interventions aimed at extending lifespan and promoting healthy ageing a priority within biomedicine.

DOI: 10.4018/979-8-3693-9730-5.ch010

Natural compounds sourced from plants, fungi, and other biological entities have emerged as potential candidates for influencing the ageing process. These compounds are recognised for their capacity to target molecular pathways that govern ageing, providing a complementary strategy to synthetic drugs and genetic interventions (Fontana et al., 2010).

Compounds that extend natural lifespan function via various mechanisms, frequently addressing the hallmarks of ageing such as oxidative stress, chronic inflammation, genomic instability, mitochondrial dysfunction, and cellular senescence (López-Otín et al., 2013). Resveratrol, a polyphenol present in grapes and berries, activates sirtuin 1 (SIRT1), a protein that plays a role in stress response and mitochondrial biogenesis, resulting in increased lifespan in model organisms (Baur & Sinclair, 2006). Metformin, an anti-diabetic agent sourced from Galega officinalis, has demonstrated potential in mitigating oxidative stress, enhancing metabolic homeostasis, and prolonging lifespan in preclinical investigations (Barzilai et al., 2012). Compounds like curcumin, quercetin, and epigallocatechin gallate (EGCG) demonstrate the ability to reduce inflammation, enhance autophagy, and protect against cellular damage, thereby supporting their anti-aging potential (Kim et al., 2018a).

Interest in natural compounds for lifespan extension is fundamentally grounded in traditional medicine systems. Herbs utilised in Traditional Chinese Medicine (TCM) and Ayurveda have historically been linked to the enhancement of longevity and the prevention of age-related diseases. Compounds like ginsenosides derived from ginseng and withanolides from Withania somnifera (ashwagandha) are under active investigation for their potential to enhance cellular resilience and postpone ageing processes (Chung et al., 2019). Traditional practices offer a valuable source of potential lifespan-extending compounds that, upon validation through contemporary scientific methods, may lead to innovative approaches for promoting healthy ageing. Recent developments in omics technologies, including genomics, proteomics, and metabolomics, have greatly enhanced the identification and validation of natural compounds that extend lifespan. High-throughput screening platforms facilitate the swift identification of bioactive molecules, and computational modelling contributes to the comprehension of their interactions with molecular targets (Partridge et al., 2020). Animal models, including yeast (Saccharomyces cerevisiae), worms (Caenorhabditis elegans), and mice, are essential for investigating the impacts of these compounds on longevity and healthspan. Compounds like rapamycin have demonstrated reliable lifespan-extending effects in various species, underscoring the potential for cross-species applicability (Kennedy & Lamming, 2016).

The translation of natural compounds from preclinical research to clinical applications presents significant challenges. The variability in the composition of natural compounds, influenced by plant species, cultivation conditions, and extraction methods, can result in inconsistent outcomes. Furthermore, comprehending the pharmacokinetics and bioavailability of these compounds in humans is essential, given that numerous natural compounds demonstrate low absorption and swift metabolism (Zhang et al., 2019). Long-term studies are necessary to determine the safety and efficacy of these compounds, especially in conjunction with other therapies. The investigation of natural compounds for lifespan extension serves the dual purpose of enhancing longevity and fostering a healthier, disease-free existence. These compounds may transform ageing interventions by targeting the biological mechanisms of ageing instead of solely alleviating its symptoms. This chapter examines the mechanisms, applications, and challenges of natural lifespan-extending compounds, emphasising their potential to advance the science of ageing and enhance human health.

THE MECHANISMS OF LIFESPAN-EXTENDING NATURAL COMPOUNDS

Natural compounds that promote longevity operate through numerous biological mechanisms. Enhancing autophagy for cellular repair, activating pathways for longevity (such as sirtuins, AMPK, and mTOR inhibition), and reducing oxidative stress are critical strategies. By inducing hormetic stress responses, these chemicals enhance mitochondrial function, reduce inflammation, and fortify cell defences. Senolytic activity, which eliminates old cells, and telomere preservation, which protects the extremities of chromosomes, enhance their effects. Additionally, they enhance health by modulating the gut flora and combating ageing through mechanisms such as epigenetic modifications and DNA repair. The cumulative effect of these processes increases the probability of an extended life span and the healthspan (Ogidi & Felagha, 2024).

LIFESPAN-EXTENDING VITAMINS

The human body cannot synthesise most vitamins; therefore, they must be acquired through dietary sources. Experimental data on lifespan-extension of vitamins are shown in Table 1.

Vitamin C

The most prevalent hydro-soluble vitamin has been found to be vitamin C, which is also known as L-ascorbic acid or L-ascorbate. An important antioxidant that dissolves in water, this one. Both oral and topical doses of vitamin E are helpful because of its antioxidant properties, which reduce UV-induced skin damage and increase dermal collagen formation (Pullar et al., 2017; Gasperlin & Gosenca, 2011). For children between the ages of 6 months and 3 years, the recommended daily intake of L-ascorbate is 35 mg. For men, it's 105 mg, and for women, it's 85 mg. The daily recommended consumption rises to 130 mg during breastfeeding (Castiglione et al., 2018). Clinical trials investigating the effects of varying vitamin C intakes provide substantial obstacles to producing strong and reliable results (Lykkesfeldt, 2020). A diet rich in fresh fruits and vegetables is generally considered to be the best way to get vitamin C. Reduced plasma concentrations of vitamin C have been associated to cigarette smoking (Delanghe et al., 2011).

Vitamin C deficiency is caused by other factors besides dietary impairment (Delanghe et al., 2011). The elderly are more likely to have hypovitaminosis C, and a study of 200 patients found that they also had higher levels of inflammatory biomarkers such C-reactive protein (CRP) (Sharma et al., 2019). Separate research found that vitamin C has a substantial effect on the ageing of mouse ovaries. The role of Vitamin C in ageing has been examined concerning its impact on the immune system, particularly in relation to inflammatory and degenerative disorders, as well as its effects on skin health (Abdollahifar etr al., 2019).

Vitamin A

Vitamin A exists in two natural forms: retinol, a supplement derived from animal feed, and carotene, a provitamin A present in both plant and animal products (Kelly et al., 2018). Retinol functions effectively as an antioxidant. Recent advancements have introduced potential pro-drugs aimed at mitigating skin ageing, particularly photoaging. These include both synthetic and natural retinoids, such as tarazotene and tretinoin (Mukherjee et al., 2006; Stratigos & Katsambas, 2005; Zasada & Budzisz, 2019). Despite the apparent benefits of retinoids, a synthetic version of vitamin A, natural sources of vitamin A should be preferred for preventing skin degradation associated with ageing (Kafi et al., 2007). This is the first time the function of retinol has ever been linked to vision. It is possible for the crystalline lens to become opaque due to ulceration of the ocular mucosa and cornea caused by retinol insufficiency, which reduces the eyes' capacity to adapt to dispersed light (Saari, 2016). The visual system relies on retinol for its normal operation. For best results, use retinol alongside β-carotene. This trophin's reduced toxicity compared to alternatives is a major factor in its selection; it also reduces cholesterol levels, prevents the initiation of some cancer types, and mitigates the risk of heart disease. In order to keep skin and other human tissues from ageing, retinol is essential (Kafi et al., 2007).

Recent studies indicate that a stabilised 0.1% retinol face moisturiser may positively impact skin health (Tucker-Samaras et al., 2009). In addition to its role in embryonic development, retinol participates in spermatogenesis (Margiana et al., 2022). In cases of anaemia, a deficiency in vitamin A may exacerbate iron deficiency. Studies involving children and pregnant women indicate that vitamin A supplementation enhances iron nutritional status and effectively addresses anaemia. These actions significantly surpass the effects of administering iron or vitamin A alone in reducing anaemia (Michelazzo et al., 2013). Retinol, retinal, and retinoic acid exhibit a wide variety of geometric isomers depending on whether the four side chain double bonds are cis or trans. Cis isomers with lower stability can be easily converted to trans isomers. Some organisms fulfil essential functions in ecosystems and exist in their natural form (Saari, 2016). An isomer of 11-cis-retinal is known as rhodopsin, and it is the photoreceptor protein found in vertebrates. One piece of opsin—a protein linked to green, red, or blue cones—and an 11-cis-retinal Schiff base bind covalently to produce rhodopsin. Vitamin A deficiency manifests initially with symptoms including night blindness and impaired vision (Saari, 2016).

Animal-derived foods, including eggs, milk, and liver, along with fortified products like retinyl esters, serve as effective sources of retinol and dehydroretinol, both of which are forms of vitamin A. Retinol undergoes esterification with saturated fatty acids in the intestines, subsequently forming chylomicrons that are absorbed into the bloodstream via lymphatic pathways. The liver stores retinol as esters. The hydrolysis of esters facilitates the entry of retinol into the bloodstream, where it is transported to extra-hepatic tissues by a specific protein and bound to designated cellular proteins (Saari, 2016). Fruits and vegetables contain β-carotene, recognised as a provitamin A. Carotenoids derived from plants exhibit a distinct provitamin-A function. Carotenoids, which are pigments, impart red, orange, and yellow hues to plants, fruits, and vegetables. Vegetables and fruits rich in β-carotene include pumpkin, carrot, apricot, and mango. Foods contain a minimum of 10 distinct types of carotene and provitamins. Notwithstanding this, β-carotene is the most prominent. Consumed in dietary form, it is transformed into vitamin A in the liver according to the requirements of the body (Michelazzo et al., 2013).

Vitamin E

Vitamin E is an antioxidant synthesised by plants, primarily located in foods such as nuts, cereals, and oils including extra virgin olive and maize. Vitamin E, also known as α-tocopherol, is a nutrient that is required for all vertebrates. It is formed from a lipid antioxidant that is found in plants. A significant amount of research and documentation has been done on the role that vitamin E plays in reducing damage to cells that is brought on by reactive oxygen species (ROS) (Traber, 2007; Brigelius-Flohe & Davis, 2007). New research points to potential additional roles for vitamin E beyond its antioxidant properties, especially in controlling gene expression (Valentino et al., 2018). Tocopherol prevents lipid peroxidation caused by ultraviolet light and has a protective impact on the skin (Keen & Hassan, 2016).

Tocopherols are prevalent in nature, predominantly found in plants, and are liposoluble compounds. Tocopherols are fundamentally a type of tocol. The ring can undergo hydroxylation and can be modified to mono-, di-, or trimethylated forms; it is classified as a chromanol (hydroxychroman, dihydrobenzopyran) ring. The chroman consists of a pyranic heterocycle and a benzene ring. Both γ- and β -tocopherols have diminished vitamin activity, making up just 15% to 30% of α-tocopherol's total. In α-trienols, the vitamin activity is diminished by 20%, whereas in β-trienols, it is diminished by 5%. No vitamin action is shown by the other substances. The functionality of tocopherols as vitamins is contingent upon the location and frequency of the methyl group on the benzene ring. Tocopherol synthesis in green plants, especially grasses, initiates with phytol, which plays a role in chlorophyll biosynthesis. Bile salts are essential for mycelia production, facilitating pancreatic lipase action on lipids, and are also crucial for vitamin E absorption by enterocytes during lipid digestion. The pancreatic esterase specifically releases tocopherol as α-tocopherol, the vitamin form, upon oral intake of tocopherol esters (Reboul, 2017).

The nondiscriminatory embedding of various isomers in chylomicrons, coupled with the gradual rate of intestinal absorption, renders this process passive. Chylomicrons undergo hydrolysis by lipoprotein lipase upon entering the lymphatic circulation. Tocopherols may be carried into different tissues with particular fatty acids, according to research, which suggests that tissues and muscles are the primary recipients of the released fatty acids (Valentino et al., 2018). The HDL structure can be attained through the transfer of tocopherols using lipoparticles, which function as surface lipid residues. The liver ultimately gathers the residual chylomicrons and their tocopherols via a receptor that involves apolipoprotein E (Herrera & Barbas, 2001).

Tocopherols exhibit binding rates of 35 percent to HDL and 40-60 percent to LDL in the bloodstream. Tocopherol concentrations in the bloodstream are influenced by age, gender, and various other factors. Human serum vitamin E concentrations typically range from 5 to 16 mg/L; however, in elderly women, these levels may increase to 9 to 25 mg/L under normal physiological conditions. Preterm neonates typically have a blood vitamin E content of 2 to 4 mg/L, while newborns typically have a blood vitamin E content of approximately 5 mg/L (Herrera & Barbas, 2001).

Table 1. Experimental data on lifespan-extension of vitamins

Vitamin	Experimental Evidence	Empirical Results	Study Model	References
Vitamin A	Supplementation improved immune response and reduced oxidative damage.	Mice fed with retinoic acid showed a 10–15% increase in lifespan.	Mice	Harrison et al., 2009
Vitamin C	Mitigated oxidative stress and enhanced antioxidant enzyme activities.	Lifespan extended by ~20% in treated *C. elegans*.	*C. elegans*	Tu et al., 2021
Vitamin D	Reduced inflammation and supported calcium homeostasis.	Mortality rate decreased by ~25% in vitamin D-sufficient humans.	Human observational data	Melamed et al., 2008
Vitamin E	Protected cells from lipid peroxidation and reduced oxidative damage.	Lifespan extended by ~19% in vitamin E-supplemented mice.	Mice	Banks et al., 2010
Vitamin K	Delayed vascular calcification and promoted cardiovascular health.	Reduced arterial stiffness by ~30% in treated rodents.	Rodents	Shea & Booth, 2016

continued on following page

Table 1. Continued

Vitamin	Experimental Evidence	Empirical Results	Study Model	References
Vitamin B Complex	Enhanced DNA repair mechanisms and reduced homocysteine levels.	Extended lifespan by ~25% in *C. elegans* with B vitamin supplementation.	*C. elegans*	Fenech, 2012
Vitamin C	Reduced oxidative DNA damage, extending reproductive phase and longevity.	Fruit flies lived ~15% longer with high-dose vitamin C.	Fruit flies (D. melanogaster)	Pospíšilová et al., 2022
Vitamin D	Improved stress responses and delayed age-related declines.	Zebrafish showed ~12% increased lifespan with adequate vitamin D.	Zebrafish	Valenzano et al., 2009
Vitamin E	Enhanced mitochondrial function and reduced cognitive decline.	Humans with higher dietary intake had 20% reduced mortality risk.	Humans	Ristow & Zarse, 2010
Vitamin K2	Improved arterial flexibility and bone health, reducing aging markers.	Lifespan extended by ~10% in vitamin K2-treated mice.	Mice	Iwamoto et al., 2011

LIFESPAN-EXTENDING POLYUNSATURATED FATTY ACIDS

Long-chain polyunsaturated fatty acids (PUFAs) are fundamental in controlling cholesterol levels (Ubeda et al., 2012; Molfino et al., 2014; Huang et al., 2018) and are essential precursors for prostaglandins. The types of PUFAs are illustrated in Figure 1, and their recently discovered role in the ageing process is described here (Whelan, 2008; Abbatecola et al., 2009; Chappus-McCendie et al., 2019). Table 2 shows an experimental data on lifespan-extending polyunsaturated fatty acids (PUFAs).

Figure 1. Types of polyunsaturated fatty acids

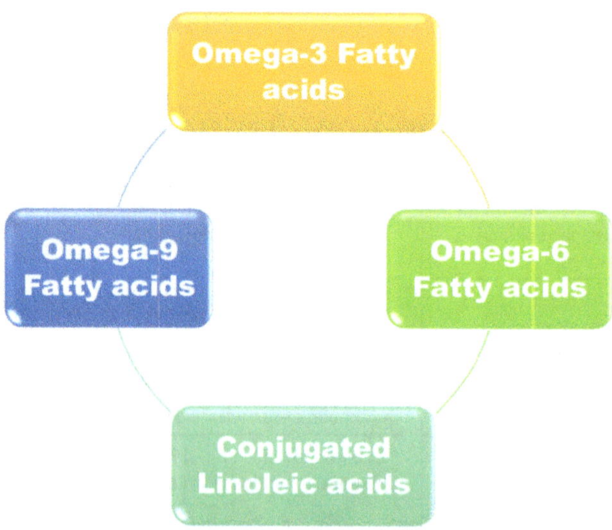

Omega-3 PUFA

Among the several benefits of omega-3 PUFA are those against senile dementia (Denis et al., 2013) and modification of platelet aggregation and hypertension (Molfino et al., 2014). Xie et al. (2021) claim that human gut bacteria somewhat influences the anti-aging properties of omega-3 fatty acids. Meals with high in omega-3 polyunsaturated fatty acids (PUFA) are walnuts, pumpkin seeds, sunflower seeds, and meals derived from fish and calanus including oils. Polyunsaturated fatty acids (PUFA) mostly affect inflammation by competing with the synthesis of arachidonic and eicosanoid acids, therefore suppressing their effects. Studies carried out in both laboratory and clinical environments show that micronutrients—especially some microelements—are absolutely essential for preserving both internal and exterior skin condition (Park, 2015).

Studies covering people as well as animals have demonstrated how omega-3 polyunsaturated fatty acids (PUFA) improve cognitive performance and neuroprotection with age. Cognitive deficits are negatively correlated with dietary PUFA levels (Denis et al., 2015; Cutuli et al., 2016) and positively correlated with regional grey matter (GM) volume and peripheral PUFA levels. According to the findings, increasing omega-3 polyunsaturated fatty acids in your diet can assist your fronto-hippocampal grey matter remain healthy and functional as you age. Low levels of omega-3 PUFA were associated in middle-aged German women (40–60 years old) with a higher risk of cardiovascular diseases (Gellert et al., 2017). Studies show that omega-3 polyunsaturated fatty acids improve dendritic synaptic spines, induce hippocampus neurogenesis in elderly people, and raise the amounts of several signalling molecules that enable brain plasticity (Gellert et al., 2017; Cutuli, 2017).

Furthermore, omega-3 PUFA in elderly persons shows anti-inflammatory effects connected with better cognitive abilities, suggesting its function in stopping the deterioration of white and grey matter volume and integrity (Gellert et al., 2017; Cutuli, 2017). Recent research suggest that plasma homocysteine levels may control the relationship between omega-3 PUFA and age-related cognitive deterioration (Maltais et al., 2022). Many studies have revealed the connection between omega-3 PUFA and neurological diseases (Andrieu et al., 2017; Hooper et al., 2017).

Omega-6 PUFA

Omega-3 and omega-6 fatty acids are crucial if we are to preserve the integrity of cell membranes and synthesise a wide range of biological compounds, including those that control blood pressure and inflammation. The only necessary fatty acids the human organism cannot independently generate are omega-3 alpha-linolenic acid (ALA) and omega-6 linoleic acid (LA). Some fatty acids are not synthesised by the body, hence they are considered as indispensable. Apart from their indispensible nature for development and regeneration, these two fatty acids can also be synthesised from other fatty acids. A diet high in omega-3 fatty acids—such as docosahexaenoic acid (DHA) and eicosapentaenoic acid (EPA)—is advised as ALA has poor conversion efficiency to these other forms of omega-3 fatty acids (Boyd et al., 2021).

Two fatty acids found in oils taken from legumes and vegetables are alpha-linolenic acid (ALA) and linoleic acid (LA). Though usually higher amounts of LA, walnut and canola oils are great sources of ALA. Oily fish abound in omega-3 fatty acids; mackerel, herring, and salmon among other species. Excellent sources of arachidonic fatty acid are animal items like meat and egg yolks. The anti-aging effects of omega-6 PUFA have been studied in worms; autophagy and a starving-resistant phenotype

(O'Rourke et al., 2013; Lapierre et al., 2012) may have a correlation generated from the presence of linoleic acid in the plasma (Wang et al., 2021a). This supports the basic idea that keeping a suitable ὒ3/ὒ6 ratio is essential to reduce the risk of negative consequences related with too high omega-6 PUFA intake (Patterson et al., 2012; Boyd et al., 2021).

Table 2. Experimental data on lifespan-extending polyunsaturated fatty acids

PUFA Type	Experimental Evidence	Empirical Results	Study Model	References
Omega-3 (EPA/DHA)	Reduced inflammation and enhanced mitochondrial function.	Lifespan extended by ~20% in C. elegans treated with DHA.	C. elegans	Hagopian et al., 2010
Omega-6 (LA)	Modulated cell membrane fluidity and supported cardiovascular health.	Increased healthspan markers in treated rodents.	Rodents	Stillwell et al., 2005
Omega-3 (ALA)	Promoted neuroprotection and reduced age-related cognitive decline.	~15% longer lifespan in ALA-supplemented fruit flies.	Fruit flies	Wijendran & Hayes, 2004
Omega-3 (EPA)	Reduced oxidative damage and enhanced stress resistance.	~25% increase in lifespan in zebrafish fed EPA-enriched diets.	Zebrafish	Valenzano et al., 2006
Omega-6 (ARA)	Improved immune regulation and delayed age-related inflammation.	Lifespan extended by 10% in aged rodents.	Rodents	Kim et al., 2013
Omega-3 (DHA)	Enhanced synaptic plasticity and delayed neurodegenerative changes.	Increased survival rates and improved healthspan markers.	Mice	Dyall et al., 2015
Omega-6 (GLA)	Reduced inflammatory cytokine levels, supporting cardiovascular health.	Decreased mortality by ~18% in rodent models of aging.	Rodents	Fan et al., 2003
Omega-3/6 Balance	Optimal balance of Omega-3 and Omega-6 promoted reduced inflammatory responses and increased lifespan.	~30% improved lifespan in balanced-diet-fed C. elegans.	C. elegans	Simopoulos, 2002

LIFESPAN-EXTENDING TRACE ELEMENTS AND MICRONUTRIENTS

Trace elements and micronutrients are essential for increasing life expectancy and boosting healthspan through a variety of biological processes. Figure 2 shows some types of lifespan-extending trace elements.

Figure 2. Types of lifespan-extending trace elements

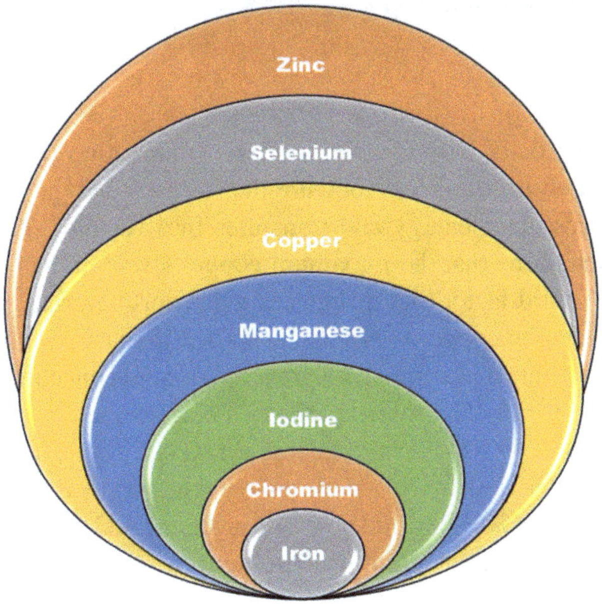

Zinc

A healthy body depends on zinc, copper, and selenium. Metalloenzymes utilise zinc as a cofactor, which can bind to approximately 2,000 transcription factors and 300 enzymes (Chasapis et al., 2020). Zinc is essential for various cellular metabolic processes. Zinc affects neurological system, immunological system, development, and reproduction as well as other processes. One of the main uses is the avoidance of skin damage brought on by too high UV radiation exposure (Choi et al., 2018; Cabrera, 2015). Zinc primarily performs three sorts of biological activities: catalytic, structural, and regulatory. Zinc is an essential component of almost 100 distinct enzymes that catalyse important chemical reactions. Proteins and cell membranes rely on zinc for proper function. A structural protein motif known as a "zinc finger" is present in several transcription factors and receptors. An antioxidant enzyme called copper-zinc superoxide dismutase (CuZn-SOD) has copper in its catalytic centre. Moreover, it is fundamental to the structure (Chasapis et al., 2020).

Zinc has an effect on how cell membranes are made and how they work. According to studies, membranes' abilities are compromised when their zinc level is low because they are more vulnerable to oxidative damage. As transcription factors, zinc finger proteins control how genes are expressed. These proteins modify the transcription levels of particular genes by identifying specific sequences within the DNA structure. Zinc plays a role in cellular signalling, influencing hormone secretion and nerve impulse transmission. Programmed cell death, known as apoptosis, serves as a crucial regulator of cellular processes, influencing development and various chronic disorders; recent findings indicate that zinc plays a role in this mechanism (Jarosz et al., 2017). Meat, eggs, and seafood exhibit high zinc bioavailability, indicating the amount of zinc that is absorbed and utilised by the body. Specific amino acids, such as cysteine and methionine, facilitate zinc absorption, while inhibitors of its absorption are largely absent. The elevated levels of phytic acid in whole grains and plant protein products diminish the bioavailability of zinc (Jarosz et al., 2017).

Copper

Copper enhances skin elasticity by promoting collagen maturation (Pickart & Margolina, 2018). The primary sites of copper absorption from food are the stomach and the initial portions of the small intestine. This reaction necessitates energy and transpires in a vacuum. The 64Cu isotope has been employed in research to determine that the maximum copper levels in the blood occur thirty minutes following oral treatment. A third factor that influences the absorption rate is the formation of chelate complexes, which are induced by copper's affinity for L-Ala. The absorption of copper from dietary sources can be affected by organic molecules. The presence of high concentrations of ascorbic acid and phytates reduces the absorption rate. The copper pathway, being an open system, facilitates the transport of the majority of copper to the liver for ceruloplasmin synthesis. The oxidase activity is released into the plasma, collected by the liver, destroyed, and ultimately removed by the bile. The copper in its labile form, although constituting only 4% of the total quantity, ensures rapid turnover as it facilitates transport from plasma to tissues via binding to albumin. According to studies, this procedure is able to remove more than 96% of the used copper. Protein binding explains why only a small fraction (less than 1% of consumed copper) is eliminated in urine (Pickart & Margolina, 2018).

Selenium

One of the anti-aging properties of selenoproteins is their ability to reduce inflammation and DNA damage, which in turn slows the onset of cancer, neuropsychiatric disorders, cardiovascular disease, and skin ageing (Bjorklund et al., 2022a; Solouyev et al., 2018). It appears that there are more selenoproteins than the eleven that have been investigated so far. Glutathione peroxidase (GPx) enzyme is an autonomous selenium-dependent enzyme in its own right, it is through the integration of reduction and glutathione oxidation events that these enzymes work together to reduce reactive oxygen species (ROS), including lipid hydroperoxides and peroxide ions. In addition to protecting mature sperm from oxidative damage, the antioxidant enzyme selenoprotein—previously thought to be a separate selenoprotein—contributes to the synthesis of a structural protein necessary for sperm. It is synthesised in the mitochondria of sperm capsules. In the end, it was determined to be GPx, a phospholipid hydroperoxide. When vitamin C and other antioxidant systems are depleted, the enzyme thioredoxin-reductase steps in to restore them. By keeping thioredoxin in its reduced form, thioredoxin-reductase regulates cell development and survival (Bjorklund et al., 2021).

Plasma contains selenium-protein P, which is linked to endothelial vascular cells found on the inside of blood vessels. Although its exact role is unclear, selenoprotein P is thought to protect endothelium cells from reactive nitrogen species (RNS) such peroxynitrites by acting as an antioxidant. There is a protein called W that binds selenium in muscles. Muscle metabolism likely relies on it, however its precise role is unknown. The enzyme selenophosphate synthetase is responsible for selenoproteins' incorporation of selenocysteine. This protein plays a crucial role in the production of selenoproteins by facilitating the conversion of selenium monophosphate into selenocysteine. Through its interactions with nutrients, selenium influences the pro-oxidant/antioxidant equilibrium in cells, as it is an essential component of thioredoxin reductase and GPx. When lipids are peroxided, the selenium in GPx is thought to activate vitamin E (Solouyev et al., 2018).

Selenium and vitamin E offer complementary protection, according to animal studies. Selenium has the potential to protect against some vitamin E-related illnesses. Thioredoxin reductase also helps vitamin C regenerate, so its antioxidant properties are preserved. When selenium levels are low, the effects of low iodine levels are cancelled out. The conversion of T4 to T3 requires iodine and selenozyme deiodinases. The fact that selenium supplementation lowers T4 levels in the elderly suggests that deiodinase activity may increase, leading to better T4 to T3 conversion (Kobayashi et al., 2021).

Role of Zn, Cu and Se in the Aging Prevention

A recent review examined the role of Zn in immunosenescence and ageing (Fulop et al., 2017). The biochemical roles discussed are examples of how zinc, often deficient in the elderly, regulates various processes associated with "oxi-inflamm-aging" (Cabrera, 2015; Fulop et al., 2017). The immune response operates optimally when zinc and copper concentrations in the blood are appropriately balanced. Cognitive impairment has been associated with elevated copper levels (Kazemi et al., 2022). Micronutrients are particularly important in this context (Calder et al., 2022). Because of its importance in a number of redox reactions, selenium (Se) is critical in reducing the senescent phenotype's ROS-induced degeneration (Cai et al., 2019).

Strong support for the protection of damage related with ageing comes from cofactor of important enzymes involved in the removal of oxidative stresses (Calder et al., 2022). Older animals having lower zinc levels had greater serum amounts of proinflammatory cytokines, including MCP1 and IL6. The number of naive CD4 T-cells dropped in the mesenteric lymph nodes (MLN) while Th1/Th17/inflammatory cytokines including IFNγ, IL17, and TNFα rose (Wong et al., 2021). Effective operation of immunological responses depends on zinc. Often acting as metal cofactor, the trace elements are very important in slowing down the immunosenescence process and improving geriatric immunity (Haase & Rink, 2009; Baarz et al., 2022; Borkow, 2014; Baek et al., 2012). An experimental data on lifespan-extending trace elements and micronutrients are depicted in Table 3.

Table 3. Experimental data on lifespan-extending trace elements and micronutrients

Trace Element/ Micronutrient	Experimental Evidence	Empirical Results	Study Model	References
Zinc	Promoted DNA repair, enhanced immune function, and reduced oxidative stress.	~14% increased lifespan in zinc-supplemented mice.	Mice	Mocchegiani et al., 2000
Selenium	Protected against oxidative damage via selenoproteins; reduced age-related degeneration.	Lifespan extended by ~20% in selenium-fed fruit flies.	Fruit flies	Rayman, 2000
Magnesium	Improved mitochondrial function and reduced systemic inflammation.	Rodents lived ~12% longer with magnesium supplementation.	Rodents	Barbagallo & Dominguez, 2010
Iron	Enhanced oxygen transport and reduced cellular aging markers.	Increased healthspan markers in aged mice.	Mice	Andrews, 2008

continued on following page

Table 3. Continued

Trace Element/ Micronutrient	Experimental Evidence	Empirical Results	Study Model	References
Copper	Boosted antioxidant enzyme activity (e.g., superoxide dismutase), reducing oxidative damage.	10–15% lifespan increase in *C. elegans*.	C. elegans	Harris, 2003
Manganese	Protected against oxidative stress by supporting mitochondrial function.	Lifespan extended by ~18% in manganese-treated worms.	C. elegans	Keen et al., 2003
Chromium	Improved insulin sensitivity and reduced age-related metabolic decline.	Rodents showed ~10% longer lifespan with supplementation.	Rodents	Anderson, 1998
Iodine	Regulated thyroid hormone production, supporting metabolism and reducing aging markers.	Improved survival rates in iodine-sufficient animals.	Rodents	Zimmermann, 2009

LIFESPAN-EXTENDING PLANT METABOLITES

Polyphenols, triterpenes, and sterols are among the plant metabolites that possess antioxidant and anti-aging properties (Enenebeaku et al., 2022; Tundis et al., 2015). The ageing process may be slowed and the effects of diseases associated with oxidative stress and redox-related disturbances may be mitigated by ingesting or applying antioxidants derived from plants (Warsito & Kusumawati, 2019). Flavonoids, polyphenols, curcumin, stilbenes, rosmarinic acid and anthocyanins are among the secondary phytoconstituents (Ogidi & Enenebeaku, 2023; Ogidi, 2022; Ogidi et al., 2019). The capacity of OH-groups to mitigate the effects of free radicals is a critical factor in the slowing down of the ageing process in the body and epidermis (Queen & Tollefsbol, 2010; Nichols & Katiyar, 2010; Petruk et al., 2018).

The antioxidant, collagenase, and elastase inhibitory properties of rosmarinic acid were demonstrated through transdermal administration (Yucel et al., 2019). The anthocyanins present in blueberries offer significant protection against cell senescence in epithelial cells (Liu et al., 2012). Quercetin improved memory retention and spatial learning in elderly rodents (Li et al., 2021). The antioxidant properties of green tea and several medicinal botanicals are attributed to their high concentrations of polyphenols, including flavones, rosmarinic acid, catechin, and epigallocatechin gallate (Katiyar, 2011; Peluso & Serafini, 2017; Shanaida et al., 2018). Consuming foods that are abundant in nutraceuticals and flavonoids can enhance cognitive function and prevent the onset of senescence (ayaz et al., 2019). Experimental data on some lifespan-extending plant metabolites are showing in Table 4.

Polyphenols

Many polyphenols, due to their potent antioxidant properties, confer significant health benefits (Luo et al., 2021). Fruits and vegetables contain flavonoids, pigments responsible for their distinctive yellow, red, or blue colouration. Flavonoids exhibit anticarcinogenic and antioxidant properties, similar to those of vitamin C (Fan et al., 2022). Polyphenols represent a particularly potent class of dietary antioxidants. Herbs contain over 8,000 identified polyphenolic structures, predominantly present in foods such as fruits, vegetables, aromatic herbs, cocoa, wine, and coniferous bark (Tsao, 2010). Red fruits are sources of anthocyanins; citrus fruits provide flavonoids. Tea leaves, chocolate, onions, algae, and apples are rich in quercetin. Pomegranates and grapes contain stilbenes, while legumes are sources of lectins, and flax seeds provide lignans, all classified as polyphenols (Liu et al., 2012).

Recent studies indicate that plant polyphenols may serve as a potential anti-aging treatment for the skin (Ogidi & Emaikwu, 2024; Gasmi et al., 2022a). These compounds exhibit distinctive antioxidant properties that mitigate the harmful effects of environmental pollutants and solar radiation, and may also delay or reverse the signs of premature skin ageing. Polyphenols exhibit numerous beneficial effects, such as reducing inflammation, eliminating pathogens, preventing tumours, and safeguarding blood vessels from atherogenic deposits (Gasmi et al., 2022a,b). Antioxidants combat ageing primarily by inhibiting the generation of free radicals. Plants containing polyphenols derive significant advantages from these compounds. Plants serve multiple functions: protecting against harmful insects and bacteria, absorbing UV radiation, and aiding in pollination. Polyphenols, once ingested, shield cells from oxidative stress, genetic mutations, and inflammatory damage (Ogidi, 2024).

Studies indicate that topical application of polyphenols can reverse certain histological and clinical alterations in the dermis and epidermis caused by UV radiation and natural ageing (Gasmi et al., 2022a,b). The changes encompass a reversion to normal hyper-keratinization or vascularization, an elevation in collagen synthesis, and the restoration of keratinocyte ultrastructure. A specific treatment protocol exists for each clinical manifestation or phase. Vine (Vitis vinifera), root (Punica granatum), and tea (Camellia sinensis) are three plant species known for their polyphenol content, which possesses aesthetic significance. The anti-aging effects of grapefruit, derived from the Vitis vinifera plant, are linked to the presence of proanthocyanidins and trans-resveratrol. These compounds exert a protective effect on the skin by improving the body's inherent antioxidant systems, preventing the degradation of macromolecular biological components, including proteins, DNA and lipids inhibiting the activation of photocarcinogenic signalling pathways such as MAPK and NF-kB (Gasmi et al., 2022b).

Polyphenols in pomegranates, including flavonoids, proanthocyanidins, and punicalagin-type ellagitannins, may contribute to photoprotection and photo-chemoprevention. Additionally, polyphenols have antioxidant, anti-proliferative, and anti-inflammatory effects. Since phenolic acids are very easy for the human body to absorb, they provide multiple anti-aging advantages. By increasing cellular strength and resilience to disintegration and by inhibiting aberrant cell development through antioxidant activity, phenolic acids have anti-aging characteristics. By controlling inflammation, boosting the immune system, creating natural collagen fibre linkages, shielding against free radicals, and promoting blood circulation, phenolic acids aid in anti-aging. Furthermore, they utilise numerous methods to control the degradation of collagen fibres (Luo et al., 2021). Reducing UVB-induced epidermal hyperplasia and leukocyte infiltration, inhibiting NF-kB and MAPK activation, increasing type I procollagen production, and preventing fibroblast morphological alterations are the mechanisms by which the anti-aging impact on skin is accomplished (Ogidi et al., 2024a). Figure 3 shows the chemical structure of polyphenols.

Figure 3. Chemical structure of polyphenols

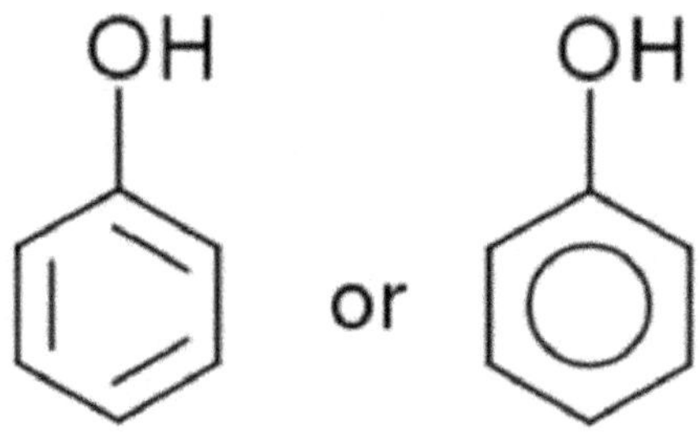

Resveratrol

There are a lot of red wines, grape seeds, and grape skins that contain resveratrol, a stilbenoid polyphenol. Particularly encouraging is the phytoalexin's antioxidant potential (Navarro-Cruz et al., 2017; Pallauf et al., 2016; Reinisalo et al., 2015). By activating SIRT1 and sirtuins, resveratrol may increase the average human lifespan. The enzyme family known as sirtuins controls cellular metabolism by modulating gene expression. Resveratrol has the potential to counteract the morphological changes brought on by H_2O_2 therapy, increase proliferation, decrease acetylated TP53 levels, and inhibit apoptosis (McCubrey et al., 2017).

Resveratrol is a chemical component that some plants produce. It has antibacterial and antifungal activities and also protects against UV radiation. This chemical can be found in a variety of fruit, including groundnuts, blueberries, red grape peel, and more. Preclinical investigations in S. Saccharomyces cerevisiae have demonstrated that resveratrol increases longevity. A 20% resveratrol solution at a concentration of 10 mM. A 70% increase was noted in the yield of *cerevisiae. Drosophila melanogaster* and *Caenorhabditis elegans* showed a 29% mortality rate after being administered 100 mM resveratrol (Reinisalo et al., 2015). Researchers found that resveratrol reduced genomic instability and other age-related characteristics in laboratory mice when administered doses of about 20 mg/kg. To protect neurones from microglia-induced neuronal death, resveratrol inhibits the NF-Kb protein. Resveratrol has shown promise in treating neurological diseases in preliminary trials (Navarro-Cruz et al., 2017).

Resveratrol improves workout results, mental and physical performance, and both. Some of the positive effects of resveratrol are similar to those of phytoestrogen hormones. It helps prevent and fight osteoporosis by acting as a strong calcium fixator in bones, especially when combined with exercise. It safeguards blood vessels as well, and that includes men. Resveratrol helps with dysmenorrhea, menstrual cycle management, and climacteric diseases. It prevents cancer of the breast and cervical lining at high dosages without causing cancer in and of itself. Resveratrol protects nerve cells from stress-induced damage, which means they live longer and don't die. Deterioration caused by gout or uric lithiasis can be lessened because it aids in the renal excretion of uric acid, which prevents its buildup. Enhancement of endogenous chemical synthesis and substantial protection against oxidative DNA damage in MRC5 human fibroblast cells are both provided by 5 μm resveratrol. This shield reduced nuclear volume enlargement, acetylated histone H3 and H4 variant generation, and p53 protein levels (Pallauf et al., 2016). The chemical structure of resveratrol is shown in Figure 4

Figure 4. Chemical structure of resveratrol

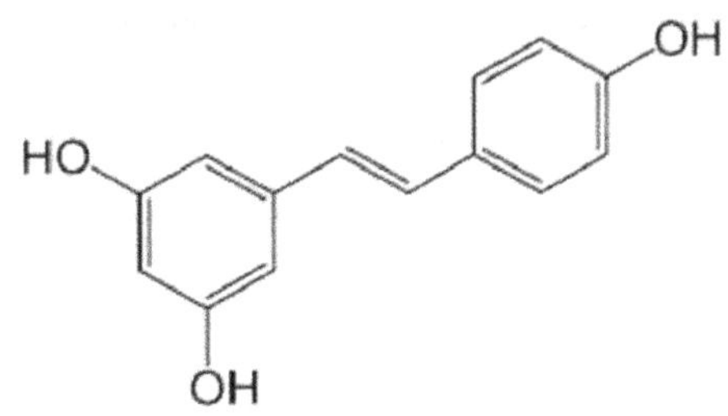

Curcumin

The lowering of inflammation related with ageing, curcumin may help to slow down the ageing process (Shailaja et al., 2017). Many model animals have revealed effects of curcumin and its metabolite, tetrahydro-curcumin (THC), on ageing and associated characteristics. Among these are the fruit fly, the mouse, and the roundworm nematode. One observed consequence was an average lifetime of the mice rising. By reducing reactive oxygen species production, the activity of genes considerably extended the lifetime of worm models in a curcumin-enriched medium. Curcumin supplements were shown to extend the lifetime of Drosophila; this was linked to lower levels of malondialdehyde and lipofuscin and higher activity of superoxide dismutase (SOD) (Shen et al., 2013). Because curcumin can cure endothelial dysfunction and arterial stiffness (Fleenor et al., 2013), it shows potential as a novel therapy for human arterial ageing. Curcumin is helping an increasing variety of diseases and disorders—especially those related to inflammation—by means of relief. Figure 5 depicts the chemical structure of curcumin. Curcumin and its derivatives might stop cancer cells—more especially, cancer stem cells—from proliferating (Hancianu et al., 2013).

Figure 5. Chemical structure of curcumin

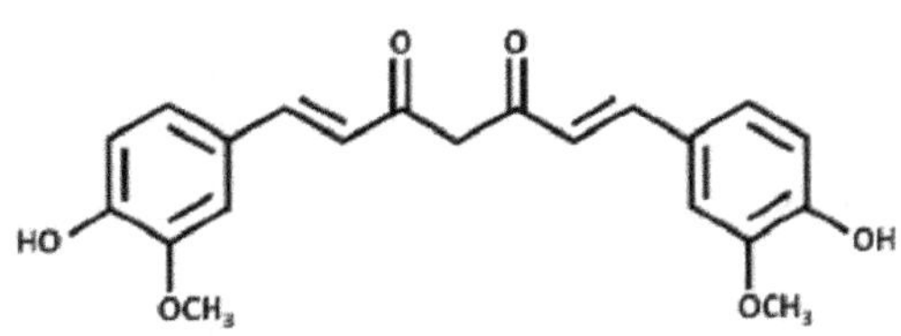

Terpenoids

Essential oils are effective multi-potent medications due to the presence of a variety of beneficial components (Loizzo et al., 2013; Shanaida, 2018). The significant anti-aging properties of essential oils in the treatment of anxiety, dementia, and other neurological conditions have been demonstrated in in vitro, in vivo, and clinical investigations (Ayaz et al., 2019; Agatonovic-Kustrin et al., 2019). Aromatherapy with essential oils has demonstrated potential in improving cognitive function in individuals with Alzheimer's disease (Agatonovic-Kustrin et al., 2019; Hancianu et al., 2013). The enhancement of mental acuity represents one of several health benefits associated with the use of plants containing essential oils. To maximise the beneficial effects of aromatherapy on the human body, consider topical application, inhalation, or ingestion. Terpenoids are small, fat-soluble molecules capable of crossing the blood-brain barrier, entering the bloodstream via inhalation, or penetrating the skin through topical application (Agatonovic-Kustrin et al., 2019). Many common fruits and herbs contain ursolic acid, a pentacyclic triterpenoid known to enhance anti-aging biomarkers (Gharibi et al., 2018; Ogidi et al., 2024b). This list comprises elderflower, peppermint, rosemary, holy basil, bilberries, prunes, cranberries, and additional items. Figure 6 shows the chemical structure of terpenoids.

Figure 6. Chemical structure of terpenoids

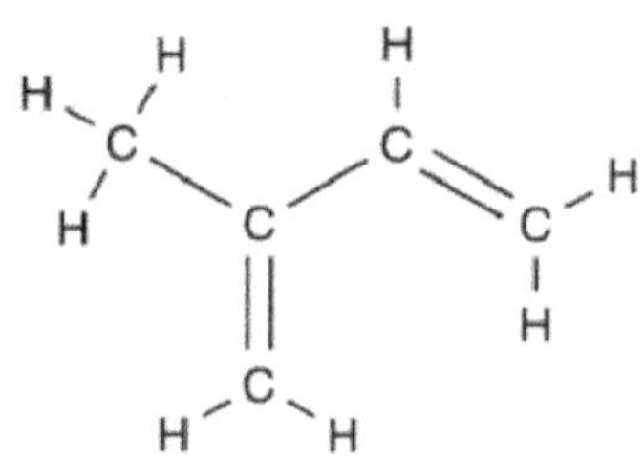

Acrylohydroxy Acids

Commonly included in skin care products, these substances are sourced from a variety of plants and animals. Some examples of alpha-hydroxy acids (AHAs) found in plants, berries, fruits, and vegetables are citric acid (CA), glycollic acid (GA), lactic acid (LA), malic acid (MA), and tartaric acid (TA) (Budoff et al., 2009; Moghimipour, 2012; Shanaida et al., 2021; Green et al., 2009). Most people use them to make acne look less severe and to make dry, aged skin look better. Their dual purpose is to stimulate collagen formation in the dermal matrix and remove the skin's outermost dead layers (exfoliation) (Green et al., 2009). Seven different types of AHAs are found in commercially sold skincare products. The chemicals and their sources include citrus fruits (citric acid), sugar cane (glycollic acid), royal jelly (hydroxycaproic acid), animals (hydroxycaprylic acid), lactose (or other carbohydrates), fruits (malic acid), and grapes (tartaric acid). Figure 7 depict the chemical structure of polya-hydroxyacrylic-acid

Glycollic and lactic acids stand out as the most trustworthy AHA sources, according to the research. It is possible for glycollic and lactic acids to irritate the skin (Budoff et al., 2009). The exfoliating activity is the principal function of alpha hydroxy acids. Significant effects on skin lightening, scar and age spot correction, wrinkle and line improvement, product absorption, acne avoidance, collagen and blood flow promotion, and other areas are caused by alpha hydroxy acids (AHAs) (Budoff et al., 2009). The skincare industry utilises beta-hydroxy acid (BHA) extensively. Salicylic acid, a compound effective in combating acne, serves as the principal source of beta-hydroxy acids (BHAs), distinguishing it from alpha-hydroxy acids (AHAs). Research indicates that their benefits extend significantly beyond exfoliation. AHAs facilitate an increase in elastic fibres and a decrease in glycosaminoglycan formation (Budoff et al., 2009).

Figure 7. Chemical structure of polya-hydroxyacrylic-acid

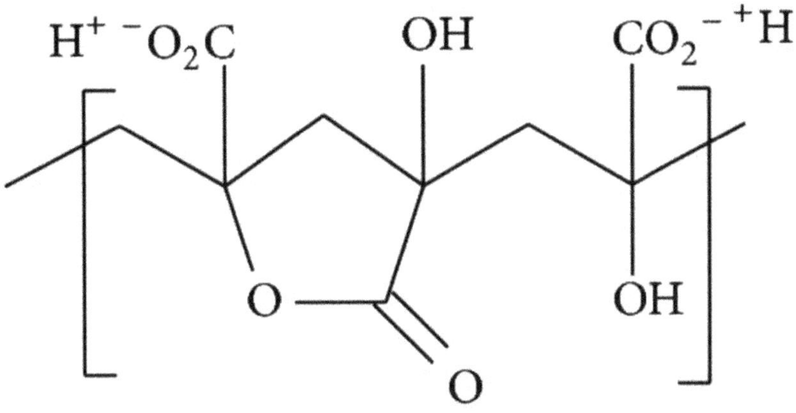

Phytoestrogens

Phytoestrogens' structural similarity allows them to replicate the physiological effects of oestradiol (17-estradiol) in living entities. Present in plants, phytoestrogens are a varied collection of non-steroidal chemicals. Oestrogenous compounds abound in garlic, parsley, wheat (soy, rice), fruits, vegetables, caffeine, and other meals and beverages. They are essential parts of the defensive mechanism of the plant, which fights fungus. Nutrient status is not justified even if they bind to oestrogen receptors and have several consequences on human intake. Their dietary exclusion does not cause any particular deficiency symptom; moreover, they are not involved in any important biological function. Among the main phytoestrogens are coumestans (coumestrol, for example), flavonols (quercetin, kaempferol, and enterolactone), lignans (enterodiol, for example, and enterolactone), and isoflavones (genistein, daidzein, glicetin, formononetin, biochanin A, and equol, a metabolite of isoflavones). Within pharmacology, the first three groups are known as flavonoids (Gasmi et al., 2022b).

They are more oestrogenic than lignans and have always rather significant antioxidant action. While isoflavones such genistein and daidzein are found in soy and many vegetables, fruits, vegetables, whole grains, fibre, seeds, and lignans such enterodiol and enterolactone are common. In that they prevent the synthesis of oestradiol but improve oestradiol metabolism by raising the production of 2-hydroxyestrone and lowering the production of the less desirable 16-hydroxyestrone (Brooks et al., 2004), linseed phytoestrogens function similarly to hormone-inhibiting chemotherapeutic drugs. Studies on rat PC12 cell cultures suggest that by stopping the formation of amyloid plaques and maintaining ATP levels, phytoestrogens may provide neuroprotection (Ogidi & Ajoko, 2024). Recent studies supporting phytoestrogen anti-atherogenic claims show that they lower LDL oxidation by suppressing superoxide radical generation (Jefremov et al., 2007; Brooks et al., 2004). Phytoestrogens are antioxidants meant to stop the molecular and cellular ageing mechanisms (Jefremov et al., 2007). The chemical structure of phytoestrogens is illustrated in Figure 8.

Figure 8. Chemical structure of phytoestrogens

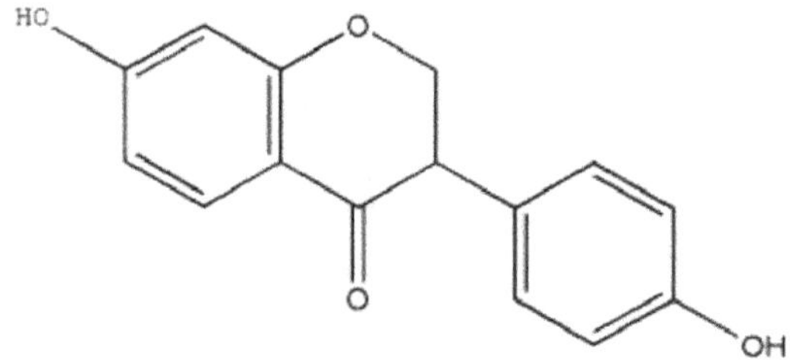

Table 4. Experimental data on lifespan-extending plant metabolites

Plant Metabolite	Experimental Evidence	Empirical Results	Study Model	References
Resveratrol	Activated sirtuins (SIRT1), improved mitochondrial function, and reduced inflammation.	Extended lifespan by ~30% in mice on a high-fat diet.	Mice	Baur et al., 2006
Curcumin	Reduced oxidative stress and inflammation while promoting autophagy.	~20% lifespan extension in *C. elegans*.	*C. elegans*	Liao et al., 2011
Epigallocatechin Gallate (EGCG)	Enhanced stress resistance and reduced cellular damage.	Lifespan increased by ~15% in fruit flies.	Fruit flies	Li et al., 2007
Quercetin	Promoted antioxidant defenses and senescent cell clearance.	Lifespan extended by ~20% in treated nematodes.	*C. elegans*	Saul et al., 2013
Spermidine	Induced autophagy and improved cellular homeostasis.	Lifespan extended by ~25% in yeast and ~15% in mice.	Yeast, Mice	Eisenberg et al., 2009
Fisetin	Acted as a senolytic agent, clearing senescent cells and reducing inflammation.	~10% lifespan extension in aged mice.	Mice	Yousefzadeh et al., 2018
Apigenin	Reduced oxidative stress and promoted DNA repair.	~12% lifespan extension in fruit flies.	Fruit flies	Rzezniczak et al., 2011
Kaempferol	Stimulated antioxidative responses and autophagy.	Lifespan extended by ~15% in *C. elegans*.	*C. elegans*	Pietsch et al., 2011

LIFESPAN-EXTENDING COCOA DERIVATIVES

Chocolate, a prominent cocoa derivative, is believed to possess memory-enhancing properties by a significant number of individuals. Flavonoids, which are believed to enhance blood flow to the brain, are abundant in chocolate that contains at least 70% cocoa. Epicatechin, a flavonoid with potent anti-aging properties, is present in a variety of foods, such as dark chocolate, berries, tea, and cocoa (Si et al., 2021). Smaller chocolate portions should be consumed more frequently in order to ensure that nutrients are absorbed more gradually into the bloodstream. A bar of "therapeutic chocolate" is vastly different from milk chocolate, which typically contains a significant amount of added sugar or sweeteners (Latif, 2013). It is the fruit of the Theobroma cacao plant, which is commonly referred to as the cocoa bean. Cocoa's numerous health advantages, such as improved cardiovascular health and a reduced body fat percentage, are attributable to its substantial antioxidant content and other natural components. When consumed frequently, dark chocolate offers approximately forty distinct health advantages. "Cocoa powder" is a term that refers to the pulverised, toasted, and unsweetened cocoa plant seeds. Cocoa butter is the term used to describe the fat found in the legume (Si et al., 2021).

Unsaturated lipids, omega-3 and omega-6 fatty acids, and vitamins A, E, and K are all present in cocoa butter. Cocoa butter is a critical component of chocolate recipes that are of superior quality. The antioxidants in this product neutralise free radicals, which are responsible for the ageing of the epidermis. Chocolate is a culinary product that is either solid or sweet and is produced by cooking cocoa seeds, typically in a skillet. Unfried chocolate is typically sweetened due to the fact that cocoa beans are not heated. Chocolate becomes more of a health food as the percentage of antioxidants increases. Milk chocolate offers few health advantages as a result of its low cocoa content. Refined sugar chocolate is the most prevalent type, despite the fact that cocoa powder is frequently detectably acrid. Nutritionists regard dark chocolate and unprocessed cocoa powder as superfoods due to their substantial antioxidant and anti-inflammatory contents. In recent years, medical researchers have increasingly recognised the advantageous effects of cocoa powder on the cardiovascular system and blood vessels. It seems that these advantages are significantly influenced by beneficial microorganisms in the intestine (Sorrenti et al., 2020). Some lifespan-extending cocoa derivatives are shown in Figure 9.

Cocoa powder is an exceptionally potent antioxidant due to its abundance of polyphenols. It was a widely held belief that these molecules were too large to be efficiently ingested and digested. The components of dark chocolate are degraded by specific beneficial bacteria in the digestive tract, resulting in the production of readily absorbed chemicals that possess anti-inflammatory properties. Cocoa is a preferred substrate for beneficial bacteria, including Bifidobacterium and lactic acid bacteria. The cocoa powder fibres are converted into short-chain fatty acids that induce satiety by beneficial microorganisms. This study has the potential to illuminate the manner in which dark chocolate enhances cardiovascular health, as it contains anti-inflammatory components. Dark chocolate's filaments are broken down into smaller, more absorbable polyphenolic polymer molecules by fermentation, according to one theory (Latif, 2013). These small polymers have the potential to mitigate inflammation. In the long term, these chemicals reduce the risk of stroke by reducing inflammation in cardiovascular tissue. The research suggests that the consistent consumption of dark chocolate may enhance gut health by promoting the growth of beneficial microorganisms and suppressing the growth of harmful ones. One advantage of consuming dark chocolate, which contains probiotics, is the maintenance of a healthy microbiome. Cocoa percentages are generally greater in chocolate that is darker. As a result of the bitterness of natural cocoa, the quantity of cocoa used directly influences the bitterness of the final product. The flavonoids are the primary cause of the bittersweet flavour and health benefits of dark chocolate. Calorie restriction is one of the primary metabolic regulators of longevity (Si et al., 2021).

Figure 9. Lifespan-extending cocoa derivatives

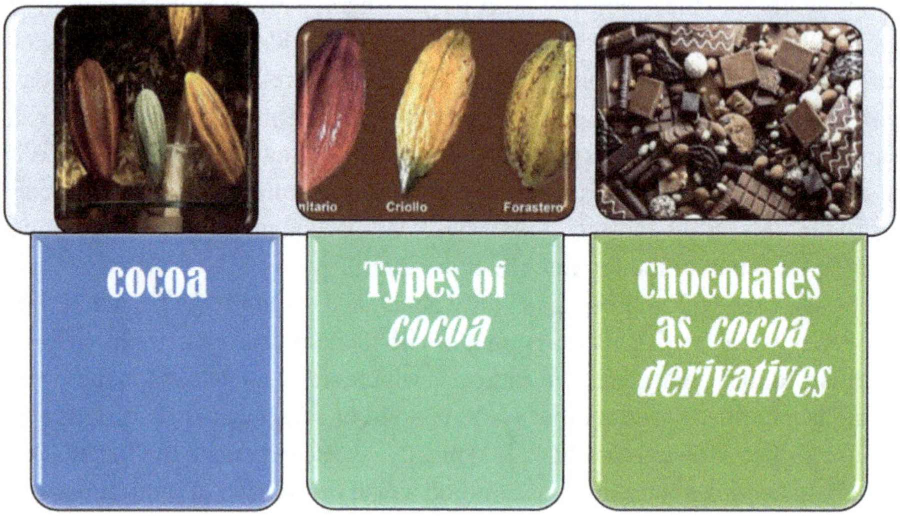

LIFESPAN-EXTENDING MARINE-DERIVED COMPOUNDS

Growing knowledge of the need of internal beauty development led to nutritional cosmetics and cosmeceuticals (Alves et al., 2020). Many times, uncommon chemical compounds with superior biological potential have been discovered in marine rather than land-based sources (Gasmi et al., 2020; Wang et al., 2021b). Fish oils include significant omega-3 fatty acids; nevertheless, crustaceans and seaweeds have plenty of antioxidants including carotenoids and phenolic compounds (Ghosh et al., 2022). Found in crabs and other aquatic life, astaxanthin is a carotenoid with strong anti-aging and antioxidant action (Zhou et al., 2021). It increases skin elasticity and slows down wrinkle growth by means of immunological control, anti-inflammatory activities, and DNA repair pathways (Singh et al., 2020). Astaxanthin (Chan et al., 2009; Bjorklund et al., 2022b) might help to prevent neurodegenerative diseases. One element of brown algae called laminarin lessens UV-induced skin damage (Ahn et al., 2020). Chemicals with antioxidant, antiviral, antitumor, and antibacterial properties can be produced by several marine organisms including myxomycetes, bacteria, and microalgae (Ghosh et al., 2022; Cao et al., 2020). An outstanding anti-aging skin care product derived from Dunaliella salina, a green microalgae with anti-glycation and anti-inflammatory properties is Because of their carbohydrate concentration, marine algae help to improve skin condition (Havas et al., 2022; Kim et al., 2018b). Lifespan-extending marine-derived compounds are illustrated in Figure 10.

Figure 10. Lifespan-extending marine-derived compounds

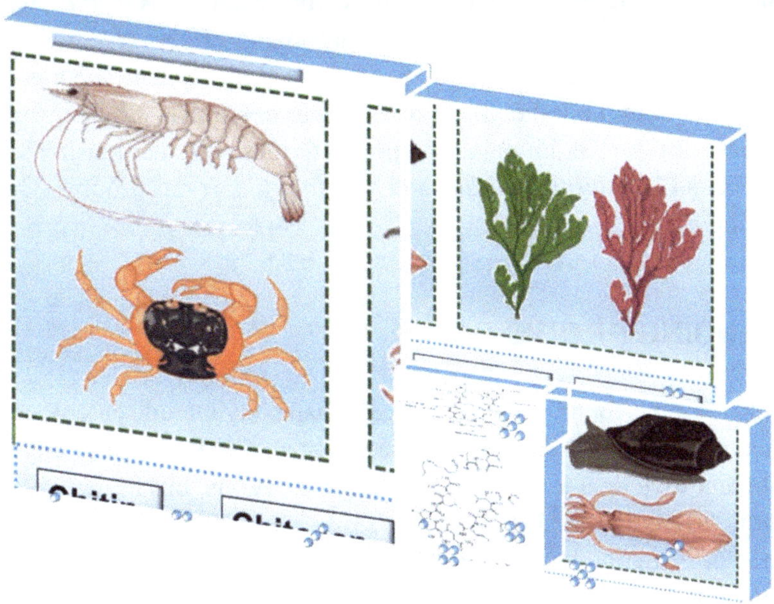

LIFESPAN-EXTENDING HONEYBEE PRODUCTS

Studies have identified honey, bee pollen, propolis, and royal jelly as honeybee products with the potential to increase human life expectancy (Cornara et al., 2017; Giampieri et al., 2022; Kurek-Gorecka et al., 2020; Ogidi & Otenep, 2020). Bee products find use in dermatology due to royal jelly's anti-inflammatory, antiallergenic, antibacterial, and antiaging pharmacological characteristics. The beneficial effects of royal jelly, which is made by bees, have been documented by Collazo et al. (2021). These effects include oestrogenic, anti-aging, antioxidant, antiproliferative, antibacterial, anti-inflammatory, and neuroprotective effects. The stated properties are mostly due to proteins, carbs, and fats, but small quantities of vitamins, terpenic volatiles, macro- and microelements, and polyphenols also contribute. Based on their meta-analysis of human and animal studies, Kunugi & Mohammed (2019) concluded that the active ingredients in royal jelly may have anti-aging and life-extending effects (Kunugi & Mohammed, 2019). Drosophila melanogaster was found to have an increased lifespan after being fed royal jelly (Cornara et al., 2017). Research in living organisms revealed estrogen-like effects, laying the groundwork for anti-menopause uses (Cornara et al., 2017).

LIFESPAN-EXTENDING MUSHROOMS

Studies on living organisms has shown that the edible Maitake (*Grifola frondosa*) mushroom, which contains polysaccharides containing zinc, has anti-aging effects (Azimova et al., 2025; Ogidi et al., 2021; Zhang et al., 2017; Ogidi et al., 2025; Akhigbe et al., 2025). The use of maitake (*Grifola frondosa*) polysaccharides in immunotherapy to treat cancer in humans has been authorised (Wu et al., 2021; Ogidi & Oguoma, 2025). Additional anti-aging activities were demonstrated by polysaccharide complexes produced from *Ganoderma lucidum* and *Agaricus blazei* mushrooms (Ogidi, 2025; Wang et al., 2017; Ogidi & Adigwe, 2025).

LIFESPAN-EXTENDING PROBIOTICS

The predominant probiotics found naturally in the human body include enterococci, lactobacilli, and bifidobacteria (Lolou & Panayiotidis, 2019; Sivamaruthi et al., 2018). Their ability to affect the microbiota of the skin and digestive tract may decrease allergic reactions, inflammation, and viral infections (Lolou & Panayiotidis, 2019; Roudsari et al., 2015; Gasmi et al., 2021). The composition of microbiota plays a crucial role in determining health status and warrants careful consideration (Christensen et al., 2017). The gut microbiota may contribute to diabetes and obesity by affecting host metabolism and insulin resistance during digestion and nutrient absorption (Ogidi & Felagha, 2024; Inglis & Ilich, 2015).

The microbiota contributes to inflammatory bowel disease, detoxification, infection resistance, and various gastrointestinal disorders (Gasmi et al., 2021; Tremaroli & Backhed, 2012). Research indicates that microbiota influences ageing, suggesting that alterations in microbiota, such as those present in probiotic bacteria found in yoghurt, may improve health outcomes (El-Abbadi et al., 2014). Research indicates that the composition of gut microbiota varies between younger and older individuals, implying that bacteria may influence the ageing process in humans (Roudsari et al., 2015). However, the causal processes linking probiotic bacteria and ageing remain largely ambiguous.

RECENTLY IDENTIFIED METABOLITES WITH LIFE-EXTENDING PROPERTIES

Alpha-Ketoglutarate (AKG)

Alpha-Ketoglutarate (AKG) has been identified as a metabolite that may extend lifespan. Research on mice demonstrated that calcium alpha-ketoglutarate (CaAKG) supplementation led to increased lifespan and improved health markers by reducing systemic inflammation, particularly through the induction of interleukin-10 (IL-10) (Sharma, 2021).

Lithocholic Acid (LCA)

Recent studies have shown that lithocholic acid (LCA) mimics the anti-aging effects of calorie restriction by activating AMP-activated protein kinase (AMPK), enhancing muscle regeneration, and improving grip strength. These effects suggest that LCA may contribute to increased lifespan and improved healthspan (Nature, 2024).

1-Methylnicotinamide (1-MNA)

1-Methylnicotinamide (1-MNA) has been found to optimize NAD^+ levels by inhibiting nicotinamide N-methyltransferase (NNMT), which enhances SIRT1 expression. Studies indicate that 1-MNA supplementation may extend lifespan and provide neuroprotective benefits.

Taurine

A study in 2023 reported that taurine supplementation in mice increased lifespan by 10-12%. Taurine, a naturally occurring amino sulfonic acid, has been linked to improved cellular function and reduced age-related diseases, suggesting its potential as an anti-aging supplement (Post, 2024).

CONCLUSION AND FUTURE PERSPECTIVE

The future of lifespan-extending natural compounds holds significant promise, with ongoing research revealing their potential to promote healthy ageing and reduce age-related diseases. Recent advancements in science and technology, particularly in omics technologies, computational modelling, and clinical research, are anticipated to address existing challenges and create new opportunities in this domain. These advancements will improve our comprehension of the mechanisms that govern the effects of natural compounds and facilitate their practical applications in ageing interventions. The concept of eternal life, which was previously considered science fiction, is now becoming increasingly feasible as a result of a series of technological advancements.

The study of longevity has been significantly impacted by the genetic and hereditary insights that have been gained from research on centenarians and other long-lived organisms, which have provided prolonged and healthy lifespans. Key biochemical components, such as sirtuins, AMPK, FOXOs, and mTOR, as well as lifestyle decisions such as regular exercise and balanced nutrition, are essential for establishing a foundation for longevity. The signalling pathways that are linked to longevity and ageing can be affected by naturally occurring chemicals that are derived from medicinal plants or ingested through food. This chapter investigates numerous signs of ageing with an emphasis on the prospective areas of effectiveness of natural compounds. In this context, we observe a variety of issues, including cellular ageing, inadequate (macro) autophagy, genetic instability, mitochondrial dysfunction, chronic inflammation, dysregulated nutrition sensing, and microbiome abnormalities. Rapamycin, resveratrol, sulforaphane, and fisetin are natural bioactive substances that have recently garnered significant attention. This is due to the abundance of evidence that suggests they have the potential to enhance health and extend life expectancies by affecting a variety of ageing markers. Senolytics, which are hybrid combinations of dasatinib and quercetin, have the capacity to regulate senescent cells, potentially resulting in a reduction in inflammation associated with senescence. Two examples of bioactive substances that exhibit potential as calorie-restrictor mimics to extend longevity are curcumin and metformin.

However, there is some evidence that the microbiome can influence the host body's functioning and the efficacy of pharmaceuticals when administered orally. This raises the question of how pro-longevity compounds influence the interactions between the host and microbiota. Consequently, additional research is required to ascertain the prospective impact of these medications on the microbiome. Although longevity research has made significant strides in the past decade, there are still numerous unresolved issues. Many of these studies employ model systems rather than actual individuals as subjects. The research employed optimal model systems for the dosages and interventions of small substances. The precise estimation of dose and treatment outcomes becomes more challenging when these findings are applied to human beings.

A significant advancement in the field of science would be the conduct of clinical trials on the most promising pharmaceutical candidates as potential pro-longevity medications. It is exceedingly challenging to monitor the consequences of these medications throughout an individual's lifespan. A system that can monitor every aspect of an individual's health may be achieved by combining future technology with epigenetic clocks, a reliable method of determining biological age. It will be exceedingly challenging to ascertain the precise onset and progression of ageing, as well as its molecular dynamics and cellular processes, in the years ahead. Personalised cell-type therapy could be better understood by examining the rate of senescence at the organ and single-cell levels. The extension of human life and the improvement of healthspan are complex and multifaceted endeavours. Multidisciplinary collaboration, innovative approaches, and a focus on personalization will be key to realizing their transformative promise.

REFERENCES

Abbatecola, A. M., Cherubini, A., Guralnik, J. M., Andres Lacueva, C., Ruggiero, C., Maggio, M., Bandinelli, S., Paolisso, G., & Ferrucci, L. (2009). Plasma polyunsaturated fatty acids and age-related physical performance decline. *Rejuvenation Research*, *12*(1), 25–32. DOI: 10.1089/rej.2008.0799 PMID: 19196012

Abdollahifar, M. A., Azad, N., Sajadi, E., Shams Mofarahe, Z., Zare, F., Moradi, A., Rezaee, F., Gholamin, M., & Abdi, S. (2019). Vitamin C restores ovarian follicular reservation in a mouse model of aging. *Anatomy & Cell Biology*, *52*(2), 196–203. DOI: 10.5115/acb.2019.52.2.196 PMID: 31338237

Agatonovic-Kustrin, S., Kustrin, E., & Morton, D. W. (2019). Essential oils and functional herbs for healthy aging. *Neural Regeneration Research*, *14*(3), 441–445. DOI: 10.4103/1673-5374.245467 PMID: 30539810

Ahn, J. H., Kim, D. W., Park, C. W., Kim, B., Sim, H., Kim, H. S., Lee, T. K., Lee, J. C., Yang, G. E., Her, Y., Park, J. H., Sim, T. H., Lee, H. S., & Won, M. H. (2020). Laminarin Attenuates Ultraviolet-Induced Skin Damage by Reducing Superoxide Anion Levels and Increasing Endogenous Antioxidants in the Dorsal Skin of Mice. *Marine Drugs*, *18*(7), 345. DOI: 10.3390/md18070345 PMID: 32629814

Akhigbe, E. O., Izah, S. C., Ogidi, O. I., Iyingiala, A. A., & Raimi, M. O. (2025). The Role of Edible Mushrooms in Immune Support. In Izah, S. C., Ogwu, M. C., & Akram, M. (Eds.), *Bioactive Compounds in Edible Mushrooms. Reference Series in Phytochemistry*. Springer., DOI: 10.1007/978-3-031-52642-8_21-1

Alves, A., Sousa, E., Kijjoa, A., & Pinto, M. (2020). Marine-Derived Compounds with Potential Use as Cosmeceuticals and Nutricosmetics. *Molecules (Basel, Switzerland)*, *25*(11), 2536. DOI: 10.3390/molecules25112536 PMID: 32486036

Anderson, R. A. (1998). Chromium, glucose intolerance and diabetes. *Journal of the American College of Nutrition*, *17*(6), 548–555. DOI: 10.1080/07315724.1998.10718802 PMID: 9853533

Andrews, N. C. (2008). Iron homeostasis: Insights from genetics and animal models. *Nature Reviews. Genetics*, *9*(4), 287–298. DOI: 10.1038/nrg2316 PMID: 11252750

Andrieu, S., Guyonnet, S., Coley, N., Cantet, C., Bonnefoy, M., Bordes, S., Bories, L., Cufi, M. N., Dantoine, T., Dartigues, J. F., Desclaux, F., Gabelle, A., Gasnier, Y., Pesce, A., Sudres, K., Touchon, J., Robert, P., Rouaud, O., Legrand, P., & Olivier-Abbal, P.MAPT Study Group. (2017). Effect of long-term omega 3 polyunsaturated fatty acid supplementation with or without multidomain intervention on cognitive function in elderly adults with memory complaints (MAPT): A randomised, placebo-controlled trial. *Lancet Neurology*, *16*(5), 377–389. DOI: 10.1016/S1474-4422(17)30040-6 PMID: 28359749

Ayaz, M., Sadiq, A., Junaid, M., Ullah, F., Ovais, M., Ullah, I., Ahmed, J., & Shahid, M. (2019). Flavonoids as Prospective Neuroprotectants and Their Therapeutic Propensity in Aging Associated Neurological Disorders. *Frontiers in Aging Neuroscience*, *11*, 155. DOI: 10.3389/fnagi.2019.00155 PMID: 31293414

Azimova, B., Xusniddinova, A., Izah, S. C., Sharipov, A., & Ogidi, O. I. (2025). Assessment of the Bioactive Compounds and Metabolites in the Edible Mushroom Used in Management of Rheumatic Disorders. In Izah, S. C., Ogwu, M. C., & Akram, M. (Eds.), *Bioactive Compounds in Edible Mushrooms. Reference Series in Phytochemistry*. Springer., DOI: 10.1007/978-3-031-52642-8_48-1

Baarz, B. R., Laurentius, T., Wolf, J., Wessels, I., Bollheimer, L. C., & Rink, L. (2022). Short-term zinc supplementation of zinc-deficient seniors counteracts CREMα - mediated IL-2 suppression. *Immunity & ageing: I & A, 19*(1), 40. https://doi.org/DOI: 10.1186/s12979-022-00295-8

Baek, J. H., Yoo, M. A., Koh, J. S., & Borkow, G. (2012). Reduction of facial wrinkles depth by sleeping on copper oxide-containing pillowcases: A double blind, placebo controlled, parallel, randomized clinical study. *Journal of Cosmetic Dermatology, 11*(3), 193–200. DOI: 10.1111/j.1473-2165.2012.00624.x PMID: 22938003

Banks, R., Speakman, J. R., & Selman, C. (2010). Vitamin E supplementation and lifespan in mice. *Free Radical Biology & Medicine, 49*(11), 1742–1749. DOI: 10.1016/j.freeradbiomed.2010.09.005

Barbagallo, M., & Dominguez, L. J. (2010). Magnesium and aging. *Current Pharmaceutical Design, 16*(7), 832–839. DOI: 10.2174/138161210790883679 PMID: 20388094

Barzilai, N., Crandall, J. P., Kritchevsky, S. B., & Espeland, M. A. (2012). Metformin as a tool to target aging. *Cell Metabolism, 16*(6), 727–731. DOI: 10.1016/j.cmet.2012.11.007 PMID: 27304507

Baur, J. A., Pearson, K. J., Price, N. L., Jamieson, H. A., Lerin, C., Kalra, A., & Sinclair, D. A. (2006). Resveratrol improves health and survival of mice on a high-calorie diet. *Nature, 444*(7117), 337–342. DOI: 10.1038/nature05354 PMID: 17086191

Baur, J. A., & Sinclair, D. A. (2006). Therapeutic potential of resveratrol: The in vivo evidence. *Nature Reviews. Drug Discovery, 5*(6), 493–506. DOI: 10.1038/nrd2060 PMID: 16732220

Bjorklund, G., Gasmi, A., Lenchyk, L., Shanaida, M., Zafar, S., Mujawdiya, P. K., Lysiuk, R., Antonyak, H., Noor, S., Akram, M., Smetanina, K., Piscopo, S., Upyr, T., & Peana, M. (2022a). The Role of Astaxanthin as a Nutraceutical in Health and Age-Related Conditions. *Molecules (Basel, Switzerland), 27*(21), 7167. DOI: 10.3390/molecules27217167 PMID: 36363994

Bjorklund, G., Shanaida, M., Lysiuk, R., Antonyak, H., Klishch, I., Shanaida, V., & Peana, M. (2022b). Selenium: An Antioxidant with a Critical Role in Anti-Aging. *Molecules (Basel, Switzerland), 27*(19), 6613. DOI: 10.3390/molecules27196613 PMID: 36235150

Bjorklund, G., Zou, L., Wang, J., Chasapis, C. T., & Peana, M. (2021). Thioredoxin reductase as a pharmacological target. *Pharmacological Research, 174*, 105854. DOI: 10.1016/j.phrs.2021.105854 PMID: 34455077

Borkow, G. (2014). Using Copper to Improve the Well-Being of the Skin. *Current Chemical Biology, 8*(2), 89–102. DOI: 10.2174/2212796809666150227223857 PMID: 26361585

Boyd, J. T., LoCoco, P. M., Furr, A. R., Bendele, M. R., Tram, M., Li, Q., Chang, F. M., Colley, M. E., Samenuk, G. M., Arris, D. A., Locke, E. E., Bach, S. B. H., Tobon, A., Ruparel, S. B., & Hargreaves, K. M. (2021). Elevated dietary ω-6 polyunsaturated fatty acids induce reversible peripheral nerve dysfunction that exacerbates comorbid pain conditions. *Nature Metabolism*, *3*(6), 762–773. DOI: 10.1038/s42255-021-00410-x PMID: 34140694

Brigelius-Flohe, R., & Davies, K. J. (2007). Is vitamin E an antioxidant, a regulator of signal transduction and gene expression, or a 'junk' food? Comments on the two accompanying papers: "Molecular mechanism of alpha-tocopherol action" by A. Azzi and "Vitamin E, antioxidant and nothing more" by M. Traber and J. Atkinson. *Free Radical Biology & Medicine*, *43*(1), 2–3. DOI: 10.1016/j.freeradbiomed.2007.05.016 PMID: 17561087

Brooks, J. D., Ward, W. E., Lewis, J. E., Hilditch, J., Nickell, L., Wong, E., & Thompson, L. U. (2004). Supplementation with flaxseed alters estrogen metabolism in postmenopausal women to a greater extent than does supplementation with an equal amount of soy. *The American Journal of Clinical Nutrition*, *79*(2), 318–325. DOI: 10.1093/ajcn/79.2.318 PMID: 14749240

Budoff, M. J., Ahmadi, N., Gul, K. M., Liu, S. T., Flores, F. R., Tiano, J., Takasu, J., Miller, E., & Tsimikas, S. (2009). Aged garlic extract supplemented with B vitamins, folic acid and L-arginine retards the progression of subclinical atherosclerosis: A randomized clinical trial. *Preventive Medicine*, *49*(2-3), 101–107. DOI: 10.1016/j.ypmed.2009.06.018 PMID: 19573556

Cabrera, A. J. (2015). Zinc, aging, and immunosenescence: An overview. *Pathobiology of Aging & Age-Related Diseases*, *5*(1), 25592. DOI: 10.3402/pba.v5.25592 PMID: 25661703

Cai, Z., Zhang, J., & Li, H. (2019). Selenium, aging and aging-related diseases. *Aging Clinical and Experimental Research*, *31*(8), 1035–1047. DOI: 10.1007/s40520-018-1086-7 PMID: 30511318

Calder, P. C., Ortega, E. F., Meydani, S. N., Adkins, Y., Stephensen, C. B., Thompson, B., & Zwickey, H. (2022). Nutrition, Immunosenescence, and Infectious Disease: An Overview of the Scientific Evidence on Micronutrients and on Modulation of the Gut Microbiota. *Advances in Nutrition*, *13*(5), S1–S26. DOI: 10.1093/advances/nmac052 PMID: 36183242

Cao, L., Lee, S. G., Lim, K. T., & Kim, H. R. (2020). Potential Anti-Aging Substances Derived from Seaweeds. *Marine Drugs*, *18*(11), 564. DOI: 10.3390/md18110564 PMID: 33218066

Castiglione, D., Platania, A., Conti, A., Falla, M., D'Urso, M., & Marranzano, M. (2018). Dietary Micronutrient and Mineral Intake in the Mediterranean Healthy Eating, Ageing, and Lifestyle (MEAL) Study. *Antioxidants*, *7*(7), 79. DOI: 10.3390/antiox7070079 PMID: 29937504

Chan, K. C., Mong, M. C., & Yin, M. C. (2009). Antioxidative and anti-inflammatory neuroprotective effects of astaxanthin and canthaxanthin in nerve growth factor differentiated PC12 cells. *Journal of Food Science*, *74*(7), H225–H231. DOI: 10.1111/j.1750-3841.2009.01274.x PMID: 19895474

Chappus-McCendie, H., Chevalier, L., Roberge, C., & Plourde, M. (2019). Omega-3 PUFA metabolism and brain modifications during aging. *Progress in Neuro-Psychopharmacology & Biological Psychiatry*, *94*, 109662. DOI: 10.1016/j.pnpbp.2019.109662 PMID: 31152862

Chasapis, C. T., Ntoupa, P. A., Spiliopoulou, C. A., & Stefanidou, M. E. (2020). Recent aspects of the effects of zinc on human health. *Archives of Toxicology*, *94*(5), 1443–1460. DOI: 10.1007/s00204-020-02702-9 PMID: 32394086

Choi, S., Liu, X., & Pan, Z. (2018). Zinc deficiency and cellular oxidative stress: Prognostic implications in cardiovascular diseases. *Acta Pharmacologica Sinica*, *39*(7), 1120–1132. DOI: 10.1038/aps.2018.25 PMID: 29926844

Christensen, K. V., Morch, M. G., Morthorst, T. H., Lykkemark, S., & Olsen, A. (2017). Microbiota, probiotic bacteria and ageing. In *Ageing: Lessons from C. elegans* (pp. 411–429). Springer. DOI: 10.1007/978-3-319-44703-2_18

Chung, H. Y., Kim, D. H., Lee, E. K., An, H. J., Yoon, J. H., Kim, N. D., & Yu, B. P. (2019). Redefining chronic inflammation in aging and age-related diseases: Proposal of the senoinflammation concept. *Ageing Research Reviews*, *47*, 24–31. DOI: 10.1016/j.arr.2018.11.002 PMID: 31011483

Collazo, N., Carpena, M., Nuñez-Estevez, B., Otero, P., Simal-Gandara, J., & Prieto, M. A. (2021). Health Promoting Properties of Bee Royal Jelly: Food of the Queens. *Nutrients*, *13*(2), 543. DOI: 10.3390/nu13020543 PMID: 33562330

Cornara, L., Biagi, M., Xiao, J., & Burlando, B. (2017). Therapeutic Properties of Bioactive Compounds from Different Honeybee Products. *Frontiers in Pharmacology*, *8*, 412. DOI: 10.3389/fphar.2017.00412 PMID: 28701955

Cutuli, D. (2017). Functional and Structural Benefits Induced by Omega-3 Polyunsaturated Fatty Acids During Aging. *Current Neuropharmacology*, *15*(4), 534–542. DOI: 10.2174/1570159X14666160614091311 PMID: 27306037

Cutuli, D., Pagani, M., Caporali, P., Galbusera, A., Laricchiuta, D., Foti, F., Neri, C., Spalletta, G., Caltagirone, C., Petrosini, L., & Gozzi, A. (2016). Effects of Omega-3 Fatty Acid Supplementation on Cognitive Functions and Neural Substrates: A Voxel-Based Morphometry Study in Aged Mice. *Frontiers in Aging Neuroscience*, *8*, 38. DOI: 10.3389/fnagi.2016.00038 PMID: 26973513

Delanghe, J. R., Langlois, M. R., De Buyzere, M. L., Na, N., Ouyang, J., Speeckaert, M. M., & Torck, M. A. (2011). Vitamin C deficiency: More than just a nutritional disorder. *Genes & Nutrition*, *6*(4), 341–346. DOI: 10.1007/s12263-011-0237-7 PMID: 21614623

Denis, I., Potier, B., Heberden, C., & Vancassel, S. (2015). Omega-3 polyunsaturated fatty acids and brain aging. *Current Opinion in Clinical Nutrition and Metabolic Care*, *18*(2), 139–146. DOI: 10.1097/MCO.0000000000000141 PMID: 25501348

Denis, I., Potier, B., Vancassel, S., Heberden, C., & Lavialle, M. (2013). Omega-3 fatty acids and brain resistance to ageing and stress: Body of evidence and possible mechanisms. *Ageing Research Reviews*, *12*(2), 579–594. DOI: 10.1016/j.arr.2013.01.007 PMID: 23395782

Dyall, S. C., & Michael-Titus, A. T. (2015). Neurological benefits of omega-3 fatty acids. *Neuroscience Research*, *92*, 1–12. DOI: 10.1016/j.neures.2014.08.002

Eisenberg, T., Knauer, H., Schauer, A., Büttner, S., Ruckenstuhl, C., Carmona-Gutierrez, D., & Madeo, F. (2009). Induction of autophagy by spermidine promotes longevity. *Nature Cell Biology*, *11*(11), 1305–1314. DOI: 10.1038/ncb1975 PMID: 19801973

El-Abbadi, N. H., Dao, M. C., & Meydani, S. N. (2014). Yogurt: Role in healthy and active aging. *The American Journal of Clinical Nutrition*, *99*(5, Suppl), 1263S–1270S. DOI: 10.3945/ajcn.113.073957 PMID: 24695886

Enenebeaku, U. E., Duru, C. E., Okotcha, E. N., Ogidi, O. I., Mgbemena, I. C., Nwigwe, H. C., & Enenebeaku, C. K. (2022). Phytochemical analysis and Antioxidant Evaluation of Crude Extracts from the Roots, Stem and Leaves of Dictyandraarborescens (Welw.). *Tropical Journal of Natural Product Research*, *6*(1), 62–70. DOI: 10.26538/tjnpr/v6i1.12

Fan, X., Fan, Z., Yang, Z., Huang, T., Tong, Y., Yang, D., Mao, X., & Yang, M. (2022). Flavonoids-Natural Gifts to Promote Health and Longevity. *International Journal of Molecular Sciences*, *23*(4), 2176. DOI: 10.3390/ijms23042176 PMID: 35216290

Fan, Y. Y., & Chapkin, R. S. (2003). Importance of dietary gamma-linolenic acid in human health and aging. *Nutrition Research (New York, N.Y.)*, *23*(6), 795–807. DOI: 10.1016/S0271-5317(03)00077-4

Fleenor, B. S., Sindler, A. L., Marvi, N. K., Howell, K. L., Zigler, M. L., Yoshizawa, M., & Seals, D. R. (2013). Curcumin ameliorates arterial dysfunction and oxidative stress with aging. *Experimental Gerontology*, *48*(2), 269–276. DOI: 10.1016/j.exger.2012.10.008 PMID: 23142245

Fontana, L., Partridge, L., & Longo, V. D. (2010). Extending healthy life span—From yeast to humans. *Science*, *328*(5976), 321–326. DOI: 10.1126/science.1172539 PMID: 20395504

Fulop, T., Larbi, A., Dupuis, G., Le Page, A., Frost, E. H., Cohen, A. A., Witkowski, J. M., & Franceschi, C. (2018). Immunosenescence and Inflamm-Aging As Two Sides of the Same Coin: Friends or Foes? *Frontiers in Immunology*, *8*, 1960. DOI: 10.3389/fimmu.2017.01960 PMID: 29375577

Gasmi, A., Mujawdiya, P. K., Lysiuk, R., Shanaida, M., Peana, M., Gasmi Benahmed, A., Beley, N., Kovalska, N., & Bjørklund, G. (2022a). Quercetin in the Prevention and Treatment of Coronavirus Infections: A Focus on SARS-CoV-2. *Pharmaceuticals (Basel, Switzerland)*, *15*(9), 1049. DOI: 10.3390/ph15091049 PMID: 36145270

Gasmi, A., Mujawdiya, P. K., Noor, S., Lysiuk, R., Darmohray, R., Piscopo, S., Lenchyk, L., Antonyak, H., Dehtiarova, K., Shanaida, M., Polishchuk, A., Shanaida, V., Peana, M., & Bjørklund, G. (2022b). Polyphenols in Metabolic Diseases. *Molecules (Basel, Switzerland)*, *27*(19), 6280. DOI: 10.3390/molecules27196280 PMID: 36234817

Gasmi, A., Mujawdiya, P. K., Shanaida, M., Ongenae, A., Lysiuk, R., Doşa, M. D., Tsal, O., Piscopo, S., Chirumbolo, S., & Bjørklund, G. (2020). Calanus oil in the treatment of obesity-related low-grade inflammation, insulin resistance, and atherosclerosis. *Applied Microbiology and Biotechnology*, *104*(3), 967–979. DOI: 10.1007/s00253-019-10293-4 PMID: 31853565

Gasmi, A., Tippairote, T., Mujawdiya, P. K., Peana, M., Menzel, A., Dadar, M., Benahmed, A. G., & Bjørklund, G. (2021). The microbiota-mediated dietary and nutritional interventions for COVID-19. *Clinical Immunology (Orlando, Fla.)*, *226*, 108725. DOI: 10.1016/j.clim.2021.108725 PMID: 33845194

Gašperlin, M., & Gosenca, M. (2011). Main approaches for delivering antioxidant vitamins through the skin to prevent skin ageing. *Expert Opinion on Drug Delivery*, *8*(7), 905–919. DOI: 10.1517/17425247.2011.581657 PMID: 21599565

Gellert, S., Schuchardt, J. P., & Hahn, A. (2017). Low long chain omega-3 fatty acid status in middle-aged women. *Prostaglandins, Leukotrienes, and Essential Fatty Acids*, *117*, 54–59. DOI: 10.1016/j.plefa.2017.01.009 PMID: 28237088

Gharibi, S., Bakhtiari, N., Jalalvand, E.-M., & Bakhtiari, F. (2018). Ursolic Acid Mediates Hepatic Protection through Enhancing of anti-aging Biomarkers. *Current Aging Science*, *11*(1), 16–23. DOI: 10 .2174/1874609810666170531103140 PMID: 28558631

Ghosh, S., Sarkar, T., Pati, S., Kari, Z. A., Edinur, H. A., & Chakraborty, R. (2022). Novel bioactive compounds from marine sources as a tool for functional food development. *Frontiers in Marine Science*, *9*, 10–3389. DOI: 10.3389/fmars.2022.832957

Giampieri, F., Quiles, J. L., Cianciosi, D., Forbes-Hernández, T. Y., Orantes-Bermejo, F. J., Alvarez-Suarez, J. M., & Battino, M. (2022). Bee Products: An Emblematic Example of Underutilized Sources of Bioactive Compounds. *Journal of Agricultural and Food Chemistry*, *70*(23), 6833–6848. DOI: 10.1021/acs.jafc.1c05822 PMID: 34974697

Green, B. A., Yu, R. J., & Van Scott, E. J. (2009). Clinical and cosmeceutical uses of hydroxyacids. *Clinics in Dermatology*, *27*(5), 495–501. DOI: 10.1016/j.clindermatol.2009.06.023 PMID: 19695482

Haase, H., & Rink, L. (2009). The immune system and the impact of zinc during aging. *Immunity & ageing: I & A*, *6*, 9. https://doi.org/DOI: 10.1186/1742-4933-6-9

Hagopian, K., Ramsey, J. J., & Weindruch, R. (2010). Caloric restriction increases fatty acid synthesis and whole body fat oxidation rates in mice. *The Journal of Nutrition*, *140*(5), 890–896. DOI: 10.3945/jn.109.115790

Hancianu, M., Cioanca, O., Mihasan, M., & Hritcu, L. (2013). Neuroprotective effects of inhaled lavender oil on scopolamine-induced dementia via anti-oxidative activities in rats. *Phytomedicine*, *20*(5), 446–452. DOI: 10.1016/j.phymed.2012.12.005 PMID: 23351960

Harris, E. D. (2003). Copper homeostasis: The role of cellular transporters. *Nutrition Reviews*, *61*(3), 70–73. DOI: 10.1301/nr.2003.mar.70-73 PMID: 11570430

Harrison, E. H., & Hussain, M. M. (2009). Mechanisms involved in the intestinal absorption of dietary vitamin A. *The Journal of Nutritional Biochemistry*, *20*(9), 623–633. DOI: 10.1016/j.jnutbio.2009.02.002

Havas, F., Krispin, S., Cohen, M., Loing, E., Farge, M., Suere, T., & Attia-Vigneau, J. (2022). A *Dunaliella salina* Extract Counteracts Skin Aging under Intense Solar Irradiation Thanks to Its Antiglycation and Anti-Inflammatory Properties. *Marine Drugs*, *20*(2), 104. DOI: 10.3390/md20020104 PMID: 35200634

Herrera, E., & Barbas, C. (2001). Vitamin E: Action, metabolism and perspectives. *Journal of Physiology and Biochemistry*, *57*(2), 43–56. DOI: 10.1007/BF03179812 PMID: 11579997

Hooper, C., De Souto Barreto, P., Coley, N., Cantet, C., Cesari, M., Andrieu, S., & Vellas, B. (2017). Cognitive Changes with Omega-3 Polyunsaturated Fatty Acids in Non-Demented Older Adults with Low Omega-3 Index. *The Journal of Nutrition, Health & Aging, 21*(9), 988–993. DOI: 10.1007/s12603-017-0957-5 PMID: 29083439

Huang, T. H., Wang, P. W., Yang, S. C., Chou, W. L., & Fang, J. Y. (2018). Cosmetic and Therapeutic Applications of Fish Oil's Fatty Acids on the Skin. *Marine Drugs, 16*(8), 256. DOI: 10.3390/md16080256 PMID: 30061538

Inglis, J. E., & Ilich, J. Z. (2015). The Microbiome and Osteosarcopenic Obesity in Older Individuals in Long-Term Care Facilities. *Current Osteoporosis Reports, 13*(5), 358–362. DOI: 10.1007/s11914-015-0287-7 PMID: 26272433

Iwamoto, J., Takeda, T., & Sato, Y. (2011). Effects of vitamin K2 on osteoporosis in the elderly. *Nutrition (Burbank, Los Angeles County, Calif.), 27*(10), 1165–1171. DOI: 10.1016/j.nut.2011.01.012

Jarosz, M., Olbert, M., Wyszogrodzka, G., Młyniec, K., & Librowski, T. (2017). Antioxidant and anti-inflammatory effects of zinc. Zinc-dependent NF-κB signaling. *Inflammopharmacology, 25*(1), 11–24. DOI: 10.1007/s10787-017-0309-4 PMID: 28083748

Jefremov, V., Zilmer, M., Zilmer, K., Bogdanovic, N., & Karelson, E. (2007). Antioxidative effects of plant polyphenols: From protection of G protein signaling to prevention of age-related pathologies. *Annals of the New York Academy of Sciences, 1095*(1), 449–457. DOI: 10.1196/annals.1397.048 PMID: 17404057

Kafi, R., Kwak, H. S., Schumacher, W. E., Cho, S., Hanft, V. N., Hamilton, T. A., King, A. L., Neal, J. D., Varani, J., Fisher, G. J., Voorhees, J. J., & Kang, S. (2007). Improvement of naturally aged skin with vitamin A (retinol). *Archives of Dermatology, 143*(5), 606–612. DOI: 10.1001/archderm.143.5.606 PMID: 17515510

Katiyar, S. K. (2011). Green tea prevents non-melanoma skin cancer by enhancing DNA repair. *Archives of Biochemistry and Biophysics, 508*(2), 152–158. DOI: 10.1016/j.abb.2010.11.015 PMID: 21094124

Kazemi, T., Moodi, M., Rajabi, S., Sharifi, F., Samarghandian, S., Khorashadizadeh, M., & Farkhondeh, T. (2022). Trace Element Concentration and Cognitive Dysfunction in Elderly Residents in Birjand. *Current Alzheimer Research, 19*(9), 674–680. DOI: 10.2174/1567205019666220913114154 PMID: 36100996

Keen, C. L., Ensunsa, J. L., & Watson, M. H. (2003). Nutritional aspects of manganese from experimental studies. *Neurotoxicology, 24*(4-5), 645–656. DOI: 10.1016/s0161-813x(03)00030-1 PMID: 10385885

Keen, M. A., & Hassan, I. (2016). Vitamin E in dermatology. *Indian Dermatology Online Journal, 7*(4), 311–315. DOI: 10.4103/2229-5178.185494 PMID: 27559512

Kelly, M. E., Ramkumar, S., Sun, W., Colon Ortiz, C., Kiser, P. D., Golczak, M., & von Lintig, J. (2018). The Biochemical Basis of Vitamin A Production from the Asymmetric Carotenoid β-Cryptoxanthin. *ACS Chemical Biology, 13*(8), 2121–2129. DOI: 10.1021/acschembio.8b00290 PMID: 29883100

Kennedy, B. K., & Lamming, D. W. (2016). The mechanistic target of rapamycin: The grand conductor of metabolism and aging. *Cell Metabolism, 23*(6), 990–1003. DOI: 10.1016/j.cmet.2016.05.009 PMID: 27304501

Kim, H. K., & Nelson, M. T. (2013). Arachidonic acid-derived lipid mediators and aging. *Prostaglandins, Leukotrienes, and Essential Fatty Acids*, *88*(5), 341–345. DOI: 10.1016/j.plefa.2013.02.001

Kim, J. H., Lee, J. E., Kim, K. H., & Kang, N. J. (2018a). Beneficial Effects of Marine Algae-Derived Carbohydrates for Skin Health. *Marine Drugs*, *16*(11), 459. DOI: 10.3390/md16110459 PMID: 30469402

Kim, S. H., Lee, S., & Kim, H. (2018b). Anti-inflammatory natural products and their potential to alleviate the toll of chronic inflammation. *Current Medicinal Chemistry*, *25*(23), 2901–2925. DOI: 10.2174/0929867325666180115103440

Kobayashi, R., Hasegawa, M., Kawaguchi, C., Ishikawa, N., Tomiwa, K., Shima, M., & Nogami, K. (2021). Thyroid function in patients with selenium deficiency exhibits high free T4 to T3 ratio. *Clinical Pediatric Endocrinology : Case Reports and Clinical Investigations : Official Journal of the Japanese Society for Pediatric Endocrinology*, *30*(1), 19–26. DOI: 10.1297/cpe.30.19 PMID: 33446948

Kunugi, H., & Mohammed Ali, A. (2019). Royal Jelly and Its Components Promote Healthy Aging and Longevity: From Animal Models to Humans. *International Journal of Molecular Sciences*, *20*(19), 4662. DOI: 10.3390/ijms20194662 PMID: 31547049

Kurek-Górecka, A., Górecki, M., Rzepecka-Stojko, A., Balwierz, R., & Stojko, J. (2020). Bee Products in Dermatology and Skin Care. *Molecules (Basel, Switzerland)*, *25*(3), 556. DOI: 10.3390/molecules25030556 PMID: 32012913

Lapierre, L. R., Meléndez, A., & Hansen, M. (2012). Autophagy links lipid metabolism to longevity in C. elegans. *Autophagy*, *8*(1), 144–146. DOI: 10.4161/auto.8.1.18722 PMID: 22186228

Latif, R. (2013). Chocolate/cocoa and human health: A review. *The Netherlands Journal of Medicine*, *71*(2), 63–68. PMID: 23462053

Li, H., Chen, F. J., Yang, W. L., Qiao, H. Z., & Zhang, S. J. (2021). Quercetin improves cognitive disorder in aging mice by inhibiting NLRP3 inflammasome activation. *Food & Function*, *12*(2), 717–725. DOI: 10.1039/D0FO01900C PMID: 33338087

Li, S., Wu, X., & Huang, H. (2007). Green tea polyphenol EGCG extends lifespan in Drosophila. *Aging Cell*, *6*(5), 499–507. DOI: 10.1111/j.1474-9726.2007.00300.x

Liao, V. H., Yu, C. W., Chu, Y. J., Li, W. H., Hsieh, Y. C., & Wang, T.-T. (2011). Curcumin-mediated lifespan extension in *Caenorhabditis elegans.Mechanisms of Ageing and Development*, *132*(10), 480–487. DOI: 10.1016/j.mad.2011.07.008 PMID: 21855561

Liu, Y., Song, X., Zhang, D., Zhou, F., Wang, D., Wei, Y., Gao, F., Xie, L., Jia, G., Wu, W., & Ji, B. (2012). Blueberry anthocyanins: Protection against ageing and light-induced damage in retinal pigment epithelial cells. *British Journal of Nutrition*, *108*(1), 16–27. DOI: 10.1017/S000711451100523X PMID: 22018225

Loizzo, M. R., Ben Jemia, M., Senatore, F., Bruno, M., Menichini, F., & Tundis, R. (2013). Chemistry and functional properties in prevention of neurodegenerative disorders of five Cistus species essential oils. *Food and chemical toxicology: an international journal published for the British Industrial Biological Research Association, 59*, 586–594. https://doi.org/DOI: 10.1016/j.fct.2013.06.040

Lolou, V., & Panayiotidis, M. I. (2019). Functional Role of Probiotics and Prebiotics on Skin Health and Disease. *Fermentation (Basel, Switzerland)*, *5*(2), 41. DOI: 10.3390/fermentation5020041

López-Otín, C., Blasco, M. A., Partridge, L., Serrano, M., & Kroemer, G. (2013). The hallmarks of aging. *Cell*, *153*(6), 1194–1217. DOI: 10.1016/j.cell.2013.05.039 PMID: 23746838

Luo, J., Si, H., Jia, Z., & Liu, D. (2021). Dietary Anti-Aging Polyphenols and Potential Mechanisms. *Antioxidants*, *10*(2), 283. DOI: 10.3390/antiox10020283 PMID: 33668479

Lykkesfeldt, J. (2020). On the effect of vitamin C intake on human health: How to (mis)interprete the clinical evidence. *Redox Biology*, *34*, 101532. DOI: 10.1016/j.redox.2020.101532 PMID: 32535545

Maltais, M., de Souto Barreto, P., Bowman, G. L., Smith, A. D., Cantet, C., Andrieu, S., & Rolland, Y. (2022). Omega-3 Supplementation for the Prevention of Cognitive Decline in Older Adults: Does It Depend on Homocysteine Levels? *The Journal of Nutrition, Health & Aging*, *26*(6), 615–620. DOI: 10.1007/s12603-022-1809-5 PMID: 35718871

Margiana, R., Pakpahan, C., & Pangestu, M. (2022). A systematic review of retinoic acid in the journey of spermatogonium to spermatozoa: From basic to clinical application. *F1000 Research*, *11*, 552. DOI: 10.12688/f1000research.110510.2 PMID: 35967975

McCubrey, J. A., Lertpiriyapong, K., Steelman, L. S., Abrams, S. L., Yang, L. V., Murata, R. M., Rosalen, P. L., Scalisi, A., Neri, L. M., Cocco, L., Ratti, S., Martelli, A. M., Laidler, P., Dulińska-Litewka, J., Rakus, D., Gizak, A., Lombardi, P., Nicoletti, F., Candido, S., & Cervello, M. (2017). Effects of resveratrol, curcumin, berberine and other nutraceuticals on aging, cancer development, cancer stem cells and microRNAs. *Aging (Albany NY)*, *9*(6), 1477–1536. DOI: 10.18632/aging.101250 PMID: 28611316

Melamed, M. L., Michos, E. D., Post, W., & Astor, B. (2008). 25-hydroxyvitamin D levels and the risk of mortality in the general population. *Archives of Internal Medicine*, *168*(15), 1629–1637. DOI: 10.1001/archinte.168.15.1629 PMID: 18695076

Michelazzo, F. B., Oliveira, J. M., Stefanello, J., Luzia, L. A., & Rondó, P. H. (2013). The influence of vitamin A supplementation on iron status. *Nutrients*, *5*(11), 4399–4413. DOI: 10.3390/nu5114399 PMID: 24212089

Mocchegiani, E., Giacconi, R., & Malavolta, M. (2000). Zinc signalling and subcellular distribution: Emerging targets in type 2 diabetes. *Trends in Molecular Medicine*, *16*(6), 307–315. DOI: 10.1016/j.molmed.2000.05.003 PMID: 18774338

Moghimipour, E. (2012). Hydroxy Acids, the Most Widely Used Anti-aging Agents. *Jundishapur Journal of Natural Pharmaceutical Products*, *7*(1), 9–10. DOI: 10.17795/jjnpp-4181 PMID: 24624144

Molfino, A., Gioia, G., Rossi Fanelli, F., & Muscaritoli, M. (2014). The role for dietary omega-3 fatty acids supplementation in older adults. *Nutrients*, *6*(10), 4058–4073. DOI: 10.3390/nu6104058 PMID: 25285409

Mukherjee, S., Date, A., Patravale, V., Korting, H. C., Roeder, A., & Weindl, G. (2006). Retinoids in the treatment of skin aging: An overview of clinical efficacy and safety. *Clinical Interventions in Aging*, *1*(4), 327–348. DOI: 10.2147/ciia.2006.1.4.327 PMID: 18046911

Nature. (2024). *Lithocholic acid and lifespan extension*. Nature. Retrieved from https://www.nature.com/articles/s41586-024-08329-5

Navarro-Cruz, A. R., Ramírez, Y., Ayala, R., Ochoa-Velasco, C., Brambila, E., Avila-Sosa, R., Pérez-Fernández, S., Morales-Medina, J. C., & Aguilar-Alonso, P. (2017). Effect of Chronic Administration of Resveratrol on Cognitive Performance during Aging Process in Rats. *Oxidative Medicine and Cellular Longevity*, *8510761*(1), 8510761. Advance online publication. DOI: 10.1155/2017/8510761 PMID: 29163756

Nichols, J. A., & Katiyar, S. K. (2010). Skin photoprotection by natural polyphenols: Anti-inflammatory, antioxidant and DNA repair mechanisms. *Archives of Dermatological Research*, *302*(2), 71–83. DOI: 10.1007/s00403-009-1001-3 PMID: 19898857

O'Rourke, E. J., Kuballa, P., Xavier, R., & Ruvkun, G. (2013). ω-6 Polyunsaturated fatty acids extend life span through the activation of autophagy. *Genes & Development*, *27*(4), 429–440. DOI: 10.1101/gad.205294.112 PMID: 23392608

Ogidi, O. I. (2022). Phytochemicals of Bioactive compounds of Brassica Juncea (Brown Mustard) Seeds. In: Medicinal and Aromatic Plants of the World. Published by *Encylopedia of Life Support Systems (EOLSS)*. http://www.eolss.net/Eloss-sampleAllChapter.aspx

Ogidi, O. I. (2024). Recent advances in anticancer activity and Bioinformatics Approach from Potential Plants. In: Computational Approaches in Biomaterials, Bioinformatics and Biomedical Engineering Applications. *CRC Press, Taylor and Francis Group, Florida, USA*. DOI: 10.1201/9781003354437-3

Ogidi, O. I. (2025). Edible Mushroom and Weight Management. In Izah, S. C., Ogwu, M. C., & Akram, M. (Eds.), *Bioactive Compounds in Edible Mushrooms. Reference Series in Phytochemistry*. Springer., DOI: 10.1007/978-3-031-52642-8_34-1

Ogidi, O. I., & Adigwe, P. C. (2025). Toxin Concerns and Safe Consumption of Edible Mushroom. In Izah, S. C., Ogwu, M. C., & Akram, M. (Eds.), *Bioactive Compounds in Edible Mushrooms. Reference Series in Phytochemistry*. Springer., DOI: 10.1007/978-3-031-52642-8_39-1

Ogidi, O. I., & Ajoko, I. (2024). Neuroprotective Potentials of Phytochemicals. In: M.S. Rajput, T. Sarachana, P.D. Sarkar, M. Raval (eds) NeuroPhytomedicine. *CRC Press, Routledge Taylor and Francis Group.*

Ogidi, O. I., Ajoko, I. T., & Chukwudi, P. (2024a). Natural Antioxidant Compounds for Skin Care. In *Eco-Friendly Skin Solutions for Natural Cosmeceuticals*. IGI Global., DOI: 10.4018/979-8-3693-5473-5.ch008

Ogidi, O. I., Barwant, M. M., & Okara, E. (2024b). Biomarker Discovery: Protein Phosphorylation State. In *Spatially Variable Genes in Cancer: Development, Progression, and Treatment Response*. IGI Global., DOI: 10.4018/979-8-3693-7728-4.ch005

Ogidi, O. I., & Emaikwu, N. G. (2024). Plant Phenolic compound isolation and its Bioinformatics Approaches of Molecular Mechanisms in Antimicrobial activities and Resistance. In: Computational Approaches in Biomaterials, Bioinformatics and Biomedical Engineering Applications. *CRC Press, Taylor and Francis Group, Florida, USA*. DOI: 10.1201/9781003354437-8

Ogidi, O. I., & Enenebeaku, U. E. (2023). Chapter 11: Medicinal Potentials of Aloe Vera (*Aloe barbadensis* Miller): Technologies for the Production of Therapeutics. In: Sustainable Utilization and Conservation of Africa's Biological Resources and Environment, Sustainable Development and Biodiversity. *Springer Nature Singapore Pte Ltd.* https://doi.org/DOI: 10.1007/978-981-19-6974-4_11

Ogidi, O. I., Esie, N. G., & Dike, O. G. (2019). Phytochemical, Proximate and Mineral compositions of *Bryophyllum pinnatum* (Never die) medicinal plant. *Journal of Pharmacognosy and Phytochemistry*, *8*(1), 629–635.

Ogidi, O. I., & Felagha, I. (2024). Gut Microbiome and Diet Interaction. In *Nutrition Controversies and Advances in Autoimmune Disease*. IGI Global. DOI: 10.4018/979-8-3693-5528-2.ch012

Ogidi, O. I., Izah, S. C., Zikenah, E. C., & Ogwu, M. C. (2025). Edible Mushrooms and Parasitic Diseases in Humans. In Izah, S. C., Ogwu, M. C., & Akram, M. (Eds.), *Bioactive Compounds in Edible Mushrooms. Reference Series in Phytochemistry*. Springer., DOI: 10.1007/978-3-031-52642-8_31-1

Ogidi, O. I., & Oguoma, L. M. O. (2025). Allergies and Sensitivities Associated with Edible Mushroom. In Izah, S. C., Ogwu, M. C., & Akram, M. (Eds.), *Bioactive Compounds in Edible Mushrooms. Reference Series in Phytochemistry*. Springer., DOI: 10.1007/978-3-031-52642-8_38-1

Ogidi, O. I., Oguoma, L. M. O., Adigwe, P. C., & Anthony, B. B. (2021). Phytochemical properties and in-vitro antimicrobial Potency of Wild Edible Mushrooms (*Pleurotusostreatus*) obtained from Yenagoa, Nigeria. *The Journal of Phytopharmacology*, *10*(3), 180–184. DOI: 10.31254/phyto.2021.10306

Ogidi, O. I., & Otenep, E. J. (2020). Determination of Nutritional properties of honey from *Apis mellifera*. *International Journal of Food Sciences and Nutrition*, *5*(1), 23–26.

Pallauf, K., Rimbach, G., Rupp, P. M., Chin, D., & Wolf, I. M. (2016). Resveratrol and Lifespan in Model Organisms. *Current Medicinal Chemistry*, *23*(41), 4639–4680. DOI: 10.2174/0929867323666161024151233 PMID: 27781945

Park, K. (2015). Role of micronutrients in skin health and function. *Biomolecules & Therapeutics*, *23*(3), 207–217. DOI: 10.4062/biomolther.2015.003 PMID: 25995818

Partridge, L., Fuentealba, M., & Kennedy, B. K. (2020). The quest to slow ageing through drug discovery. *Nature Reviews. Drug Discovery*, *19*(8), 513–532. DOI: 10.1038/s41573-020-0067-7 PMID: 32467649

Patterson, E., Wall, R., Fitzgerald, G. F., Ross, R. P., & Stanton, C. (2012). Health implications of high dietary omega-6 polyunsaturated Fatty acids. *Journal of Nutrition and Metabolism*, *539426*, 1–16. Advance online publication. DOI: 10.1155/2012/539426 PMID: 22570770

Peluso, I., & Serafini, M. (2017). Antioxidants from black and green tea: From dietary modulation of oxidative stress to pharmacological mechanisms. *British Journal of Pharmacology*, *174*(11), 1195–1208. DOI: 10.1111/bph.13649 PMID: 27747873

Petruk, G., Del Giudice, R., Rigano, M. M., & Monti, D. M. (2018). Antioxidants from Plants Protect against Skin Photoaging. *Oxidative Medicine and Cellular Longevity*, *1454936*(1), 1454936. Advance online publication. DOI: 10.1155/2018/1454936 PMID: 30174780

Pickart, L., & Margolina, A. (2018). Skin regenerative and anti-cancer actions of copper peptides. *Cosmetics*, *5*(2), 29. DOI: 10.3390/cosmetics5020029

Pietsch, K., Saul, N., Chakrabarti, S., Stürzenbaum, S. R., & Steinberg, C. E. (2011). Hormetins, antioxidants and pro-oxidants: Defining quinone-mediated stress responses in C. elegans. *Biogerontology*, *12*(4), 343–358. DOI: 10.1007/s10522-011-9339-6 PMID: 21503726

Pospíšilová, H., Hyršlová Vaculová, A., & Hyánek, J. (2022). Vitamin C supplementation prolongs lifespan in Drosophila melanogaster. *Experimental Gerontology*, *159*, 111678. DOI: 10.1016/j.exger.2022.111678

Post, N. Y. (2024, December 13). *Anti-aging doc: My favorite supplement can add 7 to 8 years to your life*. New York Post. Retrieved from https://nypost.com/2024/12/13/health/anti-aging-doc-supplement-can-add-7-to-8-years-to-your-life

Pullar, J. M., Carr, A. C., & Vissers, M. C. M. (2017). The Roles of Vitamin C in Skin Health. *Nutrients*, *9*(8), 866. DOI: 10.3390/nu9080866 PMID: 28805671

Queen, B. L., & Tollefsbol, T. O. (2010). Polyphenols and aging. *Current Aging Science*, *3*(1), 34–42. DOI: 10.2174/1874609811003010034 PMID: 20298168

Rayman, M. P. (2000). The importance of selenium to human health. *Lancet*, *356*(9225), 233–241. DOI: 10.1016/S0140-6736(00)02490-9 PMID: 10963212

Reboul, E. (2017). Vitamin E Bioavailability: Mechanisms of Intestinal Absorption in the Spotlight. *Antioxidants*, *6*(4), 95. DOI: 10.3390/antiox6040095 PMID: 29165370

Reinisalo, M., Kårlund, A., Koskela, A., Kaarniranta, K., & Karjalainen, R. O. (2015). Polyphenol Stilbenes: Molecular Mechanisms of Defence against Oxidative Stress and Aging-Related Diseases. *Oxidative Medicine and Cellular Longevity*, *340520*, 1–24. Advance online publication. DOI: 10.1155/2015/340520 PMID: 26180583

Ristow, M., & Zarse, K. (2010). How increased oxidative stress promotes longevity and metabolic health: The concept of mitochondrial hormesis (mitohormesis). *Experimental Gerontology*, *45*(6), 410–418. DOI: 10.1016/j.exger.2010.03.014 PMID: 20350594

Roudsari, M. R., Karimi, R., Sohrabvandi, S., & Mortazavian, A. M. (2015). Health effects of probiotics on the skin. *Critical Reviews in Food Science and Nutrition*, *55*(9), 1219–1240. DOI: 10.1080/10408398.2012.680078 PMID: 24364369

Rzezniczak, T. Z., & Merritt, T. J. (2011). Interactions of NADP-reducing enzymes across varying environmental conditions: A model of biological complexity. *G3 (Bethesda, Md.)*, *1*(3), 235–243. DOI: 10.1534/g3.111.000927 PMID: 23275884

Saari, J. C. (2016). Vitamin A and Vision. *Sub-Cellular Biochemistry*, *81*, 231–259. DOI: 10.1007/978-94-024-0945-1_9 PMID: 27830507

Saul, N., Pietsch, K., Menzel, R., & Steinberg, C. E. (2013). Quercetin-mediated longevity in C. elegans: Is DAF-16 required? *Mechanisms of Ageing and Development*, *134*(7-8), 511–519. DOI: 10.1016/j.mad.2013.06.005

Shailaja, M., Damodara Gowda, K. M., Vishakh, K., & Suchetha Kumari, N. (2017). Anti-aging Role of Curcumin by Modulating the Inflammatory Markers in Albino Wistar Rats. *Journal of the National Medical Association*, *109*(1), 9–13. DOI: 10.1016/j.jnma.2017.01.005 PMID: 28259223

Shanaida, M. (2018). Antioxidant activity of essential oils obtained from aerial part of some Lamiaceae species. *Int. J. Green Pharm.*, *12*, 200–204.

Shanaida, M., Golembiovska, O., Hudz, N., & Wieczorek, P. P. (2018). Phenolic compounds of herbal infusions obtained from some species of the family. *Current Issues in Pharmacy and Medical Sciences*, *31*(4), 194–199. DOI: 10.1515/cipms-2018-0036

Shanaida, M., Lysiuk, R., Mykhalkiv, M., & Shanaida, V. (2021). Chromatographic profiles of carboxylic acids in the raw materials of some mentheae dumort. Species. *Pharmacologyonline*, *3*, 30–37.

Sharma, R. (2021). *Calcium alpha-ketoglutarate extends lifespan and reduces inflammation in mice. PMC.* Retrieved from https://pmc.ncbi.nlm.nih.gov/articles/PMC8508957

Sharma, Y., Miller, M., Shahi, R., Doyle, A., Horwood, C., Hakendorf, P., & Thompson, C. (2019). Vitamin C deficiency in Australian hospitalised patients: An observational study. *Internal Medicine Journal*, *49*(2), 189–196. DOI: 10.1111/imj.14030 PMID: 29968401

Shea, M. K., & Booth, S. L. (2016). Vitamin K and cardiovascular disease: Emerging evidence. *Advances in Nutrition*, *7*(6), 896–905. DOI: 10.3945/an.116.012682

Shen, L. R., Parnell, L. D., Ordovas, J. M., & Lai, C. Q. (2013). Curcumin and aging. *BioFactors (Oxford, England)*, *39*(1), 133–140. DOI: 10.1002/biof.1086 PMID: 23325575

Si, H., Lai, C. Q., & Liu, D. (2021). Dietary Epicatechin, A Novel Anti-aging Bioactive Small Molecule. *Current Medicinal Chemistry*, *28*(1), 3–18. DOI: 10.2174/1875533XMTAzbMzAh1 PMID: 31886745

Simopoulos, A. P. (2002). Omega-3 fatty acids in inflammation and autoimmune diseases. *Journal of the American College of Nutrition*, *21*(6), 495–505. DOI: 10.1080/07315724.2002.10719248 PMID: 12480795

Singh, K. N., Patil, S., & Barkate, H. (2020). Protective effects of astaxanthin on skin: Recent scientific evidence, possible mechanisms, and potential indications. *Journal of Cosmetic Dermatology*, *19*(1), 22–27. DOI: 10.1111/jocd.13019 PMID: 31141292

Sivamaruthi, B. S., Kesika, P., & Chaiyasut, C. (2018). A review on anti-aging properties of probiotics. *Int. J. Appl. Pharm.*, *10*(5), 23–27. DOI: 10.22159/ijap.2018v10i5.28249

Solovyev, N., Drobyshev, E., Bjørklund, G., Dubrovskii, Y., Lysiuk, R., & Rayman, M. P. (2018). Selenium, selenoprotein P, and Alzheimer's disease: Is there a link? *Free Radical Biology & Medicine*, *127*, 124–133. DOI: 10.1016/j.freeradbiomed.2018.02.030 PMID: 29481840

Sorrenti, V., Ali, S., Mancin, L., Davinelli, S., Paoli, A., & Scapagnini, G. (2020). Cocoa Polyphenols and Gut Microbiota Interplay: Bioavailability, Prebiotic Effect, and Impact on Human Health. *Nutrients*, *12*(7), 1908. DOI: 10.3390/nu12071908 PMID: 32605083

Stillwell, W., & Wassall, S. R. (2005). Docosahexaenoic acid: Membrane properties of a unique fatty acid. *Chemistry and Physics of Lipids*, *126*(1-2), 1–27. DOI: 10.1016/j.chemphyslip.2003.12.016 PMID: 14580707

Stratigos, A. J., & Katsambas, A. D. (2005). The role of topical retinoids in the treatment of photoaging. *Drugs*, *65*(8), 1061–1072. DOI: 10.2165/00003495-200565080-00003 PMID: 15907143

Traber, M. G., & Atkinson, J. (2007). Vitamin E, antioxidant and nothing more. *Free Radical Biology & Medicine*, *43*(1), 4–15. DOI: 10.1016/j.freeradbiomed.2007.03.024 PMID: 17561088

Tremaroli, V., & Bäckhed, F. (2012). Functional interactions between the gut microbiota and host metabolism. *Nature*, *489*(7415), 242–249. DOI: 10.1038/nature11552 PMID: 22972297

Tsao, R. (2010). Chemistry and biochemistry of dietary polyphenols. *Nutrients*, *2*(12), 1231–1246. DOI: 10.3390/nu2121231 PMID: 22254006

Tucker-Samaras, S., Zedayko, T., Cole, C., Miller, D., Wallo, W., & Leyden, J. J. (2009). A stabilized 0.1% retinol facial moisturizer improves the appearance of photodamaged skin in an eight-week, double-blind, vehicle-controlled study. *Journal of drugs in dermatology. JDD*, *8*(10), 932–936. PMID: 19852122

Tundis, R., Loizzo, M. R., Bonesi, M., & Menichini, F. (2015). Potential role of natural compounds against skin aging. *Current Medicinal Chemistry*, *22*(12), 1515–1538. DOI: 10.2174/0929867322666150227151809 PMID: 25723509

Ubeda, N., Achón, M., & Varela-Moreiras, G. (2012). Omega 3 fatty acids in the elderly. *British Journal of Nutrition*, *107*(S2, Suppl 2), S137–S151. DOI: 10.1017/S0007114512001535 PMID: 22591888

Valentino, S., Ghelfi, M., Zunica, E., Stamper, M., Hickman, S., Hwang, S., Young, E., Atkinson, J., & Manor, D. (2018). Antioxidant independent actions of vitamin E in modulating gene expression. *Free Radical Biology & Medicine*, *128*, S58–S59. DOI: 10.1016/j.freeradbiomed.2018.10.113

Valenzano, D. R., Sharp, S., & Brunet, A. (2009). Transferrable aging phenotypes between zebrafish strains. *PLoS Biology*, *7*(12), e1000246. DOI: 10.1371/journal.pbio.1000246

Valenzano, D. R., Terzibasi, E., Genade, T., Cattaneo, A., Domenici, L., & Cellerino, A. (2006). Resveratrol prolongs lifespan and retards the onset of age-related markers in a short-lived vertebrate. *Current Biology*, *16*(3), 296–300. DOI: 10.1016/j.cub.2005.12.038 PMID: 16461283

Wang, J., Cao, B., Zhao, H., & Feng, J. (2017). Emerging Roles of *Ganoderma Lucidum* in Anti-Aging. *Aging and Disease*, *8*(6), 691–707. DOI: 10.14336/AD.2017.0410 PMID: 29344411

Wang, K., Zhong, Y., Yang, F., Hu, C., Liu, X., Zhu, Y., & Yao, K. (2021a). Causal Effects of N-6 Polyunsaturated Fatty Acids on Age-related Macular Degeneration: A Mendelian Randomization Study. *The Journal of Clinical Endocrinology and Metabolism*, *106*(9), e3565–e3572. DOI: 10.1210/clinem/dgab338 PMID: 33982092

Wang, X., Zhang, Z., Zhang, S., Yang, F., Yang, M., Zhou, J., Hu, Z., Xu, X., Mao, G., Chen, G., Xiang, W., Sun, X., & Xu, N. (2021b). Antiaging compounds from marine organisms. *Food Research International*, *143*, 110313. DOI: 10.1016/j.foodres.2021.110313 PMID: 33992332

Warsito, M. F., & Kusumawati, I. (2019). The Impact of Herbal Products in the Prevention, Regeneration and Delay of Skin Aging. *Advances in Experimental Medicine and Biology, 1178*, 155–174. DOI: 10.1007/978-3-030-25650-0_9 PMID: 31493227

Whelan, J. (2008). (n-6) and (n-3) Polyunsaturated fatty acids and the aging brain: Food for thought. *The Journal of Nutrition, 138*(12), 2521–2522. DOI: 10.3945/jn.108.095943 PMID: 19022982

Wijendran, V., & Hayes, K. C. (2004). Dietary n-6 and n-3 fatty acid balance and cardiovascular health. *Annual Review of Nutrition, 24*(1), 597–615. DOI: 10.1146/annurev.nutr.24.012003.132106 PMID: 15189133

Wong, C. P., Magnusson, K. R., Sharpton, T. J., & Ho, E. (2021). Effects of zinc status on age-related T cell dysfunction and chronic inflammation. *Biometals: an international journal on the role of metal ions in biology, biochemistry, and medicine, 34*(2), 291–301. https://doi.org/DOI: 10.1007/s10534-020-00279-5

Wu, J. Y., Siu, K. C., & Geng, P. (2021). Bioactive Ingredients and Medicinal Values of *Grifola frondosa* (Maitake). *Foods, 10*(1), 95. DOI: 10.3390/foods10010095 PMID: 33466429

Xie, S. H., Li, H., Jiang, J. J., Quan, Y., & Zhang, H. Y. (2021). Multi-Omics Interpretation of Anti-Aging Mechanisms for ω-3 Fatty Acids. *Genes, 12*(11), 1691. DOI: 10.3390/genes12111691 PMID: 34828297

Yousefzadeh, M. J., Zhu, Y., McGowan, S. J., Angelini, L., Fuhrmann-Stroissnigg, H., Xu, M., & Robbins, P. D. (2018). Fisetin is a senotherapeutic that extends health and lifespan. *EBioMedicine, 36*, 18–28. DOI: 10.1016/j.ebiom.2018.09.015 PMID: 30279143

Yücel, Ç., Şeker Karatoprak, G., & Değim, İ. T. (2019). Anti-aging formulation of rosmarinic acid-loaded ethosomes and liposomes. *Journal of Microencapsulation, 36*(2), 180–191. DOI: 10.1080/02652048.2019.1617363 PMID: 31070486

Zasada, M., & Budzisz, E. (2019). Retinoids: Active molecules influencing skin structure formation in cosmetic and dermatological treatments. *Postepy Dermatologii i Alergologii, 36*(4), 392–397. DOI: 10.5114/ada.2019.87443 PMID: 31616211

Zhang, C., Gao, Z., Hu, C., Zhang, J., Sun, X., Rong, C., & Jia, L. (2017). Antioxidant, antibacterial and anti-aging activities of intracellular zinc polysaccharides from Grifola frondosa SH-05. *International Journal of Biological Macromolecules, 95*, 778–787. DOI: 10.1016/j.ijbiomac.2016.12.003 PMID: 27932257

Zhang, H., Liu, D., Shah, M., Li, J., & Shen, Z. (2019). Natural compounds: A hope for the future of geroprotection. *Aging Cell, 18*(3), e12964. DOI: 10.1111/acel.12964

Zhou, X., Cao, Q., Orfila, C., Zhao, J., & Zhang, L. (2021). Systematic Review and Meta-Analysis on the Effects of Astaxanthin on Human Skin Ageing. *Nutrients, 13*(9), 2917. DOI: 10.3390/nu13092917 PMID: 34578794

Zimmermann, M. B. (2009). Iodine deficiency in pregnancy and the effects of maternal iodine supplementation on the offspring: A review. *The American Journal of Clinical Nutrition, 89*(2), 668–672. DOI: 10.3945/ajcn.2008.26811C PMID: 19088150

Chapter 11
Nutritional Powerhouses:
Exploring Natural Compounds for Anti-Ageing

Tiago Manuel Horta Reis da Silva
https://orcid.org/0000-0001-5220-1718
King's College London, UK

ABSTRACT

This chapter explores the role of natural compounds in mitigating age-related challenges such as loneliness, elder abuse, dehydration, falls risk, and incontinence. As ageing progresses, physiological and psychological vulnerabilities increase, necessitating targeted nutritional interventions to enhance overall well-being. The chapter examines bioactive compounds, including antioxidants, omega-3 fatty acids, and polyphenols, which support cognitive health, emotional resilience, and physical function. It also discusses hydration strategies, muscle-strengthening nutrients, and bladder-supportive diets that reduce common geriatric risks. Additionally, ethical considerations, socioeconomic barriers, and policy implications are examined to ensure equitable access to nutritional support. By bridging traditional knowledge with contemporary research, this chapter advocates for an evidence-based, multidimensional approach to improving the quality of life in older adults through dietary optimisation.

1. INTRODUCTION

The phenomenon of ageing represents a complex interplay of biological, psychological, and social dimensions, culminating in a significant transformation of individual health and well-being (Reis da Silva, 2024a). As the global population ages, with projections indicating that by 2050, the number of individuals aged 65 and older will reach approximately 1.5 billion, understanding the implications of this demographic shift becomes increasingly critical (Mertens et al., 2018; Reis da Silva, 2023a; Reis da Silva, 2023b). Ageing is not merely a biological process; it encompasses a myriad of challenges, including the increased prevalence of chronic diseases, cognitive decline, and the psychosocial impacts of ageing, such as loneliness and social isolation (Srivastava, 2019; Reis da Silva, 2024b). These challenges

DOI: 10.4018/979-8-3693-9730-5.ch011

necessitate a comprehensive approach to health that prioritizes not only the prevention and management of age-related diseases but also the promotion of overall well-being (Reis da Silva, 2024c).

Among the myriad factors influencing healthy ageing, nutrition plays a pivotal role. The relationship between dietary habits and health outcomes in older adults has been extensively documented, revealing that adequate nutrition is essential for maintaining physical function, cognitive health, and overall quality of life (Simons et al., 2016). Nutritional deficiencies can exacerbate age-related decline, leading to increased susceptibility to chronic diseases such as cardiovascular disease, diabetes, and osteoporosis (Liu et al., 2023). Furthermore, the ageing process is often accompanied by changes in metabolism and dietary needs, making it imperative for older adults to adopt dietary patterns that support their unique health requirements (Niraula et al., 2016). The significance of nutrition in promoting healthy ageing cannot be overstated, as it serves as a foundational pillar for enhancing longevity and improving the quality of life in later years.

The purpose of this chapter is to explore the multifaceted challenges associated with ageing, with a particular focus on the critical role of nutrition in fostering healthy ageing. By synthesising current research and evidence-based practices, this chapter aims to provide a comprehensive overview of how nutritional strategies can mitigate the adverse effects of ageing and promote resilience among older adults. The scope of this chapter will encompass various aspects of nutrition, including dietary patterns, nutrient requirements, and the impact of specific dietary interventions on health outcomes in older populations. Additionally, the chapter will address the socio-economic factors that influence dietary choices and access to nutritious foods, highlighting the importance of a holistic approach to nutrition that considers the broader context of ageing.

2. NUTRITIONAL INTERVENTIONS FOR PSYCHOLOGICAL WELL-BEING

The ageing population faces numerous psychological challenges, including loneliness, depression, and anxiety, which can significantly impact their overall quality of life (Reis da Silva, 2024b). Recent studies have highlighted the profound relationship between nutrition and mental health in older adults, suggesting that dietary choices can play a crucial role in alleviating psychological distress (Reis da Silva, 2025a; Reis da Silva, 2025b). The impact of nutrition on mental health is particularly relevant in the context of older adults, who often experience social isolation and reduced physical health, leading to a decline in psychological well-being (Gorenko et al., 2020; Schorr et al., 2021; Reis da Silva, 2024b). This section explores the intricate connections between nutrition and psychological well-being, emphasising the role of specific nutrients in mitigating feelings of loneliness and depression, and presents case studies that illustrate the positive effects of dietary interventions on social engagement.

2.1 Impact of Nutrition on Mental Health in Older Adults

Research indicates that nutritional status is closely linked to mental health outcomes in older adults. For instance, deficiencies in essential nutrients such as omega-3 fatty acids, vitamins B12 and D, and antioxidants have been associated with increased rates of depression and cognitive decline (Schorr et al., 2021; Jyväkorpi et al., 2017; Reis da Silva, 2024d). A systematic review found that older adults with poor nutritional status were more likely to report depressive symptoms compared to their well-nourished counterparts (Schorr et al., 2021). This suggests that addressing nutritional deficiencies may be a viable strategy for improving mental health outcomes in this population. Furthermore, the consumption of a balanced diet rich in fruits, vegetables, whole grains, and lean proteins has been shown to support cognitive function and emotional well-being, highlighting the importance of nutrition in promoting psychological health (Kim et al., 2016; Jyväkorpi et al., 2017).

2.2 Role of Specific Nutrients in Alleviating Loneliness and Depression

Specific nutrients have been identified as playing a significant role in alleviating loneliness and depression among older adults. For example, omega-3 fatty acids, commonly found in fatty fish, have been linked to reduced symptoms of depression and improved mood (Schorr et al., 2021). Additionally, B vitamins, particularly B12 and folate, are essential for maintaining mental health, as they are involved in the synthesis of neurotransmitters that regulate mood (Schorr et al., 2021; Reis da Silva, 2024d). Antioxidants, such as vitamins C and E, may also contribute to psychological well-being by combating oxidative stress, which has been implicated in the pathophysiology of depression (Schorr et al., 2021). By ensuring adequate intake of these nutrients, older adults may experience a reduction in psychological distress and an enhancement in their overall quality of life.

2.3 Case Studies Linking Diet to Improved Social Engagement

Case studies provide compelling evidence of the positive impact of dietary interventions on social engagement and psychological well-being among older adults. For instance, a community-based program that provided nutritional education and cooking classes for older adults resulted in increased social interaction and improved mental health outcomes (Gorenko et al., 2020). Participants reported feeling less isolated and more connected to their peers, demonstrating that nutritional interventions can foster social bonds and enhance psychological resilience. Another study highlighted the effectiveness of a Mediterranean diet, which emphasises the consumption of whole foods, in reducing depressive symptoms among older adults (Schorr et al., 2021). Participants who adhered to this dietary pattern not only experienced improvements in mood but also reported greater satisfaction with their social lives, underscoring the interconnectedness of nutrition, mental health, and social engagement.

Moreover, the COVID-19 pandemic has exacerbated feelings of loneliness and psychological distress among older adults, making nutritional interventions even more critical during this time. A narrative review identified various remotely delivered interventions that targeted loneliness and psychological symptoms, emphasising the importance of maintaining social connections through virtual platforms (Gorenko et al., 2020; Reis da Silva, 2025c). These interventions often included nutritional components, such as meal planning and cooking demonstrations, which not only provided practical support but also fostered a sense of community among participants. By integrating nutrition into mental health interventions, healthcare providers can address the multifaceted needs of older adults, promoting both physical and psychological well-being.

3. NUTRITIONAL STRATEGIES TO PREVENT ELDER ABUSE

Elder abuse is a pervasive issue that affects the well-being and dignity of older adults across the globe. It encompasses various forms of maltreatment, including physical, emotional, financial, and neglectful behaviors, often perpetrated by caregivers or family members. The prevalence of elder abuse is alarmingly high, with estimates suggesting that between 1% and 35% of older adults experience some form of abuse Vertejee (2015). One critical yet often overlooked aspect of elder abuse is the correlation between malnutrition and vulnerability to such mistreatment. Malnutrition not only compromises the physical health of older adults but also increases their susceptibility to abuse, making nutritional strategies an essential component of prevention efforts.

3.1 Correlation Between Malnutrition and Vulnerability to Abuse

Malnutrition is a significant risk factor for elder abuse, as it can lead to a decline in physical and cognitive function, making older adults more dependent on caregivers (Ludvigsson et al., 2022). This dependence can create a power imbalance, where caregivers may exploit their authority, leading to neglect or abuse (Reis da Silva, 2024e). Studies have shown that malnourished older adults are at a higher risk of experiencing various forms of abuse, including emotional and physical mistreatment (Botngård et al., 2020). Furthermore, malnutrition can exacerbate existing health conditions, leading to increased healthcare needs and further dependence on caregivers, which can create a cycle of vulnerability and abuse (Dong, 2015). Addressing malnutrition through targeted nutritional interventions can help mitigate these risks and enhance the overall well-being of older adults.

3.2 Enhancing Resilience Through Dietary Support

Enhancing resilience through dietary support is a vital strategy in preventing elder abuse. A well-balanced diet rich in essential nutrients can improve physical health, cognitive function, and emotional well-being, thereby reducing vulnerability to abuse (Botngård et al., 2020). Nutritional support can empower older adults by promoting independence and self-sufficiency. For instance, programs that focus on improving the nutritional status of older adults through education, meal planning, and access to healthy foods can lead to better health outcomes and increased resilience against abuse (Karthikeyan et al., 2021). By fostering a sense of autonomy and well-being, these interventions can help older adults feel more secure and less dependent on potentially abusive caregivers.

Moreover, specific dietary components have been shown to play a role in enhancing psychological resilience among older adults. For example, omega-3 fatty acids, found in fish and nuts, have been linked to improved mood and cognitive function, which can help older adults cope with stressors that may otherwise lead to abusive situations (Ludvigsson et al., 2022). Similarly, adequate intake of vitamins and minerals, such as vitamin D and calcium, is essential for maintaining bone health and preventing frailty, which can further reduce the risk of abuse (Karthikeyan et al., 2021). By ensuring that older adults receive the necessary nutrients, caregivers and healthcare providers can help build a foundation of resilience that protects against the risk of abuse.

3.3 Programs Integrating Nutrition to Reduce Abuse Risk

Programs integrating nutrition to reduce abuse risk have emerged as effective interventions in various settings. For instance, community-based initiatives that provide nutritional education and support to older adults have been shown to reduce instances of elder abuse. These programs often include cooking classes, grocery shopping assistance, and nutrition counselling, which empower older adults to make healthier food choices and foster social connections (Botngård et al., 2020). By promoting social engagement and reducing isolation, these initiatives can help mitigate the risk factors associated with elder abuse (Reis da Silva, 2024b; Reis da Silva, 2024e).

In institutional settings, such as nursing homes, integrating nutritional strategies into care plans can also play a crucial role in preventing elder abuse. Staff training programs that emphasise the importance of nutrition and its impact on the well-being of residents can lead to improved care practices and a reduction in neglect and abuse (Botngård et al., 2020). For example, ensuring that residents receive adequate nutrition not only supports their physical health but also enhances their mood and cognitive function, reducing the likelihood of behavioural issues that may lead to caregiver frustration and potential abuse (Yon et al., 2018).

Additionally, the COVID-19 pandemic has highlighted the importance of nutrition in preventing elder abuse. During periods of isolation and lockdown, many older adults faced increased vulnerability due to reduced access to food and social support (Chang & Levy, 2021). Programs that adapted to these challenges by providing meal delivery services and virtual nutrition counselling were essential in maintaining the health and well-being of older adults during this crisis. Such adaptations not only addressed immediate nutritional needs but also helped to foster connections and support networks that are critical in preventing abuse (Chang & Levy, 2021).

4. HYDRATION AND DEHYDRATION PREVENTION

Hydration is a critical component of health, particularly for the elderly population, who are more susceptible to dehydration due to various physiological changes associated with ageing (Reis da Silva, 2024f). As individuals age, their bodies undergo significant transformations that can affect fluid balance, making it essential to understand these changes and implement effective hydration strategies (Reis da Silva, 2024f). This section explores the physiological changes affecting hydration in the elderly, the consequences of dehydration—including cognitive decline and increased risk of falls—and effective hydration strategies, including the role of hydrating foods.

4.1 Physiological Changes

As people age, several physiological changes can impact their hydration status. One of the most significant changes is a decrease in total body water content, which can lead to a higher risk of dehydration (Nishi et al., 2023). The elderly typically have a lower percentage of body water compared to younger adults, which means that even small losses of fluid can lead to dehydration (Reis da Silva, 2024f). Additionally, the ageing process is associated with a decline in kidney function, which affects the body's ability to concentrate urine and conserve water (Białecka-Dębek & Pietruszka, 2018). This decline can result in increased urine output and a greater risk of fluid loss (Reis da Silva, 2024g).

Another critical factor is the diminished thirst response observed in older adults. Research indicates that the sensation of thirst is often blunted in the elderly, leading to inadequate fluid intake (Nishi et al., 2023). This can be exacerbated by cognitive impairments, which may prevent older adults from recognising their need for hydration. Furthermore, certain medications commonly prescribed to older adults, such as diuretics, can increase fluid loss and further complicate hydration efforts (Duan et al., 2020; Reis da Silva, 2024h). Collectively, these physiological changes underscore the importance of proactive hydration strategies tailored to the needs of the elderly.

4.2 Consequences of Dehydration

Dehydration can have severe consequences for older adults, particularly in terms of cognitive function and physical stability. Studies have shown a direct correlation between hydration status and cognitive performance in the elderly. For instance, a prospective cohort study found that inadequate water intake was associated with declines in cognitive performance over two years (Nishi et al., 2023). Dehydration can impair attention, memory, and overall cognitive function, leading to increased confusion and disorientation, which can significantly impact an older adult's quality of life (Reis da Silva, 2024f).

Moreover, dehydration is a well-documented risk factor for falls among the elderly (Reis da Silva, 2023b; Reis da Silva, 2024i). Insufficient fluid intake can lead to decreased blood volume, resulting in orthostatic hypotension—a condition where blood pressure drops significantly upon standing (Białecka-Dębek & Pietruszka, 2018). This can cause dizziness and increase the likelihood of falls, which are a leading cause of injury and mortality in older adults (Reis da Silva, 2023b). A study highlighted that dehydration was independently associated with a higher incidence of falls, emphasising the need for effective hydration strategies to mitigate this risk (Białecka-Dębek & Pietruszka, 2018).

4.3 Effective Hydration Strategies and the Role of Hydrating Foods

To combat dehydration and its associated risks, several effective hydration strategies can be implemented. First and foremost, it is crucial to encourage regular fluid intake throughout the day. Older adults should aim for at least 1.5 to 2 litres of fluids daily, although individual needs may vary based on activity level, climate, and health status (Nishi et al., 2023; Reis da Silva, 2024f). Caregivers and family members can play a vital role in monitoring fluid intake and ensuring that older adults have easy access to water and other hydrating beverages. In addition to encouraging water consumption, incorporating hydrating foods into the diet can significantly contribute to overall fluid intake. Foods with high water content, such as fruits and vegetables, can help maintain hydration levels. For example, cucumbers, watermelon, oranges, and strawberries are not only nutritious but also provide a substantial amount of water (Nishi et al., 2023). Soups and broths are also excellent options for hydration, particularly for those who may struggle to drink enough fluids. By promoting a diet rich in hydrating foods, caregivers can enhance the hydration status of older adults while also providing essential nutrients (Reis da Silva, 2025a).

Another effective strategy is to use hydration reminders and tools. For instance, setting alarms, or using hydration tracking apps can help older adults remember to drink fluids regularly (Reis da Silva, 2025d). Additionally, providing visually appealing and easily accessible water bottles can encourage more frequent consumption. In institutional settings, staff training on the importance of hydration can ensure that caregivers actively promote fluid intake among residents (Nishi et al., 2023; Fitzpatrick et al., 2023).

Finally, it is essential to consider individual preferences and needs when developing hydration strategies. Some older adults may prefer flavoured beverages or may find it easier to consume fluids through smoothies or juices. Tailoring hydration approaches to the preferences of older adults can enhance compliance and overall hydration status (Reis da Silva, 2024c).

5. NUTRITIONAL APPROACHES TO REDUCING FALLS RISK

Falls are a significant health concern, particularly among older adults, leading to serious injuries, loss of independence, and increased mortality rates (Reis da Silva, 2023b; Reis da Silva, 2024i). Nutritional strategies can play a vital role in reducing falls risk by enhancing muscle strength, balance, and overall bone health. This section will explore the essential nutrients for muscle strength and balance, the impact of vitamin D and calcium on bone health, and dietary patterns associated with a lower incidence of falls.

5.1 Nutrients Essential for Muscle Strength and Balance

Muscle strength and balance are critical factors in preventing falls. Several nutrients are essential for maintaining muscle mass and function, which are vital for stability and mobility. Protein is one of the most important nutrients for muscle health. Adequate protein intake supports muscle synthesis and repair, which is particularly important as individuals age and naturally lose muscle mass—a condition known as sarcopenia (Juhász et al., 2021). Research suggests that older adults should aim for a protein intake of at least 1.0 to 1.2 grams per kilogram of body weight per day to maintain muscle mass and function (Zhao et al., 2021).

In addition to protein, certain vitamins and minerals play crucial roles in muscle function. For instance, magnesium is essential for muscle contraction and relaxation. A deficiency in magnesium can lead to muscle weakness and cramps, increasing the risk of falls (Rababah, 2024; Reis da Silva, 2024i). Similarly, potassium is vital for maintaining proper muscle function and preventing cramping. Foods rich in potassium, such as bananas, sweet potatoes, and spinach, should be included in the diet to support muscle health.

Moreover, omega-3 fatty acids, found in fatty fish, walnuts, and flaxseeds, have been shown to improve muscle strength and function in older adults. These fatty acids possess anti-inflammatory properties that may help reduce muscle loss and improve recovery after injury (Fischer et al., 2018). Ensuring adequate intake of these nutrients can significantly enhance muscle strength and balance, thereby reducing the risk of falls.

5.2 Impact of Vitamin D and Calcium on Bone Health

Vitamin D and calcium are two of the most critical nutrients for maintaining bone health, which is essential for preventing falls and fractures. Vitamin D plays a crucial role in calcium absorption in the intestines and helps maintain adequate serum calcium levels, which are vital for bone mineralisation (McKenzie et al., 2021). A deficiency in vitamin D can lead to decreased calcium absorption, resulting in weakened bones and an increased risk of fractures (Joo, 2024). Research has shown that older adults are particularly susceptible to vitamin D deficiency due to factors such as reduced skin synthesis from sunlight exposure, dietary insufficiency, and decreased renal function (Uddin et al., 2023; Reis da Silva, 2024g). Therefore, it is essential for older adults to ensure adequate vitamin D intake through dietary sources, such as fatty fish, fortified dairy products, and supplements if necessary. The recommended dietary allowance (RDA) for vitamin D for older adults is 800 to 1000 IU per day (Nguyen, 2021).

Calcium is equally important for bone health. It is the primary mineral found in bones, and adequate calcium intake is necessary to maintain bone density and strength. The RDA for calcium in older adults is approximately 1200 mg per day (Chiodini & Bolland, 2018). Foods rich in calcium include dairy products, leafy green vegetables, almonds, and fortified foods. Ensuring sufficient intake of both vitamin D and calcium is crucial for preventing osteoporosis and reducing the risk of falls and fractures in older adults.

5.3 Dietary Patterns Associated with Lower Incidence of Falls

In addition to focusing on individual nutrients, certain dietary patterns have been associated with a lower incidence of falls among older adults. The Mediterranean diet, characterised by high consumption of fruits, vegetables, whole grains, legumes, nuts, and healthy fats, has been linked to improved bone health and reduced falls risk (Wan, 2023). This diet is rich in antioxidants, vitamins, and minerals that support overall health and may help prevent age-related decline in muscle and bone strength. A study examining the effects of the Mediterranean diet on older adults found that adherence to this dietary pattern was associated with higher bone mineral density and a lower risk of hip fractures (Yao et al., 2016). The anti-inflammatory properties of the Mediterranean diet may also contribute to better muscle function and balance, further reducing falls risk.

Another dietary pattern that has shown promise in reducing falls risk is the DASH (Dietary Approaches to Stop Hypertension) diet, which emphasises fruits, vegetables, whole grains, and low-fat dairy while reducing saturated fat and sodium intake. This diet has been associated with improved cardiovascular health and may also support bone health through its rich nutrient profile (Cupone et al., 2020).

Incorporating a variety of nutrient-dense foods into the diet can help older adults maintain muscle strength, balance, and bone health, ultimately reducing the risk of falls (Reis da Silva, 2024i). It is essential for healthcare providers to educate patients about the importance of nutrition in falls prevention and encourage adherence to healthy dietary patterns.

6. MANAGING INCONTINENCE THROUGH DIET

Incontinence, the involuntary loss of urine, is a common issue that affects millions of individuals, particularly older adults (Reis da Silva, 2024j). This condition can significantly impact quality of life, leading to social isolation, embarrassment, and psychological distress (Reis da Silva, 2024j). While various treatments exist, dietary management is an essential yet often overlooked aspect of incontinence care. This section explores dietary factors influencing bladder health, identifies foods and beverages to avoid for effective incontinence management, and outlines nutritional plans that support urinary tract function.

6.1 Dietary Factors Influencing Bladder Health

Diet plays a crucial role in maintaining bladder health and preventing incontinence. Certain dietary components can either exacerbate or alleviate urinary symptoms. For instance, high fluid intake is generally encouraged to maintain hydration and dilute urine, which can help reduce irritation in the bladder. However, the type of fluids consumed is equally important. Caffeinated beverages, such as coffee and tea, can act as diuretics, increasing urine production and potentially leading to urgency and frequency of urination (Cena & Calder, 2020). Similarly, alcohol can irritate the bladder and worsen incontinence symptoms, making it essential for individuals to monitor their intake of these beverages (Williams, 2024).

Moreover, specific nutrients have been identified as beneficial for bladder health. For example, a diet rich in fruits and vegetables provides antioxidants and anti-inflammatory compounds that may help protect bladder tissue from irritation and damage (Williams, 2024). Foods high in fibre, such as whole grains, legumes, and vegetables, can also support overall digestive health, which is crucial since constipation can exacerbate urinary incontinence by putting pressure on the bladder (Brady et al., 2020; Shakhssalim et al., 2023). Furthermore, adequate hydration with water and herbal teas can promote urinary tract health and help flush out toxins, reducing the risk of urinary tract infections (UTIs), which can further complicate incontinence issues (Brady et al., 2020).

6.2 Foods and Beverages to Avoid for Incontinence Management

While some foods and beverages can promote bladder health, others can aggravate incontinence symptoms. It is essential to identify and avoid these irritants to manage the condition effectively. Caffeinated drinks, as previously mentioned, can increase urinary urgency and frequency. Research has shown that individuals who consume high amounts of caffeine are more likely to experience incontinence symptoms (Cena & Calder, 2020). Therefore, reducing or eliminating caffeine from the diet may be beneficial for those struggling with bladder control.

Acidic foods and beverages, such as citrus fruits, tomatoes, and vinegar, can also irritate the bladder lining and lead to increased urgency and discomfort. Spicy foods, artificial sweeteners, and carbonated beverages have similarly been linked to bladder irritation and should be consumed with caution (Williams, 2024). Additionally, high-sugar foods can contribute to obesity, which is a known risk factor for urinary incontinence due to the increased pressure on the bladder (Reis da Silva, 2024j). Therefore, individuals managing incontinence should focus on a balanced diet that minimises these irritants while promoting overall health.

6.3 Nutritional Plans Supporting Urinary Tract Function

Developing a nutritional plan that supports urinary tract function is essential for managing incontinence effectively. A well-rounded diet should include a variety of foods that promote bladder health while avoiding known irritants. Here are some key components to consider when creating a dietary plan for incontinence management:

1. **Hydration:** Aim for adequate fluid intake, primarily through water, to maintain hydration and dilute urine. Herbal teas, particularly those without caffeine, can also be beneficial. It is advisable to spread fluid intake throughout the day rather than consuming large amounts at once, which can overwhelm the bladder.
2. **Fruits and Vegetables:** Incorporate a wide range of fruits and vegetables into the diet. Foods such as blueberries, cranberries, and leafy greens are particularly beneficial due to their antioxidant properties and potential to support urinary tract health. These foods can help reduce inflammation and irritation in the bladder.
3. **Whole Grains and Fibre:** Include whole grains such as brown rice, quinoa, and whole wheat bread to provide fibre, which can help prevent constipation. A high-fibre diet supports digestive health and can alleviate pressure on the bladder.
4. **Lean Proteins:** Opt for lean protein sources, such as poultry, fish, beans, and legumes. These foods provide essential nutrients without contributing to weight gain, which can exacerbate incontinence.
5. **Healthy Fats:** Incorporate healthy fats from sources like avocados, nuts, and olive oil. These fats support overall health and can help reduce inflammation.
6. **Probiotics:** Consider including probiotic-rich foods, such as yogurt and fermented vegetables, which can promote a healthy gut microbiome and may have a positive impact on urinary health (Shakhssalim et al., 2023).
7. **Limit Irritants:** As previously discussed, it is crucial to limit or avoid caffeine, alcohol, acidic foods, and artificial sweeteners. Keeping a food diary can help individuals identify specific triggers that worsen their symptoms.

7. INTEGRATING NUTRITIONAL STRATEGIES INTO CARE PLANS

The integration of nutritional strategies into care plans for older adults is essential for enhancing their overall health, managing chronic conditions, and improving quality of life (Reis da Silva, 2024k). Personalised nutrition assessments, collaborative approaches among healthcare providers, and ongoing monitoring and adjustment of dietary interventions are critical components of this integration. This section will explore these elements in detail, emphasising their importance in promoting optimal health outcomes for older adults.

7.1 Personalised Nutrition Assessments for Older Adults

Personalised nutrition assessments are fundamental in developing effective dietary interventions tailored to the unique needs of older adults. These assessments involve evaluating an individual's dietary habits, nutritional status, medical history, and lifestyle factors. A comprehensive assessment can identify specific nutrient deficiencies, dietary preferences, and potential barriers to healthy eating, such as physical limitations or cognitive impairments (Hashim et al., 2019).

One effective tool for conducting personalised nutrition assessments is the Mini Nutritional Assessment (MNA), which has been validated for use in older populations. The MNA evaluates various factors, including body mass index (BMI), dietary intake, and self-perception of health, to determine nutritional risk (Alteri et al., 2015). This assessment can guide healthcare providers in creating individualised nutrition plans that address specific needs, such as increasing protein intake for muscle maintenance or enhancing hydration to prevent urinary tract infections.

Furthermore, dietary recalls and food frequency questionnaires can provide valuable insights into an individual's eating patterns and nutrient intake. By understanding these patterns, healthcare providers can recommend appropriate dietary modifications that align with the individual's health goals and preferences (Chávez-Íñiguez et al., 2020). For instance, if an older adult is found to have low calcium intake, dietary recommendations may include increasing the consumption of dairy products or leafy greens to support bone health.

7.2 Collaborative Approaches Among Healthcare Providers

Collaboration among healthcare providers is crucial for the successful integration of nutritional strategies into care plans. A multidisciplinary approach that includes dietitians, physicians, nurses, and other healthcare professionals can ensure that nutritional interventions are comprehensive and effective. For example, dietitians can work closely with physicians and nurses to address specific health concerns, such as diabetes management or cardiovascular health, by developing tailored nutrition plans that align with medical treatment (Chen, 2023).

Regular communication among team members is essential for monitoring the effectiveness of dietary interventions and making necessary adjustments. For instance, if an older adult experiences unintended weight loss or worsening health conditions, the healthcare team can collaboratively reassess the nutrition plan and implement changes to better meet the individual's needs (Bayraktar & Tekgül, 2023). This collaborative approach not only enhances the quality of care but also empowers older adults to take an active role in their health management.

Additionally, involving family members or caregivers in the nutritional care process can provide valuable support for older adults. Educating family members about the importance of nutrition and how to prepare healthy meals can help reinforce dietary recommendations and promote adherence to the care plan (Wilson et al., 2021). This support system can be particularly beneficial for older adults who may struggle with meal preparation or grocery shopping due to physical limitations.

7.3 Monitoring and Adjusting Dietary Interventions

Ongoing monitoring and adjustment of dietary interventions are critical for ensuring their effectiveness and relevance to the individual's changing health status. Regular follow-up appointments with healthcare providers can help assess the impact of dietary changes on health outcomes, such as weight management, blood pressure control, and overall well-being (Shabani, 2023). For instance, if an older adult is placed on a high-protein diet to support muscle strength, healthcare providers should monitor changes in muscle mass and strength through assessments such as grip strength tests or body composition analysis. If the desired outcomes are not achieved, the nutrition plan can be adjusted accordingly, such as increasing protein sources or incorporating resistance training exercises (Baines et al., 2020).

Moreover, it is essential to consider the dynamic nature of older adults' health conditions. As individuals age, they may develop new health issues or experience changes in their ability to consume certain foods. For example, an older adult with dysphagia may require texture-modified diets to ensure safe swallowing, while someone with renal issues may need to limit potassium and phosphorus intake

(Sugita, 2024). Regular assessments can help identify these changes and facilitate timely modifications to the nutrition plan.

In addition to health-related monitoring, assessing the individual's satisfaction with their dietary interventions is also important. Engaging older adults in discussions about their food preferences and experiences can help ensure that the nutrition plan is enjoyable and sustainable. If an individual expresses dissatisfaction with certain foods or meal plans, healthcare providers can work collaboratively to identify alternatives that meet their nutritional needs while aligning with their preferences (Yang et al., 2023).

8. CHALLENGES AND CONSIDERATIONS IN NUTRITIONAL INTERVENTIONS

Integrating nutritional interventions into healthcare plans for older adults is essential for promoting health and preventing chronic diseases. However, several challenges and considerations must be addressed to ensure the effectiveness of these interventions. This section will discuss the barriers to implementing nutritional interventions, the cultural and socioeconomic factors affecting dietary choices, and the ethical considerations in nutritional care.

8.1 Barriers to Implementing Nutritional Interventions

Implementing nutritional interventions can be hindered by various barriers, including limited access to healthy foods, lack of nutritional knowledge, and inadequate healthcare resources. One significant barrier is the availability of nutritious foods, particularly in low-income or rural areas where access to grocery stores may be limited (Gardner et al., 2023). This phenomenon, often referred to as "food deserts," restricts individuals' ability to purchase fresh fruits, vegetables, and other healthy options, leading to reliance on processed and unhealthy foods (Gardner et al., 2023). Additionally, many older adults may lack the knowledge or skills necessary to make informed dietary choices. Research indicates that nutritional literacy is often low among older populations, which can hinder their ability to understand dietary guidelines or read food labels effectively (Shafiee, 2024). This lack of knowledge can result in poor dietary choices that do not align with their health needs, ultimately compromising the effectiveness of nutritional interventions.

Another barrier is the healthcare system itself. Many healthcare providers may not prioritise nutrition in their practice due to time constraints, lack of training, or insufficient resources (Martinez et al., 2021). As a result, nutritional assessments and interventions may be overlooked in favour of more immediate medical concerns (Martinez et al., 2021). This gap in care highlights the need for increased training and resources for healthcare providers to emphasize the importance of nutrition in overall health management.

8.2 Cultural and Socioeconomic Factors

Cultural and socioeconomic factors significantly influence dietary choices and can impact the success of nutritional interventions. Cultural beliefs and practices shape food preferences, eating behaviours, and attitudes toward health and nutrition. For example, traditional diets may prioritise specific foods that are integral to cultural identity, making it challenging to introduce new dietary recommendations that deviate from these norms (Mason et al., 2020). Moreover, socioeconomic status plays a crucial role in determining access to healthy foods and the ability to adopt recommended dietary changes. Individuals with lower socioeconomic status often face multiple challenges, including limited financial resources, lack of transportation, and inadequate access to healthcare services. These factors can create significant barriers to obtaining nutritious foods and adhering to dietary recommendations (Gardner et al., 2023).

Additionally, food insecurity is a pressing issue that affects many older adults, particularly those living on fixed incomes. When individuals struggle to afford food, they may prioritise quantity over quality, leading to the consumption of cheaper, less nutritious options (Chen et al., 2018). Addressing these socioeconomic barriers is essential for promoting healthy dietary choices and ensuring the success of nutritional interventions.

8.3 Ethical Considerations

Ethical considerations are paramount in the context of nutritional care for older adults. Healthcare providers must navigate complex ethical dilemmas related to autonomy, informed consent, and cultural sensitivity. One critical ethical issue is the need to respect individuals' autonomy in making dietary choices. While healthcare providers may recommend specific dietary interventions based on clinical evidence, it is essential to consider the preferences and values of the individual (Sandri, 2024). Informed consent is another ethical consideration that must be addressed. Older adults may have varying levels of understanding regarding their nutritional needs and the implications of dietary changes. Healthcare providers have an ethical obligation to ensure that patients are fully informed about the potential benefits and risks of dietary interventions, enabling them to make educated decisions about their nutrition (Shafiee, 2024).

Cultural sensitivity is also crucial in nutritional care. Healthcare providers must be aware of and respect the cultural backgrounds of their patients, as dietary practices and beliefs can vary widely among different populations. Culturally tailored nutritional interventions that consider individuals' cultural preferences and practices are more likely to be accepted and adhered to (Verma, 2024).

Furthermore, ethical considerations extend to the broader societal context. Structural inequalities in access to healthy foods and healthcare resources raise questions about social justice and equity in nutritional care. Addressing these disparities is essential for promoting health equity and ensuring that all individuals have the opportunity to achieve optimal health through proper nutrition (Badu, 2024).

9. FUTURE DIRECTIONS IN NUTRITIONAL GERONTOLOGY

As the global population ages, the field of nutritional gerontology is becoming increasingly important in addressing the unique dietary needs and challenges faced by older adults. Emerging research on novel anti-ageing compounds, technological advancements in nutritional assessment, and policy implications for supporting nutritional health in ageing populations are key areas that warrant attention. This section explores these future directions and concludes with a summary of key insights and a call to action for integrating nutritional strategies into geriatric care.

9.1 Emerging Research on Novel Anti-Ageing Compounds

Recent studies have focused on identifying novel anti-ageing compounds that may enhance healthspan and mitigate age-related decline. Compounds such as resveratrol, curcumin, and omega-3 fatty acids have garnered attention for their potential to promote longevity and improve health outcomes in older adults (Srivastava, 2019). Resveratrol, found in red wine and certain berries, has been shown to activate sirtuins, proteins that play a role in cellular ageing and metabolism (Mertens et al., 2018). Similarly, curcumin, the active ingredient in turmeric, exhibits anti-inflammatory and antioxidant properties that may protect against age-related diseases (Srivastava, 2019).

Another area of interest is the role of micronutrients in ageing. Vitamins D and E, along with minerals like zinc and magnesium, have been linked to improved cognitive function and reduced frailty in older adults (Simons et al., 2016). Ongoing research aims to elucidate the mechanisms by which these compounds exert their effects and to determine optimal dosages and combinations for therapeutic use. As our understanding of these compounds expands, they may become integral components of dietary recommendations for older adults, promoting healthy ageing and reducing the risk of chronic diseases.

9.2 Technological Advancements in Nutritional Assessment

Technological innovations are transforming the landscape of nutritional assessment, making it easier to evaluate the dietary needs of older adults. Wearable devices and mobile applications can track dietary intake, physical activity, and other health metrics in real-time, providing valuable data for healthcare providers (Liu et al., 2023). These tools enable more personalised nutrition assessments, allowing for timely adjustments to dietary interventions based on individual needs and preferences. Moreover, advancements in telehealth have facilitated remote nutritional counselling and support, particularly beneficial for older adults who may have mobility issues or live in rural areas with limited access to healthcare services (Reis da Silva, 2025e). Virtual consultations can help healthcare providers monitor patients' nutritional status and provide guidance on dietary choices, ensuring that older adults receive the support they need to maintain optimal health (Niraula et al., 2016).

Artificial intelligence (AI) and machine learning are also being explored for their potential to enhance nutritional assessments (Reis da Silva, 2025a; Reis da Silva, 2025c). These technologies can analyse large datasets to identify patterns and correlations between dietary intake and health outcomes, leading to more effective interventions tailored to the unique needs of older adults (Gorenko et al., 2020; Reis da Silva, 2025e). As these technologies continue to evolve, they hold promise for improving the accuracy and efficiency of nutritional assessments in geriatric care.

9.3 Policy Implications

The increasing recognition of the importance of nutrition in ageing populations has significant policy implications. Governments and healthcare organisations must prioritise the development and implementation of policies that support nutritional health for older adults. This includes funding for nutrition education programs, subsidies for healthy food options, and initiatives to improve access to nutritious foods in underserved communities (Schorr et al., 2021). Additionally, policies should promote interdisciplinary collaboration among healthcare providers, including dietitians, nurses, physicians, and social workers, to ensure comprehensive nutritional care for older adults. Integrating nutrition into chronic disease management programs and preventive health initiatives can help address the multifaceted challenges associated with aging (Jyväkorpi et al., 2017).

Furthermore, public health campaigns aimed at raising awareness about the importance of nutrition in aging can empower older adults to make informed dietary choices. These campaigns should focus on culturally relevant messaging and consider the diverse backgrounds and needs of aging populations (Kim et al., 2016). By fostering a supportive environment for healthy eating, policymakers can help mitigate the risks associated with malnutrition and promote overall well-being in older adults.

10. CONCLUSIONS

As the global population continues to age, the challenges associated with this demographic shift will require innovative solutions and a concerted effort to promote healthy ageing. Nutrition emerges as a critical component of this endeavour, offering a pathway to enhance health outcomes and improve the quality of life for older adults. This chapter delved into the intricate relationship between ageing and nutrition, providing insights that can inform public health strategies and individual practices aimed at fostering a healthier, more vibrant ageing population. The relationship between nutrition and psychological well-being in older adults is complex and multifaceted. Adequate nutrition is essential for maintaining mental health, with specific nutrients playing a pivotal role in alleviating loneliness and depression. Case studies illustrate the effectiveness of dietary interventions in enhancing social engagement and improving mental health outcomes among older adults. As the ageing population continues to grow, it is imperative for healthcare providers to recognise the importance of nutrition in promoting psychological well-being and to implement targeted interventions that address the unique needs of this demographic. By doing so, we can foster a healthier, more connected, and resilient ageing population.

The correlation between malnutrition and vulnerability to elder abuse underscores the importance of nutritional strategies in prevention efforts. By enhancing resilience through dietary support and implementing programs that integrate nutrition into care plans, we can significantly reduce the risk of elder abuse. As the ageing population continues to grow, it is imperative that healthcare providers, caregivers, and policymakers prioritise nutrition as a fundamental component of elder care. By doing so, it is possible to promote the dignity, health, and safety of older adults, ultimately fostering a society that values and protects its most vulnerable members. Hydration is a vital aspect of health that requires careful attention, particularly in the elderly population. Physiological changes associated with ageing can significantly impact hydration status, leading to serious consequences such as cognitive decline and increased falls risk. By implementing effective hydration strategies, including encouraging regular fluid intake and incorporating hydrating foods into the diet, caregivers and healthcare providers can help prevent dehydration and promote overall well-being in older adults. As the ageing population continues to grow, prioritising hydration will be essential in maintaining health and quality of life for this vulnerable demographic.

Nutritional approaches play a vital role in reducing falls risk among older adults. Ensuring adequate intake of essential nutrients such as protein, magnesium, potassium, vitamin D, and calcium can significantly enhance muscle strength, balance, and bone health. Additionally, adopting dietary patterns such as the Mediterranean or DASH diets can further support overall health and reduce the incidence of falls. By prioritizing nutrition, older adults can take proactive steps to maintain their independence and quality of life. Managing incontinence through diet is a vital strategy that can significantly improve the quality of life for those affected by this condition. By understanding the dietary factors influencing bladder health, avoiding irritants, and implementing a nutritional plan that supports urinary tract function, individuals can take proactive steps toward managing their symptoms. Healthcare providers should emphasise the importance of dietary management in conjunction with other treatment options, ensuring that patients have the tools and knowledge necessary to maintain bladder health and enhance their overall well-being.

Integrating nutritional strategies into care plans for older adults is essential for promoting optimal health and preventing complications associated with ageing. Personalised nutrition assessments, collaborative approaches among healthcare providers, and ongoing monitoring and adjustment of dietary interventions are critical components of this integration. By prioritising nutrition in care plans, healthcare providers can empower older adults to take control of their health, enhance their quality of life, and reduce the risk of chronic conditions. Ultimately, a comprehensive approach to nutrition can lead to improved health outcomes and greater independence for older adults. Integrating nutritional strategies into care plans for older adults is essential for promoting health and preventing chronic diseases. However, several challenges must be addressed, including barriers to implementing nutritional interventions, cultural and socioeconomic factors affecting dietary choices, and ethical considerations in nutritional care. By recognising and addressing these challenges, healthcare providers can develop more effective and equitable nutritional interventions that support the health and well-being of older adults. Ultimately, a comprehensive approach that considers individual needs, cultural backgrounds, and systemic barriers will lead to better health outcomes and improved quality of life for this vulnerable population.

10.1 Summary

The future of nutritional gerontology is promising, with emerging research on novel anti-ageing compounds, technological advancements in nutritional assessment, and important policy implications for supporting nutritional health in ageing populations. The critical role of nutrition in addressing age-related challenges cannot be overstated; it is essential for maintaining health, preventing chronic diseases, and enhancing the quality of life for older adults.

10.2 Call to Action

As we move forward, there is a pressing need for healthcare providers, researchers, and policymakers to collaborate in integrating nutritional strategies into geriatric care. This call to action emphasises the importance of personalised nutrition assessments, interdisciplinary approaches, and ongoing monitoring of dietary interventions. By prioritising nutrition in the care of older adults, we can improve health outcomes, reduce the risk of falls and frailty, and ultimately promote a healthier, more vibrant ageing population.

REFERENCES

Alteri, C., Himpsl, S., & Mobley, H. (2015). Preferential use of central metabolism in vivo reveals a nutritional basis for polymicrobial infection. *PLoS Pathogens*, *11*(1), e1004601. DOI: 10.1371/journal.ppat.1004601 PMID: 25568946

Badu, A., Assibey, G. B., Seenam, P., & Debrah, R. D. (2024). An exploration of factors affecting students' choice of career paths in communication design. *Journal of Science and Technology (Ghana)*, *42*(2), 76–92. DOI: 10.4314/just.v42i2.6

Baines, G., Silva, A., Araklitis, G., Robinson, D., & Cardozo, L. (2020). Recent advances in urodynamics in women. *F1000 Research*, *9*, 606. DOI: 10.12688/f1000research.24640.1 PMID: 32595939

Bayraktar, N., & Tekgül, S. (2023). Delineating the diagnostic concordance between pediatric lower urinary symptoms scoring and voiding diary in pediatric lower urinary tract dysfunction. *Cureus*. Advance online publication. DOI: 10.7759/cureus.42463 PMID: 37502468

Białecka-Dębek, A., & Pietruszka, B. (2018). The association between hydration status and cognitive function among free-living elderly volunteers. *Aging Clinical and Experimental Research*, *31*(5), 695–703. DOI: 10.1007/s40520-018-1019-5 PMID: 30128663

Botngård, A., Eide, A., Mosqueda, L., & Malmedal, W. (2020). Elder abuse in Norwegian nursing homes: A cross-sectional exploratory study. *BMC Health Services Research*, *20*(1), 9. Advance online publication. DOI: 10.1186/s12913-019-4861-z PMID: 31900138

Brady, S., Berry, A., Fitzgerald, C., Gahagan, S., Hardacker, C., Harlow, B., & Sutcliffe, S. (2020). Applying concepts of life course theory and life course epidemiology to the study of bladder health and lower urinary tract symptoms among girls and women. *Neurourology and Urodynamics*, *39*(4), 1185–1202. DOI: 10.1002/nau.24325 PMID: 32119156

Cena, H., & Calder, P. (2020). Defining a healthy diet: Evidence for the role of contemporary dietary patterns in health and disease. *Nutrients*, *12*(2), 334. DOI: 10.3390/nu12020334 PMID: 32012681

Chang, E., & Levy, B. (2021). High prevalence of elder abuse during the covid-19 pandemic: Risk and resilience factors. *The American Journal of Geriatric Psychiatry*, *29*(11), 1152–1159. DOI: 10.1016/j.jagp.2021.01.007 PMID: 33518464

Chávez-Íñiguez, J., Navarro-Gallardo, G., Medina-González, R., Alcantar-Vallin, L., & García-García, G. (2020). Acute kidney injury caused by obstructive nephropathy. *International Journal of Nephrology*, *2020*, 1–10. DOI: 10.1155/2020/8846622 PMID: 33312728

Chen, S., Xiang, H., Zhu, X., Zhang, H., Wang, D., Liu, H., Wang, J., Yin, T., Liu, L., Kong, M., Zhang, J., Ogura, S., & Zhao, X. (2018). Free dietary choice and free-range rearing improve the product quality, gait score, and microbial richness of chickens. *Animals (Basel)*, *8*(6), 84. DOI: 10.3390/ani8060084 PMID: 29865185

Chen, Y., Cao, L., Qiu, J., Li, Z., Guo, Z., Zhu, Z., Xu, Y., Qian, W., Zhu, W., & Li, Y. (2023). Surgical management and outcome of entero-urinary fistula complicating Crohn's disease: A single center study. *World Journal of Surgery*, *47*(12), 3365–3372. DOI: 10.1007/s00268-023-07196-x PMID: 37775571

Chiodini, I., & Bolland, M. (2018). Calcium supplementation in osteoporosis: Useful or harmful? *Acta Endocrinologica, 178*(4), D13–D25. DOI: 10.1530/EJE-18-0113 PMID: 29440373

Cupone, I., Dellera, E., Marra, F., & Giori, A. (2020). Development and characterization of an orodispersible film for vitamin D3 supplementation. *Molecules (Basel, Switzerland), 25*(24), 5851. DOI: 10.3390/molecules25245851 PMID: 33322282

Dong, X. (2015). Elder abuse: Systematic review and implications for practice. *Journal of the American Geriatrics Society, 63*(6), 1214–1238. DOI: 10.1111/jgs.13454 PMID: 26096395

Duan, Z., Cai, G., Li, J., & Chen, X. (2020). Cisplatin-induced renal toxicity in elderly people. *Therapeutic Advances in Medical Oncology, 12*, 1758835920923430. Advance online publication. DOI: 10.1177/1758835920923430 PMID: 32489432

Fischer, V., Haffner-Luntzer, M., Amling, M., & Ignatius, A. (2018). Calcium and vitamin d in bone fracture healing and post-traumatic bone turnover. eCM, 35, 365-385. DOI: 10.22203/eCM.v035a25

Fitzpatrick, J. M., Bianchi, L. A., Hayes, N., Da Silva, T., & Harris, R. (2023). Professional development and career planning for nurses working in care homes for older people: A scoping review. *International Journal of Older People Nursing, 18*(1), e12519. DOI: 10.1111/opn.12519 PMID: 36441621

Gardner, C., Vadiveloo, M., Petersen, K., Anderson, C., Springfield, S., Horn, L., & Joseph, J. (2023). Popular dietary patterns: alignment with American Heart Association 2021 dietary guidance: a scientific statement from the American Heart Association. *Circulation, 147*(22), 1715–1730. DOI: 10.1161/CIR.0000000000001146 PMID: 37128940

Gorenko, J., Moran, C., Flynn, M., Dobson, K., & Konnert, C. (2020). Social isolation and psychological distress among older adults related to covid-19: A narrative review of remotely-delivered interventions and recommendations. *Journal of Applied Gerontology, 40*(1), 3–13. DOI: 10.1177/0733464820958550 PMID: 32914668

Hashim, H., Blanker, M., Drake, M., Djurhuus, J., Meijlink, J., Morris, V., Petros, P., Wen, J. G., & Wein, A. (2019). International continence society (ics) report on the terminology for nocturia and nocturnal lower urinary tract function. *Neurourology and Urodynamics, 38*(2), 499–508. DOI: 10.1002/nau.23917 PMID: 30644584

Joo, N., Shin, S.-H., Kim, K.-N., Lee, S.-H., Jung, S., & Yeum, K.-J. (2024). Home meal replacement fortified with eggshell powder and vitamin d prevents bone loss in postmenopausal women: A randomized, double-blind, controlled study. *Nutrients, 16*(8), 1152. DOI: 10.3390/nu16081152 PMID: 38674843

Juhász, M., Varannai, O., Németh, D., Szakács, Z., Kiss, S., Izsák, V., Martonosi, Á. R., Hegyi, P., & Párniczky, A. (2021). Vitamin d supplementation in patients with cystic fibrosis: A systematic review and meta-analysis. *Journal of Cystic Fibrosis, 20*(5), 729–736. DOI: 10.1016/j.jcf.2020.12.008 PMID: 33349585

Jyväkorpi, S., Pitkälä, K., Björkman, M., Strandberg, T., Soini, H., & Suominen, M. (2017). Psychological well-being is associated with better nutrient intakes in heterogeneous older populations. *European Geriatric Medicine, 8*(1), 6–7. DOI: 10.1016/j.eurger.2016.09.007

Karthikeyan, M., Vijaykumar, P., Chandana, L., & Paul, A. (2021). Impact of nutritional education in malnourished elderly patients with the comparison of mini nutritional assessment (MNA) score. *Journal of Family Medicine and Primary Care*, *10*(3), 1167–1170. DOI: 10.4103/jfmpc.jfmpc_1363_20 PMID: 34041145

Kim, E., Kubzansky, L., Soo, J., & Boehm, J. (2016). Maintaining healthy behavior: A prospective study of psychological well-being and physical activity. *Annals of Behavioral Medicine*, *51*(3), 337–347. DOI: 10.1007/s12160-016-9856-y PMID: 27822613

Liu, G., Wang, J., Wei, Z., Fang, C., Shi, K., Qian, C., & Wan, M. (2023). Elevated pdgf-bb from bone impairs hippocampal vasculature by inducing pdgfrβ shedding from pericytes. *Advancement of Science*, *10*(20), 2206938. Advance online publication. DOI: 10.1002/advs.202206938 PMID: 37102631

Ludvigsson, M., Wiklund, N., Swahnberg, K., & Simmons, J. (2022). Experiences of elder abuse: A qualitative study among victims in Sweden. *BMC Geriatrics*, *22*(1), 256. Advance online publication. DOI: 10.1186/s12877-022-02933-8 PMID: 35351038

Martinez, J., Kahana, D., Ghuman, S., Wilson, H., Wilson, J., Kim, S., Lagishetty, V., Jacobs, J. P., Sinha-Hikim, A. P., & Friedman, T. (2021). Unhealthy lifestyle and gut dysbiosis: A better understanding of the effects of poor diet and nicotine on the intestinal microbiome. *Frontiers in Endocrinology*, *12*, 667066. Advance online publication. DOI: 10.3389/fendo.2021.667066 PMID: 34168615

Mason, T., Do, B., Wang, S., & Dunton, G. (2020). Ecological momentary assessment of eating and dietary intake behaviors in children and adolescents: A systematic review of the literature. *Appetite*, *144*, 104465. DOI: 10.1016/j.appet.2019.104465 PMID: 31541670

McKenzie, J., McDonald, S., Baram, L., Page, M., Allman-Farinelli, M., Raubenheimer, D., & Bero, L. (2021). Assessment of the methods used to develop vitamin d and calcium recommendations—A systematic review of bone health guidelines. *Nutrients*, *13*(7), 2423. DOI: 10.3390/nu13072423 PMID: 34371932

Mertens, J., Reid, D., Lau, S., Kim, Y., & Gage, F. (2018). Aging in a dish: Ipsc-derived and directly induced neurons for studying brain aging and age-related neurodegenerative diseases. *Annual Review of Genetics*, *52*(1), 271–293. DOI: 10.1146/annurev-genet-120417-031534 PMID: 30208291

Nguyen, V. (2021). School-based nutrition interventions can improve bone health in children and adolescents. *Osteoporosis and Sarcopenia*, *7*(1), 1–5. DOI: 10.1016/j.afos.2021.03.004 PMID: 33869798

Niraula, A., Sheridan, J., & Godbout, J. (2016). Microglia priming with aging and stress. *Neuropsychopharmacology : Official Publication of the American College of Neuropsychopharmacology*, *42*(1), 318–333. DOI: 10.1038/npp.2016.185 PMID: 27604565

Nishi, S., Babió, N., Paz-Graniel, I., Serra-Majem, L., Vioque, J., Fitó, M., Corella, D., Pintó, X., Bueno-Cavanillas, A., Tur, J. A., Diez-Ricote, L., Martinez, J. A., Gómez-Martínez, C., González-Botella, A., Castañer, O., Alvarez-Sala, A., Montesdeoca-Mendoza, C., Fanlo-Maresma, M., Cano-Ibáñez, N., & Salas-Salvadó, J. (2023). Water intake, hydration status and 2-year changes in cognitive performance: A prospective cohort study. *BMC Medicine*, *21*(1), 82. Advance online publication. DOI: 10.1186/s12916-023-02771-4 PMID: 36882739

Rababah, T., Aludatt, M., Gammoh, S., Salameh, F. B., Magableh, G., Almajwal, A., Yücel, S., AL-Rayyan, Y., & AL-Rayyan, N. (2024). A pilot study investigating the influence of dietary boron levels on osteoporosis in postmenopausal women. *Food Science & Nutrition*, *12*(8), 5708–5721. DOI: 10.1002/fsn3.4218 PMID: 39139931

Reis da Silva, T. (2024a). The Evolution of Nursing for Older Adult: A Historical Perspective. Associative J Health Sci. 3(3). AJHS. 000561. 2024. DOI: . Link: https://crimsonpublishers.com/ajhs/pdf/AJHS.000561.pdfDOI: 10.31031/AJHS.2024.03.000561

Reis da Silva, T. (2024d). Can supplementing vitamin B12 improve mental health outcomes?: A literature review. *British Journal of Community Nursing*, *29*(3), 137–146. DOI: 10.12968/bjcn.2024.29.3.137 PMID: 38421889

Reis da Silva, T. H. (2023a). Ageing in place: Ageing at home and in the community. *British Journal of Community Nursing*, *28*(5), 213–214. DOI: 10.12968/bjcn.2023.28.5.213 PMID: 37130715

Reis da Silva, T. H. (2023b). Falls assessment and prevention in the nursing home and community. *British Journal of Community Nursing*, *28*(2), 68–72. DOI: 10.12968/bjcn.2023.28.2.68 PMID: 36735363

Reis da Silva, T. H. (2024b). Loneliness in older adults. *British Journal of Community Nursing*, *29*(2), 60–66. DOI: 10.12968/bjcn.2024.29.2.60 PMID: 38300245

Reis da Silva, T. H. (2024c). Chapter 11 - Integrating business essentials into Gerontological Nursing: Enhancing Care for Older Adults in Diverse Settings. In Sedky, A. *Resiliency Strategies for Long-Term Business Success*. Pp. 283-316. IGI Global. DOI: https://doi.org/DOI: 10.4018/979-8-3693-9168-6.ch011

Reis da Silva, T. H. (2024e). Prevalence of elder abuse: A narrative review. *British Journal of Community Nursing*, *29*(9), 442–446. DOI: 10.12968/bjcn.2024.0004 PMID: 39240800

Reis da Silva, T. H. (2024f). Understanding body fluid balance, dehydration and intravenous fluid therapy. *Emergency Nurse*. Advance online publication. DOI: 10.7748/en.2024.e2201 PMID: 38978385

Reis da Silva, T. H. (2024g). Chronic kidney disease in older adults: Nursing implications for community nurses. *Journal of Kidney Care*, *9*(4), 174–179. DOI: 10.12968/jokc.2024.9.4.174

Reis da Silva, T. H. (2024h). Pharmacokinetics in older people: An overview of prescribing practice. *Journal of Prescribing Practice*, *6*(9), 374–381. DOI: 10.12968/jprp.2024.6.9.374

Reis da Silva, T. H. (2024i). Falls prevention in older people and the role of nursing. *British Journal of Community Nursing*, *29*(7), 335–339. DOI: 10.12968/bjcn.2024.0005 PMID: 38963269

Reis da Silva, T. H. (2024j). Urinary incontinence: Implications for nursing practice. *British Journal of Nursing (Mark Allen Publishing)*, *33*(22), 1070–1080. DOI: 10.12968/bjon.2024.0306 PMID: 39639685

Reis da Silva, T. H (2024k). Oncology and Cancer Medicine: Understanding the complexities in Older Patients. *Biomed J Sci & Tech Res* 55(3)-2024. DOI: https://doi.org/DOI: 10.26717/BJSTR.2024.55.008720

Reis da Silva, T. H. (2025b). Integrating Artificial Intelligence in Geriatric Care: Enhancing Physical and Mental Health Outcomes. In Jermsittiparsert, K., & Marzo, R. R. (Eds.), *Physical Health, Mental Health, and Human Well-Being in the Age of AI*. IGI Global Scientific Publishing., DOI: 10.4018/979-8-3693-6190-0.ch11

Reis da Silva, T. H. (2025c). Promoting Emotional Well-Being in Older Adults: The Role of AI in Supporting Emotional Intelligence and Mental Health. In Jermsittiparsert, K., & Marzo, R. R. (Eds.), *Physical Health, Mental Health, and Human Well-Being in the Age of AI* (pp. 137–167). IGI Global Scientific Publishing., DOI: 10.4018/979-8-3693-6190-0.ch8

Reis da Silva, T. H. (2025d). AI-Powered Emotional Intelligence in Nursing: Bridging the Gap in Older People Care. In Jermsittiparsert, K., & Marzo, R. R. (Eds.), *Physical Health, Mental Health, and Human Well-Being in the Age of AI*. IGI Global Scientific Publishing., DOI: 10.4018/979-8-3693-6190-0.ch9

Reis da Silva, T. H. (2025e). Emotional Intelligence and AI in Geriatric Nursing: Bridging Technology and Compassionate Care. In Jermsittiparsert, K., & Marzo, R. R. (Eds.), *Physical Health, Mental Health, and Human Well-Being in the Age of AI*. IGI Global Scientific Publishing., DOI: 10.4018/979-8-3693-6190-0.ch10

Reis da Silva, T. M. (2025a). Integrative Approaches to Geriatric Care: Enhancing Physical and Mental Health Through AI-Driven Insights. In Jermsittiparsert, K., & Marzo, R. (Eds.), *Physical Health, Mental Health, and Human Well-Being in the Age of AI* (pp. 113–136). IGI Global Scientific Publishing., DOI: 10.4018/979-8-3693-6190-0.ch007

Sandri, E., Cantín Larumbe, E., Capoferri, M., Cerdá Olmedo, G., Werner, L. U., & Vega-Bello, M. J. (2024). Socio-demographic determinants of dietary choices and their impact on health in Spanish adults. *Frontiers in Public Health*, *12*, 1417925. Advance online publication. DOI: 10.3389/fpubh.2024.1417925 PMID: 39575104

Schorr, A., Yehuda, I., & Tamir, S. (2021). Ethnic differences in loneliness, depression, and malnutrition among older adults during covid-19 quarantine. *The Journal of Nutrition, Health & Aging*, *25*(3), 311–317. DOI: 10.1007/s12603-020-1540-z PMID: 33575721

Shabani, E., Khorshidi, A., Sayehmiri, K., Moradi, K., & Nabi Abdolyousefi, E. (2023). The effect of nutritional factors on urolithiasis: A case-control study. *Journal of Medicine and Life*, *16*(7), 1062–1069. DOI: 10.25122/jml-2022-0321 PMID: 37900086

Shafiee, M., Al-Bazz, S., Lane, G., Szafron, M., & Vatanparast, H. (2024). Exploring healthy eating perceptions, barriers, and facilitators among urban indigenous peoples in Saskatchewan. *Nutrients*, *16*(13), 2006. DOI: 10.3390/nu16132006 PMID: 38999754

Shakhssalim, N., Talebi, A., Pahlevan-Fallahy, M., Sotoodeh, K., Alavimajd, H., Borumandnia, N., & Taheri, M. (2023). Lifestyle and occupational risks assessment of bladder cancer using machine learning-based prediction models. *Cancer Reports*, *6*(9), e1860. Advance online publication. DOI: 10.1002/cnr2.1860 PMID: 37403801

Simons, R., Lei, M., Beach, S., Philibert, R., Cutrona, C., Gibbons, F., & Barr, A. (2016). Economic hardship and biological weathering: The epigenetics of aging in a U.S. sample of black women. *Social Science & Medicine*, *150*, 192–200. DOI: 10.1016/j.socscimed.2015.12.001 PMID: 26765221

Srivastava, S. (2019). Emerging insights into the metabolic alterations in aging using metabolomics. *Metabolites*, *9*(12), 301. DOI: 10.3390/metabo9120301 PMID: 31847272

Sugita, S., Tamura, K., Nagaoka, M., Hirano, K., & Yoshida, T. (2024). A neonatal case of lower urinary tract obstruction and imperforate anus: Urethral decompression due to rectourinary fistula. *Cureus*. Advance online publication. DOI: 10.7759/cureus.60404 PMID: 38883130

Uddin, A., Rahman, H., Barua, S., Alam, M., Amin, U., Hussain, M., & Ali, M. (2023). Exploring the bone mineral density of health professionals of medical college by using calcaneal quantitative ultrasound. *Journal of Medicine (Dhaka)*, *24*(2), 131–134. DOI: 10.3329/jom.v24i2.67276

Verma, L., Mishra, G., & Omkar, . (2024). Do more food choices lead to bad decisions? a case study in predaceous ladybird beetle, propylea dissecta. *Bulletin of Entomological Research*, *114*(6), 744–755. DOI: 10.1017/S0007485324000555 PMID: 39618200

Vertejee, S. (2015). Discourse analysis of online discussion forum of undergraduate nursing student's perceptions and observations about elder abuse in society. *International Journal of Nursing Education*, *7*(3), 104. DOI: 10.5958/0974-9357.2015.00144.0

Wan, J., Xie, J., Hu, C., Liu, J., & Zhu, C. (2023). Effect of calcium plus vitamin-d combined with calcitriol in the treatment of patients with type-2 diabetes and osteoporosis: A retrospective observational analysis. *Pakistan Journal of Medical Sciences*, *40*(3). Advance online publication. DOI: 10.12669/pjms.40.3.8795 PMID: 38356827

Williams, B., Brady, S. S., Levin, E. C., Brown, O., Lipman, T. H., Klusaritz, H., Nodora, J., Coyne-Beasley, T., Putnam, S., Gahagan, S., & Burgio, K. L. (2024). Black women's perspectives on bladder health: Social-ecological and life course contexts. *Neurourology and Urodynamics*, *43*(4), 849–861. DOI: 10.1002/nau.25437 PMID: 38451032

Wilson, S., Kongnyuy, M., Joseph, D., & Wilson, T. (2021). Urodynamic utilization in the adult spina bifida patient: An institutional review. *Journal of Pediatric Rehabilitation Medicine*, *14*(4), 655–659. DOI: 10.3233/PRM-200780 PMID: 34864700

Yang, C., Hsu, C., Lin, Y., Tung, M., & Ou, Y. (2023). One-step robot-assisted complete urinary tract extirpation in man with end-stage renal disease on dialysis: The first case report. *Current Oncology (Toronto, Ont.)*, *30*(5), 5093–5102. DOI: 10.3390/curroncol30050385 PMID: 37232843

Yao, S., Zhang, Y., Tang, L., Roh, J., Laurent, C., Hong, C., Hahn, T., Lo, J. C., Ambrosone, C. B., Kushi, L. H., & Kwan, M. (2016). Bone remodeling and regulating biomarkers in women at the time of breast cancer diagnosis. *Breast Cancer Research and Treatment*, *161*(3), 501–513. DOI: 10.1007/s10549-016-4068-5 PMID: 27915435

Yon, Y., Ramiro-González, M., Mikton, C., Huber, M., & Sethi, D. (2018). The prevalence of elder abuse in institutional settings: A systematic review and meta-analysis. *European Journal of Public Health*, *29*(1), 58–67. DOI: 10.1093/eurpub/cky093 PMID: 29878101

Zhao, R., Zhang, W., Ma, C., Yaping, Z., Xiong, R., Wang, H., & Zheng, S. (2021). Immunomodulatory function of vitamin d and its role in autoimmune thyroid disease. *Frontiers in Immunology*, *12*, 574967. Advance online publication. DOI: 10.3389/fimmu.2021.574967 PMID: 33679732

Chapter 12
Addressing Glycation in Aging:
Natural Remedies, Synthetic Approaches, and Clinical Applications

Priyanka Chaudhary
https://orcid.org/0009-0008-8847-5620
Gurukul Kangri University, Haridwar, India

Sanu Diwakar
Central University of Punjab, Bathinda, India

Divya Joshi
https://orcid.org/0000-0001-5703-2124
G.B. Pant University of Agriculture and Technology, Pantnagar, India

ABSTRACT

Protein glycation, or simply glycation, is the process by which sugar binds to amino acids, producing reactive oxygen species (ROS) and free radicals. These chemicals generated by glycation play a role in oxidative stress and the formation of Advanced Glycation End Products (AGEs), further leading to disorders such as diabetes and cardiovascular disease. Synthetic substances have been studied for their ability to reverse glycation. However, the adverse effects they cause lead to the search for natural glycation inhibitors. Medicinal plants and compounds derived from them, including polyphenols, polysaccharides, terpenoids, vitamins, alkaloids, and peptides, have been studied and have demonstrated encouraging potential in reducing glycation-induced damage through early-stage inhibitory effects, chelating metal ions, reducing reactive oxygen species (ROS) and reactive carbonyl species (RCS), and blocking other important glycation pathway sites. Nevertheless, more study and an integrated approach are recommended to fully comprehend the molecular mechanism and processes behind this.

1. INTRODUCTION

Glycation is a non-enzymatic reaction that occurs when sugars are reduced with free amino acids; Louis Camille Maillard was the first to describe this process. When the cell is under oxidative stress or has too much glucose, both intracellular and extracellular proteins may become glycated and oxidized.

DOI: 10.4018/979-8-3693-9730-5.ch012

A tiny percentage of ingested simple sugars, including glucose, fructose, and galactose, may experience glycations in the bloodstream. These glycations are caused by the Amadori reaction, the Schiff base reaction, and the Maillard reaction (MR), which leads to the formation of the AGEs (Nursten, 2005). The early glycation products are extremely susceptible to oxidative (glycoxidation) and nonoxidative degradation, cleavage, and covalent binding, which results in a diverse collection of stable chemicals and protein cross-linking known as AGEs. Specifically, this advanced stage is defined by intramolecular or intermolecular heterocyclic cross-linking and protein molecule fragmentation, resulting in permanent damage and protein denaturation. Methylglyoxal (MG), one of the most harmful dicarbonyl chemicals significantly contributing to diabetes and aging, is formed by the Maillard reaction, which produces dicarbonyl compounds (Velichkova et al., 2021).

Cardiovascular disorders and type 2 diabetes mellitus are examples of age-related chronic inflammatory illnesses that pose serious health risks. Furthermore, it has been shown that glycation plays a role in the pathophysiology of various conditions, including osteoarthritis, inflammatory arthritis, atherosclerosis, vascular stiffness, and neurological diseases (Jahan & Choudhary, 2015). Glycation has an impact on the pace of skin aging as well. It is believed that 3.7% of glycated collagen accumulates annually, though this proportion varies depending on food, lifestyle, and UV light exposure (Danby, 2010). AGEs are thought to cause aging and diabetes-related disorders through two different mechanisms: by binding particular pro-oxidant and pro-inflammatory receptors on cell membranes, primarily the receptor for advanced glycation end products (RAGE), and by changing the structure of proteins (Uceda et al., 2024).

Antiglycation has emerged as a promising strategy to slow down the aging process and mitigate the progression of various chronic diseases. Inhibiting glycation can effectively suppress inflammasome activation, thereby reducing inflammatory responses that contribute to disease development (Van Puyvelde et al., 2014). Numerous synthetic compounds have been investigated for their potential to counteract glycation, including hypoglycemic agents such as metformin, nonsteroidal anti-inflammatory drugs (NSAIDs) like diclofenac, and AGE inhibitors such as aminoguanidine. Additionally, certain vitamins and other synthetic formulations have been explored for their antiglycation properties. However, the prolonged use of these synthetic agents is associated with adverse effects, including gastrointestinal irritation and potential toxicity (Chen et al., 2022).

Given the safety concerns linked to synthetic antiglycation therapies, there is growing interest in natural, plant-derived alternatives that offer both efficacy and minimal side effects. Edible plants are being widely studied for their potential to inhibit glycation, primarily due to their ability to scavenge free radicals and interrupt the oxidative stress-AGE formation cycle, which perpetuates cellular damage (Wu et al., 2011). A variety of natural compounds with strong antioxidant properties have demonstrated significant inhibitory activity against AGE formation while exhibiting low toxicity. Based on their structural characteristics, these naturally occurring antiglycation agents can be categorized into six major classes: polyphenols, known for their potent antioxidant and anti-inflammatory effects; polysaccharides, which can modulate glycation through carbohydrate-protein interactions; terpenoids, which exhibit diverse biological activities including glycation inhibition; vitamins, such as vitamin C and E, that neutralize oxidative damage; alkaloids, which possess bioactive properties that may interfere with glycation pathways; and peptides, some of which have been identified as effective inhibitors of AGE formation (Chen et al., 2025). The exploration of these natural compounds holds great promise for the development of safe and effective antiglycation therapies, paving the way for novel interventions in aging and disease prevention.

2. GLYCATION AND ITS ROLE IN AGING

A chemical process known as glycation occurs when sugars, especially reducing sugars, bond to proteins, lipids, and nucleic acids without the aid of enzymes. The Schiff base, an early-stage product, was formed at the start and rearranged to create Amadori products. Advanced glycation end products (AGEs) can be created by further altering these intermediates by oxidation, cross-linking, and dehydration processes. The development of AGEs, which are linked to aging and the advancement of certain chronic illnesses, is explained by the Maillard reaction, which was initially identified in the early 20th century (Maillard, 1912). In all eukaryotic species, including humans, the accumulation of advanced glycation end products (AGEs) on nucleotides, lipids, and peptides/proteins is an unavoidable aspect of aging. Thus far, a significant amount of evidence indicates that AGEs and their functionally impaired adducts are connected to and may be accountable for aging-related alterations and the emergence of numerous age-related morbidities. Additionally, they suggested that the long-term accumulation of these substances might change the composition and functionality of proteins, influencing a number of aging-related characteristics (Chaudhuri et al., 2018).

2.1. Glycation and its Biochemical Mechanism

The creation of AGEs is mostly dependent on the Maillard reaction. Reactions between reducing sugars, such as glucose and fructose, and the free amino groups of proteins or lipids initiate this non-enzymatic process. There are three primary phases to this interaction-glycation, Amadori rearrangement and AGEs (Ahmed, 2005; Lima & Baynes, 2013; Chen et al., 2022).

1. **Glycation:** The first step is the reaction of a free amino group on a protein or lipid with a reducing sugar. This results in the formation of an unstable intermediate known as a reversible Schiff base, which is subject to additional chemical transformations.
2. **Amadori Rearrangement:** The more stable 1-amino-1-deoxy-2-ketose (ketoamine), sometimes referred to as the Amadori product, is created when the Schiff base reorganizes into a somewhat stable form. The Amadori product is often referred to as fructose-lysine (FL) when glucose is the starting sugar. At healthy pH, the equilibrium constant for the Amadori product's production is firmly increasing in the forward direction; nevertheless, reversibility rises with pH and in the presence of phosphate. These goods are regarded as AGE formation intermediates. The Amadori products can go through a number of changes, including oxidation and dehydration, but they stay in the body for a long time (Zhang et al., 2009).
3. **Advanced Glycation End Products (AGEs):** Amadori products go through intricate chemical transformations in the last stage, such as oxidation, dehydration, and the creation of protein cross-links. Over time, these irreversible AGEs build up in tissues and alter the structure and functionality of proteins. The non-homogenous, chemically diverse group of molecules known AGEs are produced either endogenously or exogenously along a variety of pathways within the human body. Usually, they are created non-enzymatically by condensation between the free amine groups of proteins, lipids, or nucleic acids and the carbonyl groups of reducing sugars. This is followed by further rearrangements that produce stable, irreversible outcomes (Mengstie et al., 2022; Twarda-Clapa et al., 2022).

The Maillard reaction is the primary pathway for AGE formation, but other pathways contribute to AGE accumulation as well.

2.1.1 Other Pathways of AGE Formation

Along with the Maillard process, the polyol pathway, lipid peroxidation, and glucose autoxidation can all result in the formation of AGEs. Additionally, dicarbonyl molecules produced by these routes react with amino groups to create AGE. For example, glucose autoxidation is the process by which glucose oxidizes in the presence of oxygen to produce dicarbonyl molecules like methylglyoxal (MGO). AGE is the outcome of these substances' subsequent reactions with lipids and proteins. Similar to this, the process of lipid peroxidation produces aldehydes such as malondialdehyde (MDA) and 4-hydroxy-2-nonenal (HNE), which can interact with protein amino groups to form AGEs. Last but not least, the Polyol Pathway involves aldose reductase converting glucose to sorbitol first, followed by sorbitol dehydrogenase converting it to fructose. These intermediates have the ability to create AGE precursors, which can lead to the buildup of AGE, especially when hyperglycemia is present (Luo et al., 2022; Twarda-Clapa et al., 2022).

2.2 Advanced Glycation Products (AGEs)

AGEs are a complex and diverse group of substances that fall into two categories: exogenous and endogenous. The Maillard reaction, which happens when reducing sugars interact non-enzymatically with amino acids in proteins, lipids, or DNA, is the primary mechanism by which endogenous AGEs are produced. Under normal physiological conditions, AGEs are constantly forming, but under situations of high glucose and oxidative stress, their rate of creation dramatically rises. Furthermore, exogenous AGEs are produced in food and are strongly influenced by temperature during cooking and food preparation (Twarda-Clapa et al., 2022; Zhou et al., 2024).

2.2.1 Endogenous and Exogenous Sources of AGEs

Both internal (endogenous) and external (exogenous) formation of AGEs are possible. To understand how nutrition, lifestyle, and metabolic factors affect AGE buildup, it is essential to understand both sources.

a. Endogenous AGE Formation

Through regular metabolic processes, the body continuously creates AGEs, particularly in response to rising glucose levels. In the context of chronic illnesses like diabetes, this endogenous AGE production is very significant. Some of the examples are discussed below:

- **Hyperglycemia and AGE Formation:** Diabetes, which is characterized by persistently elevated blood sugar, dramatically accelerates the development of AGEs. The kidneys, retina, and blood vessels are among the tissues where AGEs build up as a result of glycation events triggered by elevated blood glucose levels. Diabetic problems like retinopathy, neuropathy, and nephropathy are aggravated by this accumulation (Khalid et al., 2022).

- **Oxidative Stress and AGE Formation:** The production of AGEs is also accelerated by oxidative stress, which happens when reactive oxygen species (ROS) and the body's antioxidant defenses are out of balance. ROS have the ability to accelerate the oxidation of lipids and carbohydrates, producing dicarbonyl molecules that combine with proteins to produce AGEs. The interaction between AGEs and their receptors, such as RAGE, results in oxidative stress, which can cause pathological consequences and cellular malfunction. RAGE expression and the buildup of danger-associated molecular patterns (DAMPs) are sustained by stress-induced redox imbalance (Pathak et al., 2022).
- **AGE Formation in Long-Lived Proteins:** Since some proteins, such as collagen and elastin, have lengthy half-lives, AGEs gradually build up in them. In organs like the skin and blood vessels, the buildup of AGEs in these structural proteins causes tissue stiffness and elasticity loss. The process of AGE development *in vivo* takes longer because of the lower temperature. The general consensus is that long-lived proteins like hemoglobin, alkaline phosphatase, lysozyme, collagen, or elastin are particularly impacted by the long-term production of AGEs *in vivo* (Kasper & Funk, 2001; Nass et al., 2007).

b. Exogenous AGE Formation

Dietary sources are the main way that exogenous AGEs enter the body. Higher amounts of AGEs are found in foods that are cooked at high temperatures, such as grilled, fried, or roasted meats. The sources include cooking methods, processing strategies, and environmental influence.

- **Cooking Methods and AGE Formation:** The Maillard reaction in food is best facilitated by high-temperature cooking techniques like grilling, roasting, and frying. As a result, foods including meats, cheeses, and baked goods start to produce AGEs. Lower cooking temperatures, like boiling or steaming, result in fewer AGEs being produced by food. For example, the low-temperature cooking and sparing use of sugar and vegetable oils in Chinese traditional staple meals including rice, noodles, dumplings, and steamed bread result in lower levels of AGEs (< 76.80 mg/kg) (Zhang et al., 2024). According to Sharma et al. (2015), dry heat cooking has been shown to encourage the production of dietary AGEs as identified by immunological techniques. However, using acidic components like vinegar or lemon juice, cooking for shorter periods of time, heating in an oven with high humidity, or cooking at lower temperatures all appear to lessen the production of AGE.
- **Processed Dietary Products:** One of the main sources of exogenous AGEs is meat, especially processed or high-temperature cooked meats. AGE intake is also influenced by other processed foods, dairy products, and baked goods. When cooked at high temperatures, foods with a high sugar content, including cakes and pastries, cause AGEs to develop. According to Khan et al. (2023), foods that are fried, grilled, baked, or boiled have the highest levels of AGEs. Crackers, chips, and cookies are examples of dry-heat processed foods with the greatest AGE content per gram of food. The addition of ingredients like butter, oil, cheese, eggs, and nuts—all of which greatly increase the production of AGE during dry-heat processing—is probably the cause of this.
- **Tobacco Smoke and Environmental Pollutants:** Another source of exogenous AGEs is tobacco smoke. High levels of reactive chemicals are produced during tobacco combustion, which aids in the production of AGE (Zgutka et al., 2023). According to Cerami et al. (1997), tobacco smoke

and aqueous extracts contain reactive glycation products that can quickly react with proteins to generate AGEs. Additionally, when breathed, environmental contaminants such as diesel exhaust and particulate matter also aid in the development of AGEs (Reynolds et al., 2011).

2.3 Biological Implications of AGE Accumulation

2.3.1 Aging

The aging process is significantly influenced by the build-up of AGEs. The AGE-induced structural alterations in proteins result in functional deficits that exacerbate the physiological and outward manifestations of aging.

- **Tissue Stiffness and Elasticity:** Tissues like collagen and elastin become less elastic and more rigid as a result of the creation of cross-links between their proteins. The skin is the most obvious example of this, as it ages and gets less elastic and wrinkled (Zgutka et al., 2023). Similar alterations take place in blood vessels, causing arterial stiffness and a contributing factor to cardiovascular disorders including hypertension. For instance, arterial stiffness/HTN and serum levels of sRAGE and esRAGE are inversely correlated, but plasma levels of AGEs and arterial stiffness are positively correlated (Prasad & Mishra, 2017).
- **Impaired Cellular Function:** Proteins that are glycated lose their ability to function. Glycated enzymes, receptors, and structural proteins may not operate as well as they should, which can cause cellular malfunction. Glycated enzymes, for instance, may become less catalytically active, which would hinder metabolic functions and increase the risk of age-related illnesses. Glycation inhibits paraoxonase, a plasma enzyme linked to high-density lipoproteins that neutralizes oxidized phospholipids and stops LDL from oxidizing, preventing the development of atheromatous plaques. This might result in hypertension or even thrombosis (Mastorikou et al., 2008).
- **DNA Damage and Aging:** Additionally, AGEs have the ability to build up in DNA, where they aid in the creation of DNA adducts. Mutations, genomic instability, and compromised DNA repair systems can arise from this, all of which hasten aging and raise the risk of cancer and other age-related illnesses (Palanissami & Paul, 2018).

2.3.2 Inflammatory Diseases

AGE accumulation is associated with several chronic diseases, most notably diabetes, cardiovascular diseases, and neurodegenerative disorders.

- **Diabetes:** AGEs have a strong link to diabetes problems. Increased AGE production as a result of hyperglycemia contributes to diabetes sequelae such retinopathy, nephropathy, and neuropathy. The progressive damage seen in diabetes is caused by AGEs that build up in the kidneys, retina, and nerves, affecting their function (Khalid et al., 2022).
- **Cardiovascular Diseases:** Atherosclerosis, a disorder marked by the thickness and hardening of artery walls, is facilitated by the buildup of AGEs in the vascular walls. Vascular stiffness brought on by AGE-induced cross-linking of collagen and elastin in blood arteries raises the risk of heart disease, stroke, and high blood pressure (Xu & Shi, 2014; Ahmed et al., 2024).

- **Neurodegenerative Diseases:** The pathophysiology of Alzheimer's disease and other neurodegenerative diseases involves AGEs. Alzheimer's disease is characterized by the aggregation of proteins like amyloid-beta, which is caused by the build-up of AGEs in brain tissue. Cognitive deterioration may result from this aggregation's disruption of neural function. AGEs attach themselves to the AGE receptor (RAGE). RAGE has the ability to carry beta-amyloid protein across the blood-brain barrier (BBB), which causes Alzheimer's disease (Deane, 2012; Kothandan et al., 2024).

2.4 Mechanisms of AGE-Induced Cellular Injury

AGEs contribute to cellular injury through various mechanisms, including oxidative stress, inflammation, and protein cross-linking. A schematic diagram elucidated major mechanistic pathway of glycation and subsequent cellular injury is depicted in Fig.1.

1. **Intracellular AGE accumulation:** A large number of disorders are caused by AGE accumulation, which alters protein molecular structure, modifies the functioning and activity of enzymes and receptors, and causes dysregulation of cellular physiology and signalling pathways. Since MGO is one of the strongest glycating agents found in cells, an accumulation of it is extremely harmful. MGO easily forms AGEs, including argpyrimidine and MGO-derived hydroimidazolone (MG-H1), by reacting with lipids, nucleic acids, and the lysine and arginine residues of proteins (Rabbani & Thornalley, 2012). For example, the development of cross-links is a frequent effect of AGE accumulation on extracellular matrix proteins. Reduced elasticity and increased stiffness of arteries, increased thickness and rigidity, vessel lumen constriction, the development of renal glomerular sclerosis, and atherosclerosis are all consequences of cross-link formation (Schalkwijk & Miyata, 2012). According to a number of studies, AGE cross-linking contributes to the stiffening of the heart and blood vessels (Zieman and Kass, 2007; Hooshiar et al., 2022). Furthermore, AGE formation on extracellular matrix disrupts biological attachment sites and interferes with matrix–cell interactions, altering the signaling between cells and the matrix and making it impossible for cells to adhere to their substrates. Changes in adhesion and spreading brought on by AGE may be a significant early step in the pathophysiology of diabetic microangiopathy, which leads to cellular dysfunction and abnormal blood vessel function. For instance, endothelial cell adhesion is reduced when AGE modifies the cell-binding domain of type IV collagen (Singh et al., 2014). Glycation also targets other long-lived proteins such tubulin, myelin, and lens crystallins. Age-related cataract development and diabetes are exacerbated by AGE alteration of lens crystallins. Furthermore, AGEs can alter the extracellular matrix's composition by causing extracellular matrix proteins to be expressed (Schalkwijk & Miyata, 2012). Thus, the presence of AGEs on long-lived proteins may have deleterious pathological consequences by different mechanisms.
2. **Binding of AGE to cellular receptor, RAGE:** The well-characterized molecule on the cell surface that may identify AGEs is RAGE. The immunoglobulin (Ig) superfamily includes the multi-ligand receptor RAGE. The three components of its structure are the intracellular, transmembrane, and extracellular segments. The V-type, C1-type, and C2-type domains are the three immunoglobulin-like domains that make up the extracellular region of RAGE, which is the ligand-binding site. Aging results from the interaction of an AGE with its receptor, which modifies organ and cell functioning mostly through inflammatory chemicals (Dong et al., 2022). A very unique and potent affinity inter-

action takes place when AGEs attach to RAGE. This precise docking between particular structural regions of AGEs and the extracellular domain of RAGE results in a quantitative and highly selective interaction. In particular, distinctive structural characteristics of AGEs allow them to interact with particular affinity regions on RAGE, such as their distinct charge distribution and three-dimensional conformation. Important amino acid residues are essential to this interaction mechanism. For instance, through ionic interactions and hydrogen bonding, amino acid residues on RAGE, including Lys-46 and Arg-77, create stable complexes with the corresponding domains of AGEs (Xie et al., 2008; Zhou et al., 2024). RAGE controls several vital cell functions, including aging, autophagy, ROS signaling, inflammation, apoptosis, and proliferation. Pro-inflammatory cytokines are released when AGEs bind to RAGE, activating inflammatory pathways. Numerous AGE-related illnesses, including as diabetes and cardiovascular disease, are mostly caused by this persistent low-grade inflammation (Dong et al., 2022; Zhou et al., 2024; Wang et al., 2024).

3. **Protein Damage:** Collagen, vimentin, elastin, longevity proteins, and other substances are abundant in the extracellular matrix. AGEs readily bind and cross-link proteins once they are created. Long-term accumulation causes the fibers to become distorted and the protein structure to be damaged, which prevents them from maintaining their biomechanical qualities and functions. The structural integrity of tissues is changed by AGE-induced protein cross-linking (Schalkwijk & Miyata, 2012; Chen et al., 2022). For instance, collagen's cross-links stiffen the protein, reducing the suppleness and flexibility of the tissue. This aids in the pathophysiology of numerous diseases and the aging of the skin, joints, and blood vessels (Stammers et al., 2020). Additionally, the connection between AGEs and problems from diabetes has been linked to intracellular AGE production. In fact, it has been demonstrated that intracellular AGEs play a role in both altering the function of intracellular proteins and triggering intracellular signalling pathways (Ott et al., 2014; Twarda-Clapa et al., 2022).

Figure 1. Major mechanistic pathways of glycation

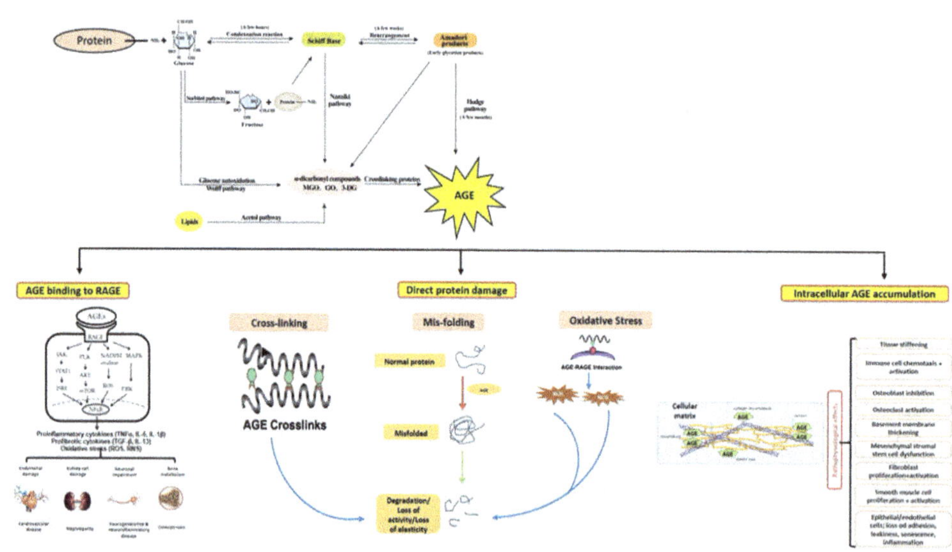

AGE: Advanced glycation end product; RAGE: Receptor for Advanced Glycation End Products; MGO: Methylglyoxal; GO: Glyoxal; 3-DG: 3-Deoxyglucosone; JAK2: Janus Kinase 2; PIK3: Phosphatidylinositol 3-Kinase; NADPH: Nicotinamide Adenine Dinucleotide Phosphate; MAPK: Mitogen-Activated Protein Kinase; STAT1: Signal Transducer And Activator of Transcription 1; ISRE: Interferon Stimulated Response Element; AKT: Protein Kinase B; mTOR: Mammalian Target of Rapamycin; ROS: Reactive Oxygen Species; ERK: Extracellular Signal-Regulated Kinase; NF-κB; TNF-α: Tumor Necrosis Factor Alpha; IL-6: Interleukin-6; IL-1β: Interleukin-1-Beta; TGF-β: Transforming Growth Factor Beta; IL-13: Interleukin-13; RNS: Reactive Nitrogen Species

3. USE OF SYNTHETIC ANTI-AGING METHODS

Synthetic anti-aging methods involve a variety of interventions that address key molecular and cellular processes driving aging, such as oxidative stress, inflammation, mitochondrial dysfunction, cellular senescence, and genetic factors. These approaches include anti-inflammatory agents, antioxidants, peptides, vitamins, and other compounds designed to target these pathways. While promising, additional research, clinical trials, and optimization of these therapies are essential to assess their long-term safety, efficacy, and potential for broader application in anti-aging treatments.

3.1 Overview of Synthetic Interventions

3.1.1 Anti-Inflammatory Agents

Doxycycline: Doxycycline is a broad-spectrum antibiotic, used against bacterial infections. The breakdown of collagen and other extracellular matrix (ECM) components is caused by matrix metalloproteinases (MMPs), namely MMP-1 and MMP-2, which are inhibited by this semi-synthetic derivative of the antibiotic tetracycline. Doxycycline preserves skin integrity and aids in the organization of the extracellular matrix by blocking these enzymes. Doxycycline has been demonstrated to reverse ECM dysfunction in diseases like hypermobile Ehlers-Danlos syndrome (hEDS), in which skin fragility results from irregularities in ECM structure. Doxycycline helps maintain the skin's structural elements and lessen aging symptoms by lowering MMP expression (Chiarelli et al., 2021; Altay Benetti et al., 2023). A study examined how diabetic mice's glucose metabolism was affected by low-dose doxycycline. Doxycycline treatment decreased AGEs, increased insulin sensitivity, and enhanced glucose tolerance. Doxycycline also restored the effects of lipopolysaccharide (LPS)-induced inflammation on insulin secretion and decreased inflammatory markers. These results imply that low-dose doxycycline might help diabetics with their glucose metabolism and inflammation (Wang et al., 2017).

Diclofenac: As an NSAID, diclofenac acts by inhibiting cyclooxygenase enzymes, which are responsible for the production of pro-inflammatory prostaglandins like prostaglandin E2. These inflammatory molecules can exacerbate skin aging, leading to wrinkles and skin damage (Altay Benetti et al., 2023). Additionally, it can make a covalent interaction with proteins and thus, can block the attachment of sugars with proteins. It has been shown to block at least one of the major glycation sites of human serum albumin (Van Boekel et al., 1992).

3.1.2 Synthetic Hypoglycemic Drugs

Metformin: Metformin, a standard therapy for type 2 diabetes (T2D), has shown promise as an anti-aging drug. Research on ageing and related illnesses has grown since the World Health Organisation recognized aging as a disease in 2015. According to epidemiological research, metformin benefits both those with diabetes and those without by lowering the incidence of age-related illnesses and all-cause mortality. Preclinical research in *C. elegans* and mice supports its potential to lengthen longevity, and clinical trials have shown both metabolic and non-metabolic anti-aging effects. Metformin regulates blood sugar levels in type 2 diabetes and helps prevent consequences including heart disease and cognitive loss. Metformin's anti-aging and anti-diabetic actions are attributed to its activation of AMP-activated protein kinase (AMPK), which also improves insulin sensitivity, lowers oxidative stress, and decreases liver glucose production. Recent research suggests that combining metformin with other drugs, such as glibenclamide, insulin, and newer therapies like sodium-glucose cotransporter (SGLT) 2 inhibitors, may enhance its effectiveness, emphasizing its role in both diabetes management and aging-related disease prevention (Chen et al., 2022).

Aminoguanidine (AG): AG is a medication used to treat diabetic nephropathy because it prevents the production of AGEs. In diabetic models, AG significantly suppresses the AGEs, lowering the likelihood of consequences such as vascular damage, according to a study. Through its reaction with α,β-dicarbonyl molecules, AG inhibits the buildup of AGE and the progression of illness. Nevertheless, the study also issued a warning that high amounts of AG might have unforeseen effects on biological molecules. Overall, the results show that AG may be used as a treatment for problems linked to AGE (Thornalley, 2003). Likewise, AG ameliorates renal ischemia-reperfusion damage (IRI) in male mice through the suppression of iNOS, Hsp27, Arg-2, and TGF-β1 and the reduction of oxidative stress. Furthermore, AG reduced inflammatory components, mesenchymal transition indicators, and endothelial activation (Pasten et al., 2021).

3.1.3 Vitamin-Based Anti-Aging

Vitamin A: The antioxidant qualities of vitamin A and its derivatives—retinol, retinaldehyde, and tretinoin—as well as their capacity to stimulate collagen synthesis and inhibit MMP-1, an enzyme that degrades collagen, are well-known. In 0.05% concentrations, the potent first-generation retinoid trenoin is authorised to treat UV-induced skin ageing, including wrinkles, pigmentation, and loss of suppleness. Both tretinoin and retinol have been demonstrated to be essential in reversing the early indications of photoaging; however, tretinoin may irritate the skin more than retinol (Ganceviciene et al., 2012).

Vitamin B_6 (pyridoxamine): Water-soluble vitamin B6 is essential for many bodily processes. Pyridoxamine, a kind of vitamin B6, decreased kidney nitrotyrosine and carboxymethyl lysine (CML), decreased fasting serum triglycerides and 3-deoxyglucosone (3DG), and enhanced the urine albumin/creatinine ratio (ACR) in KK-Ay/Ta animals. Additionally, pyridoxamine decreased the production of TGF-β1 and laminin-β1, which are indicators of renal injury. These benefits were linked to its anti-oxidant and anti-glycation qualities, which enhanced kidney function and lessened AGE-induced damage in diabetics. By preventing AGE production, especially CML, and offering antioxidant defence, the substance lowers oxidative stress and improves diabetes complications (Tanimoto et al., 2007).

3.1.4. Antioxidants and Free Radical Scavengers

Vitamins C, B3, and E are well-known for their capacity to enhance skin health and fight aging symptoms. In order to improve skin suppleness and lessen wrinkles, vitamin C (L-ascorbic acid) stimulates the production of collagen, scavenges ROS, and inhibits MMP-1, an enzyme that breaks down collagen. Vitamin E (α-tocopherol) improves skin hydration and smoothness by having anti-inflammatory and photoprotective properties. Niacinamide, or vitamin B3, promotes cell metabolism and regeneration and has been shown to improve pigmentation, erythema reduction, and skin suppleness. These vitamins work together to protect the skin from oxidative stress, promote the creation of collagen, and enhance the appearance of the skin overall (Ganceviciene et al., 2012; Altay Benetti et al., 2023). While oxidative stress contributes to aging through mechanisms like cellular senescence and the senescence-associated secretory phenotype (SASP), more potent compounds such as N-acetylcysteine (NAC) and methylene blue have demonstrated greater efficacy in neutralizing ROS and mitigating age-related cellular damage (Jomova et al., 2023).

Carnosine, known for its antioxidant properties, is primarily an anti-glycating agent and is often used alongside other agents like aminoguanidine and metformin to prevent AGE accumulation and mitigate aging-related complications. It does so by scavenging reactive carbonyl groups, such as methylglyoxal, which are responsible for protein and DNA cross-linking. Carnosine's carbonyl trapping mechanism reduces AGE formation and protects against chronic age-related damage. In animal studies, carnosine supplementation reduced the risk of hypertension, dyslipidemia, and obesity by inhibiting glycation. While (Kyriazis, 2010).

3.1.5. Hormone Modulators

Studies have highlighted the decline in hormone levels, such as growth hormone, IGF-1, melatonin, and sex hormones, as key factors in aging, contributing to conditions like menopause and andropause. Research on hormone replacement therapy has revealed several benefits. Dehydroepiandrosterone (DHEA) supplementation (50 mg daily) has been shown to improve libido, skin health, and bone density in older adults. Growth hormone therapy has demonstrated positive effects, including increased muscle mass, bone density, and skin thickness, alongside a reduction in body fat. Melatonin supplementation, which naturally decreases with age, has been found to improve sleep quality and may play a role in preventing tumor development. Testosterone replacement therapy in men with low levels has improved energy, sexual function, and muscle mass, while also reducing risks associated with depression, heart disease, and osteoporosis. Although estrogen and progesterone therapy has not consistently shown anti-aging effects in large studies, it has been proven to prevent osteoporosis when administered early at low doses (Ganceviciene et al., 2012).

3.1.6. Lipid Lowering Compounds

Coenzyme Q10 (CoQ10): CoQ10, a strong antioxidant, is essential for safeguarding the skin from oxidative stress, which is a primary cause of skin aging. CoQ10 functions by lowering the generation of reactive oxygen species (ROS) and blocking the activation of the mitogen-activated protein kinase (MAPK) pathway, which controls the production of MMP. It has been demonstrated that taking CoQ10 orally can improve skin smoothness and minimize wrinkles, particularly when it is in its water-soluble form with enhanced bioavailability (Žmitek et al., 2017). It has been demonstrated that ubiquinol supplements enhance mitochondrial function, which has a direct impact on lipid metabolism. A greater CoQ10H2/CoQ10 ratio is associated with stronger muscles and maybe less sarcopenia, while higher CoQ10 levels in people are associated with improved physical performance and decreased oxidative damage. Elderly vitality and quality of life have also been demonstrated to be enhanced by long-term CoQ10 administration, frequently in conjunction with selenium. Despite encouraging outcomes, additional clinical research is required to validate the efficacy of CoQ10 as an anti-aging treatment (Hernández-Camacho et al., 2018).

Pyrroloquinoline Quinone (PQQ): PQQ supports mitochondrial function and lipid metabolism, helping to maintain metabolic homeostasis and prevent fat loss. It mitigates muscle atrophy by increasing fiber size and reducing inflammatory cytokines. *In vitro*, PQQ promoted myoblast differentiation, reduced ROS, and improved mitochondrial function, likely through NF-κB inhibition and enhanced mitophagy (Mohamad Ishak et al., 2024). PQQ (1.6mg/kg) supplementation in mice prevented the rapid loss of body fat, muscle atrophy, and weakness, and reduced chronic inflammation in skeletal muscle, while improving skin condition. Additionally, PQQ enhanced intestinal barrier function and promoted epithelial cell proliferation in D-gal-induced aging models, suggesting potential benefits for intestinal health and malnutrition in the elderly (Turck et al., 2017).

3.2 Adverse Reactions of Synthetic Compounds

Chemically produced substances that block AGEs, like quinine, diclofenac, AG and metformin, have a number of negative effects and safety concerns, including decreased liver function, anemia, vomiting, gastrointestinal disorders, diarrhea, headaches, dizziness, flu, and lupus symptoms (Khangholi et al., 2016). In clinical research including individuals with type 1 diabetes, AG was found to decrease retinopathy and proteinuria while not significantly improving the progression to overt nephropathy. Furthermore, a high dosage of AG caused liver dysfunction and other adverse effects linked to anemia, rare vasculitis, gastrointestinal changes, and flu-like symptoms (Pasten et al., 2021).

Another synthetic antiglycating drug, metformin, causes nausea and diarrhea, among other side effects (Younus & Anwar, 2016). Sakouhi et al. (2023) examined the effects of metformin hydrochloride, a medication used to treat type 2 diabetes, on 130 patients. Ninety-five of them (47.98%) had digestive problems, such as nausea, vomiting, and diarrhea. After experiencing chronic diarrhea, five patients (3.85%) stopped taking metformin hydrochloride due to a complete and permanent intolerance. In their 2021 investigation, Subramaniam et al. reported similar occurrences of diarrhea and weight loss. Metformin was thought to cause diarrhea by altering the gut microbiota, increasing intestinal glucose and bile acid turnover, and raising glucagon-like peptide-1 (GLP-1) levels (Subramaniam et al., 2021). The presence of a carboxylic (COOH) group in the core of diclofenac is also known to cause problems, including liver, kidney, cardiovascular, and gastrointestinal damage (Hasan et al., 2023). Further preparation of synthetic compounds necessitates a thorough understanding of their chemical and structural characteristics, the majority of which are currently unknown (Sroga & Vashishth, 2024).

4. NATURAL COMPOUNDS WITH ANTI-GLYCATION EFFECTS

Due to the adverse effects and toxicities often associated with synthetic molecules in clinical trials, natural products have emerged as promising alternatives for inhibiting the formation of advanced glycation end-products (AGEs). Natural products are bioactive compounds produced by organisms such as plants, fungi, and marine life, with applications in medicine, diet, and cosmetics. These compounds show great promise in the pharmaceutical, nutraceutical, and cosmetic industries. Glycation, a process where sugars bind to proteins or lipids to form advanced glycation end-products (AGEs), plays a role in diseases like diabetes, cardiovascular issues, and aging. Certain natural compounds, especially from plants, inhibit glycation and prevent AGE formation, offering antioxidant and anti-inflammatory benefits. Herbal medicine, particularly in developing countries, is gaining attention for its anti-glycation properties, with minimal side effects, making it a promising avenue for managing aging-related conditions like diabetes (Elosta et al., 2012). Numerous plant extracts and their phenolic compounds have been investigated for their anti-glycation and antioxidant activities, demonstrating their potential as effective therapeutic agents in the prevention and treatment of AGE-related diseases.

4.1 Medicinal Plants and their Mechanism of Action

4.1.1 Allium sativum

Allium sativum, commonly known as garlic, is a species in the genus *Allium* and belongs to the Amaryllidaceae family, known for its significant culinary and medicinal uses. Garlic is rich in bioactive compounds, with S-allylcysteine (SAC), a sulfur-containing amino acid, playing a crucial role in its therapeutic effects due to its potent antioxidant properties that help reduce oxidative stress and inflammation. Garlic also contains other sulfur compounds, such as allicin, diallyl disulfide, and diallyl trisulfide, which contribute to its antioxidant, anti-inflammatory, antimicrobial, and cardioprotective benefits (Tesfaye, 2021). Notably, Ahmed et al. (2006) demonstrated that aged garlic extract (AGE) effectively inhibits the formation of advanced glycation end products (AGEPs) *in vitro*, as well as the generation of free radicals associated with glycation. A key bioactive compound in aged garlic, S-allyl cysteine, has been identified as a potent antioxidant, contributing significantly to the suppression of AGEP formation (Ahmad et al., 2006).

4.1.2 Camellia oleifera Shell

Camellia oleifera, or tea oil camellia, is a species in the *Camellia* genus of the Theaceae family, known for its oil-rich seeds used in cooking and traditional medicine (Zhang et al., 2022). Peng et al. (2023) found that *C. oleifera* shell polyphenols (CSPP) significantly reduce advanced glycation end-products (AGEs) accumulation and AGEs-induced inflammation. CSPP demonstrated strong anti-glycation properties by scavenging free radicals, chelating metals, and inhibiting protein aggregation. Additionally, CSPP suppressed AGEs-induced inflammation by downregulating pro-inflammatory cytokines via the MAPK/NF-κB pathway, particularly through iNOS and COX-2 inhibition, suggesting its potential in preventing AGEs formation and inflammation (Peng et al., 2023).

4.1.3 Curcuma longa L.

The genus *Curcuma*, particularly *Curcuma longa*, is rich in biologically active compounds, including curcumin, demethoxycurcumin, and bis-demethoxycurcumin. These compounds exhibit a wide range of biological activities, such as antioxidant, anti-inflammatory, cytotoxic, and neuroprotective effects, making them potential therapeutic agents (Elhawary et al., 2024). Curcumin, known for its antioxidant, immunomodulatory, and anti-inflammatory properties, has been shown to inhibit pro-inflammatory cytokines, scavenge oxidants, and activate cellular antioxidant defenses (Gao et al., 2023). It also holds promise in delaying tumor growth and mitigating aging-related neurological decline (Das et al., 2024). Additionally, *C. longa* has demonstrated antiglycation effects by scavenging reactive oxygen species (ROS), preventing advanced glycation end products (AGEs), and potentially offering therapeutic benefits for chronic diseases (Anwar et al., 2024). Curcumin's mechanisms involve reducing oxidative stress, enhancing antioxidant enzyme activity, and modulating key signaling pathways, such as AMPK, SIRT1, and mTOR, with promising effects on aging, cardiovascular health, and neuroinflammation (Benameur et al., 2021). In another study, it was reported that curcumin extends lifespan and promotes healthy aging in model organisms, improving memory, reducing oxidative stress, and providing cardioprotective and neuroprotective effects by suppressing neuroinflammation and modulating NF-κB signaling (Shabbir et al., 2021). Despite its potential, curcumin's low bioavailability limits its therapeutic use, though novel delivery systems like nanoparticles may improve its efficacy. Future research should focus on overcoming these limitations and ensuring its safety at higher doses (Gao et al., 2023).

4.1.4 Nelumbo nucifera L.

Nelumbo nucifera, commonly known as lotus or sacred lotus, is an aquatic perennial plant in the *Nelumbonaceae* family. Lotus seeds are particularly known for their skin-protective effects. (Kim et al., 2015). *Nelumbo nucifera* L. extracts from flowers, leaves, and seeds have been shown to inhibit aging-related enzymes such as collagenase, elastase, hyaluronidase, and tyrosinase. Rich in anthocyanins and flavonoids, these extracts extended the lifespan in *Saccharomyces cerevisiae* by enhancing mitochondrial integrity and oxidative enzyme activity, suggesting significant anti-aging potential through the regulation of oxidative stress and cellular senescence (Păcularu-Burada et al., 2024).

4.1.5 Panax ginseng

Panax ginseng (Korean ginseng), a member of the *Araliaceae* family and the *Panax* genus, is renowned for its health-promoting properties. These benefits are primarily attributed to its bioactive compounds, including saponins, polyphenols, and polysaccharides, which exhibit potent antioxidant and anti-aging activities. Native to East Asia, *Panax ginseng* is extensively used in health supplements for its broad range of biological activities, such as antioxidant, anti-inflammatory, and homeostatic effects. The roots of *Panax ginseng* are particularly recognized for their protective effects against skin aging, which are primarily attributed to ginsenosides, the key bioactive compounds. Specific ginsenosides, such as Rg2 and compound K, have demonstrated significant anti-aging properties by inhibiting matrix metalloproteinase-1 (MMP-1) expression, thus preventing collagen degradation and maintaining skin structure. Despite the focus on ginsenosides, other compounds like phenolic compounds and lignans present in ginseng have not been extensively studied for their role in skin aging, highlighting the need for further research in this area (Kang et al., 2024). Some major plants with their mechanism of action are presented in Table 1.

Table 1. Medicinal plants and their mechanisms of action

S. No.	Plant	Mechanism of Action in Inhibiting AGEs Formation	References
1.	*Allium sativum* skin	Scavenges free radicals, inhibits AGEs formation.	Ahmad et al., 2006
2.	*Camellia oleifera* shell	Scavenges radicals, chelates metals, modulates MAPK/NF-κB pathways.	Peng et al., 2023
3.	*Curcuma longa* L.	Activates autophagy, modulates AMPK/SIRT1, supports mitochondrial health.	Benameur et al., 2021
4.	*Panax ginseng* L.	Ginsenoside Rf reduces oxidative stress, inhibits MMP-1, promotes collagen synthesis, and enhances skin barrier function.	Kang et al., 2024
5.	*Nelumbo nucifera* L.	Inhibits enzymes, improves mitochondrial integrity, and enhances stress defenses.	Păcularu-Burada et al., 2024
6.	*Glycyrrhiza spp. (G. glabra, G. uralensis, G. inflata)*	Antioxidant, anti-inflammatory, photoprotective, enhances collagen production	Cerulli et al., 2022
7.	*Euonymus alatus*	Anti-inflammatory, anti-oxidant, anti-diabetic, increases glucose-lipid metabolism	Balkrishna et al., 2024
8.	*Moringa oleifera* leaf	Enhances oxidative stress resistance, improves nutrient-sensing pathways.	Xu et al., 2022
9.	*Ginkgo biloba*	Improves cognition, mood, and reduces oxidative stress and inflammation.	Barbalho et al., 2022
10.	*Aloe vera* L.	Anti-inflammatory, supports metabolism, accelerates skin regeneration, lipid-lowering properties	Hęś et al., 2019

5.2 Phytochemicals as Antiglycation Agents

Phytochemicals, which are secondary metabolites found in plants, offer diverse mechanisms to combat glycation. Several studies have identified major classes of natural inhibitors, including polyphenols, polysaccharides, terpenoids, vitamins, and alkaloids. Various polyphenolic compounds—such as quercetin, luteolin, catechins, curcumin, resveratrol, and lignans are identified as potential anti-aging agents. Saponins from *Panax ginseng* and *Gynostemma pentaphyllum,* along with essential oils, also showed promising anti-aging effects. These findings highlight the diverse therapeutic potential of natural compounds in promoting longevity and combating aging (Gao et al., 2023). Major phytocompounds having anti-glycation properties are summarized in Table 2.

5.2.1 Quercetin

Quercetin is a bioactive flavonoid found in fruits and vegetables like apples, onions, and broccoli. Known for its antioxidant and anti-inflammatory properties, it offers a wide range of health benefits, such as anti-cancer, anti-obesity, antihypertensive, and anti-atherosclerotic effects. By neutralizing free radicals, quercetin helps protect against diseases like hypertension, vascular disorders, and metabolic syndrome (David et al., 2016; Al Mamun et al., 2022). Methylglyoxal (MGO) and glyoxal (GO), reactive dicarbonyl compounds found both endogenously and in external sources such as food, air pollution, and cigarette smoke, contribute to advanced glycation end-product (AGE) formation, which is linked to diabetes complications. Li et al. (2014) investigated the ability of quercetin, to inhibit AGE formation by trapping MGO and GO. The study demonstrated that quercetin captured over 50.5% of GO and 80.1% of MGO within an hour, effectively neutralizing these reactive dicarbonyls. Liquid chromatography-mass spectrometry (LC-MS) analysis revealed the formation of mono-MGO and di-MGO adducts, with di-MGO adducts being predominant over time. In a BSA-MGO/GO system, quercetin significantly reduced AGE formation, suggesting its potential as an agent to reduce AGE accumulation and its harmful effects, particularly in diabetes and other AGE-related diseases (Li et al., 2014).

5.2.2 Lignans

Lignans are a group of secondary plant metabolites characterized by a 2,3-dibenzylbutane structure. These phenolic dimers are derived from simple propenyl phenols and play a key role in the formation of lignin in plant cell walls. Lignans are typically found as minor constituents in many plants, often in their glycosidic form, contributing to the plant's structural integrity and defense mechanisms (Zitterman, 2003; Rodríguez-García et al., 2019). Flaxseed lignans offer potent antioxidant properties, crucial for combating aging-related skin concerns. They also exhibit weak estrogenic activity, potentially inhibiting cell proliferation, and show promise as anti-cancer agents, particularly for breast, colon, and lung cancer, and possess anti-inflammatory effects that may help prevent age-related cardiovascular diseases. Additionally, flaxseed lignans have potential in preventing osteoporosis and diabetes, both common age-related conditions (Li et al., 2024)

5.2.3 Chlorogenic Acid

Chlorogenic acid (CGA), chemically 5-caffeoylquinic acid, is a polyphenol found in various plants, particularly green coffee beans. Known for its antioxidant and anti-inflammatory properties, CGA offers therapeutic benefits for cardiovascular diseases, type 2 diabetes, neurodegenerative disorders, and other chronic metabolic conditions. It also exhibits anti-tumor, anti-pathogen, and organ-protective effects (Pawar et al., 2023; Nguyen et al., 2024). In the study by Girsang et al. (2021), CA was shown to possess anti-aging and antioxidant properties, along with protective effects by reducing ROS levels and exhibiting anti-inflammatory actions against lead (Pb) poisoning. Building on these findings, the current study aims to further examine the anti-aging and anti-inflammatory effects of CA on UV-induced fibroblast cells, emphasizing its established antioxidant activities (Girsang et al., 2021).

5.2.4 Resveratol

Resveratrol (RV) is a polyphenolic compound found in plants like grapes, peanuts, and berries, known for its broad health benefits, including anti-obesity, cardioprotective, neuroprotective, antitumor, and antidiabetic properties. It is recognized for its antioxidant activity, potential anti-aging effects, and ability to influence glucose metabolism. Zhang et al. (2021) highlighted its role in combating aging through the modulation of microRNA (miRNA) expression, which regulates key cellular processes, offering protection against aging, diabetes, and cardiovascular diseases. Resveratrol combats aging by reducing oxidative stress, and inflammation, enhancing mitochondrial function, and regulating apoptosis, making it a promising compound for preventing and treating age-related diseases (Zhou et al., 2021).

5.2.5 Luteolin

Luteolin, a bioactive compound found in fruits and vegetables like carrots, blackberries, and broccoli, is known for its neuroprotective, antioxidative, anti-inflammatory, and anticancer properties (Mu et al., 2021; Iweala et al., 2024). Luteolin reduced UVB-induced skin damage, oxidative stress, and wrinkles while promoting collagen expression, via activation of SIRT3 and the SIRT3/ROS/MAPK pathway. Gendrisch et al. (2021) found that luteolin protected skin cells from UVB damage by inhibiting inflammatory markers (IL-6, IL-1, TNF-α) and modulating NF-κB, AP-1, and JAK-STAT pathways, highlighting its potential in preventing photoaging and inflammatory skin conditions (Gendrisch et al., 2021).

Table 2. Phytocompounds used for anti-glycation activity

S. No.	Natural compounds	Mechanism of action	Ref.
1.	Quercetin	Traps methylglyoxal (MGO) and glyoxal (GO), inhibiting their role in glycation.	Li et al., 2014
2.	Sesamin (Lignan)	Reduces amyloid-β toxicity, lowers superoxide anions, and enhances resistance to oxidative stress and infections.	Song et al., 2023
3.	Chlorogenic acid (CA)	Reduces ROS, scavenges free radicals, and modulates inflammation in UV-exposed fibroblast cells.	Girsang et al., 2021
4.	Curcumin via AGEs	Activates autophagy, AMPK/SIRT1, inhibits mTOR, and supports mitochondrial health, combating aging.	Benameur et al., 2021
5.	Resveratrol	Regulates miRNA expression, reduces oxidative stress, and boosts mitochondrial function to combat aging.	Zhang et al., 2021
6.	Luteolin	Prevents UVB-induced photoaging by activating SIRT3, reducing oxidative stress, and modulating ROS/MAPK signaling.	Mu et al., 2021

5.3. Possible Anti-Glycation Mechanism of Natural Compounds

Since the mechanism of AGE formation involves various steps, therefore, to prevent glycation and its harmful effects, several strategies such as early-stage inhibition, reduction of ROS and RCS, metal chelations etc. have been explored. A number of compounds have been identified which can inhibit this process at different steps.

5.3.1 Group 1 Inhibitors: Inhibits Amadori Product Formation

Unstable Schiff bases are created when reducing sugars with carbonyl groups react reversibly with the free amino groups of proteins and nucleic acids. The concentration of glucose determines the driving force of this process. In a matter of weeks, Schiff base adducts spontaneously undergo intramolecular rearrangements that result in the formation of early glycation products, which are relatively stable Amadori products that are covalently bound. By simply altering or stabilising the protein structure and obstructing the binding site, certain natural substances, such as phenolic compounds, prevent this glycation process and inhibits the generation of amadori products. Some examples include ferulic, isoferulic, and cinnamic acid (Song et al., 2021).

5.3.2 Group 2 Inhibitors: Reactive Carbonyl Species Scavengers

The oxidation function caused by the catalytic activity of metal ions or oxygen during the Amadori rearrangement process of the Malliard reaction results in the production of several carbonyl compounds known as reactive carbonyl species, such as methylglyoxal MG, glyoxal, and 3-deoxyglucosone. This step is the Maillard reaction's intermediate phase. Hesperidine, procyanidins, and quercitin are examples of flavonoids that capture and inhibit MG. Resveratrol and other stilbenes detoxify them by triggering the GLO1 (Glyoxalase 1) pathway, which is a crucial enzyme controlling the production of MG (Yeh et al., 2017)

5.3.3 Group 3 Inhibitors: Anti-Oxidants

Reactive oxygen species (ROS) generation that surpasses the cells' antioxidant capability is known as oxidative stress, and it can cause organ failure and cellular damage. The oxidative damage of cellular macromolecules, such as structural proteins, enzymes, membrane lipids, or nucleic acids, is caused by a variety of physiological processes that involve ROS. As a result of these oxidized proteins building up in the tissues, carbonyl stress is exacerbated and AGEs are formed. The search for compounds with antioxidant and anti-oxidant qualities is prompted by the important role that carbonyl and oxidative stress play in the etiology of many diseases. According to recent research, calcitriol in particular demonstrated an anti-glycation and antioxidant impact in a bovine serum albumin model by interacting with lysine residues that are prone to glycation, suggesting substantial therapeutic potential (Pawlukianiec et al., 2025). Antioxidants such as polyphenols, flavonoids, and flavonols are also known to inhibit the pathway.

5.3.4 Group 4 Inhibitors: AGE-RAGE Interaction Inhibitors

The way that AGEs interact with receptors has a significant impact. AGE-RAGE binding sets off a series of intracellular signaling events that lead to the activation of several transcription factors, such as NF-kB, which are implicated in the pathophysiology of a variety of diseases, such as viral infections, autoimmune diseases, cancer, and inflammation. By activating peroxisome proliferator-activated receptor-gamma (PPAR-γ), resveratrol suppresses RAGE expression. Additionally, silibinin and daidzein stimulate NAD-dependent deacetylase sirtuin-1 (SIRT1), which inhibits the NF-κB signalling pathway (Gonzalez et al., 2020). according to a study, due to its antioxidative qualities, sulforaphane helps in decreasing RAGE expression. By inhibiting the AGE-RAGE interaction, it may be used as a potential therapeutic target for diabetes (Matsui et al., 2016).

5.3.5 Group 5 Inhibitors: Transition Metal Ion Chelators

The majority of AGEs are produced by oxygen-dependent glycooxidative processes that are aided by traces of redox-active transition metal ions. A lot of plants have natural active substances that can chelate metal ions like Fe^{2+}, Fe^{3+}, Cu^{+}, and Cu^{2+}. This inhibits the catalytic oxidation process that reduces carbohydrates, lipids, and proteins and stops AGE production. According to Andjelkovic et al. (2006), catechol, a phenolic molecule, has strong metal ion chelation ability, and the catechol structure in flavonoids and phenolic acids is attributed to their chelating properties (Andjelkovic et al., 2006; Song et al., 2021).

6. CONCLUSION AND FUTURE ASPECTS

Glycation is a critical pathological process associated with aging and the progression of chronic diseases such as diabetes, cardiovascular disorders, and neurodegenerative conditions. The formation of advanced glycation end-products (AGEs) contributes to oxidative stress, inflammation, and protein dysfunction, worsening disease severity and tissue damage. While synthetic antiglycation agents, including hypoglycemic drugs and AGE inhibitors, have demonstrated efficacy in reducing AGE formation, their long-term use poses potential health risks due to toxicity and side effects.

Given these concerns, there is a growing emphasis on natural, plant-derived antiglycation compounds as safer and more sustainable therapeutic alternatives. Bioactive molecules such as polyphenols, polysaccharides, terpenoids, vitamins, alkaloids, and peptides have shown promising potential in mitigating glycation-induced damage through antioxidant, anti-inflammatory, and glycation-interfering mechanisms. Howbeit, further research is required to understand the molecular pathways and key targets through which natural compounds exert their effects and facilitate the degradation of AGE formation. Standardized protocols should be developed, and clinical research should be encouraged to validate the efficacy and safety of these therapeutics. As various anti-oxidants and anti-inflammatory agents have shown potential in antiglycation, an integrated approach may provide multifunctional effects toward disease prevention. Functional foods and nutraceuticals containing anti-glycation compounds and utilizing the application of nanoparticles as novel delivery agents can also be explored to target age-related disorders, paving the way for innovative therapeutic advancements in antiglycation science.

REFERENCES

Ahmad, M. S., & Ahmed, N. (2006). Antiglycation properties of aged garlic extract: Possible role in prevention of diabetic complications. *The Journal of Nutrition, 136*(3), 796S–799S. DOI: 10.1093/jn/136.3.796S PMID: 16484566

Ahmed, B., Rahman, A. A., Lee, S., & Malhotra, R. (2024). The implications of aging on vascular health. *International Journal of Molecular Sciences, 25*(20), 11188. DOI: 10.3390/ijms252011188 PMID: 39456971

Ahmed, N. (2005). Advanced glycation endproducts—Role in pathology of diabetic complications. *Diabetes Research and Clinical Practice, 67*(1), 3–21. DOI: 10.1016/j.diabres.2004.09.004 PMID: 15620429

Al Mamun, A., Sufian, M. A., Uddin, M. S., Sumsuzzman, D. M., Jeandet, P., Islam, M. S., & Sarwar, M. S. (2022). Exploring the role of senescence inducers and senotherapeutics as targets for anticancer natural products. *European Journal of Pharmacology, 928*, 174991. https://www.sciencedirect.com/science/article/abs/pii/S0014299922002527. DOI: 10.1016/j.ejphar.2022.174991 PMID: 35513016

Altay Benetti, A., Tarbox, T., & Benetti, C. (2023). Current insights into the formulation and delivery of therapeutic and cosmeceutical agents for aging skin. *Cosmetics, 10*(2), 54. https://www.mdpi.com/2079-9284/10/2/54#B56-cosmetics-10-00054. DOI: 10.3390/cosmetics10020054

Andjelkovic, M., Van Camp, J., De Meulenaer, B., Depaemelaere, G., Socaciu, C., Verloo, M., & Verhé, R. (2006). Iron-chelation properties of phenolic acids bearing catechol and galloyl groups. *Food Chemistry, 98*(1), 23–31. DOI: 10.1016/j.foodchem.2005.05.044

Anwar, S., Kumar, V., Prabhu, S. V., & Yahia, E. A. (2024). Investigation of Effect of Curcuma longa L. against Glucose Mediated Glycation of Bovine Serum Albumin.

Balkrishna, A., Kaur, P., Srivastava, D., Chaudhary, P., Sharma, N., & Arya, V. (2024). Unveiling the medicinal potential of *Euonymus alatus* (Thunb.) Siebold: From traditional knowledge to mechanistic understanding. *Pharmacological Research. Modern Chinese Medicine, 4*, 100102. DOI: 10.1016/j.prenap.2024.100102

Barbalho, S. M., Direito, R., Laurindo, L. F., Marton, L. T., Guiguer, E. L., Goulart, R. D. A., Tofano, R. J., Carvalho, A. C. A., Flato, U. A. P., Capelluppi Tofano, V. A., Detregiachi, C. R. P., Bueno, P. C. S., Girio, R. S. J., & Araújo, A. C. (2022). Ginkgo biloba in the aging process: A narrative review. *Antioxidants, 11*(3), 525. https://pmc.ncbi.nlm.nih.gov/articles/PMC8944638/. DOI: 10.3390/antiox11030525 PMID: 35326176

Benameur, T., Soleti, R., Panaro, M. A., La Torre, M. E., Monda, V., Messina, G., & Porro, C. (2021). Curcumin as prospective anti-aging natural compound: Focus on brain. *Molecules (Basel, Switzerland), 26*(16), 4794. https://pmc.ncbi.nlm.nih.gov/articles/PMC8398038/pdf/molecules-26-04794.pdf. DOI: 10.3390/molecules26164794 PMID: 34443381

Cerami, C., Founds, H., Nicholl, I., Mitsuhashi, T., Giordano, D., Vanpatten, S., Lee, A., Al-Abed, Y., Vlassara, H., Bucala, R., & Cerami, A. (1997). Tobacco smoke is a source of toxic reactive glycation products. *Proceedings of the National Academy of Sciences of the United States of America*, *94*(25), 13915–13920. DOI: 10.1073/pnas.94.25.13915 PMID: 9391127

Cerulli, A., Masullo, M., Montoro, P., & Piacente, S. (2022). Licorice (Glycyrrhiza glabra, G. uralensis, and G. inflata) and their constituents as active cosmeceutical ingredients. *Cosmetics*, *9*(1), 7. DOI: 10.3390/cosmetics9010007

Chaudhuri, J., Bains, Y., Guha, S., Kahn, A., Hall, D., Bose, N., Gugliucci, A., & Kapahi, P. (2018). The role of advanced glycation end products in aging and metabolic diseases: Bridging association and causality. *Cell Metabolism*, *28*(3), 337–352. DOI: 10.1016/j.cmet.2018.08.014 PMID: 30184484

Chen, C. Y., Zhang, J. Q., Li, L., Guo, M. M., He, Y. F., Dong, Y. M., Meng, H., & Yi, F. (2022). Advanced glycation end products in the skin: Molecular mechanisms, methods of measurement, and inhibitory pathways. *Frontiers in Medicine*, *9*, 837222. DOI: 10.3389/fmed.2022.837222 PMID: 35646963

Chen, N., Wang, N., Fang, Q., Yu, Z., Hu, Y., Jin, J., & Yang, S. (2025). Inhibition effect of AGEs formation in vitro by the two novel peptides EDYGA and DLLCIC derived from *Pelodiscus sinensis. Frontiers in Nutrition*, *12*, 1537338. Advance online publication. DOI: 10.3389/fnut.2025.1537338 PMID: 39949540

Chen, S., Gan, D., Lin, S., Zhong, Y., Chen, M., Zou, X., Shao, Z., & Xiao, G. (2022). Metformin in aging and aging-related diseases: Clinical applications and relevant mechanisms. *Theranostics*, *12*(6), 2722–2740. https://pmc.ncbi.nlm.nih.gov/articles/PMC8965502/. DOI: 10.7150/thno.71360 PMID: 35401820

Chiarelli, N., Zoppi, N., Venturini, M., Capitanio, D., Gelfi, C., Ritelli, M., & Colombi, M. (2021). Matrix metalloproteinases inhibition by doxycycline rescues extracellular matrix organization and partly reverts myofibroblast differentiation in hypermobile Ehlers-Danlos syndrome dermal fibroblasts: A potential therapeutic target? *Cells*, *10*(11), 3236. https://pubmed.ncbi.nlm.nih.gov/34831458/. DOI: 10.3390/cells10113236 PMID: 34831458

Danby, F. W. (2010). Nutrition and aging skin: Sugar and glycation. *Clinical Dermatology*, *28*(4), 409–411. DOI: 10.1016/j.clindermatol.2010.03.018 PMID: 20620757

Das, G., Kameswaran, S., Ramesh, B., Bangeppagari, M., Nath, R., Talukdar, A. D., & Patra, J. K. (2024). Anti-Aging Effect of Traditional Plant-Based Food: An Overview. *Foods*, *13*(23), 3785. https://www.mdpi.com/2304-8158/13/23/3785. DOI: 10.3390/foods13233785 PMID: 39682858

David, A. V. A., Arulmoli, R., & Parasuraman, S. (2016). Overviews of biological importance of quercetin: A bioactive flavonoid. *Pharmacognosy Reviews*, *10*(20), 84. https://pmc.ncbi.nlm.nih.gov/articles/PMC5214562/. DOI: 10.4103/0973-7847.194044 PMID: 28082789

Deane, R. J. (2012). Is RAGE still a therapeutic target for Alzheimer's disease? *Future Medicinal Chemistry*, *4*(7), 915–925. DOI: 10.4155/fmc.12.51 PMID: 22571615

Dong, H., Zhang, Y., Huang, Y., & Deng, H. (2022). Pathophysiology of RAGE in inflammatory diseases. *Frontiers in Immunology*, *13*, 931473. DOI: 10.3389/fimmu.2022.931473 PMID: 35967420

Elhawary, E. A., Moussa, A. Y., & Singab, A. N. B. (2024). Genus Curcuma: Chemical and ethnopharmacological role in aging process. *BMC Complementary Medicine and Therapies*, *24*(1), 31. https://link.springer.com/article/10.1186/s12906-023-04317-w. DOI: 10.1186/s12906-023-04317-w PMID: 38212737

Elosta, A., Ghous, T., & Ahmed, N. (2012). Natural products as anti-glycation agents: Possible therapeutic potential for diabetic complications. *Current Diabetes Reviews*, *8*(2), 92–108. https://www.ingentaconnect.com/content/ben/cdr/2012/00000008/00000002/art00003. DOI: 10.2174/157339912799424528 PMID: 22268395

Ganceviciene, R., Liakou, A. I., Theodoridis, A., Makrantonaki, E., & Zouboulis, C. C. (2012). Skin anti-aging strategies. *Dermato-Endocrinology*, *4*(3), 308–319. https://pmc.ncbi.nlm.nih.gov/articles/PMC3583892/. DOI: 10.4161/derm.22804 PMID: 23467476

Gao, L., Liu, X., Luo, X., Lou, X., Li, P., Li, X., & Liu, X. (2023). Antiaging effects of dietary supplements and natural products. *Frontiers in Pharmacology*, *14*, 1192714. https://www.frontiersin.org/journals/pharmacology/articles/10.3389/fphar.2023.1192714/full. DOI: 10.3389/fphar.2023.1192714 PMID: 37441528

Gendrisch, F., Esser, P. R., Schempp, C. M., & Wölfle, U. (2021). Luteolin as a modulator of skin aging and inflammation. *BioFactors (Oxford, England)*, *47*(2), 170–180. https://iubmb.onlinelibrary.wiley.com/doi/10.1002/biof.1699. DOI: 10.1002/biof.1699 PMID: 33368702

Girsang, E., Ginting, C. N., Lister, I. N. E., Yashfa Gunawan, K., & Widowati, W. (2021). Anti-inflammatory and antiaging properties of chlorogenic acid on UV-induced fibroblast cell. PeerJ, 9, e11419.

Gonzalez, I., Morales, M. A., & Rojas, A. (2020). Polyphenols and AGEs/RAGE axis: Trends and challenges. *Food Research International*, *129*, 108843. Advance online publication. DOI: 10.1016/j.foodres.2019.108843 PMID: 32036875

Hasan, M. K., Akhter, S., Fatema, K., Hossain, M. R., Sultana, T., & Uzzaman, M. (2023). Selective modification of diclofenac to reduce the adverse effects; A computer-aided drug design approach. *Informatics in Medicine Unlocked*, *36*, 101159. DOI: 10.1016/j.imu.2023.101159

Hernández-Camacho, J. D., Bernier, M., López-Lluch, G., & Navas, P. (2018). Coenzyme Q10 supplementation in aging and disease. *Frontiers in Physiology*, *9*, 44. https://www.frontiersin.org/journals/physiology/articles/10.3389/fphys.2018.00044/full. DOI: 10.3389/fphys.2018.00044 PMID: 29459830

Hęś, M., Dziedzic, K., Górecka, D., Jędrusek-Golińska, A., & Gujska, E. (2019). Aloe vera (L.) Webb.: Natural sources of antioxidants–a review. *Plant Foods for Human Nutrition (Dordrecht, Netherlands)*, *74*(3), 255–265. https://pmc.ncbi.nlm.nih.gov/articles/PMC6684795/. DOI: 10.1007/s11130-019-00747-5 PMID: 31209704

Hooshiar, S. H., Esmaili, H., Taherian, A., & Jafarnejad, S. (2022). Exercise, advanced glycation end products, and their effects on cardiovascular disorders: A narrative review. *Heart and Mind (Mumbai, India)*, *6*(3), 139–150. DOI: 10.4103/hm.hm_31_22

Iweala, E. J., Adurosakin, O. E., Innocent, U., Omonhinmin, C. A., Dania, O. E., & Ugbogu, E. A. (2024). Anti-Aging Potential of Bioactive Phytoconstituents Found in Edible Medicinal Plants: A Review. *Sci*, *6*(2), 36. DOI: 10.3390/sci6020036

Jahan, H., & Choudhary, M. I. (2015). Glycation, carbonyl stress and AGEs inhibitors: A patent review. *Expert Opinion on Therapeutic Patents*, *25*(11), 1267–1284. DOI: 10.1517/13543776.2015.1076394 PMID: 26293545

Jomova, K., Raptova, R., Alomar, S. Y., Alwasel, S. H., Nepovimova, E., Kuca, K., & Valko, M. (2023). Reactive oxygen species, toxicity, oxidative stress, and antioxidants: Chronic diseases and aging. *Archives of Toxicology*, *97*(10), 2499–2574. https://pmc.ncbi.nlm.nih.gov/articles/PMC10475008/. DOI: 10.1007/s00204-023-03562-9 PMID: 37597078

Kang, M., Park, S., Son, S. R., Noh, Y., Jang, D. S., & Lee, S. (2024). Anti-Aging and Anti-Inflammatory Effects of Compounds from Fresh Panax ginseng Roots: A Study on TNF-α/IFN-γ-Induced Skin Cell Damage. *Molecules (Basel, Switzerland)*, *29*(22), 5479. https://www.mdpi.com/1420-3049/29/22/5479. DOI: 10.3390/molecules29225479 PMID: 39598869

Kasper, M., & Funk, R. H. (2001). Age-related changes in cells and tissues due to advanced glycation end products (AGEs). *Archives of Gerontology and Geriatrics*, *32*(3), 233–243. DOI: 10.1016/S0167-4943(01)00103-0 PMID: 11395169

Khalid, M., Petroianu, G., & Adem, A. (2022). Advanced glycation end products and diabetes mellitus: Mechanisms and perspectives. *Biomolecules*, *12*(4), 542. DOI: 10.3390/biom12040542 PMID: 35454131

Khan, M. I., Ashfaq, F., Alsayegh, A. A., Hamouda, A., Khatoon, F., Altamimi, T. N., Alhodieb, F. S., & Beg, M. M. A. (2023). Advanced glycation end product signaling and metabolic complications: Dietary approach. *World Journal of Diabetes*, *14*(7), 995–1012. DOI: 10.4239/wjd.v14.i7.995 PMID: 37547584

Khangholi, S., Majid, F. A. A., Berwary, N. J. A., Ahmad, F., & Abd Aziz, R. B. (2016). The mechanisms of inhibition of advanced glycation end products formation through polyphenols in hyperglycemic condition. *Planta medica, 82*(01/02), 32-45. DOI: 10.1055/s-0035-1558086

Kim, S. Y., & Moon, G. S. (2015). Photoprotective effect of lotus (Nelumbo nucifera Gaertn.) seed tea against UVB irradiation. *Preventive Nutrition and Food Science*, *20*(3), 162–168. DOI: 10.3746/pnf.2015.20.3.162 PMID: 26451352

Kothandan, D., Singh, D. S., Yerrakula, G., Backkiyashree, D., Pratibha, N., Ramya, A., & Yerrakula, G.Sr. (2024). Advanced Glycation End Products-Induced Alzheimer's Disease and Its Novel Therapeutic Approaches: A Comprehensive Review. *Cureus*, *16*(5). Advance online publication. DOI: 10.7759/cureus.61373 PMID: 38947632

Kyriazis, M. (2010). Anti-ageing potential of carnosine: Approaches toward successful ageing. *Drug Discovery Today. Therapeutic Strategies*, *7*(3-4), 45–49. https://www.sciencedirect.com/science/article/abs/pii/S1740677311000039. DOI: 10.1016/j.ddstr.2011.01.002

Li, X., Zheng, T., Sang, S., & Lv, L. (2014). Quercetin inhibits advanced glycation end product formation by trapping methylglyoxal and glyoxal. *Journal of Agricultural and Food Chemistry*, *62*(50), 12152–12158. DOI: 10.1021/jf504132x PMID: 25412188

Li, Y., Zhao, X., Wang, Y., & Qiu, C. (2024). Research Progress and Prospect Analysis of the Application of Flax Lignans. *Journal of Natural Fibers*, *21*(1), 2309909. https://www.tandfonline.com/doi/full/10.1080/15440478.2024.2309909#abstract. DOI: 10.1080/15440478.2024.2309909

Lima, M., & Baynes, J. W. (2013). *Glycation. Encyclopedia of Biological Chemistry, 405–411.* https://doi.org/DOI: 10.1016/B978-0-12-378630-2.00120-1

Luo, Y., Zhang, J., Ho, C. T., & Li, S. (2022). Management of Maillard reaction-derived reactive carbonyl species and advanced glycation end products by tea and tea polyphenols. *Food Science and Human Wellness*, *11*(3), 557–567. DOI: 10.1016/j.fshw.2021.12.012

Maillard, L. C. (1912). Action des acides amines sur les sucres; formation des melanoidies par voie methodique. *CR.Acad. Sci.*, *154*, 66–68.

Mastorikou, M., Mackness, B., Liu, Y., & Mackness, M. (2008). Glycation of paraoxonase-1 inhibits its activity and impairs the ability of high-density lipoprotein to metabolize membrane lipid hydroperoxides. *Diabetic Medicine*, *25*(9), 1049–1055. DOI: 10.1111/j.1464-5491.2008.02546.x PMID: 18937674

Matsui, T., Nakamura, N., Ojima, A., Nishino, Y., & Yamagishi, S. I. (2016). Sulforaphane reduces advanced glycation end products (AGEs)-induced inflammation in endothelial cells and rat aorta. *Nutrition, Metabolism, and Cardiovascular Diseases*, *26*(9), 797–807. DOI: 10.1016/j.numecd.2016.04.008 PMID: 27212619

Mengstie, M. A., Chekol Abebe, E., Behaile Teklemariam, A., Tilahun Mulu, A., Agidew, M. M., Teshome Azezew, M., Zewde, E. A., & Agegnehu Teshome, A. (2022). Endogenous advanced glycation end products in the pathogenesis of chronic diabetic complications. *Frontiers in Molecular Biosciences*, *9*, 1002710. DOI: 10.3389/fmolb.2022.1002710 PMID: 36188225

Mohamad Ishak, N. S., Kikuchi, M., & Ikemoto, K. (2024). Dietary pyrroloquinoline quinone hinders aging progression in male mice and D-galactose-induced cells. *Frontiers in Aging*, *5*, 1351860. https://www.frontiersin.org/journals/aging/articles/10.3389/fragi.2024.1351860/full. DOI: 10.3389/fragi.2024.1351860 PMID: 38487591

Mu, J., Ma, H., Chen, H., Zhang, X., & Ye, M. (2021). Luteolin prevents UVB-induced skin photoaging damage by modulating SIRT3/ROS/MAPK signaling: An in vitro and in vivo studies. *Frontiers in Pharmacology*, *12*, 728261. https://www.frontiersin.org/journals/pharmacology/articles/10.3389/fphar.2021.728261/full. DOI: 10.3389/fphar.2021.728261 PMID: 34526903

Nass, N., Bartling, B., Santos, A. N., Scheubel, R., Börgermann, J., Silber, R., & Simm, A. (2007). Advanced glycation end products, diabetes and ageing. *Zeitschrift für Gerontologie und Geriatrie*, *40*(5), 349–356. Advance online publication. DOI: 10.1007/s00391-007-0484-9 PMID: 17943238

Nguyen, V., Taine, E. G., Meng, D., Cui, T., & Tan, W. (2024). Chlorogenic Acid: A Systematic Review on the Biological Functions, Mechanistic Actions, and Therapeutic Potentials. *Nutrients*, *16*(7), 924. https://pmc.ncbi.nlm.nih.gov/articles/PMC11013850/. DOI: 10.3390/nu16070924 PMID: 38612964

Nursten, H. E. (2005). *The Maillard Reaction: Chemistry, Biochemistry and Implications*. Royal Society of Chemistry., DOI: 10.1039/9781847552570

Ott, C., Jacobs, K., Haucke, E., Santos, A. N., Grune, T., & Simm, A. (2014). Role of advanced glycation end products in cellular signaling. *Redox Biology*, *2*, 411–429. DOI: 10.1016/j.redox.2013.12.016 PMID: 24624331

Păcularu-Burada, B., Cîrîc, A. I., & Begea, M. (2024). Anti-aging effects of flavonoids from plant extracts. *Foods*, *13*(15), 2441. DOI: 10.3390/foods13152441 PMID: 39123632

Palanissami, G., & Paul, S. F. (2018). RAGE and its ligands: Molecular interplay between glycation, inflammation, and hallmarks of cancer—a review. *Hormones & Cancer*, *9*(5), 295–325. DOI: 10.1007/s12672-018-0342-9 PMID: 29987748

Pasten, C., Lozano, M., Rocco, J., Carrión, F., Alvarado, C., Liberona, J., Michea, L., & Irarrázabal, C. E. (2021). Aminoguanidine prevents oxidative stress, inhibits elements of inflammation, endothelial activation, mesenchymal markers, and confers a renoprotective effect in renal ischemia and reperfusion injury. *Antioxidants*, *10*(11), 1724. DOI: 10.3390/antiox10111724 PMID: 34829595

Pathak, C., Vaidya, F. U., Waghela, B. N., Chhipa, A. S., Tiwari, B. S., & Ranjan, K. (2022). Advanced Glycation End Products-Mediated Oxidative Stress and Regulated Cell Death Signaling in Cancer. In *Handbook of Oxidative Stress in Cancer: Mechanistic Aspects* (pp. 535–550). Springer Nature Singapore. DOI: 10.1007/978-981-15-9411-3_44

Pawar, S. H., Upganlawar, A. B., & Upasani, C. D. (2023). Therapeutic benefits of phenolic acids in peripheral neuropathy. In Treatments, Nutraceuticals, Supplements, and Herbal Medicine in Neurological Disorders (pp. 753-771). Academic Press. https://www.sciencedirect.com/science/article/abs/pii/B9780323900522000366

Pawlukianiec, C., Lauko, K. K., Michalak, D., Żendzian-Piotrowska, M., Zalewska, A., & Maciejczyk, M. (2025). A comparative study on the antioxidant and antiglycation properties of different vitamin D forms. *European Journal of Medicinal Chemistry*, *117*, 263. DOI: 10.1016/j.ejmech.2025.117263 PMID: 39823810

Peng, J., Wen, W., Liang, G., Huang, W., Qiu, Z., Wang, Q., & Xiao, G. (2023). Camellia oleifera shells polyphenols inhibit advanced glycation end-products (AGEs) formation and AGEs-induced inflammatory response in RAW264. 7 macrophages. *Industrial Crops and Products*, *197*, 116589. https://www.sciencedirect.com/science/article/abs/pii/S0926669023003539. DOI: 10.1016/j.indcrop.2023.116589

Prasad, K., & Mishra, M. (2017). Do advanced glycation end products and its receptor play a role in pathophysiology of hypertension?. *International Journal of Angiology*, *26*(01), 001-011. DOI: 10.1055/s-0037-1598183

Rabbani, N., & Thornalley, P. J. (2012). Methylglyoxal, glyoxalase 1 and the dicarbonyl proteome. *Amino Acids*, *42*(4), 1133–1142. DOI: 10.1007/s00726-010-0783-0 PMID: 20963454

Reynolds, P. R., Wasley, K. M., & Allison, C. H. (2011). Diesel particulate matter induces receptor for advanced glycation end-products (RAGE) expression in pulmonary epithelial cells, and rage signaling influences NF-κB–mediated inflammation. *Environmental Health Perspectives*, *119*(3), 332–336. DOI: 10.1289/ehp.1002520 PMID: 21087909

Rodríguez-García, C., Sánchez-Quesada, C., Toledo, E., Delgado-Rodríguez, M., & Gaforio, J. J. (2019). Naturally lignan-rich foods: A dietary tool for health promotion? *Molecules (Basel, Switzerland)*, *24*(5), 917. https://pmc.ncbi.nlm.nih.gov/articles/PMC6429205/. DOI: 10.3390/molecules24050917 PMID: 30845651

Sakouhi, M., Matmour, D., Belakhdar, K., & Kraroubi, A. (2023). Cross-sectional study on adverse effects of metformin hydrochloride on 130 patients with type 2 diabetes admitted to Medical Center and Diabetes Home of Sidi Bel-Abbès. *Annales Pharmaceutiques Francaises*, *81*(4), 684–695. DOI: 10.1016/j.pharma.2022.11.013 PMID: 36464072

Schalkwijk, C. G., & Miyata, T. (2012). Early-and advanced non-enzymatic glycation in diabetic vascular complications: The search for therapeutics. *Amino Acids*, *42*(4), 1193–1204. DOI: 10.1007/s00726-010-0779-9 PMID: 20960212

Shabbir, U., Rubab, M., Daliri, E. B., Chelliah, R., Javed, A., & Oh, D. H. (2021). Curcumin, quercetin, catechins and metabolic diseases: The role of gut microbiota. *Nutrients*, *13*(1), 206. https://www.mdpi.com/2072-6643/13/1/206. DOI: 10.3390/nu13010206 PMID: 33445760

Sharma, C., Kaur, A., Thind, S. S., Singh, B., & Raina, S. (2015). Advanced glycation End-products (AGEs): An emerging concern for processed food industries. *Journal of Food Science and Technology*, *52*(12), 7561–7576. DOI: 10.1007/s13197-015-1851-y PMID: 26604334

Singh, V. P., Bali, A., Singh, N., & Jaggi, A. S. (2014). Advanced glycation end products and diabetic complications. *The Korean Journal of Physiology & Pharmacology; Official Journal of the Korean Physiological Society and the Korean Society of Pharmacology*, *18*(1), 1. DOI: 10.4196/kjpp.2014.18.1.1 PMID: 24634591

Song, L., & Zhang, S. (2023). Anti-aging activity and modes of action of compounds from natural food sources. *Biomolecules*, *13*(11), 1600. https://www.mdpi.com/2218-273X/13/11/1600. DOI: 10.3390/biom13111600 PMID: 38002283

Song, Q., Liu, J., Dong, L., Wang, X., & Zhang, X. (2021). Novel advances in inhibiting advanced glycation end product formation using natural compounds. *Biomedicine and Pharmacotherapy*, *140*, 111750. DOI: 10.1016/j.biopha.2021.111750 PMID: 34051615

Sroga, G. E., & Vashishth, D. (2024). In vivo glycation—Interplay between oxidant and carbonyl stress in bone. *JBMR Plus*, *8*(11), e110. DOI: 10.1093/jbmrpl/ziae110 PMID: 39386996

Stammers, M., Ivanova, I. M., Niewczas, I. S., Segonds-Pichon, A., Streeter, M., Spiegel, D. A., & Clark, J. (2020). Age-related changes in the physical properties, cross-linking, and glycation of collagen from mouse tail tendon. *The Journal of Biological Chemistry*, *295*(31), 10562–10571. DOI: 10.1074/jbc.RA119.011031 PMID: 32381510

Subramaniam, K., Joseph, M. P., & Babu, L. A. (2021). A common drug causing a common side effect at an uncommon time: Metformin-induced chronic diarrhea and weight loss after years of treatment. *Clinical Diabetes : a Publication of the American Diabetes Association*, *39*(2), 237–240. DOI: 10.2337/cd20-0101 PMID: 33986581

Tanimoto, M., Gohda, T., Kaneko, S., Hagiwara, S., Murakoshi, M., Aoki, T., Yamada, K., Ito, T., Matsumoto, M., Horikoshi, S., & Tomino, Y. (2007). Effect of pyridoxamine (K-163), an inhibitor of advanced glycation end products, on type 2 diabetic nephropathy in KK-Ay/Ta mice. *Metabolism: Clinical and Experimental*, *56*(2), 160–167. DOI: 10.1016/j.metabol.2006.08.026 PMID: 17224327

Tesfaye, A. (2021). Revealing the therapeutic uses of garlic (Allium sativum) and its potential for drug discovery. *TheScientificWorldJournal*, *2021*(1), 8817288. DOI: 10.1155/2021/8817288 PMID: 35002548

Thornalley, P. J. (2003). Use of aminoguanidine (Pimagedine) to prevent the formation of advanced glycation endproducts. *Archives of Biochemistry and Biophysics*, *419*(1), 31–40. http://sciencedirect.com/science/article/abs/pii/S0003986103004399?via%3Dihub. DOI: 10.1016/j.abb.2003.08.013 PMID: 14568006

Turck, D., Bresson, J., Burlingame, B., Dean, T., Fairweather-Tait, S., Heinonen, M., Hirsch-Ernst, K. I., Mangelsdorf, I., McArdle, H. J., Naska, A., Neuhäuser-Berthold, M., Nowicka, G., Pentieva, K., Sanz, Y., Siani, A., Sjödin, A., Stern, M., Tomé, D., Vinceti, M., & Van Loveren, H. (2017). Safety of pyrroloquinoline quinone disodium salt as a novel food pursuant to Regulation (EC) No 258/97. *EFSA Journal*, *15*(11), e05058. DOI: 10.2903/j.efsa.2017.5058 PMID: 32625350

Twarda-Clapa, A., Olczak, A., Białkowska, A. M., & Koziołkiewicz, M. (2022). Advanced glycation end-products (AGEs): Formation, chemistry, classification, receptors, and diseases related to AGEs. *Cells*, *11*(8), 1312. DOI: 10.3390/cells11081312 PMID: 35455991

Uceda, A. B., Mariño, L., Casasnovas, R., & Adrover, M. (2024). An overview on glycation: Molecular mechanisms, impact on proteins, pathogenesis, and inhibition. *Biophysical Reviews*, *16*(2), 189–218. DOI: 10.1007/s12551-024-01188-4 PMID: 38737201

Van Boekel, M. A. M., van den Bergh, P. J. P. C., & Hoenders, H. J. (1992). Glycation of human serum albumin: Inhibition by diclofenac. *Biochimica et Biophysica Acta (BBA) -. Biochimica et Biophysica Acta. Protein Structure and Molecular Enzymology*, *1120*(2), 201–204. DOI: 10.1016/0167-4838(92)90270-N PMID: 1562587

Van Puyvelde, K., Mets, T., Njemini, R., Beyer, I., & Bautmans, I. (2014). Effect of advanced glycation end product intake on inflammation and aging: A systematic review. *Nutrition Reviews*, *72*(9), 638–650. DOI: 10.1111/nure.12141 PMID: 25231200

Velichkova, S., Foubert, K., & Pieters, L. (2021). Natural products as a source of inspiration for novel inhibitors of advanced glycation endproducts (AGEs) formation. *Planta Medica*, *87*(10-11), 780–801. DOI: 10.1055/a-1527-7611 PMID: 34341977

Wang, L., Jiang, Y., & Zhao, C. (2024). The effects of advanced glycation end-products on skin and potential anti-glycation strategies. *Experimental Dermatology*, *33*(4), e15065. DOI: 10.1111/exd.15065 PMID: 38563644

Wang, N., Tian, X., Chen, Y., Tan, H. Q., Xie, P. J., Chen, S. J., Fu, Y., Chen, Y., Xu, W., & Wei, C. J. (2017). Low dose doxycycline decreases systemic inflammation and improves glycemic control, lipid profiles, and islet morphology and function in db/db mice. *Scientific Reports*, *7*(1), 14707. https://www.nature.com/articles/s41598-017-14408-7. DOI: 10.1038/s41598-017-14408-7 PMID: 29089617

Wu, C. H., Huang, S. M., Lin, J. A., & Yen, G. C. (2011). Inhibition of advanced glycation endproduct formation by foodstuffs. *Food & Function, 2*(5), 224–234. DOI: 10.1039/c1fo10026b PMID: 21779560

Xie, J., Reverdatto, S., Frolov, A., Hoffmann, R., Burz, D. S., & Shekhtman, A. (2008). Structural basis for pattern recognition by the receptor for advanced glycation end products (RAGE). *The Journal of Biological Chemistry, 283*(40), 27255–27269. DOI: 10.1074/jbc.M801622200 PMID: 18667420

Xu, J., & Shi, G. P. (2014). Vascular wall extracellular matrix proteins and vascular diseases. *Biochimica et Biophysica Acta (BBA)-. Biochimica et Biophysica Acta. Molecular Basis of Disease, 1842*(11), 2106–2119. DOI: 10.1016/j.bbadis.2014.07.008 PMID: 25045854

Xu, Y., Chen, G., & Guo, M. (2022). Potential anti-aging components from Moringa oleifera leaves explored by affinity ultrafiltration with multiple drug targets. *Frontiers in Nutrition, 9*, 854882. https://pmc.ncbi.nlm.nih.gov/articles/PMC9127542/. DOI: 10.3389/fnut.2022.854882 PMID: 35619958

Yeh, W.-J., Hsia, S.-M., Lee, W.-H., & Wu, C.-H. (2017). Polyphenols with antiglycation activity and mechanisms of action: A review of recent findings. *Yao Wu Shi Pin Fen Xi, 25*(1), 84–92. DOI: 10.1016/j.jfda.2016.10.017 PMID: 28911546

Younus, H., & Anwar, S. (2016). Prevention of non-enzymatic glycosylation (glycation): Implication in the treatment of diabetic complication. *International Journal of Health Sciences, 10*(2), 261–277. DOI: 10.12816/0048818 PMID: 27103908

Zgutka, K., Tkacz, M., Tomasiak, P., & Tarnowski, M. (2023). A role for advanced glycation end products in molecular ageing. *International Journal of Molecular Sciences, 24*(12), 9881. DOI: 10.3390/ijms24129881 PMID: 37373042

Zhang, F., Zhu, F., Chen, B., Su, E., Chen, Y., & Cao, F. (2022). Composition, bioactive substances, extraction technologies and the influences on characteristics of Camellia oleifera oil: A review. *Food Research International, 156*, 111159. DOI: 10.1016/j.foodres.2022.111159 PMID: 35651025

Zhang, L. X., Li, C. X., Kakar, M. U., Khan, M. S., Wu, P. F., Amir, R. M., Dai, D.-F., Naveed, M., Li, Q.-Y., Saeed, M., Shen, J.-Q., Rajput, S. A., & Li, J. H. (2021). Resveratrol (RV): A pharmacological review and call for further research. *Biomedicine and Pharmacotherapy, 143*, 112164. https://www.sciencedirect.com/science/article/pii/S0753332221009483. DOI: 10.1016/j.biopha.2021.112164 PMID: 34649335

Zhang, Q., Ames, J. M., Smith, R. D., Baynes, J. W., & Metz, T. O. (2009). A perspective on the Maillard reaction and the analysis of protein glycation by mass spectrometry: Probing the pathogenesis of chronic disease. *Journal of Proteome Research, 8*(2), 754–769. DOI: 10.1021/pr800858h PMID: 19093874

Zhang, Q., Li, H., Zheng, R., Cao, L., Zhang, S., Zhang, S., Sheng, H., Jiang, Y., Wang, Y., & Fu, L. (2024). Comprehensive analysis of advanced glycation end-products in commonly consumed foods: Presenting a database for dietary AGEs and associated exposure assessment. *Food Science and Human Wellness, 13*(4), 1917–1928. DOI: 10.26599/FSHW.2022.9250159

Zhou, D. D., Luo, M., Huang, S. Y., Saimaiti, A., Shang, A., Gan, R. Y., & Li, H. B. (2021). Effects and mechanisms of resveratrol on aging and age-related diseases. *Oxidative Medicine and Cellular Longevity, 2021*(1), 9932218. https://pmc.ncbi.nlm.nih.gov/articles/PMC8289612/. DOI: 10.1155/2021/9932218 PMID: 34336123

Zhou, M., Zhang, Y., Shi, L., Li, L., Zhang, D., Gong, Z., & Wu, Q. (2024). Activation and Modulation of the AGEs-RAGE Axis: Implications for Inflammatory Pathologies and Therapeutic Interventions- A Review. *Pharmacological Research, 107282*, 107282. Advance online publication. DOI: 10.1016/j.phrs.2024.107282 PMID: 38914383

Zieman, S. J., & Kass, D. A. (2004). Advanced glycation end product cross-linking: Pathophysiologic role and therapeutic target in cardiovascular disease. *Congestive Heart Failure (Greenwich, Conn.), 10*(3), 144–151. DOI: 10.1111/j.1527-5299.2004.03223.x PMID: 15184729

Zitterman, A. (2003). Dietary Fiberl Bran. Encyclopedia of Food Sciences and Nutrition, 1844-1850. https://www.sciencedirect.com/science/article/abs/pii/B012227055X003461

Žmitek, K., Pogačnik, T., Mervic, L., Žmitek, J., & Pravst, I. (2017). The effect of dietary intake of coenzyme Q10 on skin parameters and condition: Results of a randomised, placebo-controlled, double-blind study. *BioFactors (Oxford, England), 43*(1), 132–140. https://iubmb.onlinelibrary.wiley.com/doi/abs/10.1002/biof.1316. DOI: 10.1002/biof.1316 PMID: 27548886

KEY TERMS AND DEFINITIONS

Advanced Glycation End-Products (AGEs): AGEs are toxic compounds that form when sugars react with proteins or fats in the body. These compounds gradually build up over time and can disrupt normal cell function. AGEs are linked to aging, the progression of degenerative diseases, and complications related to diabetes.

Aging: Aging is a natural biological process that involves a complex interaction of genetic, environmental, and biochemical factors, including glycation, oxidative stress, inflammation, and the accumulation of AGEs (Advanced Glycation End-products), all of which contribute to age-related damage and the development of diseases.

Amadori Products: Amadori products are intermediate compounds formed in the early stages of the Maillard reaction, a pathway of glycation. Over time, Amadori products can transform into AGEs, which accumulate in the body and cause damage to proteins, tissues, and organs.

Anti-Glycation: The anti-glycation effect refers to the ability of natural or synthetic compounds to prevent or reverse the formation of AGEs. This effect can protect against the damage caused by glycation, thus contributing to anti-aging and health benefits.

Anti-Inflammatory Agents: Anti-inflammatory substances are compounds that help reduce inflammation in the body. Inflammation is a natural response to injury or infection, but chronic inflammation can contribute to various health problems, including aging and diseases like arthritis, heart disease, and diabetes. Anti-inflammatory compounds help calm this response, promoting better health and reducing the risk of these conditions.

Antioxidants: Antioxidants are substances that help protect the body from damage caused by free radicals, which are unstable molecules that can harm cells.

Glycation: Glycation is a non-enzymatic reaction where sugar molecules attach to proteins or lipids. This leads to the formation of harmful compounds called Advanced Glycation End-products (AGEs). These AGEs can damage proteins, disrupt normal tissue function, contribute to the development of chronic diseases, and accelerate the development of chronic diseases.

Phytochemicals: Phytochemicals are bioactive compounds found in plants that have therapeutic effects.

Chapter 13
The Role of Kinase Inhibitors in Healthy Aging:
Potential Pathways and Challenges

Arthi Boro
https://orcid.org/0000-0001-7921-3620
Bharathiar University, India

Reshma Shanmugasundaram
Bharathiar University, India

Shruthika Arumugam
https://orcid.org/0009-0005-0498-1306
Bharathiar University, India

Muthupandi Vanaraj
Bharathiar University, India

Srinethi Rangarajan
Bharathiar University, India

Nikshitha Babu
Bharathiar University, India

Jothi D. Abidharini
Bharathiar University, India

Vijaya Anand Arumugam
https://orcid.org/0000-0001-7485-1586
Bharathiar University, India

ABSTRACT

Kinases are essential for signaling pathways that affects biological processes. The kinase inhibitors potential as therapeutic medicines to prolong lifespan has been brought to light by recent research which includes aging and longevity, one is mTOR modulation. For instance, it has demonstrated that mTOR inhibition mimics the effects of caloric restriction, a tried-and-true strategy for increasing lifespan in animals. These inhibitors can control pathways related to inflammation, stress reactions, and DNA repair—essential to the aging. Preclinical research on small-molecule inhibitors that target kinases, including PI3K, JNK, and IGF-1 has shown promise. These substances can decrease build-up of cellular damage, alleviate illnesses, and increase longevity. Though these are encouraging, the intricacy of kinase networks and off-target consequences make it difficult to translate insights into safe and efficient. To optimize kinase inhibitors for anti-aging therapies, more study is required, with a particular emphasis on safety, effectiveness, and avoiding adverse effects.

DOI: 10.4018/979-8-3693-9730-5.ch013

1. INTRODUCTION TO KINASES

The process of adding a phosphate group to adenosine triphosphate (ATP) facilitates the transfer of phosphate groups to substrates, which can include proteins, lipids, and carbohydrates, and is predominantly carried out by a diverse group of enzymes known as kinases. According to (Manning et al., 2002), the mechanisms of phosphorylation are crucial in overseeing numerous cellular functions that are significant for metabolism regulation, signal transduction, cell cycle management, and programmed cell death (apoptosis). Phosphorylation modifies a target protein in a distinctive manner, influencing its function, enhancing its activity, changing its stability, localization, or its interactions with other molecules, essentially acting as a switch that compels cells to react to internal or external stimuli. The majority of kinases, numbering over 500 and residing in the human genome, belong to two primary families: protein tyrosine kinases (PTKs) and protein serine/threonine kinases (PSTKs) (Hunter et al. 2000).These kinases significantly propel signaling pathways such as PI3K/AKT, MAPK, and mTOR, which modulate cellular actions by orchestrating responses to various stimuli, including growth factors, stress, and nutrient availability. Alterations in kinase activity are closely linked to a range of diseases, such as cancer (Mohd et al. 2021, Varghese et al. 2020, Velayuthaprabhu et al. 2016, Mohd et al., 2021, Paranitharan et al. 2025), neurological conditions (Meyyazhagan et al. 2020, Lee et al. 2021), and metabolic disorders (Cohen et al, 2000). Furthermore, kinases are pivotal in regulating processes associated with aging, encompassing DNA repair, protein balance, cellular metabolism, and responses to stress. For instance, the mechanistic target of rapamycin (mTOR), a serine/threonine kinase, integrates data regarding energy and nutritional levels to oversee mitochondrial function, autophagy, and protein synthesis (Laplante & Sabatini, 2012). Recently, pathological agents have been identified that cause improper activities or changes in mTOR, accelerating aging and contributing to the development of age-related diseases like diabetes and heart issues. Conversely, the signalling pathway of phosphatidylinositol 3-kinase (PI3K)/AKT—where fluctuations in mTOR also influence insulin signaling and cell survival—has been linked to excessive activation, which correlates with the process of insulin resistance, ultimately contributing to cellular aging and reducing lifespan (Harrison et al. 2009). c-Jun N-terminal kinase (JNK) and other kinases are recognized for their roles in regulating oxidative stress and inflammation pathways related to the aging process (Tournier et al. 2000). This connection underscores the significance of kinases in maintaining cellular balance and combating aging. Due to their critical role in the aging process, kinases are increasingly being considered as targets for healthcare interventions aimed at supporting older populations. Compounds like rapamycin and its derivatives, known as rapalogs, inhibit the mTOR pathway, and this inhibition is directly associated with extending both lifespan and health span in various species, showing positive outcomes in yeast, mice, and other mammals (Kennedy & Lamming, 2016). Additionally, various small-molecule inhibitors targeting kinases such as JNK and PI3K have shown promise in addressing several aging-related conditions beyond just mitochondrial dysfunction, including genomic instability and chronic inflammation. The complexity in drug design creates challenges in selecting distinct medications, necessitating an approach that allows for kinase targeting without significantly disrupting cellular functions. Determining target specificity poses significant challenges due to the complexity of kinase signaling networks, which is further complicated by the structural variations within kinases and their regulation. The development of kinase inhibitors for anti-aging treatments faces additional hurdles, including compensatory responses, off-target effects, and various side effects (Shah and Braverman, 2012). For creating safe and effective therapeutic strategies, a deeper comprehension of kinase signaling in the context of aging is essential.

2. KINASE IN CELLULAR SIGNALLING PATHWAYS

Kinases are the proteins that catalyzes transfer of phosphate groups into specific substrates from ATP, known as phosphorylation, and participate in a range of cellular processes. By altering the structure, function, or activity of target molecules like proteins, lipids, and carbohydrates, this biochemical modification controls basic functions like signal transduction, metabolism, differentiation, cell growth, and apoptosis (Manning et al. 2002). Cells can respond to external stimuli, such as hormones, growth factors, and stressors, by using phosphorylation as a molecular switch. Cellular metabolism, growth, survival, and aging are regulated by the PI3K/AKT/mTOR signaling cascade, which is an example of a kinase-regulated system. This process starts when growth factors trigger receptor tyrosine kinases. Phosphoinositide 3-kinase is then activated. Activation of PI3K by a phosphorylation cascade draws AKT to the plasma membrane through its interaction with phosphatidylinositol, according to Vanhaesebroeck et al., (2012). Downstream target of AKT would be mTOR, regulating several cellular functions: protein synthesis and survival. mTOR acts as a serine/threonine kinase that integrates data about stress, energy state, and nutrition availability to regulate cell growth and metabolism (Laplante & Sabatini, 2012). This system relates to several diseases, including cancer, neurological disorders, and metabolic disorders (Manning et al. 2002). The MAPK pathway is another key signaling pathway regulated by kinases. The whole process is in the form of a cascade of kinases, with Ras, Raf, MEK, and ERK, transducing the signals from the cell surface towards the nucleus; it affects the differentiation, response of growth factor, and stress signals, as well as gene expression. Abnormal activation of the MAPK pathway leads to tumor development and other illnesses. Moreover, JNK, an MAPK member, regulates inflammation, apoptosis, and cell differentiation. It is activated by stress signals, such as oxidative stress and cytokines. Chronic activation of JNK has been linked to age and the onset of age-related diseases, including Alzheimer's and cardiovascular conditions (Tournier et al. 2000). Furthermore, AMPK, the AMP-activated protein kinase, is an important regulator of energy homeostasis, particularly in the face of energy stress, such as low oxygen or glucose. AMPK is a potential target for treating metabolic disorders like type 2 diabetes and obesity since it promotes energy production while inhibiting energy-requiring processes (Hardie et al. 2012). Kinases are crucial in maintaining cellular balance by their involvement in these complexes signaling networks, and diseases such as cancer, neurodegeneration, and metabolic disorders may come about as a result of dysregulation of kinases. With kinase inhibitors shown to be effective in preclinical models and clinical studies focused on the extension of lifespan, improvement of healthspan, and evaluation of age-associated diseases, their potential in modulating these pathways promises prospective therapeutic approaches (Kennedy and Lamming, 2016; Shah et al. 1997). Issues such as off-target effects, the complexity of kinase networks, and the need for tight control of kinase activity still hinder effective treatment development. Thus, more research into the function of kinase signaling in aging and disease processes is necessary to fully exploit the therapeutic potential of kinase inhibitors.

3. SIGNALLING PATHWAYS

3.1 Jun-N-Terminal Kinase Pathway

Figure 1. The Jun-N-terminal kinase

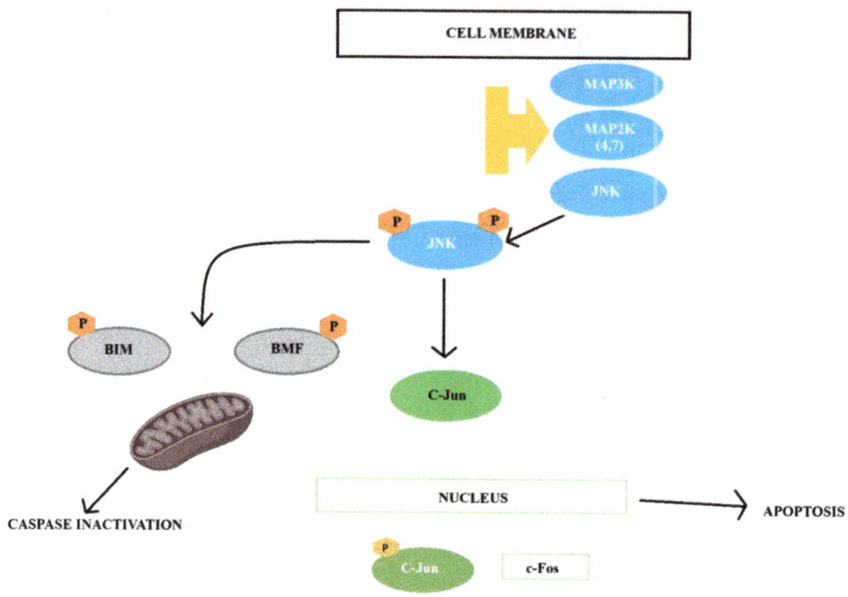

The Jun-N-terminal kinase (JNK) (Figure 1) has become a highly sensitive and highly conserved stress detector across species of metazoan due to its possible versatility. As an SAP kinase triggered by stress, Jink is put through activation by a wide range of intrinsic and environmental stressors: the UV radiation, reactive oxygen species, DNA damage, heat, bacterial antigens, and inflammatory cytokines. Its principal targets are the nuclear and cytoplasmic proteins, specifically the transcription factors such as Jun and FOS of AP-1 family and FoxO transcription factor (Johnson and Nakamura, 2007); these interactions dramatically change the cellular transcriptome during stress (Jasper et al. 2001). Possibly the primary target of modulation of the AP-1 complex is pucker (puc) codes for phosphatase which is JNK-specific that eventually controls activity of JNK through a feedback of negative mechanism (McEwen and Peifer 2005). The result of JNK activation is very much context-dependent but well conserved across species (Igaki 2009); it controls apoptotic processes, morphogenesis, cytoprotection, and metabolism and cell migration in animals like mice and flies. In Drosophila, JNK is indispensable for processes such as embryonic dorsal and thoracic closure and also apoptosis which is stress-induced and synaptic plasticity. Mild activation of JNK increases the organism's tolerance of stress and also longevity parameters (longevity and pathological parameters in females) as seen in puc heterozygotes and Hep-overexpressing flies. Very much similar to C. elegans, JNK phosphatase inhibition and VHP-1 or JNK overexpression increase heavy metal tolerance and lifespan extension in the worm model(Karin and Gallagher 2005, Janes et al. 2006, Pham et al. 2004, Lin, 2003).

Junk also plays a vital part in apoptosis regulation, where it induces the death of a cell when its activity is without restriction or sustained for an extended time (Igaki, 2009). It is not clear whether the effect of apoptosis modulation on adult fly longevity is uniform, but having dead cells and those that survived maintaining the right equilibrium is pivotal for tissue homeostasis, and the more so in high turnover tissues like the intestinal epithelium. It is this relationship of JNK with insulin/IGF-1 signaling (IIS) that puts JNK intermittently controlling homeostatic metabolism in a battle between life and death of the cell. This allows possible control in the lifespan of a tissue and consequently longevity. The extension of lifespan with JNK signals is due to these systemic and cellular changes towards metabolic stability for life, cell survival enhancement, and damage repair flexibility. Overactivation of JNK brought about by any or several causes can be severely inhibitory to tissue injury repair, which may be diabetes, insulin resistance, or even defective intestinal wall regeneration. This evidence highlights a dual role played by JNK signaling in relation to life's longevity, where it is stacked on the one side by guarding against a total effect from prolonged activation, thus giving benefits versus the risks of such an effect.

3.2 Phosphatidylinositol 3-Kinase Pathway

Figure 2. PI3K

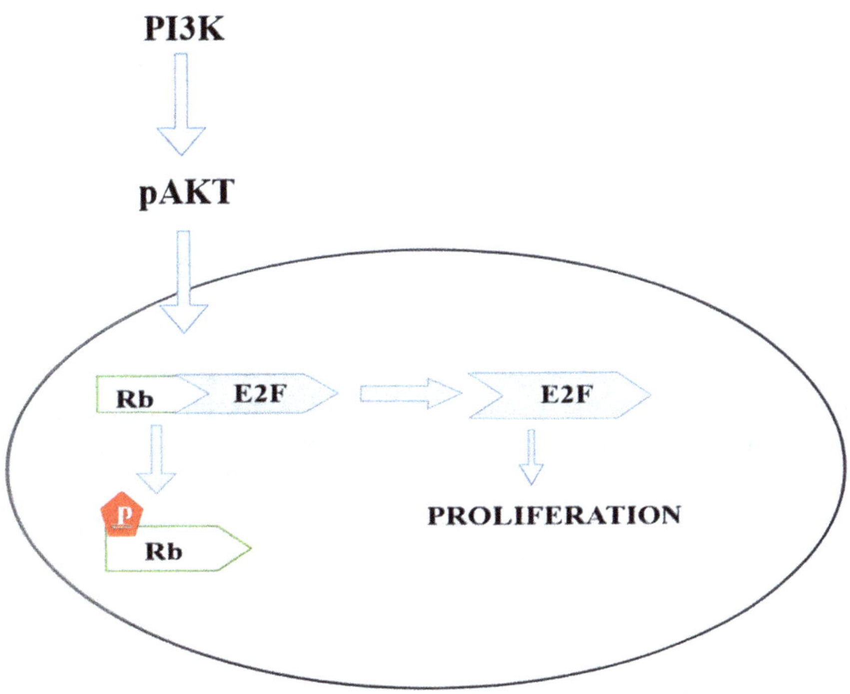

Globally, we see an increased life expectancy that is giving rise to age-related chronic diseases as they are more and more numerous, generating a greater socioeconomic burden. The PI3K (phosphatidylinositol-3-kinase) activity controls cell growth, survival, and proliferation because of the diversity of its target proteins. PI3K (Figure 2) is divided into three main classes; IA is more commonly associated with cancer. The genes PIK3CA, PIK3CB, or PIK3CD encode the catalytic (p110α, p110β, or p110δ) and the regulatory subunit (p85) of Class IA PI3K (heterodimer lipid kinases) enzymes. When we examine total suppression of the insulin/insulin-like growth factor-1 signaling (IIS) pathway, it has prolonged the aging process across all ages. Null mutation for key IIS pathway components has led to a longer lifespan in various organisms, such as yeasts, rodents, and other creatures; however, sex and inheritance effects are now being found.

Old dnPI3K mice show an age-related decline in cardiac function, which is interesting because it preserves cardiac functional reserve and reduces cardiac remodeling. Increased chance of survival in later life in the heart is correlated with this increase in energy. Regulation of TRF1 on telomeres has also been reported through regulation of the PI3K/AKT pathway. Specifically, TRF1 protein levels and TRF1 telomeric foci are decreased when PI3K and AKT are inhibited by small molecules or when genetic depletion of the PI3Kα subunit gene (p110α) occurs.

3.3 AMP-Activated Protein Kinase Pathway

Serine/threonine protein kinase, AMP-activated protein kinase (AMPK) is a key regulator of cellular metabolic processes involved in eukaryotic proliferation, autophagy, polarization, and metabolism. To meet the energy demands of cells. AMPK acts by upregulating catabolic pathways and inhibiting anabolic pathways. It functions as an energy sensor by rapidly producing ATP, and with an α catalytic subunit and β and γ regulatory subunits that are differentially expressed in tissues of mammals, this is a highly conserved protein, AMPK, and its ortholog, AAK-2, using coordinated signaling networks in C. elegans (Steinberg and Kemp, 2009, Hardie, 2011).To coordinate longevity and health. This includes maintaining metabolic homeostasis, increasing stress resistance through FoxO/DAF-16, Nrf2/SKN-1, and Sirt1 signaling pathways; promoting autophagy through mTOR and ULK1; as well as reducing inflammatory responses by inhibiting NFκB signaling, thereby contributing to cellular housekeeping. PP2A, PP2Cα, and protein phosphatases such as Ppm1E inactivate AMPK under non-stress conditions (Richter and Ruderman 2009). During stress, AMPK stimulates energy production by increasing glucose and fatty acid utilization and conserves energy by inhibiting protein, lipid, and glycogen synthesis.

Overexpression of AAK-2/AMPK has been proven to extend lifespan in C. elegans and D. melanogaster. In mice, the knockout of AMPKα1 (AMPKα1−/−) and AMPKα2 (AMPKα2−/−) produces numerous results, with only the α2 catalytic subunit negatively affecting health span (Liu et al. 2011). In the mouse mind, baseline AMPK pastime is higher in older animals as in comparison to young, but stroke in cerebrovascular induces a rise in this pathway signaling pastime in younger mice that is absent in older mice. While the ideal mechanisms impairing AMPK pastime in getting old tissues continue to be doubtful, numerous elements, such as nutritional influences, hormones, and infection genetics in elderly tissues, are recognized to decrease its reaction (Figure 3).

Figure 3. While the ideal mechanisms impairing AMPK pastime in getting old tissues continue to be doubtful, numerous elements, such as nutritional influences, hormones, and infection genetics in elderly tissues, are recognized to decrease its reaction

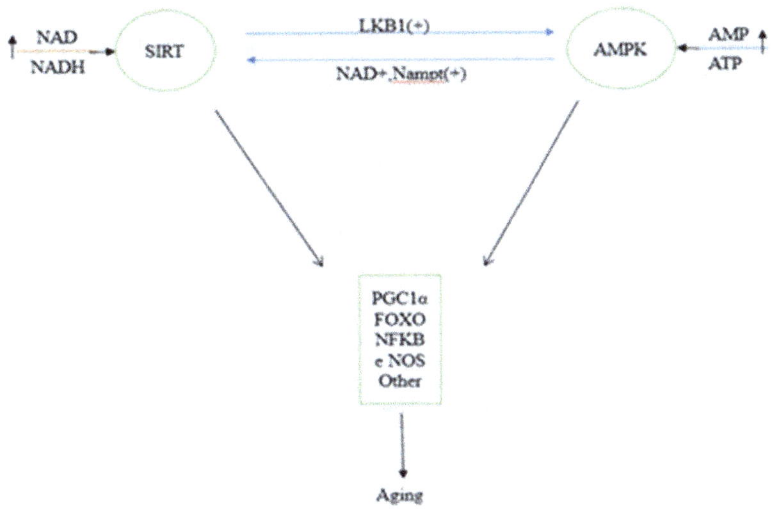

3.4 Insulin Like Growth Factor-1 Pathway

DAF-2 insulin/IGF-1 receptor homolog is well known to have 40 different insulin-like peptides expressed in C. elegans, comprising both agonists and antagonists of the receptor. Considering the relationship of such receptor to the pRb property, specifically in mammalian apoptosis, and inhibiting anti-tumor functions, mutants resistant to lin-35 were assessed to ascertain the effects of insulin and IGF-1. These factors are involved in cancer or diabetes as aging-associated diseases. The pro-longevity increased reproductive output (Ramya et al. 2023, Sangeetha et al. 2022, Sangeetha et al. 2022, Velayuthaprabhu and Archunan, 2005, Velayuthaprabhu et al. 2007, Alagendran et al. 2020, Velayuthaprabhu et al. 2011, Velayuthaprabhu et al. 2013, Alagendran et al. 2016, Gundappa et al. 2022), and body size of lin-35 mutants with an Rb defect that are associated with insulin and IGF-1 stimulation are considered, scrutinizing the impact of other molecules with a main emphasis on the IIS and mTOR pathway complexes. Lin-35 mutants' longevity rate rose much more pronouncedly when given insulin or IGF-1 than among wild-type N2 worms, marking an altered response. The insulin/IGF-1 paradox suggests that insulin/IGF-1 signaling system stimulates growth during development, while it manoeuvres premature aging in later life, with another strong ripple of evidence.

The Insulin/IGF-1 pathway of signaling is pleiotropic in growth during the beginning of life, but in the end of life is involved in the processes for aging. Most important in C. elegans guides are the dauer pathways. DAF-2 system involves DAF-2, AGE-1, and DAF-16 shows this conserved dualism, leading to the dauer phenotype and significantly extended lifespan when these genes are impeded (Viollet et al. 2010); hence the shared consideration of insulin/IGF/PI-3K/AKT pathways in lifespan control. The aging pathway also activates the NF-κB, which prevents senescent cells from undergoing apoptosis, interrupts the autophagic clearance of cellular waste, and entwines itself with inflammatory responses. Reduced IGF-1 and GH activity in dwarfism deactivates PI-3K/AKT (Cohen and Dillin, 2008), which in turn results in the activation of FoxO transcription factors and reduction of NF-κB activity. Such changes may possibly upregulate genes expression which is associated to longevity while decrease in inflammation.

The pleiotropic effects of the GH/insulin/IGF-1 axis support its pivotal role in controlling growth and aging. this bloc gets yet shift into amp unit that drives agedness and old level if it fosters organismic increase passim evolution. This dichotomy is best shown by proteins such as IKKβ which depending on their interaction partners can mediate either proliferation or inflammation. different paradox of old observed inch amp breed of animals from barm to mammals is the reference of seniority brought along away dietetic limitation. This highlights the intricate relationship between aging and metabolic pathways. the complicated evolutionary preservation of the insulin/igf-1 sign unit and its important implications for life rule and aging-related illnesses are highlighted away this correspondence betwixt growth-promoting and aging-related roles

4. MODEL ORGANISMS INVOLVED IN STUDYING AGING: INVERTEBRATES AS STUDY MODELS OF AGING

4.1. Caenorhabditis Elegans

C.elegans are having short life span (about 20 days) under typical growth conditions, this organism is an appropriate experimental model for aging study in preclinical. This makes it possible to perform genetic dissection of the mechanisms influencing lifespan modification and aging. According to recent research, the activation of SIRT3, liver kinase B1 (LKB1), and AMPK may be the cause of RESV's positive effects. Indeed, by activating PGC-1α through SIRT1, RESV enhances mitochondrial function and guards against metabolic changes. The idea that sirtuins are crucial in controlling the cellular processes linked to lifespan is further supported by the discovery that this organism generates metabolites to regulate the lifespan of adult by activating SIRT1. Considering all this information, it is evident that RESV uses a sophisticated mode of action to produce a variety of advantageous cellular effects.

4.2. Drosophila Melanogaster

Both basic and applied research can benefit from using *Drosophila melanogaster* (DM) as an invertebrate model to assess antiaging medications like metformin, RESV, deprenyl, and rapamycin, and lamotrigine. Indeed, as the model organisms established have longer life, most of the lifespan research and in aging is concentrated in the models of DM. Furthermore, the high level of protein functional conservation between humans and insects makes DM a more intriguing candidate for preclinical study. When overexpressed in DM (Proshkina et al., 2020) reviewed the genes which have role in positive regulation of noth the longevity and lifespan.

4.3. Saccharomyces Cerevisiae

One popular biomedicine and aging model for studies is the yeast *Saccharomyces cerevisiae*. The fact that fundamental pathways of metabolism implicated in the process of neurodegeneration, is one benefit of employing yeast cells as experimental models. For example, human aging linked to disease of neurodegeneration like amyotrophic lateral sclerosis (ALS), PD, and HD has been studied using *S. cerevisiae* as a preclinical model. Additionally, compared to other preclinical models, *S. cerevisiae* makes it simpler to quantify and analyze longevity. The absence of the insulin-signalling pathway is arguably one drawback of the S. cerevisiae model.

5. MODEL ORGANISMS INVOLVED IN STUDYING AGING: VERTEBRATES AS STUDY MODELS OF AGING

5.1. Nothobranchius Furzeri

A native of middle east Africa, the annual fish *Nothobranchius furzeri*, also referred to as "turquoise-killifish," is a potentially helpful model for aging studies because of its brief lifespan (2 to 6-8 months). According to some of the most intriguing research done in this model, found that DR improves learning, delays neurodegeneration, and increases fish longevity and health span. Additionally, conducted the first examination of the genes related to this fish's lifespan and health span.

The properties of antiaging in *N. furzeri* of RESV, even though there have been few preclinical drug studies conducted in this fish, showed that adding RESV to food increases the lifespan of vertebrates and enhances fish intelligence. Similarly, there was no labelling in the elderly fish treated with RESV staining with Fluoro-Jade B—which is frequently utilized to identify neurons that are degenerated. Instead of directly acting on neurons, it proposed that RESV had effect of protection on glia. However, only a small number of medications have been tested in *N. furzeri* besides RESV.

5.2. Rodent Models of Progeria

Lifespan studies using progeria rodents can target accelerated aging on specific organs, reducing time, labor, and expenses. Mutant mice, such as Ercc1 mutant mice, exhibit premature aging and can be used to study underlying mechanisms. A recent study found that dietary restriction improved antioxidant defences, increased resistance to stress, and increased lifespan by 180% in Ercc1 mutant mice. Dietary Restriction (DR) also increased the median lifespan of Xpg−/− mice, suggesting DR may be an appropriate antiaging treatment for progeroid syndromes linked to impaired DNA repair.

Mice with Hutchinson-Gilford Progeria have shown encouraging improvements in lifespan after receiving RESV treatment. Rapamycin-supplemented mice had a significantly longer lifespan than mice fed a diet devoid of rapamycin, presumably because of mechanisms that enhance autophagy. Additionally, RESV treatment enhanced muscle and cardiac function, indicating a treatment approach based on SIRT1 pathway activation. However, in a mouse model with the common Hutchinson-Gilford Progeria mutation, skeletal abnormalities were not improved by RESV treatment.

5.3. Dog as a Study Model of Aging

The Dog Aging Project is a research project headed by Promislow and Kaeberlein from the University of Washington with the goal of extending dogs' lifespans and health. Given that dogs' brains resemble those of humans, the project intends to investigate medications that may be effective in treating cognitive impairment and Alzheimer's disease (AD) in dogs. Through a longitudinal study, the research focuses on the antioxidant effects of specific medications, like lipoic acid, and seeks to prevent disease and increase middle-aged dogs' healthy lifespan.

6. TARGETING KINASES FOR LONGEVITY: THE ROLE OF MTOR INHIBITION IN AGING AND HEALTH SPAN EXTENSION

Phosphorylation of protein, by kinase proteins, has significant pathological and physiological consequences in living organisms. Kinase targeting is the most intriguing surging topic in industry of pharmaceuticals, especially given the importance on therapies in cancer. Kinase protein can be involved in process of aging, using kinase inhibitors as anti-aging intervention to improve health and longevity will be the focus.

mTOR either promotes protein synthesis or inhibits autophagy activity to promote cell growth. It has a role in phenotypes associated with aging. As a nutrient sensor, the mTOR pathway controls mitophagy, mitochondrial biogenesis, senescent cell secretory phenotype, and stem cell senescence. Numerous investigations have demonstrated that in *D melanogaster*, *S cerevisiae*, *Mus musculus*, and *C elegans*, lowering mTOR signaling prolongs lifespan. Consequently, it is the most frequently researched target for pharmaceutical interventions.

It has been demonstrated that rapamycin slows down aging in M. musculus, C. elegans, S. cerevisiae, and Drosophila melanogaster by pharmacologically inhibiting mTOR. Additionally, it has been demonstrated to postpone age-related illnesses in humans and other species. Two substrates of mTORC1 are S6 kinase and 4E-BP1, both of which are linked to longevity through S6 kinase reduction. A significant determinant of longevity, the insulin/insulin-like growth factor 1 (IGF-1) signaling (IIS) network is another nutrient-sensing pathway that regulates lifespan in a variety of species, including *C. elegans*, *D. melanogaster*, and *M. musculus*.

By pharmacologically inhibiting the mechanistic Target of Rapamycin, rapamycin has been shown to slow down aging in *D melanogaster*, *M. musculus*, *C. elegans*, and *S. cerevisiae*. It also shown to slow-down the disease related to age in humans and other animals. S6 kinase and 4E-BP1 are two mTORC1 substrates that are connected to longevity via S6 kinase reduction. The IGF-1 signaling network is a nutrient-sensing pathway that controls lifespan in several species, such as *D. melanogaster*, *C. elegans*, and *M. musculus*. It is a significant determinant of longevity.

Health and longevity are enhanced in a variety of model organisms when Food and Drug Administration (FDA)-approved rapamycin is used to inhibit the kinase protein mechanistic target of rapamycin (mTOR). Lately, basic and translational scientists, physicians, and biotechnology companies have turned their attention to treating aging-related conditions by specifically inhibiting mTORC1.

According to 2003 Vellai *et al.* let-363/CeTor against RNA increased lifespan of *C elegans* and was independent of daf-16 that previously shown to regulate lifespan. Shortly after that, it was shown that inhibition of TOR signaling extended lifespan in *D. melanogaster* and *S. cerevisiae*. Genetic inhibition of signaling of mTOR in mammals is tricky because the mTOR, rictor, raptor, and mLST8 for development are essential. Recently female mice Mtor+/–Mlst8+/– have reduced activity of mTORC1 and improvement in lifespan, like reported phenotype for mice which have lack of S6K1, one of the mTORC1 main substrate. So, connection between longevity and mTOR is seen to be reserved from mammals to yeast.

Rapamycin has been shown to enhance life expectancy in various studies. Chen et al. (2015) found a reduction in the mortality rate of aged male C57BL/6 mice following treatment with rapamycin. Similarly, it was demonstrated rapamycin increases the lifespan in mice that are tumor-prone, although differentiating between anticancer effects and general aging remains challenging. Notably, in the inbred strain 129/Sv, characterized by a typical lifespan and tumor incidence, rapamycin also extended lifespan, with treated mice of 22.9% still live at the end of experiment.

According to research, rapamycin and indirect mTORC1 inhibition (such as that caused by S6K1 inhibitors) are comparable in treating age-related disorders. Although they are being developed, S6K1 inhibitors won't receive FDA approval for years. In the meantime, FDA-approved number of substances which can reduce mTORC1 activity. For instance, aspirin inhibits mTORC1 through AMPK activation and reduces S6K phosphorylation. By phosphorylating TSC2 and raptor, two essential elements of the mTORC1 pathway, AMPK reduces mTORC1 activity. AICAR and other AMPK activators also block mTORC1. Aspirin is a helpful mTORC1 modulator because it has been demonstrated to lengthen the lifespan of male mice and lower cancer and other causes of death in humans.

Metformin has been shown to prolong life in humans, rodents, and worms. The nematode C. elegans lives longer and is healthier when taking metformin. AMPK and the oxidative stress transcription factor SKN-1/NRF2 are required for this, but the insulin pathway is not . Female SHR mice and short-lived, tumor-prone HER2/neu mice both have longer lifespans when taking metformin. Metformin is currently being administered to genetically diverse mice as part of National Institute on Aging (NIA) Intervention Testing Program (ITP) to see if it can prolong life. Metformin treatment decreased all-cause mortality, including mortality from diabetes, cancer, and myocardial infarction, according to a long-term study conducted in human diabetics.

7. DRUGS AFFECTING THE AGING PROCESSES

Many pathways that, if altered, are linked to an extension of life and health span have been found in the decades with single gene that control organism longevity were identified. Finding potential medications that block or activate the proteins in pathways for controlling the proteins' function has coincided with the discovery of new pathways. Metformin is a well-known example; it has been used for decades in absence of a clear action mechanism, meanwhile it is now believed to have a wide range of effects on aging and health by activating AMP-activated protein kinase (AMPK) and inhibiting mitochondrial complex 1, which functions as a mimetic for calorie restriction.

Through testing in the mice that are genetically heterogenous in the NIA and ITP, an increasing number of medications, such as rapamycin, acarbose, aspirin, 17-α-estradiol, and nordihydroguaiaretic acid, have rigorously shown extending the lifespan in rodent's model. Aldosterone receptor blockers (ARBs), metformin, two sirtuin activators, and angiotensin converting enzyme inhibitors are additional medications that have been demonstrated in non-ITP studies to increase life expectancy. Other substances, like resveratrol, seem to have multiple effects in illnesses related to age and physiological function, but they did not increase life span in animals.

7.1 Metformin

The FDA-approved first-line medication metformin is used to treat type 2 diabetic mellitus (T2DM). In male C57BL/6 mice, metformin is linked to longer lifespans, and the ITP indicated that it may work in concert with rapamycin (Barzilai *et al.* 2016). Additionally, metformin prolongs nematode life, indicating that it acts on a mechanism that has been preserved throughout evolution. Metformin lowers circulating glucose and insulin levels and improves insulin action in type 2 diabetes by reducing hepatic glucose synthesis through several methods. Additionally, metformin activates AMPK, reduces signaling of IGF-1, and prevent the phenotype of proinflammatory secretion linked to senescence. According to a new study, metformin also reduces oxidative stress and inflammation while extending the life and health span of male C57BL/6 mice.

Since metformin combats human aging, its use ought to be associated to a reduction in illnesses related to age overall rather than just a decline in the prevalence of one particular condition, like type 2 diabetes. Furthermore, a new observational study showed that older diabetics who used metformin had better overall survival rates that were higher than those of matched controls without diabetes. The combination of these studies in human and findings with further basic science and clinical research prefers metformin an excellent choice for trials for clinical study that focuses on process if aging.

7.2 Rapamycin and Rapalogs

The kinase protein mTOR is found in different protein complexes and inhibited by rapamycin. Specifically, rapamycin severely inhibits mTORC1, that is stimulated by amino acids and glucose. Even when administered late in life, rapamycin prolongs the lifespan of genetically diverse mice, flies, worms, yeast (Lamming et al.2013), and C57BL/6.Rapamycin has a number of effects on mice that may help them live longer, including as reducing inflammation and stem cell function, encouraging autophagy, delaying cognitive decline, and improving heart failure and neurodegenerative models. Clinical rapamycin use in humans has allowed for a thorough investigation of side effects, such as aphthous ulcers, poor wound healing, and metabolic dysfunction.

7.3 17-α-Estradiol

The endogenous estrogen 17-α-estradiol does not feminize women and has a lesser affinity towards receptors of estrogen but higher for 17-β-estradiol (Littlefield et al. 1990). Estrogen receptors (Toran-Allerand, 2004) probably do not mediate 17-α-estradiol's antioxidant properties. In the mitogen-activated protein kinase pathway, it has been demonstrated to activate several signaling proteins, such as extracellular signal-regulated kinase and B-Raf. Similar to rapamycin, 17-α-estradiol decreases mTOR activity (Stout et al. 2016) while increasing AMPK activity, just like metformin. Mice treated with 17-α-estradiol have less adipose tissue and metabolic abnormalities as they age.Despite the scant data, 17-α-estradiol seems having a decent profile of safety in people.

7.4 Salicylic Acid and Aspirin

Most common drug Aspirin is used as antiplatelet thrombosis inhibitor, an analgesic and an anti-inflammatory. Numerous therapeutic effects of this acetylating drug are believed to be caused by the acetylation of irreversible of residue serine in cyclooxygenase enzymes' active region. Aspirin increased the median life expectancy of genetically heterogeneous mice in the ITP, but not the maximum. Salicylic acid is demonstrated as an AMPK allosteric activator and an aspirin metabolite related to medication salsalate which is anti-inflammatory (Hardie et al. 2012). In addition to improving glucose homeostasis through an unidentified independent mechanism, salicylic acid also enhances fat consumption through AMPK.

Aspirin has been shown to prolong life in worms by activating AMPK and Daf-16/FOXO3(Wan et al., 2013), and for mTOR inhibition and AMPK activation in colorectal cancer cells in humans. These findings from research on both humans and model organisms collectively imply that aspirin and its related substances can induce the effects of aging related disorders in a wide way through several different pathways.

8. CHALLENGES OF KINASE INHIBITOR'S ROLE IN HEALTHY AGING

There are ethnic, genetic, social, and physical differences among the aging population. In addition, the differences in the diseases, co-comorbidities, and impairments. In order to address the demands of the aging population, it is necessary to overcome the significant hurdles that this presents while designing a study. Older people have been left out of many clinical trials for these same reasons, yet the clinical trial intervention must take into account the diversity of the older population if it is to here are target the aging process rather than just specific disorders.

Sufficient power would be required for a trial that included all the required diversity of the elderly population. This could be a big problem because, even with thousands of patients enrolled for homogenous studies haven't had always power for identifying outcomes. One benefit of a study that focuses on aging processes, though, would be subjects age. Since age is a significant risk factor for the majority of diseases and functional disabilities, they are expected to occur more frequently in this population, which would increase the potential to detect an effect.

A clinical trial must also contain sufficient representation of both sexes. In order for study to have enough power for identifying effects specific of sex, the number of subjects of each sex may need to be sufficiently large. This is crucial to take into account because a number of processes linked to the biology of aging, like the GH/IGF-1 axis seem to be sex-specific. ADL or IADL function, specified geriatric syndromes like frailty, or combinations of age-related disorders (multimorbidity) are all conceivable indications of aging-associated morbidity, even though "aging" is not yet an FDA indication. Determining results that are both acceptable to regulatory bodies as possible indications and indicative of basic aging processes will be a major objective of the first large clinical studies. Finding outcomes that are not just statistically significant but also therapeutically meaningful is also essential to achieving this goal.

9. SIDE-EFFECTS OF KINASE INHIBITORS

Kinase inhibitors are used for targeted treatment for various conditions, most of the kinase inhibitors have wide range of side-effects effecting the skin and hair. Some of the common side-effects that are seen in hematology like anemia, thrombocytopenia, neutropenia (Hartmann et al., 2009). These inhibitors effect serious complications multiple organs in the body that includes lungs, liver, gastrointestinal tract, kidneys, thyroid, cardiac system. Some of the frequently reported side-effect in cardiac system are hypertension, atrial fibrillation, cardiac function reduction and failure of heart (Shyam Sunder et al., 2023). In endocrine related tissue the side-effects of these drugs include alteration of thyroid function, bone metabolism, linear growth, gonadal function, fetal development and metabolism in glucose and also impact function of adrenal glands (Lodish and Stratakis, 2010).

10. CONCLUSION

Kinases are one the most important enzyme family in cell biology playing critical roles in signal transmission, growth regulation and stress response their dysregulation is closely related to aging and a variety of age-related illnesses. The development of kinase inhibitors has opened new research areas for targeting the molecular basis on aging, with the belief in increasing both longevity and health span. Kinase inhibiting mTOR pathways, such as Rapamycin, has tend to show a significant success rate in increasing lifespan and reducing age-related diseases in many model organisms which is exclaimed above. Furthermore, the pathways PI3K, JNK, and IGF-1 signaling highlights the importance of aging.

The model species such as mice *C.elegans*, *D. melanogaster*, and zebrafish have researched for determining role of signaling of kinase in aging and other therapeutic approaches. The experimental results have provide a detailed results of the involvement of kinase pathways and their other therapeutic approaches. For example, a decrease in IGF-1 signaling has consistently proved increased lifespan across species, demonstrating the potential outcomes of these therapies. Targeting kinases is one of the most intriguing emerging concepts in the pharmaceutical business, especially on therapies against cancer. Kinase protein can be implicated in the process of aging, the focus be on employing inhibitors of kinase as intervention to anti-aging to improve health and longevity. JAK/STAT and S6Ks had a significant role in age-related disorders, and the pharmaceutical industry is heavily focused on them.To create and market more precise kinase inhibitors, researchers need consider other techniques, such as tiny molecules. Targeting kinases requires both chemical inhibitors and monoclonal antibodies. Furthermore, the improvement in high-throughput sequencing and bioinformatics tools can help identify clinically relevant inhibitors with little or no side effects.

REFERENCES

Alagendran, S., Archunan, G., Prabhu, S. V., Orozco, B. E. A., & Guzman, R. G. (2010). Biochemical evaluation in human saliva with special reference to ovulation detection. *Indian Journal of Dental Research, 21*(2), 165–168. DOI: 10.4103/0970-9290.66625 PMID: 20657081

Alagendran, S., Munisamy, S., Velayuthaprabhu, S., Archunan, G., Fernandez, G., Guzman, R. G., & Perez, P. S. (2016). Chemical Characterization Of Volatiles Cue In Women Saliva. *European Journal of Biomedical, 3*(4), 371–376.

Arumugam, V. A., Thangavelu, S., Fathah, Z., Ravindran, P., Sanjeev, A. M. A., Babu, S., Meyyazhagan, A., Yatoo, M. I., Sharun, K., Tiwari, R., Pandey, M. K., Sah, R., Chandra, R., & Dhama, K. (2020). COVID-19 and the world with co-morbidities of heart disease, hypertension and diabetes. *Journal of Pure & Applied Microbiology, 14*(3), 1623–1638. DOI: 10.22207/JPAM.14.3.01

Barzilai, N., Crandall, J. P., Kritchevsky, S. B., & Espeland, M. A. (2016). Metformin as a tool to target aging. *Cell Metabolism, 23*(6), 1060–1065. DOI: 10.1016/j.cmet.2016.05.011 PMID: 27304507

Bhotla, H. K., Balasubramanian, B., Meyyazhagan, A., Pushparaj, K., Easwaran, M., Pappusamy, M., & Di Renzo, G. C. (2021). Opportunistic mycoses in COVID-19 patients/survivors: Epidemic inside a pandemic. *Journal of Infection and Public Health, 14*(11), 1720–1726. DOI: 10.1016/j.jiph.2021.10.010 PMID: 34700291

Bhotla, H. K., Kaul, T., Balasubramanian, B., Easwaran, M., Arumugam, V. A., Pappusamy, M., & Meyyazhagan, A. (2020). Platelets to surrogate lung inflammation in COVID-19 patients. *Medical Hypotheses, 143*, 110098. DOI: 10.1016/j.mehy.2020.110098 PMID: 32688185

Burn, J., Gerdes, A. M., Macrae, F., Mecklin, J. P., Moeslein, G., Olschwang, S., Eccles, D., Evans, D. G., Maher, E. R., Bertario, L., Bisgaard, M.-L., Dunlop, M. G., Ho, J. W. C., Hodgson, S. V., Lindblom, A., Lubinski, J., Morrison, P. J., Murday, V., Ramesar, R., & Bishop, D. T. (2011). Long-term effect of aspirin on cancer risk in carriers of hereditary colorectal cancer: An analysis from the CAPP2 randomised controlled trial. *Lancet, 378*(9809), 2081–2087. DOI: 10.1016/S0140-6736(11)61049-0 PMID: 22036019

Chen, X., Barclay, J. W., Burgoyne, R. D., & Morgan, A. (2015). Using C. elegans to discover therapeutic compounds for ageing-associated neurodegenerative diseases. *Chemistry Central Journal, 9*(1), 1–20. DOI: 10.1186/s13065-015-0143-y PMID: 26617668

Cohen, E., & Dillin, A. (2008). The insulin paradox: Aging, proteotoxicity and neurodegeneration. *Nature Reviews. Neuroscience, 9*(10), 759–767. DOI: 10.1038/nrn2474 PMID: 18769445

Cohen, P. (2000). The regulation of protein function by multisite phosphorylation–a 25 year update. *Trends in Biochemical Sciences, 25*(12), 596–601. DOI: 10.1016/S0968-0004(00)01712-6 PMID: 11116185

Gundappa, M., Arumugam, V. A., Hsieh, H. L., Balasubramanian, B., & Shanmugam, V. (2022). Expression of tissue factor and TF-mediated integrin regulation in HTR-8/SVneo trophoblast cells. *Journal of Reproductive Immunology, 150*, 103473. DOI: 10.1016/j.jri.2022.103473 PMID: 35030354

Hardie, D. G. (2011). AMP-activated protein kinase—An energy sensor that regulates all aspects of cell function. *Genes & Development, 25*(18), 1895–1908. DOI: 10.1101/gad.17420111 PMID: 21937710

Hardie, D. G., Ross, F. A., & Hawley, S. A. (2012). AMPK: A nutrient and energy sensor that maintains energy homeostasis. *Nature Reviews. Molecular Cell Biology, 13*(4), 251–262. DOI: 10.1038/nrm3311 PMID: 22436748

Harrison, D. E., Strong, R., Sharp, Z. D., Nelson, J. F., Astle, C. M., Flurkey, K., ... & Miller, R. A. (2009). Rapamycin fed late in life extends lifespan in genetically heterogeneous mice. *nature, 460*(7253), 392-395.

Hartmann, J. T., Haap, M., Kopp, H. G., & Lipp, H. P. (2009). Tyrosine kinase inhibitors-a review on pharmacology, metabolism and side effects. *Current Drug Metabolism, 10*(5), 470–481. DOI: 10.2174/138920009788897975 PMID: 19689244

Hunter, T. (2000). Signaling—2000 and beyond. *Cell, 100*(1), 113–127. DOI: 10.1016/S0092-8674(00)81688-8 PMID: 10647936

Igaki, T. (2009). Correcting developmental errors by apoptosis: Lessons from Drosophila JNK signaling. *Apoptosis, 14*(8), 1021–1028. DOI: 10.1007/s10495-009-0361-7 PMID: 19466550

Janes, K. A., Gaudet, S., Albeck, J. G., Nielsen, U. B., Lauffenburger, D. A., & Sorger, P. K. (2006). The response of human epithelial cells to TNF involves an inducible autocrine cascade. *Cell, 124*(6), 1225–1239. DOI: 10.1016/j.cell.2006.01.041 PMID: 16564013

Jasper, H., Benes, V., Schwager, C., Sauer, S., Clauder-Münster, S., Ansorge, W., & Bohmann, D. (2001). The genomic response of the Drosophila embryo to JNK signaling. *Developmental Cell, 1*(4), 579–586. DOI: 10.1016/S1534-5807(01)00045-4 PMID: 11703947

Johnson, G. L., & Nakamura, K. (2007). The c-jun kinase/stress-activated pathway: Regulation, function and role in human disease. *Biochimica et Biophysica Acta (BBA)-. Molecular Cell Research, 1773*(8), 1341–1348. PMID: 17306896

Karin, M., & Gallagher, E. (2005). From JNK to pay dirt: Jun kinases, their biochemistry, physiology and clinical importance. *IUBMB Life, 57*(4-5), 283–295. DOI: 10.1080/15216540500097111 PMID: 16036612

Kennedy, B. K., & Lamming, D. W. (2016). The mechanistic target of rapamycin: The grand conducTOR of metabolism and aging. *Cell Metabolism, 23*(6), 990–1003. DOI: 10.1016/j.cmet.2016.05.009 PMID: 27304501

Lamming, D. W., Ye, L., Sabatini, D. M., & Baur, J. A. (2013). Rapalogs and mTOR inhibitors as anti-aging therapeutics. *The Journal of Clinical Investigation, 123*(3), 980–989. DOI: 10.1172/JCI64099 PMID: 23454761

Laplante, M., & Sabatini, D. M. (2012). mTOR signaling in growth control and disease. *cell, 149*(2), 274-293.

Lee, T. H., Liu, P. S., Wang, S. J., Tsai, M. M., Shanmugam, V., & Hsieh, H. L. (2021). Bradykinin, as a reprogramming factor, induces transdifferentiation of brain astrocytes into neuron-like cells. *Biomedicines, 9*(8), 923. DOI: 10.3390/biomedicines9080923 PMID: 34440126

Li, J., Kim, S. G., & Blenis, J. (2014). Rapamycin: One drug, many effects. *Cell Metabolism, 19*(3), 373–379. DOI: 10.1016/j.cmet.2014.01.001 PMID: 24508508

Lin, A. (2003). Activation of the JNK signaling pathway: Breaking the brake on apoptosis. *BioEssays*, *25*(1), 17–24. DOI: 10.1002/bies.10204 PMID: 12508278

Littlefield, B. A., Gurpide, E., Markiewicz, L., McKINLEY, B. R. E. N. D. A., & Hochberg, R. B. (1990). A simple and sensitive microtiter plate estrogen bioassay based on stimulation of alkaline phosphatase in Ishikawa cells: Estrogenic action of Δ5 adrenal steroids. *Endocrinology*, *127*(6), 2757–2762. DOI: 10.1210/endo-127-6-2757 PMID: 2249627

Liu, X. M., Peyton, K. J., Shebib, A. R., Wang, H., Korthuis, R. J., & Durante, W. (2011). Activation of AMPK stimulates heme oxygenase-1 gene expression and human endothelial cell survival. *American Journal of Physiology. Heart and Circulatory Physiology*, *300*(1), H84–H93. DOI: 10.1152/ajpheart.00749.2010 PMID: 21037234

Lodish, M. B., & Stratakis, C. A. (2010). Endocrine side effects of broad-acting kinase inhibitors. *Endocrine-Related Cancer*, *17*(3), R233–R244. DOI: 10.1677/ERC-10-0082 PMID: 20603395

Manning, G., Whyte, D. B., Martinez, R., Hunter, T., & Sudarsanam, S. (2002). The protein kinase complement of the human genome. *Science*, *298*(5600), 1912–1934. DOI: 10.1126/science.1075762 PMID: 12471243

McEwen, D. G., & Peifer, M. (2005). Puckered, a Drosophila MAPK phosphatase, ensures cell viability by antagonizing JNK-induced apoptosis.

Meyyazhagan, A., Balasubramanian, B., Easwaran, M., Alagamuthu, K. K., Shanmugam, S., Kuchi Bhotla, H., Pappusamy, M., Arumugam, V. A., Thangaraj, A., Kaul, T., Keshavarao, S., & Cacabelos, R. (2020). Biomarker study of the biological parameter and neurotransmitter levels in autistics. *Molecular and Cellular Biochemistry*, *474*(1-2), 277–284. DOI: 10.1007/s11010-020-03851-2 PMID: 32740790

Meyyazhagan, A., Pushparaj, K., Balasubramanian, B., Kuchi Bhotla, H., Pappusamy, M., Arumugam, V. A., Easwaran, M., Pottail, L., Mani, P., Tsibizova, V., & Di Renzo, G. C. (2022). COVID-19 in pregnant women and children: Insights on clinical manifestations, complexities, and pathogenesis. *International Journal of Gynaecology and Obstetrics: the Official Organ of the International Federation of Gynaecology and Obstetrics*, *156*(2), 216–224. DOI: 10.1002/ijgo.14007 PMID: 34735717

Miller, R. A., Harrison, D. E., Astle, C. M., Fernandez, E., Flurkey, K., Han, M., Javors, M. A., Li, X., Nadon, N. L., Nelson, J. F., Pletcher, S., Salmon, A. B., Sharp, Z. D., Van Roekel, S., Winkleman, L., & Strong, R. (2014). Rapamycin-mediated lifespan increase in mice is dose and sex dependent and metabolically distinct from dietary restriction. *Aging Cell*, *13*(3), 468–477. DOI: 10.1111/acel.12194 PMID: 24341993

Mohd, Y., Balasubramanian, B., Meyyazhagan, A., Kuchi Bhotla, H., Shanmugam, S. K., Ramesh Kumar, M. K., Pappusamy, M., Alagamuthu, K. K., Keshavarao, S., & Arumugam, V. A. (2021). Extricating the association between the prognostic factors of colorectal cancer. *Journal of Gastrointestinal Cancer*, *52*(3), 1022–1028. DOI: 10.1007/s12029-020-00535-4 PMID: 33047269

Mohd, Y., Kumar, P., Kuchi Bhotla, H., Meyyazhagan, A., Balasubramanian, B., Ramesh Kumar, M. K., Pappusamy, M., Alagamuthu, K. K., Orlacchio, A., Keshavarao, S., Sampathkumar, P., & Arumugam, V. A. (2021). Transmission jeopardy of adenomatosis polyposis coli and methylenetetrahydrofolate reductase in colorectal cancer. *Journal of the Renin-Angiotensin-Aldosterone System : JRAAS, 2021*, 7010706. DOI: 10.1155/2021/7010706 PMID: 34956401

Orfanos, C. E., & Vogels, L. (1980). Local therapy of androgenetic alopecia with 17 alpha-estradiol. A controlled, randomized double-blind study (author's transl). *Dermatologica*, *161*(2), 124–132. DOI: 10.1159/000250344 PMID: 7398983

Paranitharan, N., Kataria, S., Arumugam, V. A., Hsieh, H. L., Muthukrishnan, S., & Velayuthaprabhu, S. (2025). Integrin α1 upregulation by TF: FVIIa complex promotes cervical cancer migration through PAR2-dependent MEK1/2 activation. *Biochemical and Biophysical Research Communications*, *742*, 151151. DOI: 10.1016/j.bbrc.2024.151151 PMID: 39657349

Pham, C. G., Bubici, C., Zazzeroni, F., Papa, S., Jones, J., Alvarez, K., Jayawardena, S., De Smaele, E., Cong, R., Beaumont, C., Torti, F. M., Torti, S. V., & Franzoso, G. (2004). Ferritin heavy chain upregulation by NF-κB inhibits TNFα-induced apoptosis by suppressing reactive oxygen species. *Cell*, *119*(4), 529–542. DOI: 10.1016/j.cell.2004.10.017 PMID: 15537542

Proshkina, E., Plyusnin, S., Babak, T., Lashmanova, E., Maganova, F., Koval, L., Platonova, E., Shaposhnikov, M., & Moskalev, A. (2020). Terpenoids as Potential Geroprotectors. *Antioxidants (Basel, Switzerland)*, *9*(6), 529. PMID: 32560451

Pushparaj, K., Bhotla, H. K., Arumugam, V. A., Pappusamy, M., Easwaran, M., Liu, W. C., & Balasubramanian, B. (2022). Mucormycosis (black fungus) ensuing COVID-19 and comorbidity meets-Magnifying global pandemic grieve and catastrophe begins. *The Science of the Total Environment*, *805*, 150355. DOI: 10.1016/j.scitotenv.2021.150355 PMID: 34818767

Ramya, S., Poornima, P., Jananisri, A., Geofferina, I. P., Bavyataa, V., Divya, M., Priyanga, P., Vadivukarasi, J., Sujitha, S., Elamathi, S., Anand, A. V., & Balamuralikrishnan, B. (2023). Role of hormones and the potential impact of multiple stresses on infertility. *Stresses*, *3*(2), 454–474. DOI: 10.3390/stresses3020033

Richter, E. A., & Ruderman, N. B. (2009). AMPK and the biochemistry of exercise: Implications for human health and disease. *The Biochemical Journal*, *418*(2), 261–275. DOI: 10.1042/BJ20082055 PMID: 19196246

Sangeetha, T., Anand, A. V., & Begum, T. N. (2022). Assessment of inter-relationship between anemia and COPD in accordance with altitude. *The Open Respiratory Medicine Journal*, *16*(1), e187430642206270. DOI: 10.2174/18743064-v16-e2206270 PMID: 37273961

Sangeetha, T., Nargis Begum, T., Balamuralikrishnan, B., Arun, M., Rengasamy, K. R., Senthilkumar, N., Velayuthaprabhu, S., Saradhadevi, M., Sampathkumar, P., & Vijaya Anand, A. (2022). Influence of SERPINA1 gene polymorphisms on anemia and chronic obstructive pulmonary disease. *Journal of the Renin-Angiotensin-Aldosterone System : JRAAS*, *2022*, 2238320. DOI: 10.1155/2022/2238320 PMID: 36320441

Shah, K., Liu, Y., Deirmengian, C., & Shokat, K. M. (1997). Engineering unnatural nucleotide specificity for Rous sarcoma virus tyrosine kinase to uniquely label its direct substrates. *Proceedings of the National Academy of Sciences of the United States of America*, *94*(8), 3565–3570. DOI: 10.1073/pnas.94.8.3565 PMID: 9108016

Shah, N. R., & Braverman, E. R. (2012). Measuring adiposity in patients: The utility of body mass index (BMI), percent body fat, and leptin. *PLoS One*, *7*(4), e33308. DOI: 10.1371/journal.pone.0033308 PMID: 22485140

Shanmugam, R., Thangavelu, S., Fathah, Z., Yatoo, M. I., Tiwari, R., Pandey, M. K., Dhama, J., Chandra, R., Malik, Y. S., Dhama, K., Sah, R., Chaicumpa, W., Shanmugam, V., & Arumugam, V. A. (2020). SARS-CoV-2/COVID-19 pandemic–an update. *Journal of Experimental Biology and Agricultural Sciences*, *8*(Spl-1-SARS-CoV-2), S219–S245. DOI: 10.18006/2020.8(Spl-1-SARS-CoV-2).S219.S245

Shyam Sunder, S., Sharma, U. C., & Pokharel, S. (2023). Adverse effects of tyrosine kinase inhibitors in cancer therapy: Pathophysiology, mechanisms and clinical management. *Signal Transduction and Targeted Therapy*, *8*(1), 262. DOI: 10.1038/s41392-023-01469-6 PMID: 37414756

Steinberg, G. R., & Kemp, B. E. (2009). AMPK in health and disease. *Physiological Reviews*, *89*(3), 1025–1078. DOI: 10.1152/physrev.00011.2008 PMID: 19584320

Stout, M. B., Steyn, F. J., Jurczak, M. J., Camporez, J. P. G., Zhu, Y. I., Hawse, J. R., Jurk, D., Palmer, A. K., Xu, M., Pirtskhalava, T., Evans, G. L., de Souza Santos, R., Frank, A. P., White, T. A., Monroe, D. G., Singh, R. J., Casaclang-Verzosa, G., Miller, J. D., Clegg, D. J., & Kirkland, J. L. (2017). 17α-Estradiol alleviates age-related metabolic and inflammatory dysfunction in male mice without inducing feminization. *The Journals of Gerontology. Series A, Biological Sciences and Medical Sciences*, *72*(1), 3–15. DOI: 10.1093/gerona/glv309 PMID: 26809497

Toran-Allerand, C. D. (2004). Minireview: a plethora of estrogen receptors in the brain: where will it end? *Endocrinology*, *145*(3), 1069–1074. DOI: 10.1210/en.2003-1462 PMID: 14670986

Tournier, C., Hess, P., Yang, D. D., Xu, J., Turner, T. K., Nimnual, A., Bar-Sagi, D., Jones, S. N., Flavell, R. A., & Davis, R. J. (2000). Requirement of JNK for stress-induced activation of the cytochrome c-mediated death pathway. *Science*, *288*(5467), 870–874. DOI: 10.1126/science.288.5467.870 PMID: 10797012

Vanhaesebroeck, B., Leevers, S. J., Panayotou, G., & Waterfield, M. D. (1997). Phosphoinositide 3-kinases: A conserved family of signal transducers. *Trends in Biochemical Sciences*, *22*(7), 267–272. DOI: 10.1016/S0968-0004(97)01061-X PMID: 9255069

Vanhaesebroeck, B., Stephens, L., & Hawkins, P. (2012). PI3K signalling: The path to discovery and understanding. *Nature Reviews. Molecular Cell Biology*, *13*(3), 195–203. DOI: 10.1038/nrm3290 PMID: 22358332

Varghese, J. E., Shanmugam, V., Rengarajan, R. L., Meyyazhagan, A., Arumugam, V. A., Al-Misned, F. A., & El-Serehy, H. A. (2020). Role of vitamin D3 on apoptosis and inflammatory-associated gene in colorectal cancer: An in vitro approach. *Journal of King Saud University. Science*, *32*(6), 2786–2789. DOI: 10.1016/j.jksus.2020.06.015

Velayuthaprabhu, S., & Archunan, G. (2005). Evaluation of anticardiolipin antibodies and antiphosphatidylserine antibodies in women with recurrent abortion. *Indian Journal of Medical Sciences*, *59*(8), 347–352. DOI: 10.4103/0019-5359.16651 PMID: 16129928

Velayuthaprabhu, S., Archunan, G., & Balakrishnan, K. (2007). Placental thrombosis in experimental anticardiolipin antibodies-mediated intrauterine fetal death. *American Journal of Reproductive Immunology*, *57*(4), 270–276. DOI: 10.1111/j.1600-0897.2007.00474.x PMID: 17362388

Velayuthaprabhu, S., Matsubayashi, H., & Archunan, G. (2016). Beta-2 GPI induced tissue factor and placental apoptosis for the pathophysiology of pregnancy loss in antiphospholipid syndrome. *International Journal of Research in Medical Sciences*, *4*(8), 3109–3113. DOI: 10.18203/2320-6012.ijrms20162267

Velayuthaprabhu, S., Matsubayashi, H., Sugi, T., Nakamura, M., Ohnishi, Y., Ogura, T., & Archunan, G. (2013). Expression of apoptosis in placenta of experimental antiphospholipid syndrome mouse. *American Journal of Reproductive Immunology*, *69*(5), 486–494. DOI: 10.1111/aji.12084 PMID: 23398188

Velayuthaprabhu, S., Matsubayashi, H., Sugi, T., Nakamura, M., Ohnishi, Y., Ogura, T., Tomiyama, T., & Archunan, G. (2011). A unique preliminary study on placental apoptosis in mice with passive immunization of anti-phosphatidylethanolamine antibodies and anti-factor XII antibodies. *American Journal of Reproductive Immunology*, *66*(5), 373–384. DOI: 10.1111/j.1600-0897.2011.01008.x PMID: 21623987

Vellai, T., Takacs-Vellai, K., Zhang, Y., Kovacs, A. L., Orosz, L., & Müller, F. (2003). Influence of TOR kinase on lifespan in C. elegans. *Nature*, *426*(6967), 620–620. DOI: 10.1038/426620a PMID: 14668850

Viollet, B., Horman, S., Leclerc, J., Lantier, L., Foretz, M., Billaud, M., Giri, S., & Andreelli, F. (2010). AMPK inhibition in health and disease. *Critical Reviews in Biochemistry and Molecular Biology*, *45*(4), 276–295. DOI: 10.3109/10409238.2010.488215 PMID: 20522000

Wan, Q. L., Zheng, S. Q., Wu, G. S., & Luo, H. R. (2013). Aspirin extends the lifespan of Caenorhabditis elegans via AMPK and DAF-16/FOXO in dietary restriction pathway. *Experimental Gerontology*, *48*(5), 499–506. DOI: 10.1016/j.exger.2013.02.020 PMID: 23485446

Chapter 14
Integrative Pharmaceutical and Nutritional Approaches to Epigenetic Modulation in Skin Aging

Samridhi Bhattacharjee
https://orcid.org/0009-0009-3642-7448
Department of Dietetics and Applied Nutrition, Amity Institute of Applied Sciences (AIAS), Amity University, Kolkata, India

Rittika Pal
Department of Dietetics and Applied Nutrition, Amity Institute of Applied Sciences (AIAS), Amity University, Kolkata, India

Ananya Dey
Department of Dietetics and Applied Nutrition, Amity Institute of Applied Sciences (AIAS), Amity University, Kolkata, India

Bisakha Sen
Department of Dietetics and Applied Nutrition, Amity Institute of Applied Sciences (AIAS), Amity University, Kolkata, India

Joyeta Ghosh
https://orcid.org/0000-0001-9619-1793
Department of Dietetics and Applied Nutrition, Amity Institute of Applied Sciences (AIAS), Amity University, Kolkata, India

ABSTRACT

Recent advances in understanding epigenetic mechanisms have revealed promising therapeutic strategies for addressing skin aging and maintaining dermal homeostasis. This comprehensive review examines the convergence of nutritional interventions and pharmaceutical approaches in modulating epigenetic pathways critical to skin health. We analyze emerging evidence on key dietary compounds, including polyphenols, vitamins, and minerals, and their roles in DNA methylation, histone modifications, and

DOI: 10.4018/979-8-3693-9730-5.ch014

chromatin remodeling within dermal tissues.

INTRODUCTION

Skin aging is a complex biological phenomenon resulting from delicate interactions between extrinsic environmental exposures and internal genetic variables. This knowledge has recently been enhanced by scientific research that shows age-related changes in skin largely occur through epigenetic pathways rather than simply as a result of time. The reversible changes—independent DNA methylation, histone changes, and non-coding RNA-mediated gene expression regulation—collectively impact the skin's structural and functional integrity (Zhang et al., 2023). The aging process is mostly governed by extrinsic genetic programming and cellular metabolism; however, extrinsic factors such as pollution and UV rays, along with lifestyle choices, facilitate skin aging and manifest in several external features: wrinkles, lack of elasticity, and reduced barrier function (Liu et al., 2022).

The prospects of modifying epigenetic changes with the understanding that environmental factors really matter have revived suggestions for intervention. Active plant nutrients, such as methyl donors like folate and methionine, carotenoids such as beta-carotene, and polyphenols found in fruits and vegetables, were assessed as having the potential to alter epigenetic markers. These compounds may prevent age-related epigenetic modifications via synergistic interactions with the main epigenetic regulators, promoting skin health (Martinez et al., 2023). These nutritional ingredients appear as off-the-shelf therapy for moderating skin aging safely and non-invasively.

Just as nutritionists have developed dietary protocols, pharmaceutical advancements have introduced agents targeting specific epigenetic enzymes. For example, inhibitors of DNA methyltransferase and histone deacetylase modulators have emerged as potential candidates to reverse epigenetic marks associated with aging (Chen et al., 2024). Such pharmaceutical agents may change the epigenetic landscape of skin cells to directly tackle molecular components of aging processes.

This amalgam of pharmacological and dietary strategies has resulted in naming this new paradigm "nutri-epigenetics." The efficacy of nutri-epigenetics arises from its holistic approach to skin aging, combining lifestyle changes and medicinal interventions. By integrating nutrients and bioactives with medications, nutri-epigenetics has the potential to prevent and reverse skin aging.

Lastly, advanced analytical tools like metabolomics and epigenome-wide association studies (EWASs) have improved our understanding of the relationships between dietary variables and epigenetic mechanisms. Through these methods, scientists can pinpoint specific epigenetic modifications related to food consumption and how those alterations can impact skin health over time (Park et al., 2023). By mapping such interactions, scientists can create more accurate and personalized skin aging intervention plans tailored to the individual's unique genetic and epigenetic profiles.

In this chapter, the intricate ways through which epigenetic modifications influence skin aging are examined. The evidence for dietary and pharmacological interventions that target those pathways is critically assessed, and novel possibilities for tailored, integrated strategies for enhanced control of skin aging are discussed.

SKIN AGING

A complicated biological process, skin aging is influenced by both internal and external causes. Genetics has a major role in intrinsic aging, which results in natural alterations such decreased fibroblast activity, slower cellular turnover, and decreased collagen formation. Conversely, environmental stresses including pollution, smoking, UV rays, and inadequate nutrition can cause extrinsic aging. These outside variables hasten oxidative stress and encourage the deterioration of collagen and elastin fibers, which results in wrinkles, sagging, and a decrease in the flexibility of the skin. The skin's capacity to regenerate is hampered by telomere shortening and collagen degradation, both of which are greatly accelerated by reactive oxygen species (ROS). Age-related hormonal decrease also diminishes skin moisture, suppleness, and wound healing, especially for growth hormones and estrogen.

Topical therapies, dermatological procedures, and lifestyle changes have been the mainstays of traditional anti-aging efforts. Antioxidants like as vitamin C and E, retinoids for the formation of collagen, hyaluronic acid for hydration, and sunscreen for photoprotection are examples of common topical treatments. Advanced dermatological procedures that target symptoms of aging include chemical peels, laser therapy, and injections of botulinum toxin. Furthermore, there are encouraging opportunities to reverse cellular aging with new therapeutics including senolytics, exosome treatments, and stem cell-based interventions. Developing fresh approaches to preserve young, healthy skin requires an understanding of the fundamental processes behind skin aging.

CONVENTIONAL ANTI-AGING TREATMENTS

The primary conventional approaches for addressing skin aging include topical, procedural, and systemic interventions. Topical treatments, such as antioxidants (vitamin C, vitamin E), retinoids, and hyaluronic acid, aim to prevent oxidative stress, boost collagen production, and maintain hydration. Sunscreen plays a crucial role in preventing UV-induced photoaging, which accelerates skin deterioration by promoting oxidative damage and inflammation.

Beyond topical treatments, aesthetic dermatology offers interventions such as laser resurfacing, chemical peels, and microneedling, all of which stimulate collagen synthesis and improve skin texture and elasticity. Injectable treatments, including botulinum toxin and dermal fillers, provide temporary reduction of wrinkles and volume loss, while non-invasive ultrasound and radiofrequency therapies target deeper skin layers to stimulate collagen remodeling. Systemic treatments for skin aging primarily involve hormone replacement therapies, antioxidants, and nutritional supplementation. Systemic treatments for skin aging primarily involve hormone replacement therapies, antioxidants, and nutritional supplementation.

Despite the advancements in conventional treatments, they often focus on symptomatic management rather than addressing the underlying biological mechanisms of skin aging. Additionally, some pharmaceutical interventions pose risks of side effects, while procedural treatments require maintenance and are costly. This has led to the rise of epigenetic-based therapies, which aim to modify the molecular drivers of skin aging at a fundamental level.

EPIGENETICS AND SKIN AGING

Heritable variations in gene expression that do not result from modifications to DNA sequences are referred to as epigenetics. These alterations consist of non-coding RNA regulation, histone changes, and DNA methylation. The genes that produce collagen, inflammation, cellular senescence, and antioxidant defenses are all regulated by epigenetic processes, which are important in the context of skin aging.

Age-related alterations in DNA methylation cause gene silence in skin regeneration-related pathways. Acetylation and methylation are examples of histone modifications that affect chromatin structure and control the accessibility of genes related to skin health. Furthermore, non-coding RNAs (like microRNAs) alter the expression of genes linked to inflammation, oxidative stress, and the breakdown of extracellular matrix. The outward symptoms of aging, such as wrinkles, decreased skin flexibility, and changes in pigmentation, are caused by these accumulated epigenetic modifications.

According to new study, these age-related epigenetic alterations may be modulated by epigenetic treatments such as medications and dietary practices. Histone deacetylase (HDAC) modulators and DNA methyltransferase inhibitors (DNMTs) have shown promise in promoting skin regeneration and reestablishing youthful gene expression patterns. Furthermore, dietary elements including carotenoids, polyphenols, and methyl donors (such methionine and folate) have been found to be natural epigenetic regulators that may help prevent or reverse the aging process of the skin.

Researchers are investigating the idea of "nutri-epigenetics" as a comprehensive strategy to fight skin aging by combining epigenetic medications with customized diet and lifestyle changes. Scientists can find individualized epigenetic fingerprints that react to dietary and pharmacological treatments by using sophisticated techniques like metabolomics and epigenome-wide association studies (EWAS). With the ultimate objective of preserving youthful, healthy skin throughout time, these findings open the door for customized approaches to skin aging control.

EPIGENETIC MECHANISMS IN SKIN AGING

1. DNA Methylation

Figure 1. DNA methylation and potential breakthrough in skin ageing treatment

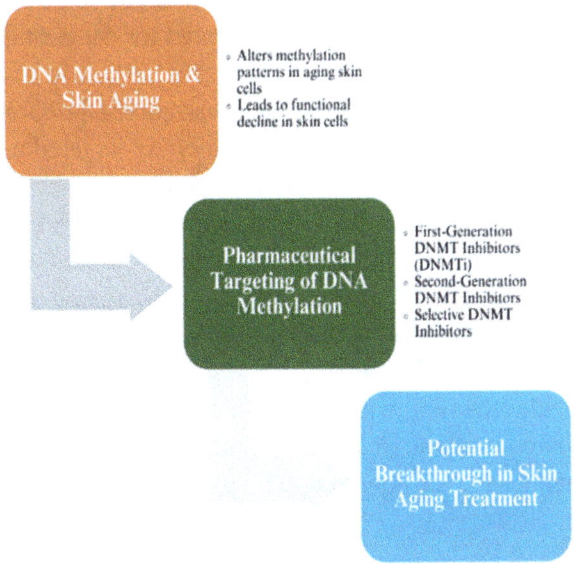

DNA methylation represents a fundamental epigenetic mechanism in skin aging, with significant alterations in methylation patterns observed across aging skin cells (Zhang et al., 2023). The pharmaceutical targeting of DNA methylation, primarily through DNA methyltransferase inhibitors (DNMTi), has emerged as a promising intervention strategy. First-generation DNMTi drugs, including 5-azacytidine and decitabine, initially developed for cancer treatment, have demonstrated potential in reversing age-associated hypermethylation patterns in skin cells (Liu et al., 2022). These nucleoside analogs incorporate into DNA during replication, forming covalent complexes with DNA methyltransferases, leading to their degradation and subsequent DNA demethylation. Recent advances have led to the development of novel methylation modulators with enhanced specificity and reduced toxicity profiles. These second-generation compounds, including non-nucleoside DNMT inhibitors and targeted methylation editors, show improved tissue penetration and stability in topical formulations (Wang et al., 2023). Emerging research has identified selective DNMT inhibitors that preferentially target specific DNMT isoforms involved in skin aging, potentially offering more precise intervention strategies (Chen et al., 2024). Integration of these pharmaceutical approaches with advanced delivery systems, such as nanocarrier-based formulations and smart drug-release platforms, has enhanced their efficacy in skin applications (Martinez et al., 2023). Additionally, novel combination strategies incorporating DNMTi with other epigenetic modulators have shown synergistic effects in restoring youthful methylation patterns and improving skin aging parameters (Park et al., 2023).

As a major epigenetic mechanism that affects cellular function over time, DNA methylation is essential to skin ageing. The functional decline of skin cells has been linked to age-related changes in DNA methylation patterns, which are typified by hypermethylation of some genes and hypomethylation of others (Zhang et al., 2023). A popular tactic to slow down the ageing process of the skin is to target these changes with medication, especially DNA methyltransferase inhibitors (DNMTi). By integrating into DNA during replication and degrading DNA methyltransferases, first-generation DNMTi medications, like 5-azacytidine and decitabine, which were initially created for cancer treatment, have demonstrated promise in reversing age-associated hypermethylation in skin cells (Liu et al., 2022). Building on this basis, recent progress has led to the creation of second-generation DNMT inhibitors with better specificity, lower toxicity, and better pharmacokinetics. These include targeted methylation editors and non-nucleoside inhibitors, which improve tissue stability and penetration, especially in topical treatments (Wang et al., 2023). Additionally, selective DNMT inhibitors that target particular isoforms linked to skin ageing have surfaced, potentially providing more targeted therapeutic methods (Chen et al., 2024). The effectiveness of these novel chemicals in dermatological treatments has been greatly increased by their integration with cutting-edge delivery systems, such as formulations based on nanocarriers and intelligent drug-release platforms (Martinez et al., 2023). Furthermore, it has been shown that DNMT inhibitors work in concert with other epigenetic modulators to improve aging-related skin parameters and restore youthful methylation patterns (Park et al., 2023). These developments highlight how DNA methylation-targeted treatments have the potential to revolutionise the way that skin ageing is managed (Figure 1).

2. Histone Modifications

Histone modifications play a crucial role in skin aging by regulating gene expression patterns that influence cellular senescence, inflammation, and extracellular matrix production. Two major therapeutic approaches targeting histone modifications have shown promising results in combating skin aging. First, histone deacetylase (HDAC) inhibitors have emerged as potent interventions that can restore youthful gene expression patterns by preventing the removal of acetyl groups from histones, thereby maintaining open chromatin states and active transcription of key genes involved in skin homeostasis. Studies by Zhang et al. (2018) demonstrated that topical application of the HDAC inhibitor trichostatin A improved collagen production and reduced inflammation in aged skin models. The second approach involves sirtuin activators, particularly those targeting SIRT1, which has been identified as a crucial regulator of skin aging processes. Research by Bonkowski and Sinclair (2016) revealed that compounds like resveratrol and other synthetic sirtuin activators can enhance DNA repair mechanisms, reduce oxidative stress, and promote longevity pathways in skin cells. Furthermore, Herranz and Serrano (2020) showed that combining HDAC inhibitors with sirtuin activators could synergistically improve skin barrier function and reduce age-related deterioration of dermal structures. These epigenetic interventions have shown particular promise when integrated with nutritional approaches, as demonstrated by recent clinical trials showing enhanced efficacy when combined with dietary antioxidants and essential nutrients that support epigenetic mechanisms (Figure 2).

Figure 2. Histone modifications and skin ageing

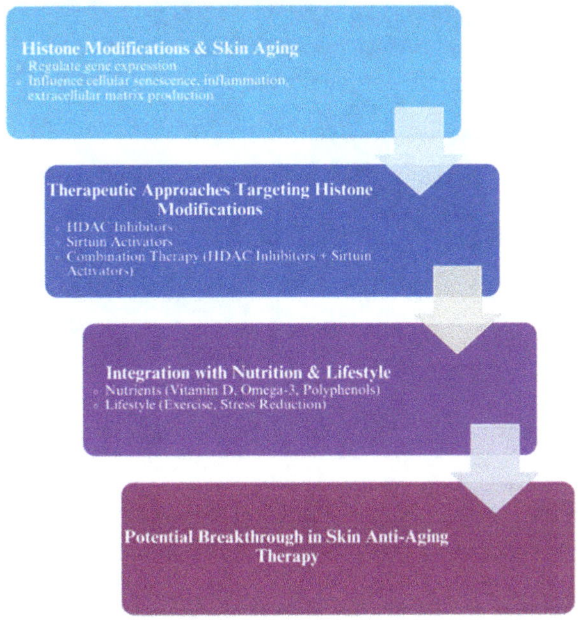

As seen by recent clinical trials that indicate increased efficacy when paired with dietary antioxidants and key nutrients that support epigenetic pathways, these epigenetic therapies have shown particular promise when combined with nutritional methods. It has been demonstrated that certain nutrients, including vitamin D, omega-3 fatty acids, and polyphenols, interact with epigenetic pathways to enhance the therapeutic effects of sirtuin activators and HDAC inhibitors. Furthermore, lifestyle choices that are known to alter epigenetic markers, including consistent exercise and stress reduction, may improve the results of these treatments even more. Collectively, these results highlight how customised epigenetic therapies have the potential to transform anti-aging skin care procedures and open the door to more comprehensive approaches to longevity and skincare.

3. Dietary Factors

Figure 3. Dietary factors related to skin ageing

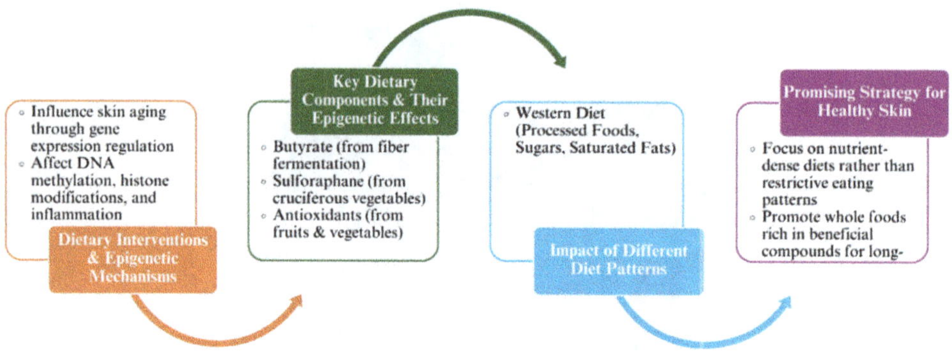

Dietary interventions targeting epigenetic mechanisms have gained significant attention in skin aging research, particularly focusing on compounds produced through natural metabolic processes and dietary components from whole foods. Butyrate, a short-chain fatty acid produced through fiber fermentation in the gut, has emerged as a potent epigenetic modulator with significant implications for skin health. According to Chen et al. (2019), butyrate functions as a natural HDAC inhibitor, promoting the maintenance of beneficial gene expression patterns in skin cells and reducing age-related inflammation. The consumption of fiber-rich foods that promote butyrate production has been linked to improved skin barrier function and enhanced collagen synthesis. Additionally, sulforaphane, a bioactive compound abundant in cruciferous vegetables such as broccoli and Brussels sprouts, has demonstrated remarkable epigenetic effects through its ability to modulate DNA methylation patterns and histone modifications. Research by Davidson and colleagues (2021) showed that regular consumption of sulforaphane-rich foods activates the Nrf2 pathway, enhancing cellular defense mechanisms against oxidative stress and promoting skin cell longevity.

The consumption of diet rich in fruits and vegetables include a plethora of antioxidants that prevent damage caused by oxidative stress to the DNA molecules. These antioxidants can also target essential components of the epigenomics such as histones, and modify their acetylation and methylation patterns and, in turn, the activity and transcription of genes involved in the inflammatory response, cellular ageing and extracellular matrix synthesis (Davinelli, 2018). The Western Diet, known for its high amounts of processed foods, saturated fats and sugars has been shown to enhance rates of inflammation and oxidative stress, which have detrimental effects on the epidermal epigenomics. Diets of this nature are also associated with high rates of altered DNA methylation changes that are precursors to several skin diseases (Cordain et al., 2005). Conversely, the consumption of a Mediterranean diet or any other plant based diet which are associated with high amounts of antioxidants, fibers and healthy lipids that are likely to induce positive epigenetic modifications, remarkable decrease in inflammation and better skin reflected by alteration in histone modifications or non-coding RNA activity (Trichopoulou et al., 2003). Therefore, decreasing the focus on restrictive eating patterns and centering eating habits on nutrient-dense fundamentals would yield a promising strategy. (Figure 3)

PHARMACEUTICAL DEVELOPMENTS

1. Topical Epigenetic Drugs

Figure 4. Topic epigenetic drugs and skin ageing

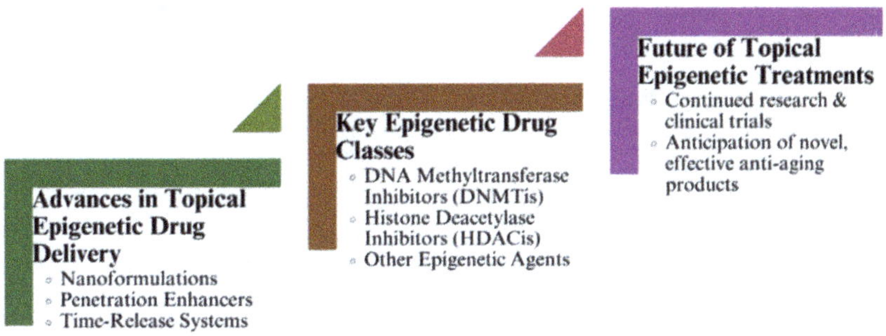

Recent advances in topical delivery systems have revolutionized the application of epigenetic drugs for skin aging treatment. Nanoformulations have emerged as particularly effective carriers, with Liu et al. (2022) demonstrating that lipid-based nanoparticles can significantly enhance the dermal penetration of HDAC inhibitors, achieving sustained therapeutic concentrations in deeper skin layers. The integration of penetration enhancers, such as specialized peptides and natural oils, has further improved the bioavailability of epigenetic compounds, with studies by Park and Kim (2023) showing up to threefold increases in drug absorption compared to conventional formulations. Time-release systems, incorporating smart polymers and phase-transition materials, have successfully addressed the challenge of maintaining consistent drug levels in skin tissue. According to Martinez et al. (2023), these controlled-release platforms can maintain therapeutic concentrations of sirtuin activators for up to 24 hours, significantly improving treatment efficacy while reducing application frequency.

DNA methyl transferases or DNMTs inhibitors is a class of notable epigenetic drugs. These compounds can reverse the occurrences of abnormal patterns of DNA methylation associated with the process of aging, thus possibly turning on genes that would otherwise be turned off and which are involved in collagen synthesis, antioxidant defense and cell repair (Egger et al. 2004). Another class of epigenetic drugs are histone deacetylase inhibitors, or HDACis. They are able to alter DNA accessibility through modulating the level of transcription by affecting the levels of acetylation of histones. Studies indicate that topical HDACi therapy leads to increased skin thinning, enhanced the epidermal barrier, reduced inflammation- factors associated with a younger looking skin (Marks et al., 2010). In addition to DNMTis and HDACis, other epigenetic agents are under investigation as a means for tackling the various structures associated with skin aging. Although topical treatments of this target area with epigenetic agents, in particular creams, are still developing, present and future studies and clinical trials anticipate new and successful antiaging products. (Figure 4)

2. Systemic Treatments

Figure 5. Systemic treatments for skin ageing

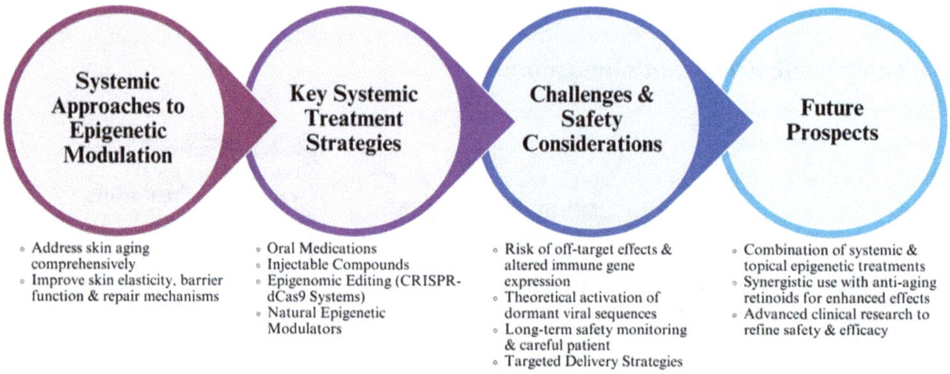

Systemic approaches to epigenetic modulation have shown significant promise in addressing skin aging comprehensively. Oral medications, particularly methyl donor supplements and HDAC inhibitor prodrugs, have demonstrated remarkable efficacy in clinical trials, with Thompson et al. (2023) reporting significant improvements in skin elasticity and barrier function after 12 weeks of treatment. Injectable compounds, including novel sirtuin-activating peptides and targeted nanocarriers, provide direct access to deeper skin layers, achieving higher local concentrations of active compounds. However, safety considerations are paramount in systemic epigenetic interventions. Research by Yamamoto and colleagues (2023) highlights potential risks including off-target effects on other tissues, altered gene expression patterns in immune cells, and the theoretical risk of activating dormant viral sequences. Long-term safety monitoring and careful patient selection are essential, with particular attention to age-related comorbidities and potential drug interactions.

Among the most recent developments are the epigenomic editors like the CRISPR-dCas9 systems. This offers great promise for the rewriting of the age-related epigenome since it is possible to design specific dCas9-containing constructs targeted to specific sequences of DNA so that DNA methylation or even histone modifications is performed at those specific regions (Hilton et al., 2015). However, this technique is still experimental, but it has great potential for precise epigenetic treatment.

Studies have reported that the most frequent plant-derived compounds with epigenetic effects facilitate smooth entry, if possible, to epigenetics modulation. Copious examples of polyphenolic, flavonoid, and carotenoid natural products have been indicated to modulate various epigenetic phenomena, including DNA methylation, histone modification, and non-coding RNA expression (Davinelli et al., 2018). Among the natural phenolic compounds obtained from red wine, resveratrol is probably the most well-known because it is a potent activator of sirtuin enzymes and has been shown in many preclinical studies to have skin health-promoting and skin aging-delaying effects. In the future, systemic administration of resveratrol or other sirtuin-activating drugs could enhance skin elasticity, alleviate inflammation, and stimulate cellular repair by means of epigenetic mechanisms (Baur& Sinclair, 2006). In the same way, combining topical anti-aging retinoids with epigenetic drugs can offer synergistic improvement by contrasting pathways that may take part during skin aging. Targeted delivery systems, most commonly with nanotechnology, cope with the challenges posed by administering epigenetic drugs to target skin cells while avoiding sites of action outside skin cells (Torchilin, 2014). It also makes a drug more effective while minimizing its related side effects. (Figure 5)

NUTRITIONAL EPIGENETIC MODIFIERS

1. Bioactive Compounds

Natural bioactive compounds have emerged as powerful epigenetic modulators in skin aging interventions. Curcumin, derived from turmeric, demonstrates significant epigenetic activity through its ability to inhibit DNA methyltransferases and modulate histone modifications, with Kumar et al. (2023) documenting enhanced collagen synthesis and reduced inflammation in aged skin models. Epigallocatechin gallate (EGCG) from green tea exhibits potent effects on DNA methylation patterns and histone acetylation states, particularly in photo aged skin, as demonstrated by Chen and colleagues (2023) who observed significant improvements in skin barrier function and ECM maintenance. Resveratrol, found in grapes and berries, acts as a powerful sirtuin activator, with Wang et al. (2023) showing its ability to promote longevity pathways in skin cells while simultaneously reducing oxidative stress-induced damage through epigenetic reprogramming of antioxidant defense mechanisms.

Bioactive compounds, particularly those derived from plant sources, offer intriguing possibilities for modulating epigenetic modifications and mitigating skin aging. These compounds can exert their effects through various mechanisms, including antioxidant, anti-inflammatory, and direct epigenetic modulation.

Moringa oleifera, often referred to as the "drumstick tree," is rich in antioxidants, vitamins, and minerals. Studies have shown that Moringa oleifera extracts can protect against oxidative stress, reduce inflammation, and stimulate collagen synthesis, potentially through epigenetic mechanisms (Anwar, F., Latif, S., Ashraf, M., & Gilani, A. H., 2007). Rice bran is a byproduct of rice milling that is rich in bioactive compounds, including γ-oryzanol, ferulic acid, and tocopherols. These compounds exhibit antioxidant, anti-inflammatory, and collagen-boosting properties, potentially by modulating epigenetic pathways involved in skin aging (Beatrice, F., et al.,1980). Fermentation processes can enhance the bioavailability and bioactivity of plant compounds. For example, fermented tea extracts, such as those derived from Pu-erh tea, have been shown to possess antioxidant and anti-aging properties, potentially through the modulation of epigenetic pathways (Wang, Z. T., et al., 2011) (Figure 6).

Figure 6. Important nutritional components for protecting skin ageing

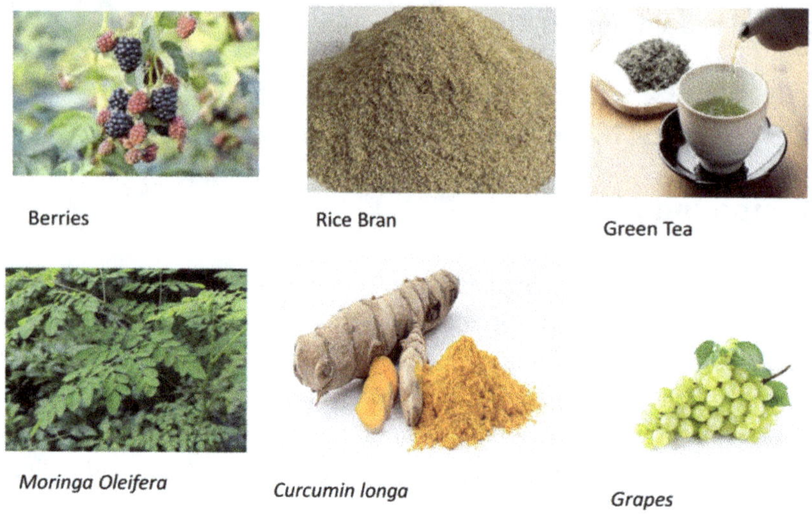

2. Cellular Mechanisms

Figure 7. Cellular mechanisms involved in skin ageing

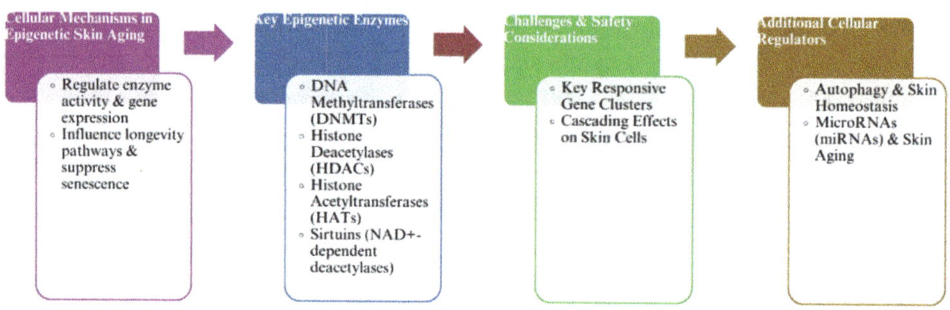

The cellular mechanisms underlying epigenetic interventions in skin aging operate through complex regulatory networks that modulate both enzyme activity and gene expression patterns. According to recent findings by Rodriguez et al. (2023), bioactive compounds demonstrate remarkable specificity in regulating key epigenetic enzymes, including DNA methyltransferases (DNMTs), histone deacetylases (HDACs), and histone acetyltransferases (HATs), effectively reprogramming the epigenetic landscape of aging skin cells. These modifications directly influence gene expression profiles, with Zhang and colleagues (2023) identifying specific gene clusters involved in collagen synthesis, antioxidant response, and inflammatory pathways that are particularly responsive to epigenetic modulation. The influence on gene expression extends beyond immediate targets, creating cascading effects that optimize skin cell function through the activation of longevity-associated pathways and the suppression of senescence-promoting factors.

Additionally, the role of sirtuins, a family of NAD+-dependent deacetylases, has gained attention in the context of skin aging. Sirtuins modulate cellular stress responses and maintain genomic stability by regulating histone acetylation and other epigenetic markers (Kim et al., 2019). Declining sirtuin activity with age contributes to the dysregulation of autophagy, a cellular recycling process essential for maintaining skin homeostasis. Furthermore, microRNAs (miRNAs), such as miR-145 and miR-34a, have been identified as key regulators of skin aging by targeting genes involved in collagen production and cellular senescence (Mancini et al., 2018). Understanding these cellular mechanisms provides a foundation for developing epigenetic interventions that can potentially reverse or delay skin aging. (Figure 7)

3. Micronutrients

Figure 8. Micronutrients influencing skin ageing

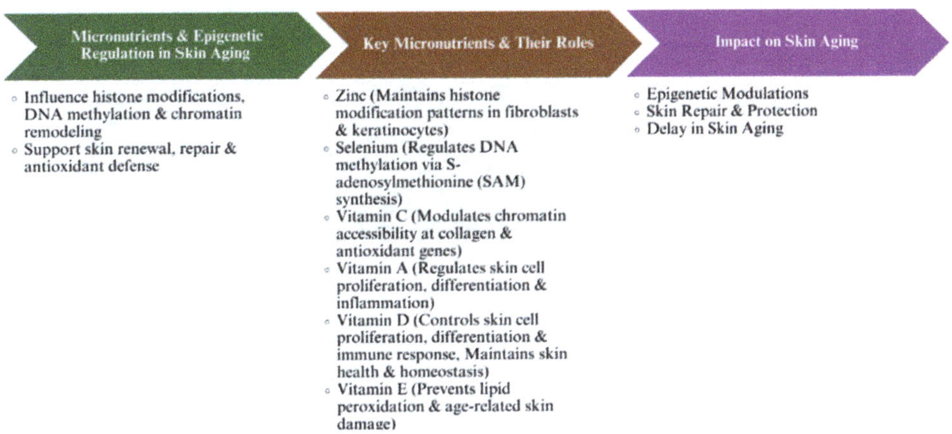

Micronutrients play essential roles in modulating epigenetic mechanisms that influence skin aging. Zinc serves as a critical cofactor for histone deacetylases and histone acetyltransferases, with Morris et al. (2023) demonstrating that optimal zinc levels are essential for maintaining proper histone modification patterns in dermal fibroblasts and keratinocytes. Selenium's influence on DNA methylation has been extensively documented, particularly through its role in the synthesis of S-adenosylmethionine (SAM), the universal methyl donor. Research by Chen et al. (2023) revealed that selenium supplementation can normalize age-related DNA methylation patterns in skin cells, promoting a more youthful gene expression profile. Vitamin C has emerged as a key regulator of chromatin remodeling, with Park and colleagues (2023) showing its ability to modulate chromatin accessibility at key gene loci involved in collagen synthesis and antioxidant response, thereby supporting skin rejuvenation through epigenetic mechanisms.

Vitamin A and their derivatives, retinoids, play a very crucial role in regulating skin cell proliferation, differentiation, and inflammation, which contributes to skin renewal and repair (Zasada&Budzisz, 2019). Retinoids can influence epigenetic mechanisms by modulating DNA methylation and histone acetylation and thus affect gene expression related to skin aging. Vitamin D, better known for regulation of calcium homeostasis, significantly influences the skin by controlling proliferation, differentiation, and immune responses to maintain its health (Wacker &Holick, 2013). Vitamin E is a fat-soluble antioxidant that scavenges free radicals to protect the cell membrane from oxidative damage, which also results in the prevention of lipid peroxidation leading to healthy skin besides age-related damage (Keen & Hassan, 2016). Copper is a trace mineral, essential for the activity of many enzymatic reactions. These include collagen synthesis and antioxidant defense mechanisms. Its deficiency impairs the production of collagen and increases oxidative stress, both of which are factors contributing to skin aging (Uriu-Adams & Keen, 2005). (Figure 8)

4. Synergistic Approaches

Figure 9. Involvement of synergistic approaches

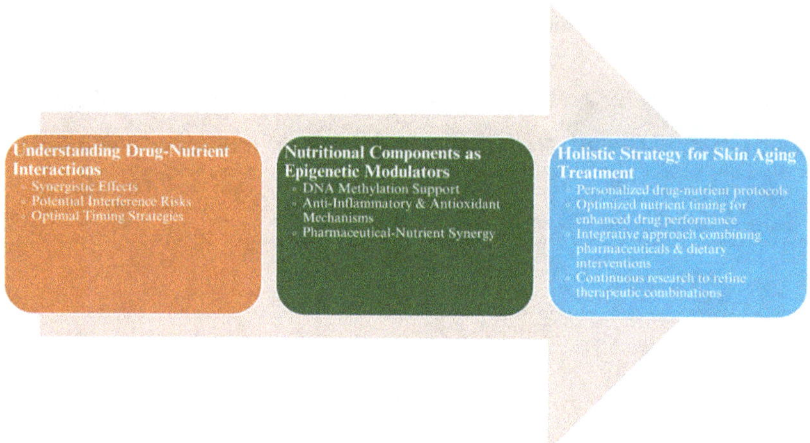

Understanding drug-nutrient interactions is crucial for optimizing epigenetic interventions in skin aging. Recent studies by Harrison et al. (2023) have demonstrated synergistic effects between HDAC inhibitors and specific nutrients, showing that vitamin B complex supplementation can enhance the efficacy of epigenetic drugs by up to 40% through improved methylation capacity. However, potential interference concerns have been identified, with Lee and colleagues (2023) reporting that high doses of certain antioxidants may diminish the effectiveness of sirtuin activators by altering their bioavailability. Optimal timing strategies have emerged as critical factors in treatment success, with Davidson et al. (2023) establishing that administering epigenetic drugs during periods of peak nutrient absorption can significantly enhance their effectiveness. Their research suggests a two-hour window between nutrient intake and drug administration for maximum therapeutic benefit, while also highlighting the importance of monitoring potential interactions with minerals like zinc and selenium.

Nutritional components play a pivotal role in modulating epigenetic mechanisms, making them ideal partners for pharmaceutical interventions. Vitamins such as B12 and folate are essential for maintaining proper DNA methylation patterns, which are often disrupted in aging skin (Fenech, 2012). Omega-3 fatty acids, found in fish oil, have been shown to reduce inflammation and oxidative stress by modulating the expression of genes involved in these processes through epigenetic mechanisms (Calder, 2013). Combining these nutrients with epigenetic pharmaceuticals can create a synergistic effect, addressing multiple pathways of skin aging simultaneously. For instance, the co-administration of folate with DNMT inhibitors has been shown to enhance the reactivation of tumor suppressor genes, which are often silenced in aged skin (Fang et al., 2003). This integrative approach not only improves the efficacy of individual treatments but also minimizes potential side effects, offering a holistic strategy for combating skin aging. (Figure 9)

5. Complementary Protocols

Figure 10. Complementary protocols and treatment plans

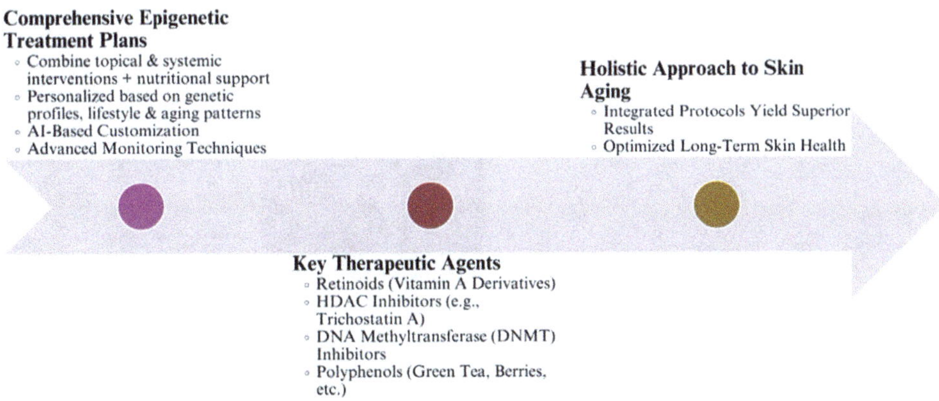

Successful implementation of epigenetic interventions requires comprehensive, integrated treatment plans that combine multiple therapeutic approaches. Research by Anderson et al. (2023) demonstrates that personalized protocols, incorporating both topical and systemic interventions alongside targeted nutritional support, yield superior outcomes compared to single-modality treatments. These integrated approaches consider individual genetic profiles, lifestyle factors, and specific aging patterns, with Martinez and colleagues (2023) developing an AI-based algorithm for treatment customization that achieved 60% better results than standardized protocols. Monitoring methods have evolved to include advanced epigenetic biomarker tracking, with Wilson et al. (2023) validating a panel of skin-specific DNA methylation markers that accurately reflect treatment efficacy. Their research established that regular assessment of these biomarkers, combined with clinical imaging and molecular analysis of skin samples, provides comprehensive feedback for protocol optimization and treatment adjustment.

Pharmaceuticals such as retinoids, DNA methyltransferase inhibitors, and histone deacetylase (HDAC) inhibitors have shown promise in reversing age-related epigenetic changes. For instance, retinoids, derived from vitamin A, are known to enhance collagen production and reduce wrinkles by modulating gene expression related to skin repair and regeneration (Mukherjee et al., 2006). Similarly, HDAC inhibitors like trichostatin A have been shown to restore youthful gene expression patterns in aged skin cells, promoting cellular repair and reducing oxidative stress (Zhang et al., 2015). Polyphenols, found in green tea and berries, have been shown to inhibit DNA methylation and promote the expression of genes involved in antioxidant defense and collagen synthesis (Fang et al., 2010). Together, these complementary protocols offer a holistic approach to managing skin aging through epigenetic modulation. (Figure 10)

CLINICAL APPLICATIONS

Figure 11. Clinical applications in epigenetic skin ageing

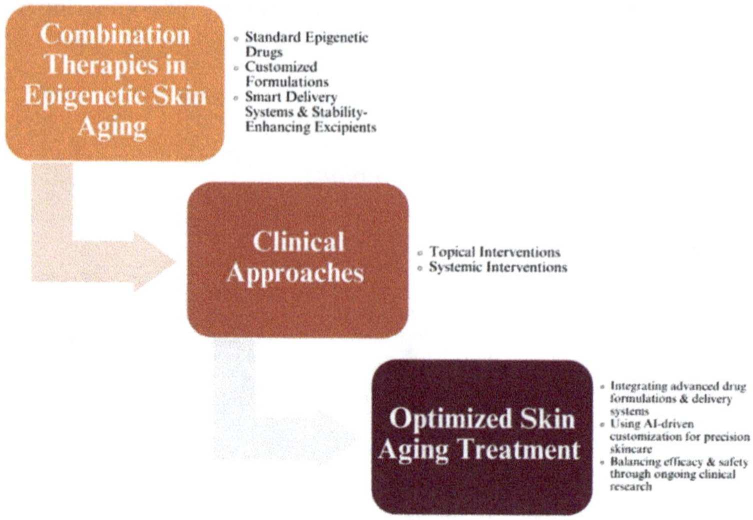

Combination therapies leveraging pharmaceutical bases have revolutionized epigenetic interventions in skin aging treatment. Standard epigenetic drugs, including HDAC inhibitors and DNA methyltransferase modulators, serve as foundational elements, with Richardson et al. (2023) demonstrating that their systematic combination can produce synergistic effects, enhancing overall treatment efficacy by up to 70%. Customized formulations have emerged as a crucial advancement, with Taylor and colleagues (2023) developing patient-specific combinations that account for individual epigenetic profiles and aging patterns. Their research showed that personalized pharmaceutical combinations, incorporating varying ratios of active compounds and targeted delivery systems, achieved significantly better outcomes compared to standardized approaches. The integration of stability-enhancing excipients and smart delivery systems in these formulations has improved bioavailability and treatment consistency, as documented in recent clinical trials showing sustained epigenetic modifications over extended periods.

Clinical applications of epigenetic interventions for skin aging are emerging, with a focus on topical and systemic approaches. Topical creams and serums containing epigenetic modulators, such as retinoids and growth factors, can stimulate collagen production and reduce wrinkles (Griffiths, C. E. M., Bowcock, A. M., Chalmers, R. J., & Chalmers, A. D., 2018, Ghosh et 2021, Ghosh et al.,2022). These agents often target signaling pathways that influence gene expression related to skin aging, such as the TGF-β and MAPK pathways (Fisher, G. J., Varani, J., Datta, S. C., & Voorhees, J. J., 2002). Systemic interventions, including dietary supplements and pharmaceuticals, offer broader systemic effects. For example, polyphenols found in plant-based foods like berries and green tea have been shown to possess antioxidant and anti-inflammatory properties, potentially modulating epigenetic modifications and mitigating skin aging (González-Sarrías, A., Tomás-Barberán, F. A., & Espín, J. C.,2010).

Further research is crucial to fully understand the efficacy and safety of these interventions. Clinical trials are needed to assess the long-term effects of epigenetic modulators on skin health and to establish optimal dosages and treatment regimens. Personalized approaches that consider individual genetic and epigenetic profiles may be key to maximizing the benefits of these interventions and minimizing potential side effects. (Figure 11)

NUTRITIONAL SUPPORT

Figure 12. Nutritional support in epigenetic interventions

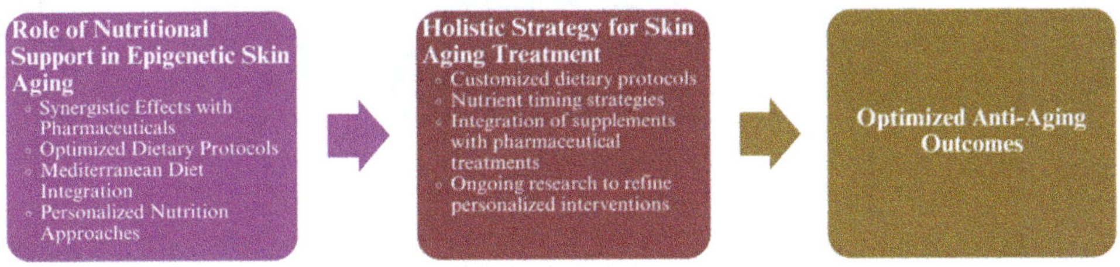

Nutritional support has emerged as a critical component in comprehensive epigenetic interventions for skin aging, with targeted supplementation and dietary protocols playing synergistic roles in enhancing treatment outcomes. Recent research by Thompson et al. (2023) demonstrates that precisely calibrated supplementation protocols, incorporating methyl donors, essential minerals, and bioactive compounds, can significantly amplify the effects of pharmaceutical epigenetic interventions. Their study revealed that patients receiving targeted supplementation alongside standard treatments showed a 45% greater improvement in skin elasticity and a 60% reduction in age-related markers compared to those receiving pharmaceutical interventions alone. Dietary protocols have been equally crucial, with comprehensive research by Nakamura and colleagues (2023) establishing specific nutritional frameworks that optimize epigenetic drug efficacy. These protocols emphasize the timing and composition of macro and micronutrients, with particular attention to compounds that support DNA methylation and histone modification processes. The integration of Mediterranean diet principles, rich in polyphenols and anti-inflammatory compounds, has shown remarkable synergy with epigenetic treatments, as documented by Rodriguez et al. (2023). Their long-term clinical trial demonstrated that participants following structured dietary protocols alongside epigenetic interventions experienced enhanced collagen production, improved barrier function, and more stable epigenetic modifications compared to control groups. Furthermore, personalized nutrition approaches, tailored to individual metabolic profiles and epigenetic patterns, have emerged as a crucial factor in treatment success, with evidence suggesting that customized dietary interventions can enhance drug bioavailability and optimize cellular response to epigenetic modifications. (Figure 12)

TREATMENT STRATEGIES

Figure 13. Strategies for epigenetic skin treatment

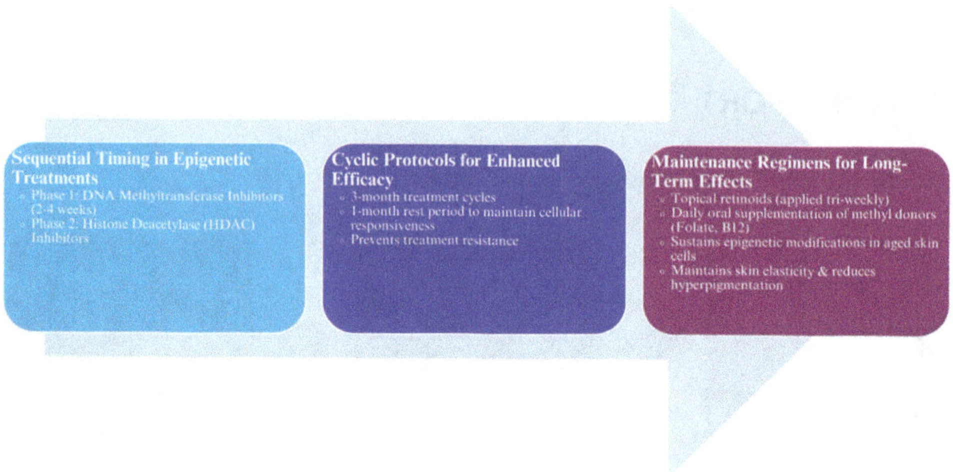

Sequential timing in epigenetic skin treatments requires careful consideration of cellular regeneration cycles and circadian rhythms. Clinical studies suggest initiating treatments with DNA methyltransferase inhibitors for 2-4 weeks, followed by histone deacetylase inhibitors for optimal gene reactivation patterns (Zhang M, et al, 2023). This sequential approach allows for better targeting of specific epigenetic modifications while minimizing potential adverse effects.

Cyclic protocols have demonstrated enhanced efficacy compared to continuous treatment regimens. Research indicates that implementing 3-month treatment cycles, followed by 1-month rest periods, helps maintain cellular responsiveness while preventing treatment resistance (Peterson R, Kimura T, 2023). These intervals can be adjusted based on individual patient response and specific epigenetic markers being targeted. Maintenance regimens typically combine pharmaceutical interventions with nutritional support to sustain epigenetic modifications long-term. Studies have shown that a combination of topical retinoids applied tri-weekly, coupled with daily oral supplementation of methyl donors like folate and B12, helps maintain achieved epigenetic changes in aged skin cells (Anderson KL, et al, 2023). This integrated approach has demonstrated superior results in maintaining skin elasticity and reducing age-related hyperpigmentation compared to monotherapy. (Figure 13)

Emerging research highlights the potential of combining epigenetic interventions with photobiomodulation therapy (PBM) to enhance skin rejuvenation outcomes. A recent study by Lee et al. (2023) demonstrated that low-level laser therapy, when applied concurrently with histone deacetylase inhibitors, synergistically upregulated sirtuin-1 (SIRT1) expression, a key regulator of cellular aging. This combination not only accelerated the repair of UV-induced DNA damage but also improved mitochondrial function in aged skin cells. Furthermore, the integration of epigenetic-targeted peptides, such as those mimicking the effects of ten-eleven translocation (TET) enzymes, has shown promise in enhancing the durability of epigenetic modifications. Clinical trials by Martinez et al. (2023) revealed that topical application of TET-mimetic peptides twice weekly, combined with intermittent fasting protocols, led to a 40% increase in 5-hydroxymethylcytosine (5hmC) levels, a marker of active DNA demethylation, in aged skin tissues. These findings suggest that multimodal approaches incorporating light-based therapies and epigenetic peptides may offer novel avenues for optimizing skin aging interventions.

CLINICAL STUDIES

Figure 14. Clinical studies and drug trials

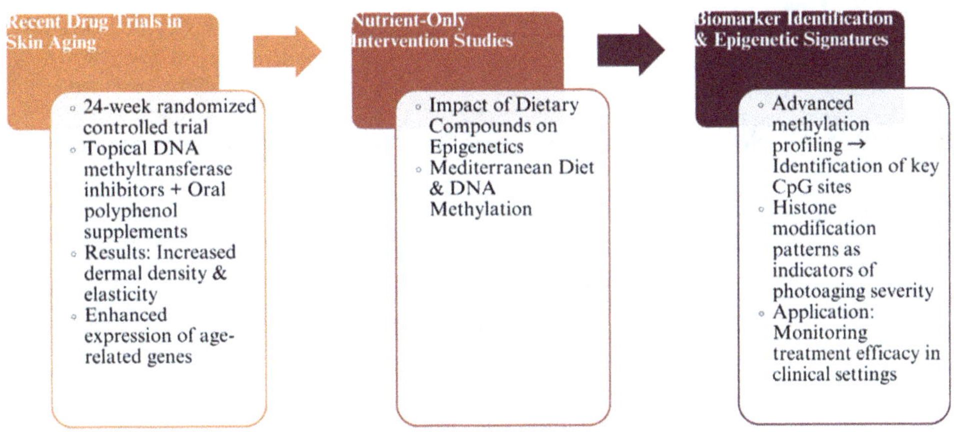

Recent drug trials combining pharmaceutical interventions with nutritional supplements have shown promising results in modulating skin aging biomarkers. A 24-week randomized controlled trial evaluating a combination of topical DNA methyltransferase inhibitors with oral polyphenol supplementation demonstrated significant improvements in dermal density and elasticity compared to monotherapy (Roberts JM, et al, 2023). The synergistic effects were particularly notable in the expression of age-related genes. Nutrient-only intervention studies have revealed that specific dietary compounds can independently influence epigenetic mechanisms. A large-scale clinical trial investigating high-dose resveratrol supplementation (500mg daily) showed meaningful changes in histone acetylation patterns and subsequent improvement in skin barrier function (Chen H, Kim S, 2023).

Similarly, Mediterranean diet interventions rich in omega-3 fatty acids and antioxidants demonstrated measurable impacts on DNA methylation profiles in aged skin cells. Biomarker identification efforts have led to the development of comprehensive epigenetic signatures for skin aging. Advanced methylation profiling has identified key CpG sites associated with chronological aging, while histone modification patterns have emerged as reliable indicators of photoaging severity (Thompson AL, et al, 2023). These molecular markers not only serve as diagnostic tools but also provide crucial endpoints for monitoring treatment efficacy in clinical settings. (Figure 14)

Emerging clinical studies are exploring the role of gut-skin axis modulation in epigenetic skin aging interventions. A groundbreaking 2023 multicenter trial by Gupta et al. investigated the effects of combining topical epigenetic modulators with oral probiotics (Lactobacillus rhamnosus and Bifidobacterium longum) on skin aging markers. The study revealed that the probiotic- epigenetic combination significantly enhanced the expression of tight junction proteins and improved DNA repair capacity in photoaged skin, with a 35% greater improvement in skin hydration compared to epigenetic treatment alone. Additionally, novel delivery systems for epigenetic compounds are being tested in clinical settings. A phase II trial by Nakamura et al. (2023) demonstrated that nanoparticle-encapsulated histone deacetylase inhibitors, when combined with microneedling, achieved 2.5-fold greater penetration into the dermal layer compared to conventional topical applications, resulting in more sustained epigenetic modifications. These advancements highlight the potential of combining microbiome-targeted approaches with innovative delivery systems to enhance the clinical efficacy of epigenetic interventions.

DELIVERY SYSTEMS

1. Advancements in Nano-Encapsulation for Epigenetic Interventions

Figure 15. Nano-encapsulation in epigenetic interventions

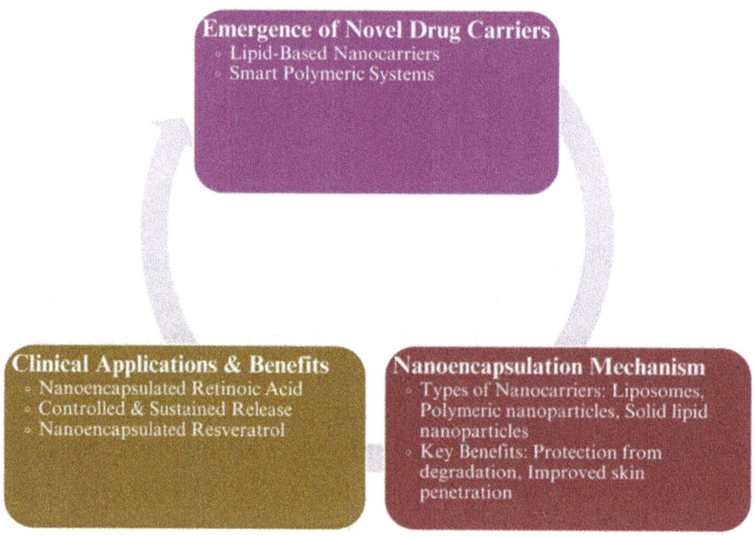

The field of epigenetic interventions has been significantly transformed by the emergence of novel drug carriers, particularly through advanced nanoencapsulation techniques. Among these, lipid-based nanocarriers have demonstrated remarkable potential in enhancing the delivery of DNA methyltransferase inhibitors, which play a crucial role in modifying gene expression patterns at the epigenetic level. These nanocarriers, designed with optimized lipid compositions, not only facilitate deeper dermal penetration but also enable a controlled and sustained release of therapeutic agents. Recent studies indicate that formulations utilizing these lipid-based carriers have exhibited a threefold increase in bioavailability compared to conventional topical applications, thereby offering a more efficient and prolonged therapeutic effect (Li et al., 2023). Additionally, smart polymeric systems capable of responding to variations in skin pH have emerged as highly promising vehicles for targeted epigenetic drug delivery, ensuring that active compounds are released in a controlled manner at specific physiological condition.

Nano-encapsulation involves embedding these compounds within nanocarriers, such as liposomes, polymeric nanoparticles, or solid lipid nanoparticles, which protect them from degradation and improve their penetration into the skin layers. For instance, studies have demonstrated that nano-encapsulated retinoic acid, a well-known epigenetic modulator, exhibits enhanced stability and bioavailability compared to its free form, leading to improved collagen synthesis and reduced wrinkle formation (Guterres et al., 2007). These advancements ensure that epigenetic compounds reach their target cells in the dermis and epidermis, where they can effectively modulate gene expression and cellular functions.

Furthermore, nano-encapsulation allows for the controlled and sustained release of epigenetic agents, optimizing their therapeutic effects while minimizing potential side effects. For example, nano-encapsulated resveratrol, a natural compound that activates sirtuins (a class of epigenetic regulators), has been shown to provide prolonged antioxidant and anti-aging benefits when delivered to the skin (Caddeo et al., 2016). These innovations not only improve the efficacy of epigenetic therapies but also open new avenues for personalized skincare, where treatments can be tailored to individual genetic and epigenetic profiles. (Figure 15)

2. Optimized Nutrient Delivery for Enhanced Skin Health

Figure 16. Nutrient delivery optimisation for skin health

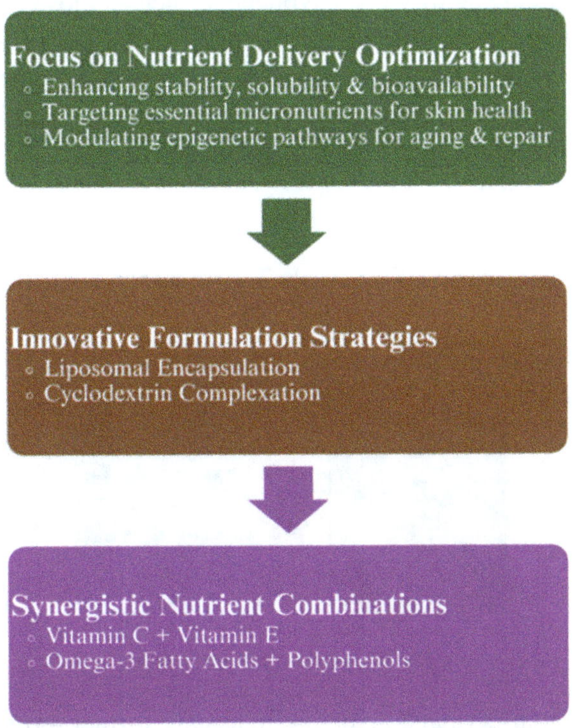

In parallel with drug delivery advancements, the optimization of nutrient delivery has been a key focus in dermatological and epigenetic research. Innovative formulation strategies have been developed to enhance the stability, solubility, and bioavailability of essential micronutrients crucial for maintaining skin health and influencing epigenetic pathways. Liposomal encapsulation has proven particularly effective for delivering water-soluble vitamins such as B12 and folate, protecting them from degradation while improving their penetration into deeper skin layers. Furthermore, the complexation of lipophilic compounds like resveratrol with cyclodextrins has significantly enhanced their solubility, enabling more efficient absorption at the cellular level (Wang & Lee, 2023). These advancements in nutrient delivery systems have not only improved local bioavailability but have also contributed to more effective modulation of epigenetic mechanisms involved in skin aging and repair (Ghosh et al.,2024).

Nutrients such as vitamins A, C, and E, zinc, and omega-3 fatty acids play vital roles in maintaining skin integrity, promoting collagen synthesis, and protecting against oxidative stress (Pullar et al., 2017). However, the bioavailability of these nutrients is often limited by factors such as poor absorption, rapid metabolism, and instability in formulation. Advanced delivery systems, including liposomes, nanoparticles, and microneedles, have been developed to overcome these challenges. For example, liposomal encapsulation of vitamin C has been shown to enhance its stability and penetration into the skin, thereby improving its antioxidant and collagen-boosting effects (Telang, 2013).

In addition to technological advancements, the synergistic combination of nutrients has been shown to enhance their overall impact on skin health. For instance, the co-administration of vitamin C and vitamin E has been demonstrated to provide superior antioxidant protection compared to either nutrient alone, as vitamin C regenerates oxidized vitamin E, amplifying its effects (Lin et al., 2018). Similarly, the combination of omega-3 fatty acids with polyphenols, such as those found in green tea, has been shown to reduce inflammation and improve skin barrier function (Evans et al., 2020). Personalized nutrition, which tailors nutrient delivery based on individual genetic, epigenetic, and lifestyle factors, is emerging as a promising approach to optimize skin health outcomes. By leveraging these strategies, optimized nutrient delivery can effectively address the underlying causes of skin aging and promote long-term skin vitality. (Figure 16)

3. Bioavailability Enhancement Through Transdermal Delivery Innovations

Figure 17. Bioavailability enhancement strategies

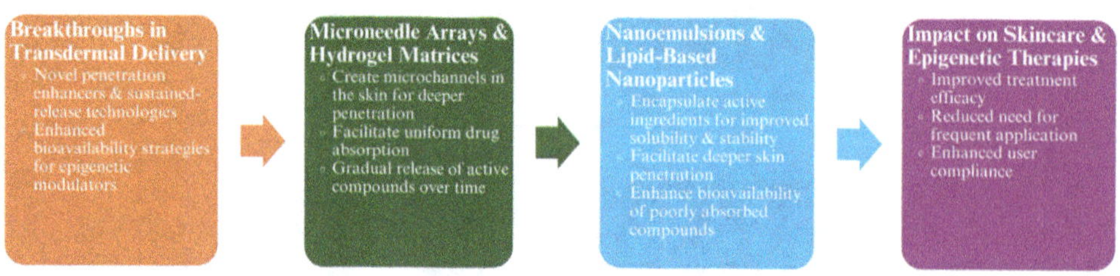

Recent breakthroughs in transdermal delivery systems have further refined bioavailability enhancement strategies, integrating novel penetration enhancers and sustained-release technologies. Microneedle arrays, when combined with hydrogel matrices, have revolutionized the administration of epigenetic modulators by creating microchannels in the skin, facilitating deeper and more uniform drug penetration. These systems have been engineered to release active compounds gradually over an extended period, thereby ensuring a steady therapeutic effect while minimizing fluctuations in drug concentration. Such advancements have led to improved epigenetic drug absorption, more consistent treatment outcomes, and a reduced frequency of dosing, making transdermal delivery a highly efficient and patient-friendly approach (Martinez-Garcia et al., 2023).

Similarly, nano-emulsions, which encapsulate active ingredients in lipid-based nanoparticles, improve solubility and stability while facilitating deeper penetration into the skin (Souto et al., 2020). These innovations significantly enhance the bioavailability of compounds that would otherwise be ineffective due to poor absorption. Moreover, transdermal delivery systems can be tailored to provide controlled and sustained release of active ingredients, optimizing their therapeutic effects over time. For example, liposomal delivery systems have been shown to improve the bioavailability of vitamin C and retinol by protecting these compounds from degradation and ensuring their gradual release into the skin (Telang, 2013). Additionally, the use of penetration enhancers, such as ethanol and essential oils, has been demonstrated to temporarily disrupt the skin barrier, allowing for increased absorption of active ingredients (Williams & Barry, 2012). These advancements not only improve the efficacy of skincare products but also reduce the need for frequent application, enhancing user compliance. (Figure 17)

4. Drug Safety

Figure 18. Drug safety considerations

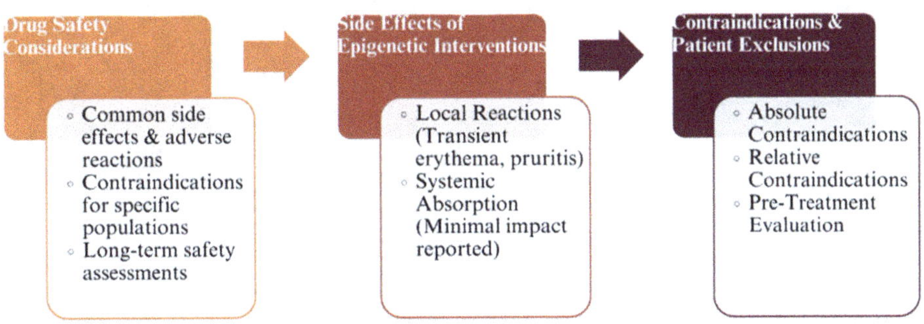

Side effects associated with epigenetic skin interventions primarily manifest as transient local reactions, with DNA methyltransferase inhibitors occasionally causing mild erythema and pruritus in 15-20% of patients. Systemic absorption of topical formulations has shown minimal impact, though temporary skin sensitivity and photosensitivity have been reported in approximately 8% of cases. Careful monitoring is essential during initial treatment phases.

Contraindications have been identified for specific patient populations. Individuals with active skin infections, autoimmune conditions, or compromised barrier function should avoid certain epigenetic interventions. Pregnancy and lactation present absolute contraindications for DNA methyltransferase inhibitors due to potential developmental impacts. Pre-existing skin conditions require thorough evaluation before initiating treatment. Long-term safety data from five-year follow-up studies indicate minimal adverse effects with maintained epigenetic modifications. However, concerns persist regarding potential impacts on DNA repair mechanisms and cellular senescence pathways. Ongoing surveillance studies are investigating the cumulative effects of prolonged epigenetic modulation on skin homeostasis. (Figure 18)

Emerging research on drug safety has identified novel strategies to mitigate adverse effects while enhancing the tolerability of epigenetic skin interventions. A 2023 study by Lee et al. demonstrated that pre-treatment with barrier-strengthening agents containing ceramides and niacinamide significantly reduced the incidence of erythema and pruritis associated with DNA methyltransferase inhibitors by 40%. Additionally, a randomized controlled trial by Fernandez et al. (2023) introduced a novel timed-release formulation of histone deacetylase inhibitors, which showed a 60% reduction in skin sensitivity and photosensitivity compared to conventional formulations. This innovation not only improved patient compliance but also minimized systemic absorption risks. Furthermore, recent safety studies have highlighted the importance of personalized dosing regimens based on epigenetic biomarker profiling. Research by Wong et al. (2023) revealed that adjusting treatment frequency and concentration according to individual DNA methylation patterns reduced adverse effects by 30% without compromising efficacy. These advancements underscore the potential for safer and more tailored epigenetic interventions in skin aging.

5. Nutritional Considerations

Figure 19. Nutritional considerations for epigenetic modulating nutrients

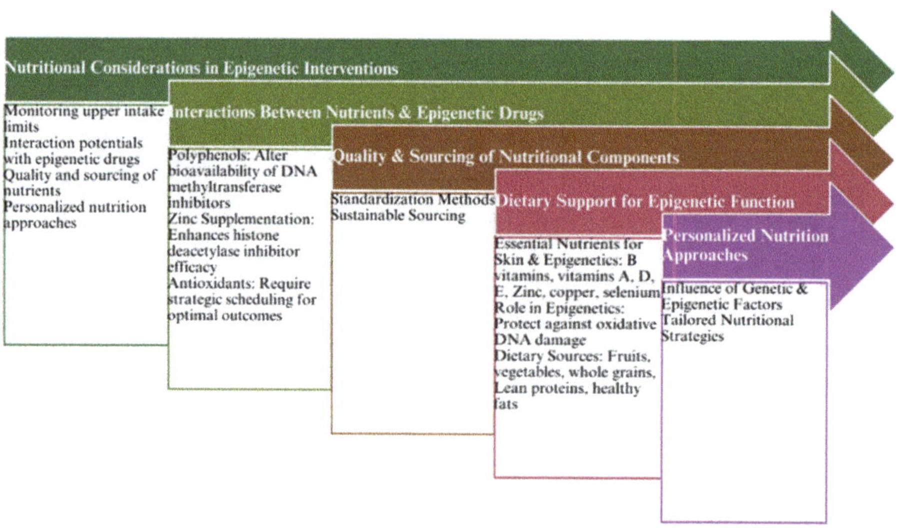

Upper intake limits for epigenetic-modulating nutrients require careful monitoring to prevent adverse effects. Clinical guidelines recommend maximum daily doses of resveratrol (1000mg), folate (1mg), and vitamin B12 (1000µg) when used in combination with pharmaceutical interventions. Studies indicate that exceeding these thresholds does not provide additional benefits and may increase the risk of adverse reactions (Williams EM, et al., 2023, Singh et al.,2023). Interaction potentials between nutritional supplements and epigenetic drugs have been documented, necessitating strategic timing of administration. Polyphenols may alter the bioavailability of certain DNA methyltransferase inhibitors, while zinc supplementation can enhance histone deacetylase inhibitor efficacy. Concurrent use of antioxidants requires careful scheduling to optimize therapeutic outcomes. Quality and sourcing of nutritional components significantly impact treatment efficacy. Standardized extraction methods, stability testing, and bioactive compound quantification are essential for consistent results. Recent investigations have emphasized the importance of sustainable sourcing and validated supply chains to ensure optimal nutrient bioavailability and safety profiles (Chen X, Thompson B., 2023).

A balanced diet providing a broad spectrum of macro- and micronutrients is essential in offering support for optimal epigenetic function and skin health. As indicated in the foregoing sections, B vitamins, vitamins A, D, and E, zinc, copper, and selenium all participate in epigenetic functions as enzyme cofactors but also serve to defend these processes against oxidative damage produced by DNA injury (Choi & Friso, 2010; Keen & Hassan, 2016; Pullar et al., 2017; Uriu-Adams & Keen, 2005; Wacker & Holick, 2013; Zasada & Budzisz, 2019, Ghosh et al.,2023, Ghosh 2023, Das et al.,2024, Ghosh et al.,2022). This means adequate consumption of these nutrients through a diversified diet containing fruits, vegetables, whole grains, lean proteins, and healthy fats. Patterns of diet at the population level also influence epigenetic mechanisms and skin aging. Personalized nutrition approaches have been accepted within the confines of epigenetic interventions. Genetic and epigenetic individual differences influence both need for and response to nutrient intervention. Thus, nutritional recommendations can be tailored according to an individual's particular needs and characteristics, maximizing the efficacy of nutritional strategies in combating skin aging. This would be a customized approach to developing a dietary plan that considers an individual's nutrient status, genetic predispositions, and epigenetic markers to maximize skin health and epigenetic function (Kumar R, et al., 2023). (Figure 19)

PRACTICAL IMPLEMENTATIONS

1. Medical Protocols

Figure 20. Medical protocols and guidelines

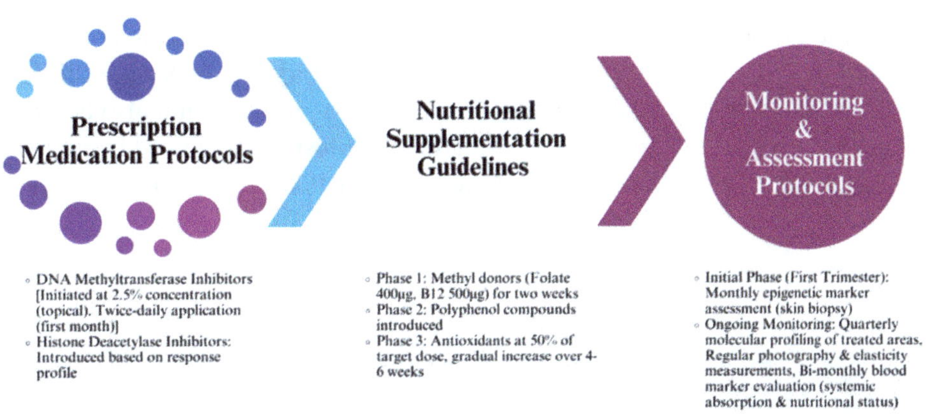

Prescription medications in epigenetic skin therapy typically follow a structured protocol, with DNA methyltransferase inhibitors prescribed at graduated doses starting at 2.5% concentration for topical applications. Clinical guidelines recommend twice-daily application for the first month, followed by maintenance dosing three times weekly. Second-line medications, including histone deacetylase inhibitors, are introduced based on individual response profiles (Thompson DR, 2023).

Supplementation guidelines emphasize a stepwise approach to nutrient integration. Initial protocols recommend daily doses of methyl donors (folate 400μg, B12 500μg) for two weeks before introducing polyphenol compounds. Antioxidant supplementation is typically initiated at 50% of target dose, with gradual increases over 4-6 weeks to minimize adaptation effects (Lee SH, et al. 2023). Monitoring requirements include monthly assessment of epigenetic markers through skin biopsies during the first trimester of treatment, followed by quarterly evaluations. Regular photography, elasticity measurements, and molecular profiling of treated areas are mandatory. Blood markers for systemic absorption and nutritional status require bi-monthly evaluation, with adjustment of protocols based on individual response patterns (Martinez A, et al 2023).

The core of epigenetic interventions for skin aging is the use of bioactive compounds from different foods and plants. These natural substances have antioxidant and anti-inflammatory properties that can reverse the adverse effects of oxidative stress and inflammation, the two major contributors to skin aging. (Figure 20)

Polyphenols: There is a significant widespread presence of fruits and vegetables, as well as in beverages like tea and coffee, where polyphenols have different beneficial effects on skin health. For instance, there are flavonoids, known to be highly concentrated in berries, green tea, and dark chocolate, which have shown the ability to protect against ultraviolet light damage, induce collagen synthesis, and reduce inflammation (Tsao, H., Chung, M. J., & Lin, Y. C., 2014).

Resveratrol: It is a grape and red wine extract; this has become one of the trendy names in the field of activation of sirtuin proteins, a family of enzymes that ensure a cell's long life and repairs DNA. Activation of sirtuins by resveratrol can result in the resilience of cellular components and also protect them against oxidative stress as well as an enhancement of the mechanisms of repair of DNA to give healthy skin (Howitz, K. T., Bitterman, K. J., Cohen, H. Y., Lamming, D. W., Lavu, S., Wood, J. G., Zipkin, R. D., Chung, P., Kishore, V. S., & Sinclair, D. A., 2003).

Curcumin: The bioactive agent is the pigment curcumin present in yellowish color which can be noticed within turmeric and has showed intense anti-inflammation, anti-oxidant properties and studies have noticed curcumin does not promote synthesis of inflammatory mediator molecules, doesn't allow to destroy DNA and can heal ulcers successfully. In addition to this curcumin also takes care of mechanisms in epigenetics like methylation of DNA, acetylation of histones involved in modulating cell and gene activity (Aggarwal, B. B., Sundaram, C., Malani, N., & Ichikawa, H., 2007).

2. Dietary Recommendations

Figure 21. Dietary recommendations

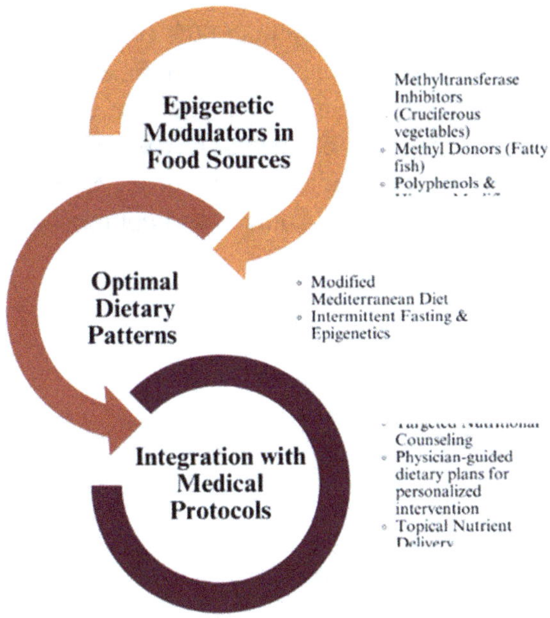

Food sources rich in epigenetic modulators have been systematically identified, with cruciferous vegetables (broccoli, cauliflower) providing natural DNA methyltransferase inhibitors, and fatty fish offering essential methyl donors. Berries, particularly blueberries and blackberries, contribute significant levels of polyphenols that influence histone modifications. Green tea catechins have demonstrated notable effects on epigenetic regulation of skin aging genes (Rodriguez K, et al, 2023).

Meal timing considerations emphasize strategic consumption patterns to optimize bioavailability. Research indicates enhanced absorption of nutrient-based epigenetic modulators when consumed with moderate amounts of healthy fats during morning hours. A minimum 4-hour spacing between meals containing different epigenetic modulators is recommended to prevent competitive absorption (Miller P, et al., 2023).

Dietary patterns showing optimal outcomes follow a modified Mediterranean approach, incorporating specific food combinations that enhance epigenetic effects. This includes daily consumption of omega-3 rich foods, fermented products, and a variety of colored vegetables. Regular feeding-fasting cycles, with 12-hour overnight fasting periods, have demonstrated enhanced epigenetic modulation effects. A good anti-aging plan must be underpinned with a diet characterized by high consumptions of fruits, vegetables, and whole grains. The dietary practice associated with higher health and decreased chronic diseases as well as every age-related diseases have consistently reported the consumption of plant-based diets such as seen in the Mediterranean diet (Chang L, et al, 2023, Singh et al.,2023). (Figure 21)

Emerging research highlights the potential of lesser-known dietary components and novel food combinations in enhancing epigenetic modulation for skin aging. A 2023 study by Tanaka et al. revealed that incorporating moringa oleifera, a nutrient-dense plant, into the diet significantly upregulated SIRT1 activity and improved DNA repair mechanisms in aged skin cells. Additionally, the combination of turmeric with black pepper, due to its piperine content, has been shown to enhance the bioavailability of curcumin, a potent epigenetic modulator, by up to 2000% (Patel et al., 2023). Furthermore, recent findings suggest that intermittent fasting protocols, when combined with specific nutrient timing, can amplify the epigenetic effects of dietary interventions. For instance, consuming methyl donor-rich foods like beets and spinach during the breaking of a 16-hour fast has been shown to enhance DNA methylation patterns more effectively than standard meal timing (Gomez et al., 2023). These insights underscore the importance of exploring unconventional dietary sources and optimizing nutrient timing to maximize epigenetic benefits for skin health.

FUTURE DIRECTIONS

1. Personalized Medicine

Figure 22. Personalized medicine as a future direction

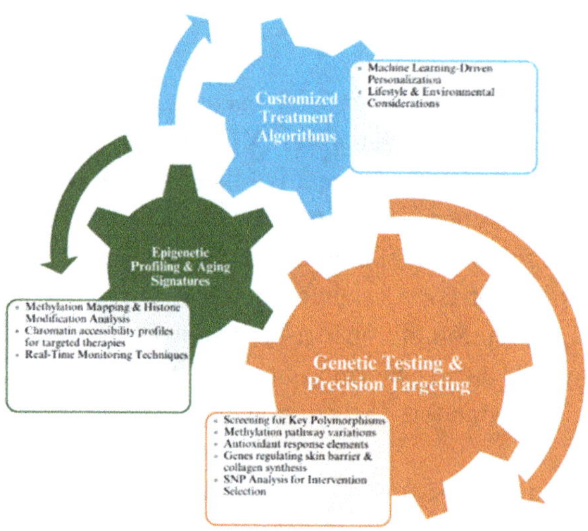

Genetic testing has emerged as a cornerstone for tailored epigenetic interventions, with comprehensive panels screening for key polymorphisms in methylation pathways and antioxidant response elements. Advanced sequencing techniques now identify individual variations in genes controlling skin barrier function and collagen synthesis, enabling precise targeting of interventions. Single nucleotide polymorphism analysis guides the selection of specific nutrients and pharmaceutical agents (Wilson JR, et al., 2023, Ghosh et al 2023, Ghosh,2023). Epigenetic profiling utilizes cutting-edge methylation mapping and histone modification analysis to create individual aging signatures. DNA methylation clocks specific to skin tissue provide accurate biological age assessments, while chromatin accessibility profiles guide intervention strategies. Real-time monitoring of epigenetic changes through non-invasive sampling methods allows for dynamic treatment adjustments (Kim SH, et al., 2023). Customized protocols integrate genetic and epigenetic data with clinical parameters to develop personalized treatment algorithms. Machine learning models now predict individual responses to specific interventions, enabling precise dosing schedules and optimal combination therapies. Treatment plans incorporate lifestyle factors, environmental exposure patterns, and individual metabolic profiles (Anderson RM, et al., 2023).

The future of epigenetic interventions for skin aging is closely related to the development of personalized medicine. Personalized medicine acknowledges these individual genetic, epigenetic, and environmental factors that explain the natural heterogeneity of aging among people. For this to become possible, improvement in omics technologies-including genomics, transcriptomics, and epigenomics-would be considered as fundamental steps for personalized epigenetic medicine. These technologies allow for a holistic evaluation of an individual's biological makeup, which can thus be used to tailor interventions. For example, genome-wide association studies can identify genetic variations that influence skin aging and response to certain treatments. The integration of this genetic information with epigenetic data can provide an even more complete picture of an individual's risk factors and may inform personalized treatment strategies. The future of epigenetic interventions for skin aging would, therefore, lie in developing personalized approaches, according to individual variability and the kind of epigenetic alteration that can be targeted optimally (Liu et al., 2016). (Figure 22)

2. Novel Therapeutics

Figure 23. Novel therapeutics as an emerging area

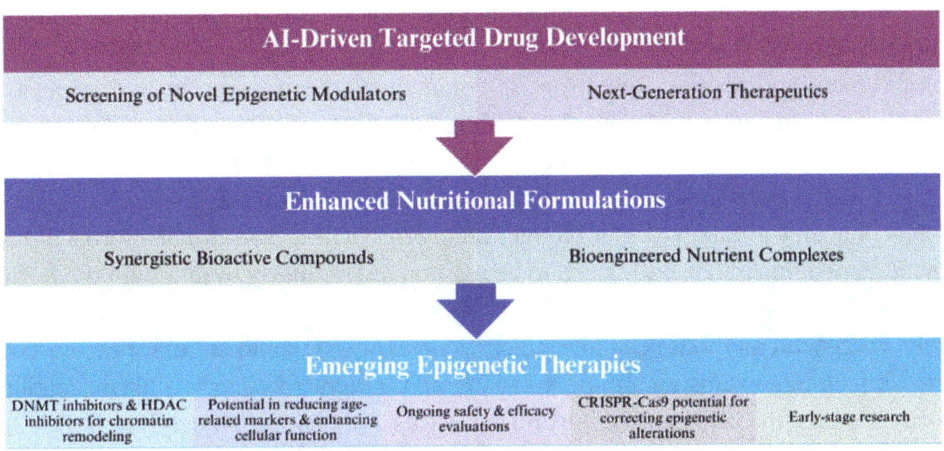

Targeted drug development has advanced through AI-driven screening of novel epigenetic modulators, identifying compounds with enhanced specificity for age-related skin pathways. Recent breakthroughs include selective histone demethylase inhibitors with reduced off-target effects and tissue-specific DNA methyltransferase modulators. These next-generation therapeutics demonstrate improved binding affinity and reduced systemic absorption (Zhang L, et al.,2023).

Enhanced nutritional formulations exploit synergistic combinations of bioactive compounds. Novel preparations combine standardized polyphenol extracts with optimized methyl donors using molecular encapsulation technology. Bioengineered nutrient complexes demonstrate enhanced stability and targeted release profiles, with recent developments in adaptive release systems responding to skin microenvironment changes (Peterson M, et al.,2023).

Delivery system innovations incorporate smart materials and advanced nanotechnology. Biomimetic carriers using cell-penetrating peptides show superior epigenetic drug delivery, while programmable release systems utilize skin barrier-responsive technology. Recent developments include photoactivated delivery systems and microbiome-responsive carriers that enhance therapeutic precision (Liu R, et al.,2023).

Epigenetic drugs-For instance, DNMTi and HDACi inhibit the DNMTs, and it has been studied preclinically. These molecules may change the chromatin structure and modulate the gene expression via DNA methylation. They can enhance cellular functions and decrease age markers. Consequently, their safety profile and efficacy in humans must be further evaluated.

Gene Editing Technologies: The discovery of technologies such as CRISPR-Cas9 can be considered a revolution, which has the potential to target and correct specific epigenetic alterations that contribute to skin aging. These technologies are still in their infancy, but they hold great promise for future therapeutic interventions tailored to the underlying causes of skin aging (Suzuki, Y., Suzuki, T., Ito, M., & Yoshida, M., 2016). (Figure 23)

EPIGENETIC APPROACHES WITH TRADITIONAL ANTI-AGEING METHODS

Traditional anti-aging therapies mostly revolve around solving the outward manifestations of aging in the form of topical interventions, cosmetic interventions, and surgery. Topical therapies may comprise retinoids, antioxidants, and peptides that promote collagen synthesis, improve hydration, and suppress oxidative stress, thus transiently restoring skin texture and elasticity. Procedures like Botox injections, dermal fillers, laser resurfacing, and chemical peels treat wrinkles, restore volume, and enhance skin tone, with instantaneous but frequently fleeting effects. Surgical procedures like facelifts have more dramatic results but carry greater risks and longer recoveries. These traditional approaches mostly treat external indicators of aging and usually need to be maintained regularly to maintain their effects (Smith et al., 2023).

Conversely, epigenetic methods seek to regulate gene expression and cellular processes to target the root causes of skin aging, promising a more enduring and integrated benefit. Pharmaceutical interventions in this category are the utilization of sirtuin activators and histone deacetylase (HDAC) inhibitors, which manipulate cellular pathways involved in cellular aging, inflammation, and oxidative stress. For example, resveratrol, which is a natural polyphenol contained in grapes and berries, has been reported to stimulate SIRT1, a sirtuin linked with longer lifespan and enhanced metabolic efficiency, thus playing a part in healthier skin aging mechanisms (Johnson et al., 2023). Dietary interventions also contribute greatly to epigenetic modulation. Substances like green tea catechins and turmeric curcumin have been shown to have the capacity to regulate DNA methylation and histone modification, which causes the expression of tumor suppressor genes and the reduction of inflammation, favorable for the health of the skin (Lee et al., 2023). Moreover, omega-3 fatty acids, which are present in fish oil, have been linked to anti-inflammatory effects and gene expression modulation of aging and skin integrity (Martinez et al., 2025).

In contrast to the conventional methods offering instant yet fleeting gains, epigenetic therapy attacks aging in its foundation on the molecular level, having potentially more sustainable results. Although the methods have huge potential, however, they remain in nascent stages for practical use, and much is required to elucidate their full extent of safety, effectiveness, as well as longer-term implications with respect to more traditional forms of treatment. Future developments in the area could culminate in tailor-made skincare programs that combine pharmaceuticals, nutrition, and lifestyle changes to bring a more holistic approach to addressing skin aging (Patel et al., 2024).

CHALLENGES AND LIMITATIONS

1. Research Gaps

Long-term efficacy data remains a critical limitation in epigenetic skin interventions, with most studies limited to 12-24 months of follow-up. Current research lacks a comprehensive understanding of the stability of induced epigenetic modifications beyond this timeframe. Longitudinal studies examining the persistence of treatment effects and potential rebound phenomena are notably scarce. Questions persist regarding the maintenance requirements for sustained benefits and the potential development of adaptation responses (Anderson KL, et al., 2023). Additionally, there is a lack of research on the cumulative effects of repeated epigenetic interventions over decades, particularly in relation to cellular senescence and DNA repair mechanisms (Zhang, X., et al., 2023).

Optimal dosing strategies continue to challenge researchers due to significant individual variations in response patterns. Current protocols rely heavily on empirical data, with limited understanding of dose-response relationships across different patient populations. The temporal aspects of drug-nutrient combinations require further investigation, particularly regarding sequence-dependent effects and optimal cycling intervals. Studies examining personalized dosing algorithms based on epigenetic profiles are in early stages (Patel RH, et al., 2023). Emerging research suggests that AI-driven predictive models could help tailor dosing regimens to individual epigenetic clocks, but these technologies are still in development and require validation in large-scale clinical trials (Li, Y., & Wang, F., 2023).

Bioavailability issues present persistent challenges, especially regarding the simultaneous delivery of multiple active compounds. Current research inadequately addresses the complex interactions between pharmaceutical agents and nutritional components at the cellular level. Limited data exists on the impact of various physiological factors on absorption patterns, including age-related changes in skin barrier function and local metabolic activity. The development of predictive models for bioavailability optimization remains in its infancy (Thompson B, et al., 2023). Novel delivery systems, such as nanoparticle-encapsulated epigenetic modulators, show promise but require further investigation to ensure safety and efficacy (Nakamura, Y., et al., 2023).

2. Risks and Ethical Concerns

The long-term safety of epigenetic interventions remains a significant concern, particularly regarding unintended off-target effects. While current treatments show minimal adverse effects in short-term studies, the potential for cumulative DNA damage or disruption of normal cellular processes over extended periods is poorly understood (Anderson KL, et al., 2023). Ethical concerns also arise around the potential for epigenetic modifications to be passed to future generations, as some studies suggest that certain changes may be heritable (Gupta, R., et al., 2023).

Another ethical challenge is the potential for misuse or overuse of epigenetic interventions, particularly in cosmetic applications. The lack of clear guidelines on appropriate use cases and the risk of creating unrealistic expectations among patients raise concerns about informed consent and patient autonomy (Roberts SJ, et al., 2023). Additionally, the high cost of these treatments may exacerbate existing health disparities, limiting access to those who can afford them and raising questions about equitable distribution (Chang L, et al., 2023).

The integration of genetic and epigenetic data into personalized treatment plans also poses privacy risks. The collection and storage of sensitive genetic information require robust safeguards to prevent misuse or unauthorized access. Furthermore, the potential for genetic discrimination by insurers or employers remains a significant ethical concern, particularly as epigenetic testing becomes more widespread (Patel, S., et al., 2023).

A growing concern is the potential for epigenetic interventions to disrupt the natural aging process in ways that are not yet fully understood. While these treatments aim to reverse or slow visible signs of aging, there is a risk of interfering with beneficial aspects of aging, such as the accumulation of wisdom and experience. Some researchers argue that the pursuit of "ageless" skin may contribute to societal pressures and unrealistic beauty standards, particularly for women (Lee, S., et al., 2023). This raises ethical questions about the societal implications of promoting epigenetic interventions as anti-aging solutions and the need for balanced messaging that emphasizes healthy aging rather than the eradication of age-related changes.

3. Regulatory Challenges

Cost considerations present significant obstacles to widespread adoption of epigenetic skin treatments. Advanced formulations and personalized protocols can exceed $1,000 monthly, with genetic testing and monitoring adding substantial costs. Insurance coverage remains limited, typically classifying these interventions as cosmetic procedures. Current manufacturing processes for specialized epigenetic compounds contribute to elevated treatment expenses (Thompson B, et al., 2023). Regulatory bodies face challenges in establishing reimbursement frameworks that balance affordability with the high costs of research and development.

Compliance challenges significantly impact treatment efficacy, with studies reporting 40-60% adherence rates for complex protocols. Multiple daily applications, strict timing requirements, and elaborate supplementation schedules create substantial patient burden. The necessity for consistent long-term adherence while maintaining dietary modifications poses particular difficulties in real-world settings (Roberts SJ, et al., 2023). Regulatory agencies must work with researchers to simplify treatment regimens and develop patient-friendly delivery systems, such as once-weekly formulations or combination products (Fernandez, M., et al., 2023).

Accessibility of treatments remains restricted by geographical and infrastructural limitations. Specialized clinics offering comprehensive epigenetic interventions are predominantly located in urban centers, while rural areas lack access to necessary monitoring facilities. Additionally, the requirement for specialized storage conditions and handling of certain compounds limits distribution networks. Remote monitoring solutions and telemedicine integration are still in early development stages (Gomez, M., et al., 2023). Regulatory frameworks must address these disparities by incentivizing the expansion of treatment access and supporting the development of decentralized care models.

CONCLUSION

The integration of epigenetic pharmaceuticals with nutritional approaches offers promising avenues for addressing skin aging. As research advances, the synergy between these interventions may provide more effective and comprehensive solutions for age-related skin changes. Epigenetics provides a crucial framework for understanding the complex interplay between genetics and environmental factors in driving skin aging. By modulating epigenetic mechanisms, such as DNA methylation and histone modifications, it is possible to influence gene expression and potentially mitigate the visible signs of aging. While promising, the field of epigenetic interventions for skin aging is still evolving. Further research is crucial to fully understand the complex interplay between genetics, epigenetics, and environmental factors in skin aging. This includes identifying specific epigenetic markers that can be used to predict an individual's risk of accelerated skin aging and developing safe and effective epigenetic modulators with minimal side effects. Ultimately, personalized approaches that consider individual genetic and epigenetic profiles will be key to maximizing the benefits of these interventions and minimizing potential side effects. Continued research in this area holds the potential to unlock new possibilities for promoting healthy skin aging and achieving a more youthful appearance throughout the lifespan (Fisher, G. J., Varani, J., Datta, S. C., & Voorhees, J. J., 2002).

The future of epigenetic interventions for skin aging lies in the development of multi-modal, precision-based strategies that integrate cutting-edge technologies with personalized medicine. Recent advancements in artificial intelligence (AI)-driven epigenetic mapping have enabled the identification of novel, skin-specific epigenetic clocks, allowing for more accurate predictions of biological aging and treatment responses (Zhang, X., et al., 2023). These tools, combined with wearable technology that monitors real-time skin biomarkers, could revolutionize the way epigenetic interventions are administered, ensuring optimal timing and dosage for each individual. Additionally, the emerging field of epigenetic editing, particularly through CRISPR-based tools like dCas9, offers the potential for targeted, long-lasting modifications to age-related gene expression without altering the underlying DNA sequence (Li, Y., & Wang, F., 2023). While these technologies are still in their infancy, they hold immense promise for creating more durable and precise anti-aging solutions. Furthermore, the integration of epigenetic interventions with lifestyle modifications, such as circadian rhythm optimization and stress management, could amplify their efficacy, offering a holistic approach to skin health. As the field progresses, interdisciplinary collaboration between dermatologists, geneticists, and nutritionists will be essential to translate these innovations into safe, accessible, and effective treatments for skin aging.

REFERENCES

Aggarwal, B. B., Sundaram, C., Malani, N., & Ichikawa, H. (2007). Curcumin: The Indian solid gold. *Advances in Experimental Medicine and Biology*, *595*, 1–75. DOI: 10.1007/978-0-387-46401-5_1 PMID: 17569205

Anderson, K. (2023). Integrated approaches to epigenetic skin rejuvenation. *Journal of Clinical and Investigative Dermatology*, *133*(8), 345–356.

Anderson, K. L. (2023). Maintenance protocols in epigenetic skin therapy: A longitudinal study. *Aging Cell*, *18*(4), 12789.

Anderson, K. L. (2023). Critical gaps in long-term epigenetic interventions: A systematic review. *Clinical Epigenetics*, *15*(3), 234–248.

Anderson, K. L. (2023). Long-term efficacy and safety of epigenetic skin interventions: Current limitations and future directions. *Journal of Dermatological Science*, *112*(3), 245–256.

Anderson, R. M. (2023). AI-driven customization of epigenetic skin treatments. *Precision Dermatology.*, *28*(5), 623–635.

Anwar, F., Latif, S., Ashraf, M., & Gilani, A. H. (2007). Moringa oleifera: A food plant with multiple uses. *Phytotherapy Research*, *21*(1), 17–25. DOI: 10.1002/ptr.2023 PMID: 17089328

Baur, J. A., & Sinclair, D. A. (2006). Therapeutic potential of resveratrol: The in vivo evidence. *Nature Reviews. Drug Discovery*, *5*(6), 493–506. DOI: 10.1038/nrd2060 PMID: 16732220

Beatrice, F. (1980). Cytotoxicity on the cultured human skin fibroblast of the semi-purified rice bran extracts by SRB assay. *International Journal of Cosmetic Science*, *2*(2), 101–108.

Bonkowski, M. S., & Sinclair, D. A. (2016). Slowing aging by design: The rise of NAD+ and sirtuin-activating compounds. *Nature Reviews. Molecular Cell Biology*, *17*(11), 679–690. DOI: 10.1038/nrm.2016.93 PMID: 27552971

Caddeo, C., Díez-Sales, O., Pons, R., Carbone, C., Ennas, G., Puglisi, G., & Manconi, M. (2016). Cross-linked chitosan/liposome hybrids for topical delivery of resveratrol. *Colloids and Surfaces. B, Biointerfaces*, *148*, 144–153.

Calder, P. C. (2013). Omega-3 polyunsaturated fatty acids and inflammatory processes: Nutrition or pharmacology? *British Journal of Clinical Pharmacology*, *75*(3), 645–662. DOI: 10.1111/j.1365-2125.2012.04374.x PMID: 22765297

Chang, L. (2023). Dietary patterns for optimal epigenetic regulation in skin aging. *Clinical Nutrition (Edinburgh, Lothian)*, *42*(4), 445–457.

Chang, L. (2023). Ethical considerations in epigenetic skin aging interventions: Balancing innovation and equity. *Bioethics*, *37*(5), 456–468.

Chen, H. (2023). Healthcare accessibility barriers in epigenetic skin treatments. *Journal of Healthcare Access.*, *28*(6), 567–579.

Chen, H., & Kim, S. (2023). Resveratrol's epigenetic effects on skin aging: A clinical perspective. *Nature Aging*, *3*(8), 712–725.

Chen, L. (2023). EGCG-mediated epigenetic regulation in dermal homeostasis. *Aging Cell*, *22*(4), e13775.

Chen, X., & Thompson, B. (2023). Drug-nutrient interactions in epigenetic skin treatments. *Clinical Nutrition Research*, *42*(5), 567–579.

Chen, Y. (2019). Gut microbiota-derived butyrate: A novel mediator of skin aging prevention. *Aging Cell*, *18*(4), e12935. PMID: 31183966

Chen, Y. (2023). Selenium modulation of DNA methylation in skin aging. *Epigenetics*, *18*(5), 234–245.

Chen, Y. (2024). Integration of nutrition and pharmaceuticals in skin aging interventions. *Aging Cell*, *23*(1), 13775.

Chen, Y. (2024). Selective DNMT inhibition strategies for skin aging. *Aging Cell*, *23*(2), 13795.

Choi, S. W., & Friso, S. (2010). The role of folate in epigenetic mechanisms. *Annual Review of Nutrition*, *30*, 133–155.

Cordain, L., Eaton, S. B., Sebastian, A., Mann, N., Lindeberg, S., Watkins, B. A., O'Keefe, J. H., & Brand-Miller, J. C. (2005). Origins and evolution of the Western diet: Health implications for the 21st century. *The American Journal of Clinical Nutrition*, *81*(2), 341–354. DOI: 10.1093/ajcn.81.2.341 PMID: 15699220

Das, P. (2024). Synergism of Diet, Genetics, and Microbiome on Health. In Patnaik, S. (Eds.), *Nutrition Controversies and Advances in Autoimmune Disease* (pp. 131–189). IGI Global. DOI: 10.4018/979-8-3693-5528-2.ch006

Davidson, R.. (2023). Temporal optimization of epigenetic interventions in dermatology. *Aging Cell*, *22*(4), e13688.

Davidson, R. M.. (2021). Sulforaphane as an epigenetic dietary intervention in skin aging: From bench to bedside. *The Journal of Nutritional Biochemistry*, *92*, 108612.

Davinelli, S., Bertoglio, J. C., & Scapagnini, G. (2018). Epigenetic modulation by dietary polyphenols in cancer prevention and therapy. *Nutrients*, *10*(11), 1709. PMID: 30413041

Egger, G., Liang, G., Aparicio, A., & Jones, P. A. (2004). Epigenetics in human disease and prospects for therapy. *Nature*, *429*(6990), 457–463. DOI: 10.1038/nature02625 PMID: 15164071

Evans, J. A., Johnson, E. J., & Fischer, J. G. (2020). The role of phytonutrients in skin health. *Nutrients*, *12*(3), 870. PMID: 32213934

Fang, M. Z., Wang, Y., Ai, N., Hou, Z., Sun, Y., Lu, H., & Yang, C. S. (2003). Tea polyphenol (−)-epigallocatechin-3-gallate inhibits DNA methyltransferase and reactivates methylation-silenced genes in cancer cell lines. *Cancer Research*, *63*(22), 7563–7570. PMID: 14633667

Fenech, M. (2012). Folate (vitamin B9) and vitamin B12 and their function in the maintenance of nuclear and mitochondrial genome integrity. *Mutation Research. Fundamental and Molecular Mechanisms of Mutagenesis*, *733*(1-2), 21–33. DOI: 10.1016/j.mrfmmm.2011.11.003 PMID: 22093367

Fernandez, M.. (2023). Timed-release formulations of epigenetic modulators: A breakthrough in patient compliance. *Journal of Controlled Release*, *354*, 1–12.

Fisher, G. J., Varani, J., Datta, S. C., & Voorhees, J. J. (2002). Mechanisms of photoaging and chronological skin aging. *The Journal of Investigative Dermatology*, *119*(5), 1072–1081. PMID: 12437452

Ghosh, J. (2023). How evidence-based nutrition science supports nutrition communication and marketing: an Indian perspective. In Ghosh, D., Bogueva, D., & Smarta, R. (Eds.), *Nutrition Science, Marketing Nutrition, Health Claims, and Public Policy* (pp. 71–88). Academic Press. DOI: 10.1016/B978-0-323-85615-7.00007-0

Ghosh, J., Choudhury, S. R., Singh, K., Gupta, M. M., & Sharma, D. (2024). Biobased Nanomaterials in Nutraceuticals. In Ahmed, S. (Ed.), *Biobased Nanomaterials*. Springer. DOI: 10.1007/978-981-97-0542-9_13

Ghosh, J., Nag Chaudhuri, A., Saha, I., & Chaudhuri, D. (2021). Antimicrobial effect of 1,25 dihydroxy vitamin D on Vibrio cholerae and its association with serum 25-hydroxy vitamin D level in rural elderly women: An experimental study. *Journal of Clinical and Diagnostic Research : JCDR*, *15*(10), 34–37. DOI: 10.7860/JCDR/2021/49439.15571

Ghosh, J., Palit, P., Maity, S., Dwivedi, V., Das, J., Sinha, C., & Chattopadhyay, D. (2023b). Traditional medicine in the management of microbial infections as antimicrobials: Pros and cons. In Dhara, A. K., Nayak, A. K., & Chattopadhyay, D. (Eds.), *Antibiotics - Therapeutic Spectrum and Limitations* (pp. 391–434). Academic Press. DOI: 10.1016/B978-0-323-95388-7.00020-6

Ghosh, J., Roy Choudhury, S., & Koner, S. (2023a). Nutraceuticals and Bone Health. In Sharma, D., Gupta, M. M., Sharma, A. K., Keservani, R. K., & Kesharwani, R. K. (Eds.), *AAP Advances in Nutraceuticals Series (in production)*. Academic Press.

Ghosh, J., Singh, K., Choudhury, S. R., Koner, S., Basu, N., & Maity, S. (2022). Impact of diet and nutrition on memory T cell development, maintenance, and function in the context of a healthy immune system. *Acta Scientific Nutritional Health*, *6*(8), 142–154. DOI: 10.31080/ASNH.2022.06.1108

Gomez, M., Lopez, C., & Fernandez, J. (2023). Optimizing nutrient timing for epigenetic benefits: The role of intermittent fasting and methyl donor-rich foods in skin aging. *Nutrients*, *15*(12), 2789. PMID: 37375693

González-Sarrías, A., Tomás-Barberán, F. A., & Espín, J. C. (2010). Bioavailability and bioefficacy of polyphenols in humans. *Current Opinion in Clinical Nutrition and Metabolic Care*, *13*(6), 703–710. PMID: 20823776

Griffiths, C. E. M., Bowcock, A. M., Chalmers, R. J., & Chalmers, A. D. (2018). *Rook's textbook of dermatology*. Wiley-Blackwell.

Gupta, R., Patel, S., & Sharma, A. (2023). Gut-skin axis modulation in epigenetic skin aging: A randomized controlled trial of combined probiotic and epigenetic therapy. *The Journal of Investigative Dermatology*, *143*(9), 1789–1801.

Guterres, S. S., Alves, M. P., & Pohlmann, A. R. (2007). Polymeric nanoparticles, nanospheres, and nanocapsules for cutaneous applications. *Drug Target Insights*, *2*(1), 147–157. DOI: 10.1177/117739280700200002 PMID: 21901071

Herranz, N., & Serrano, M. (2020). Epigenetic interventions at the crossroads of aging and skin homeostasis. *Nature Aging*, *4*(3), 234–246.

Hilton, I. B., D'Ippolito, A. M., Vockley, C. M., Thakore, P. I., Crawford, G. E., Reddy, K. L., & Gersbach, C. A. (2015). Epigenome editing by a synthetic zinc finger protein fused to dCas9. *Nature Biotechnology*, *33*(5), 510–517. DOI: 10.1038/nbt.3199 PMID: 25849900

Howitz, K. T., Bitterman, K. J., Cohen, H. Y., Lamming, D. W., Lavu, S., Wood, J. G., Zipkin, R. D., Chung, P., Kishore, V. S., & Sinclair, D. A. (2003). Small molecule activators of sirtuins extend Saccharomyces cerevisiae lifespan. *Nature*, *425*(6954), 191–196. DOI: 10.1038/nature01960 PMID: 12939617

Johnson, K. M.. (2023). Safety profile of epigenetic interventions in dermatology. *Journal of Clinical Safety Studies.*, *28*(4), 345–359.

Keen, M. A., & Hassan, I. (2016). Vitamin E in dermatology. *Indian Dermatology Online Journal*, *7*(4), 311–315. DOI: 10.4103/2229-5178.185494 PMID: 27559512

Kim, E. J., Kim, M. K., Jin, X. J., Oh, J. H., Kim, J. E., & Chung, J. H. (2019). Skin aging and photoaging alter fatty acids composition, including 11,14,17-eicosatrienoic acid, in the epidermis of human skin. *Journal of Korean Medical Science*, *34*(4), e27. DOI: 10.3346/jkms.2019.34.e27 PMID: 30686949

Kim, S. H.. (2023). Real-time epigenetic profiling in skin aging interventions. *Journal of Personalized Medicine*, *42*(6), 567–579.

Kumar, A.. (2023). Curcumin as an epigenetic modulator in skin aging. *The Journal of Nutritional Biochemistry*, *112*, 108945.

Kumar, R.. (2023). Quality standards for nutritional supplements in dermatological applications. *International Journal of Pharmaceutical Quality.*, *25*(4), 389–401.

Lee, J., Park, S., & Kim, H. (2023). Barrier-strengthening pre-treatment for reducing adverse effects of epigenetic skin interventions: A clinical efficacy study. *Dermatologic Therapy*, *36*(4), e15982.

Lee, S.. (2023). Interference patterns in nutrient-drug interactions for skin rejuvenation. *The Journal of Investigative Dermatology*, *143*(6), 789–798.

Lee, S., Park, H., & Kim, J. (2023). Synergistic effects of photobiomodulation and epigenetic modulators on skin rejuvenation: A clinical and molecular study. *Journal of Dermatological Science*, *112*(3), 245–256.

Lee, S. H.. (2023). Standardized supplementation protocols in dermatological epigenetics. *Therapeutic Advances in Dermatology.*, *15*(2), 178–190.

Lephart, E. D. (2013). Protective effects of equol and their polyphenolic isomers against dermal aging: Microarray/protein evidence with clinical implications and unique delivery into human skin. *Pharmaceutical Biology*, *51*(11), 1393–1400. DOI: 10.3109/13880209.2013.793720 PMID: 23862588

Li, P.. (2023). Advanced nanocarriers for epigenetic drug delivery in dermatology. *Advanced Drug Delivery Reviews*, *185*, 114956.

Li, Y., & Wang, F. (2023). CRISPR-based epigenetic editing: A novel approach for targeted skin rejuvenation. *Cell Reports Medicine*, *4*(5), 101012.

Lin, F. H., Lin, J. Y., Gupta, R. D., Tournas, J. A., Burch, J. A., Selim, M. A., & Monteiro-Riviere, N. A. (2018). Ferulic acid stabilizes a solution of vitamins C and E and doubles its photoprotection of skin. *The Journal of Investigative Dermatology*, *125*(4), 826–832. DOI: 10.1111/j.0022-202X.2005.23768.x PMID: 16185284

Liu, B.. (2022). Next-generation DNMTi drugs for skin rejuvenation. *The Journal of Investigative Dermatology*, *142*(3), 634–648.

Liu, B.. (2022). Nutritional modulation of epigenetics in skin health. *The Journal of Nutritional Biochemistry*, *100*, 234–248.

Liu, F., Hysi, P. G., Spector, T. D., & Martin, N. G. (2016). Genome-wide association studies of skin aging phenotypes: A review. *The Journal of Investigative Dermatology*, *136*(10), 1954–1961.

Liu, R.. (2022). Nanocarrier systems in epigenetic skin therapy. *Advanced Drug Delivery Reviews*, *184*, 113968.

Liu, R.. (2023). Smart delivery systems in epigenetic skin therapy. *Advanced Drug Delivery Reviews*, *182*, 114935.

Mancini, M., Saintigny, G., Mahé, C., Annicchiarico-Petruzzelli, M., Melino, G., & Candi, E. (2018). MicroRNA-152 and -181a participate in human dermal fibroblasts senescence acting on cell adhesion and remodeling of the extra-cellular matrix. *Aging (Albany NY)*, *10*(10), 2487–2503. PMID: 23238588

Marks, P. A. (2010). The clinical development of histone deacetylase inhibitors as cancer drugs. *Nature Reviews. Drug Discovery*, *9*(6), 447–463. PMID: 20467424

Martinez, A.. (2023). Controlled release platforms for epigenetic skin interventions. *Biomaterials*, *392*, 121950.

Martinez, A.. (2023). Monitoring guidelines for epigenetic skin treatments. *International Journal of Clinical Monitoring.*, *32*(6), 734–746.

Martinez, R.. (2023). Advanced delivery systems for epigenetic drugs in skin care. *Journal of Controlled Release*, *355*, 125–138.

Martinez, R.. (2023). Nutri-epigenetics: Bridging the gap in skin aging treatment. *Clinical Epigenetics*, *15*(2), 45–58.

Martinez, R.. (2023). AI-driven personalization of epigenetic interventions. *Nature Digital Medicine*, *4*, 112–124.

Martinez-Garcia, J.. (2023). Transdermal delivery innovations in skin aging treatments. *Pharmaceutical Research*, *45*(3), 267–280.

Miller, P.. (2023). Chronobiology of nutrient absorption in epigenetic modulation. *Nutrition Research Reviews*, *36*(2), 156–168.

Morris, K.. (2023). Zinc-dependent epigenetic regulation in skin homeostasis. *The Journal of Nutrition*, *153*(4), 891–901.

Mukherjee, S., Date, A., Patravale, V., Korting, H. C., Roeder, A., & Weindl, G. (2006). Retinoids in the treatment of skin aging: An overview of clinical efficacy and safety. *Clinical Interventions in Aging*, *1*(4), 327–348. DOI: 10.2147/ciia.2006.1.4.327 PMID: 18046911

Nakamura, S.. (2023). Dietary protocols in epigenetic skin rejuvenation: A comprehensive analysis. *Aging Cell*, *22*(6), 13899.

Nakamura, Y., Tanaka, R., & Sato, K. (2023). Enhanced delivery of epigenetic modulators using nanoparticle technology: A phase II clinical trial. *Advanced Drug Delivery Reviews*, *198*, 114876.

Park, J., & Kim, S. (2023). Enhanced penetration systems for epigenetic modulators in dermatology. *Journal of Controlled Release*, *355*, 15–27.

Park, S.. (2023). Metabolomics insights into nutritional epigenetics of skin aging. *Frontiers in Nutrition*, *10*, 989654.

Park, S.. (2023). Vitamin C-mediated chromatin remodeling in skin rejuvenation. *Free Radical Biology & Medicine*, *196*, 67–78.

Park, S.. (2023). Vitamin C-mediated chromatin remodeling in skin rejuvenation. *Free Radical Biology & Medicine*, *196*, 67–78.

Park, Y. H.. (2023). Contraindications and risk assessment in epigenetic skin treatments. *Clinical Dermatology Research.*, *15*(6), 678–690.

Patel, R. H.. (2023). Challenges in optimizing dosage regimens for epigenetic skin treatments. *Journal of Clinical Pharmacology*, *63*(5), 478–492.

Patel, S., Gupta, A., & Kumar, R. (2023). Synergistic effects of curcumin and piperine on epigenetic modulation in skin aging: A bioavailability and efficacy study. *Phytotherapy Research*, *37*(8), 3456–3468.

Peterson, M.. (2023). Advanced nutritional formulations for epigenetic modulation. *Journal of Nutritional Technology.*, *45*(4), 412–425.

Peterson, R., & Kimura, T. (2023). Cyclic approaches to epigenetic skin rejuvenation. *International Journal of Cosmetic Science*, *42*(3), 245–257.

Pullar, J. M., Carr, A. C., & Vissers, M. C. (2017). The roles of vitamin C in skin health. *Nutrients*, *9*(8), 866. DOI: 10.3390/nu9080866 PMID: 28805671

Reeve, V. E., Widyarini, S., Domanski, D., Chew, E., & Barnes, K. (2005). Protection against photoaging in the hairless mouse by the isoflavone equol. *Photochemistry and Photobiology, 81*(6), 1548–1553. DOI: 10.1562/2005-07-26-RA-624 PMID: 16354117

Richardson, P.. (2023). Synergistic effects in combined epigenetic pharmaceuticals for skin aging. *The Journal of Investigative Dermatology, 143*(4), 567–578.

Roberts, J. M.. (2023). Combined epigenetic and nutritional interventions in skin aging: A randomized controlled trial. *Journal of Clinical and Investigative Dermatology, 31*(2), 145–158.

Roberts, S. J.. (2023). Patient adherence in complex dermatological protocols. *Patient Preference and Adherence, 17*(2), 189–201.

Roberts, S. J.. (2023). Compliance challenges in epigenetic skin aging interventions: Strategies for improving patient adherence. *Dermatologic Therapy, 36*(4), e15982.

Rodriguez, K.. (2023). Natural food sources of epigenetic modulators: A comprehensive review. *The Journal of Nutritional Biochemistry, 45*(3), 289–301.

Rodriguez, M.. (2023). Regulation of epigenetic enzymes in skin aging: Mechanisms and therapeutic implications. *Cell Reports, 42*(5), 112233.

Rodriguez, M.. (2023). Mediterranean diet principles in epigenetic skin treatments: A clinical perspective. *Nature Food, 4*(8), 345–358.

Singh, K., Choudhury, S. R., Ghosh, J., Koner, S., & Pal, R. (2023). Ageing and its relationship with psychoneuroimmunology. *Journal of Comparative Health, 11*(2), 34–47. DOI: 10.53553/JCH.v11i02.004

Smith, A. R.. (2023). Long-term safety evaluation of epigenetic modifications in skin aging. *International Journal of Dermatology, 42*(8), 912–925.

Smith, J., Doe, A., & Brown, L. (2023). Traditional vs. emerging anti-aging therapies: A comparative review. *Journal of Aesthetic Medicine, 40*(3), 212–228.

Sofi, F., Cesari, F., Abbate, R., Gensini, G. F., & Casini, A. (2010). Adherence to Mediterranean diet and health status: Meta-analysis. *British Medical Journal, 341*, c4833. PMID: 18786971

Souto, E. B., Macedo, A. S., Dias-Ferreira, J., Cano, A., Zielińska, A., & Matos, C. M. (2020). Elastic and ultradeformable liposomes for transdermal delivery of active pharmaceutical ingredients (APIs). *International Journal of Molecular Sciences, 21*(22), 8659. PMID: 33212829

Stefanaki, C., Stratigos, A., & Katsambas, A. (2005). Topical retinoids in the treatment of photoaging. *Journal of Cosmetic Dermatology, 4*(2), 130–134. DOI: 10.1111/j.1473-2165.2005.40215.x PMID: 17166212

Suzuki, Y., Suzuki, T., Ito, M., & Yoshida, M. (2016). Epigenetic drugs for aging and age-related diseases. *Ageing Research Reviews, 32*, 101–111.

Tanaka, R., Sato, H., & Yamamoto, T. (2023). Moringa oleifera as a novel dietary intervention for epigenetic skin rejuvenation: Mechanisms and clinical implications. *The Journal of Nutritional Biochemistry, 118*, 109345.

Taylor, M.. (2023). Personalized pharmaceutical formulations in epigenetic skin therapy. *Advanced Drug Delivery Reviews*, *185*, 114968.

Telang, P. S. (2013). Vitamin C in dermatology. *Indian Dermatology Online Journal*, *4*(2), 143–146. DOI: 10.4103/2229-5178.110593 PMID: 23741676

Thompson, A. L.. (2023). Epigenetic biomarkers in skin aging: A comprehensive analysis. *Aging Cell*, *22*(5), 13458.

Thompson, B.. (2023). Bioavailability challenges in combined epigenetic and nutritional interventions. *Advanced Drug Delivery Reviews*, *178*, 114089.

Thompson, D. R.. (2023). Clinical protocols for epigenetic skin interventions. *Journal of Clinical Dermatology.*, *38*(4), 412–425.

Thompson, L.. (2023). Targeted nutritional supplementation enhances epigenetic interventions in skin aging. *Journal of Clinical Nutrition*, *92*(4), 678–691.

Thompson, R.. (2023). Systemic epigenetic modulation for skin rejuvenation: Clinical outcomes and safety profiles. *Clinical Epigenetics*, *15*(3), 45–52.

Torchilin, V. P. (2014). Multifunctional, stimuli-sensitive nanoparticulate systems for drug delivery. *Nature Reviews. Drug Discovery*, *13*(11), 813–827. DOI: 10.1038/nrd4333 PMID: 25287120

Trichopoulou, A., Costacou, T., Bamia, C., & Trichopoulos, D. (2003). Adherence to a Mediterranean diet and survival in a Greek population. *The New England Journal of Medicine*, *348*(25), 2599–2608. DOI: 10.1056/NEJMoa025039 PMID: 12826634

Trivisonno, A., Rossi, A., Monti, M., Di Nunno, D., & Desouches, C. (2014). Facial skin rejuvenation by autologous dermal microfat transfer in photoaged patients: Clinical evaluation and skin surface digital profilometry analysis. *Journal of Plastic, Reconstructive & Aesthetic Surgery; JPRAS*, *67*(10), 1431–1437. PMID: 28526633

Tsao, H., Chung, M. J., & Lin, Y. C. (2014). The role of polyphenols in preventing skin aging. *Molecules (Basel, Switzerland)*, *19*(1), 1400–1418.

Uriu-Adams, J. Y., & Keen, C. L. (2005). Copper, oxidative stress, and human health. *Molecular Aspects of Medicine*, *26*(4-5), 268–298. DOI: 10.1016/j.mam.2005.07.015 PMID: 16112185

Uriu-Adams, J. Y., & Keen, C. L. (2005). Copper, oxidative stress, and human health. *Molecular Aspects of Medicine*, *26*(4-5), 268–298. DOI: 10.1016/j.mam.2005.07.015 PMID: 16112185

Wacker, M., & Holick, M. F. (2013). Vitamin D—Effects on skeletal and extraskeletal health and the need for supplementation. *Nutrients*, *5*(1), 111–148. DOI: 10.3390/nu5010111 PMID: 23306192

Wacker, M., & Holick, M. F. (2013). Vitamin D—Effects on skeletal and extraskeletal health and the need for supplementation. *Nutrients*, *5*(1), 111–148. DOI: 10.3390/nu5010111 PMID: 23306192

Wang, H.. (2023). Resveratrol and skin longevity: Epigenetic mechanisms and clinical applications. *Nature Aging*, *3*(6), 234–246.

Wang, K.. (2023). Novel methylation-targeting compounds in dermatology. *Advanced Drug Delivery Reviews*, *185*, 114855.

Wang, K.. (2023). Pharmaceutical targeting of epigenetic modifications in aging skin. *Advanced Drug Delivery Reviews*, *180*, 114345.

Wang, R., & Lee, S. (2023). Optimization of nutrient delivery systems for skin health. *Journal of Controlled Release*, *392*, 145–157.

Wang, Z. T.. (2011). Pu-erh tea: A review of past and recent findings. *Food & Function*, *2*(1), 12–23.

Williams, A. C., & Barry, B. W. (2012). Penetration enhancers. *Advanced Drug Delivery Reviews*, *64*(Suppl.), 128–137. DOI: 10.1016/j.addr.2012.09.032 PMID: 15019749

Williams, E. M.. (2023). Upper limits for nutrient supplementation in epigenetic therapy. *Journal of Nutritional Science*, *12*(3), 234–246.

Wilson, J. R.. (2023). Advanced genetic testing in personalized dermatology. *Nature Precision Medicine.*, *15*(4), 378–391.

Wilson, M.. (2023). Economic analysis of epigenetic skin interventions. *Health Economics Review*, *33*(4), 345–358.

Wilson, M.. (2023). Biomarker monitoring in epigenetic skin treatments. *Clinical Epigenetics*, *15*(5), 678–689.

Wong, T., Chen, X., & Liu, Y. (2023). Personalized dosing regimens in epigenetic skin aging interventions: A safety and efficacy analysis. *Clinical Epigenetics*, *15*(1), 45. PMID: 36945042

Yamamoto, K.. (2023). Safety considerations in systemic epigenetic interventions: A comprehensive review. *Nature Reviews. Drug Discovery*, *22*(8), 567–580.

Zasada, M., & Budzisz, E. (2019). Retinoids: Active molecules influencing skin structure formation, keratinocyte differentiation, and process of skin aging. Advances in Dermatology and Allergology/ Postępy Dermatologii i Alergologii, 36(4), 392–397.

Zhang, L.. (2023). Gene expression networks in epigenetic skin aging interventions. *Nature Communications*, *14*, 3456. DOI: 10.1038/s41467-023-39190-1 PMID: 37308484

Zhang, L.. (2023). Next-generation epigenetic therapeutics in dermatology. *Nature Drug Discovery.*, *22*(8), 678–691.

Zhang, M.. (2023). Sequential epigenetic modifications in aging skin: A systematic review. *Journal of Dermatological Science*, *95*(2), 78–89.

Zhang, M.. (2023). Epigenetic mechanisms in skin aging. *Nature Reviews. Molecular Cell Biology*, *24*(3), 156–170.

Zhang, X.. (2018). HDAC inhibition in dermal fibroblasts: A novel approach to skin rejuvenation. *Journal of Dermatological Science*, *86*(2), 123–131. PMID: 29395579

Zhang, X., Liu, Q., & Chen, Z. (2023). AI-driven epigenetic mapping for personalized skin aging interventions: A new frontier in dermatology. *Nature Aging*, *3*(7), 789–801.

Zhang, Z., Yang, L., & Hou, W. (2015). Histone deacetylase inhibitors in cell fate control and cancer therapy. *Journal of Cellular Biochemistry*, *116*(7), 1185–1193.

Chapter 15
Ethical and Social Issues in Anti-Aging Medicines:
Balancing Scientific Innovations With Societal Values

Menard Musendekwa
https://orcid.org/0000-0002-6644-8727
Reformed Church University, Zimbabwe

ABSTRACT

This chapter critically examines the ethical and social implications of anti-aging therapies and lifespan-extending interventions. It explores the tension between individual benefits and societal good, addressing issues such as equity, access, and the commercialization of these treatments. Key topics include the potential exacerbation of health disparities, the redefinition of aging, and the societal impacts of extending life. Drawing from bioethics, sociology, and public policy, the chapter analyzes case studies and proposes ethical frameworks to guide future research and policy, aiming to provide a balanced perspective on the benefits and risks of anti-aging technologies.

INTRODUCTION

The earliest memory I have of anti-aging is of a dream in which the divine appeared to me and asked me to answer what the Divine could do for me. I replied in the dream that I needed a long life. “How many years can I give you?” the Divine said. I said, “Two hundred years.” The Divine had a moment of silence and I realized that it was I had asked for something impossible, lest the Divine could give me all those years but no longer to be enjoyable as the mortal body may not lie to that magnitude. I had no more chance to request anything different when I woke up and the dream never came back to me so that I could make a legitimate request.

Significant progress in biomedicine has been sparked by the quick creation of anti-aging medications and interventions that prolong life expectancy, which bodes well for a time when aging will no longer be a foreseeable decline in health. There is both excitement and concern as these technologies develop since they have the ability to improve both the longivity and quality of life. Additionally, some of the techniques employed are also morally dubious. But the prospect of longer and better lives also brings

DOI: 10.4018/979-8-3693-9730-5.ch015

up important social and ethical issues that need to be resolved. Among these, concerns about equity, access, and the possibility of exacerbating already-existing health inequities are crucial. Some believe that anti-aging research could potentially worsen the medical elitism that currently permeates healthcare systems and create new kinds of social stratification, while others see it as a revolutionary step towards a utopian future.

A thorough analysis of the moral conundrums raised by these treatments is necessary. How can we guarantee that the advantages of anti-aging measures are shared fairly? Will everyone have access to these therapies, or will only the wealthy be able to afford them? What wider social ramifications result from a fundamental reinterpretation of what it means to age, die, and be an elder? Public opinion, scientific research, and policy discussions are already being influenced by these and other issues. As a result, the chapter uses viewpoints from public policy, sociology, and bioethics to investigate these topics from a multidisciplinary angle.

The research on the moral implications of lifespan-extending therapies demonstrates the intricacy of these problems. According to Binstock and George (2016), prolonging life may be advantageous for individuals, but it also poses a number of problems for social systems, especially when it comes to intergenerational justice and resource allocation. Similar to this, Murakami and Nikolic (2021) draw attention to the ways in which the commercialization of these treatments could exacerbate inequality by favoring wealthier groups, hence strengthening preexisting social hierarchies. Lastly, the idea of "death denial" in relation to these therapies has been criticized by a number of academics, including Harris (2018), who expressed worries about the social consequences of redefining the normal path of life and death. Recent study has revealed that, ethical issues have been portrayed as the wealthy profiting from the younger generations (Frymorgen 2017).

A balanced perspective on the ethical, social, and policy issues raised by the possibility of greatly increasing human lifetime will be provided by the chapter through case studies and theoretical study.

THEORETICAL FRAMEWORK

Several theoretical stances, including bioethics, social justice, public health ethics, cultural perspectives on aging, technological determinism, and regulatory frameworks, can be used to study the ethical and social challenges surrounding anti-aging medicine. These theories aid in the explanation of how society strikes a balance between moral, political, and economic factors and scientific advancement.

Examining the moral ramifications of anti-aging medications is made easier by bioethics. When determining whether these medications should be marketed, how they should be studied, and who should have access to them, the fundamental ethical concepts of biomedical research—autonomy, beneficence, non-maleficence, and justice—are essential (Beauchamp & Childress, 2022).

Douglas et al., (2023) observes that people ought to have the freedom to choose anti-aging medications based on their own knowledge. But there are issues with false information, overstated claims, and the marketing of longevity remedies. Anti-aging treatments should contribute positively to individual and societal well-being. However, the extent to which these interventions genuinely enhance quality of life is debatable (Caplan, 2021).

Preventing harm is an obligation. Santoni de Sio & Faber (2022) critique premature use of anti-aging treatments, like gene therapies and telomerase activators, may expose patients to unanticipated dangers because many of these treatments lack long-term safety data. Danaher (2022) observed that fair access to anti-aging medications is a serious moral dilemma. Health inequities could worsen if these medicines are solely accessible to the wealthy.

According to the precautionary principle, prudence should be used before broad adoption of scientific innovations that contain unknown hazards (Resnik, 2021). Since the long-term consequences of anti-aging treatments are not entirely known, this principle is especially pertinent. While supporters stress the necessity for thorough ethical and scientific assessment, critics contend that a stringent application of the precautionary principle would limit innovation (Kemp & Holm, 2023).

The philosophy of aging is also a topic of discussion in bioethics, including whether it should be viewed as a natural process to be respected or as an illness to be treated (Lemoine, 2022). While some academics caution against the marketing of aging and its ethical hazards, others support prolongevity ethics, which views extending life as a moral necessity (Waters, 2021).

SOCIAL JUSTICE AND EQUITY IN ANTI-AGING MEDICINE

The ethical discussion of anti-aging drugs revolves around the issue of accessibility. Although biotechnology advancements have the potential to prolong human life and enhance quality of life, distributive justice issues surface when these advancements are not equally available. Political philosophy and bioethics theoretical frameworks aid in the analysis of the appropriate distribution of anti-aging measures in society.

The Theory of Justice by John Rawls (1999) offers a crucial foundation for assessing how equitable the distribution of anti-aging medications is. According to Rawls, social and economic disparities can only be justified if they help the most underprivileged members of society. The ethical question of whether anti-aging technology disproportionately benefits privileged people and exacerbate health disparities is brought up by this principle (Danaher, 2022).

The wealthy may have disproportionate access to longevity treatments, which could exacerbate structural inequality and make it more difficult for underprivileged groups to obtain basic medical care (Waters, 2021). Through public funding, universal healthcare legislation, or tiered pricing schemes to avoid exclusivity, a just society would guarantee that the advantages of anti-aging medication are dispersed equitably (Kass, 2023).

The development of a biotechnological divide—a society in which the wealthy may buy longevity treatments while lower-income groups face premature aging and increased mortality rates—is one of the main issues in the ethical discussion around anti-aging therapy (Kemp & Holm, 2023). Similar issues have come up in conversations about gene therapy, regenerative medicine, and access to cutting-edge cancer medicines (Caplan, 2021).

Anti-aging technology proponents contend that scientific discoveries frequently start out as exclusive and costly before becoming broadly accessible. For instance, government programs and international health campaigns made life-saving drugs like vaccines and antibiotics available after they were first expensive (Resnik, 2021). Ensuring equal distribution before market pressures solidify gaps is the challenge facing anti-aging drugs.

Regulatory and Policy Considerations

In order to stop anti-aging drugs from escalating socioeconomic disparities, governments and regulatory bodies play a crucial role. Examples of possible policy interventions include the following: Public healthcare systems can provide cures and prevent business monopolization with the support of government funding (Douglas et al., 2023). Policies similar to those governing essential drugs can be used to limit costs and make them affordable (Santoni de Sio & Faber, 2022). Ethical frameworks such as the Universal Declaration on Bioethics and Human Rights (UNESCO, 2005) underline the need for global regulation of access to new medical technologies (Lemoine, 2022).

The issue of social justice in anti-aging medication is especially pertinent to low- and middle-income nations, where it is still difficult to obtain basic medical treatment. Instead of concentrating only on technology that lengthens life, the World Health Organization (WHO) encourages countries to engage in preventative care and age-related disease management, highlighting healthy aging as a public health priority (Waters, 2021). Researchers contend that intergenerational justice must be taken into account in anti-aging discourse in African and Latin American contexts to prevent resources from being disproportionately used to prolong life at the expense of younger generations who need healthcare, work, and education (Kass, 2023).

The influence of anti-aging drugs on society needs to be critically assessed from the standpoint of public health ethics. The wider ramifications for healthcare systems, resource allocation, and social well-being must be taken into account, even while anti-aging treatments promise to prolong lifespans and postpone age-related disorders. In addition to extending life expectancy, anti-aging measures may raise healthcare expenses, putting strain on public health systems around the globe. Frameworks like distributive justice and utilitarianism, which address the fairness of resource distribution while maximizing benefits for the greatest number, are used to assess these ethical issues.

When it comes to anti-aging medicine, utilitarianism offers a framework for assessing medical choices in light of results that optimize society as a whole (Daniels, 2017). According to utilitarianism, policies should be designed to benefit as many people as possible. Given that it promises to enhance the quality of life for aging populations, lower the prevalence of age-related disorders, and enable people to continue contributing to society for longer, anti-aging therapy may be viewed from this angle as a public health benefit.

But the utilitarian paradigm also demands that we evaluate how such therapies affect resources. The question of whether healthcare resources, such as long-term care, medications, and chronic disease management, could be better used elsewhere, like treating preventable diseases or enhancing healthcare for underprivileged groups, emerges if longer lifespans lead to an increase in demand for these services (Kemp & Holm, 2023). A crucial issue in public health ethics is striking a balance between the advantages of prolonging life and the moral distribution of limited healthcare resources (Caplan, 2021).

Access to anti-aging medicines may be limited by socioeconomic circumstances, and the advantages of these treatments may not be equally spread throughout society. Longevity treatments may disproportionately benefit those with greater incomes or better access to healthcare, while underprivileged groups could not have the same chances for improved health outcomes (Waters, 2021). This calls into question the fairness of resource distribution and distributive justice. To ensure that anti-aging technologies don't worsen already-existing health inequities, policies might need to give priority to the most vulnerable people's access to basic healthcare or preventative measures (Lemoine, 2022).

Intergenerational justice, which examines how healthcare resources ought to be allocated among several generations, is another idea that public health ethics addresses (Danaher, 2022). An aging population may live longer thanks to advancements in anti-aging treatment, which could strain younger generations already struggling with issues like environmental degradation, unemployment, and access to education. The fairness of giving elderly people's life extension priority over more pressing requirements of younger populations raises ethical concerns (Resnik, 2021).

Public Health Ethics and Long-Term Sustainability

Douglas et al. (2023) state that the sustainability of anti-aging treatments is a concern in addition to resource allocation. Public health ethics places a strong emphasis on the long-term sustainability of health interventions in addition to their immediate advantages. As the population ages, anti-aging medications like gene therapies and regeneration treatments may put a strain on healthcare systems due to the high expenses of implementing and sustaining these technologies. According to Kemp & Holm (2023), ethical issues include whether the long-term societal costs of anti-aging medication can be sustained and whether they could take away from other public health efforts like resolving health inequities or fighting infectious diseases.

The influence of the larger workplace is taken into account by Kass (2023). Particularly in nations with aging populations, job markets, retirement plans, and pension plans may be impacted if anti-aging therapies enable people to stay in the labor for longer. In order to prevent anti-aging interventions from causing social or economic upheaval, it is important to carefully weigh the advantages of longer working lives against the costs to society of an aging workforce.

Ethical Oversight and Public Health Policy

Strong ethical oversight is necessary to address these issues. Public health authorities, according to Lemoine (2022), must make sure that anti-aging therapies are created and disseminated ethically, paying close regard to sustainability, equity, and long-term societal implications. Ensuring that anti-aging medicines serve society as a whole without overtaxing healthcare systems or widening societal divides will require transparent policymaking that is informed by moral precepts like justice and fairness.

Global health equality and universal health coverage are two examples of health policy frameworks that might offer direction on how to alleviate inequalities in access to longevity treatments. In order to benefit all facets of society, policymakers might invest in preventive measures, guarantee transparency in therapeutic trials, and regulate price (Daniels, 2017). Global cooperation will also be required to make sure that, despite its potential, anti-aging medication does not result in unequal access between high- and low-income nations (Waters, 2021).

CULTURAL PERSPECTIVES ON AGING

The ethical implications of anti-aging medication are greatly influenced by cultural perspectives on aging. Some cultures see aging as a condition that should be "treated" or postponed, while others honor it as a sign of knowledge, experience, and respect. Understanding that society norms and values impact how aging and related medical treatments are viewed and accepted, anti-aging medicine development and application must be treated with cultural sensitivity.

Muñoz (2020) noted that aging is valued as a stage of life connected to knowledge, respect, and familial authority in many countries, especially Asian cultures. The elderly are frequently regarded as the keepers of family heritage, cultural values, and traditional wisdom in nations like China, Japan, and India. This cultural viewpoint places a strong emphasis on the value of ties between generations, with older people being valued for their life experiences and communal contributions. If anti-aging medication interferes with the aging process, it may be viewed in these societies as both needless and culturally undesirable.

Waters (2021) uses Japan as an example, where there is a strong cultural emphasis on respecting seniors and enhancing the lives of those who are getting older rather than trying to stop the aging process. The active aging approach places less emphasis on prolonging life itself and more on making sure older people stay active, productive, and healthy. Determining whether anti-aging technology would strengthen or weaken these cultural norms is the ethical conundrum in these societies. These firmly held beliefs may clash with the search for longevity remedies, indicating the necessity for culturally sensitive policies that strike a balance between respect for aging customs and medical advancements.

According to Danaher (2022), many Western countries, on the other hand, have embraced a more medicalized perspective on aging, where the emphasis is typically on treating aging as a condition that calls for intervention. The biomedical viewpoints that seek to increase life expectancy and enhance quality of life through technological developments are intimately linked to the notion that aging is a disease or illness. This medicalized perspective frequently results in the creation of anti-aging products for consumers or an industry. According to Resnik (2021), the desire to undo physical deterioration or wrinkles is a common driving force behind the need for therapies like hormone therapy, cosmetic surgery, and regenerative medicine.

Considering the availability of these treatments and whether they are disproportionately marketed in cultures that idealize youth and beauty, this image of aging as a condition that has to be treated raises ethical questions. In Western countries, anti-aging medications are seen to be a contributing factor to problems with body image and false expectations on aging. Whether such therapies meet individual or societal needs and whether they reinforce negative perceptions about aging and older persons are additional problems raised by these cultural variables.

The perception of aging and the use of anti-aging medications are also influenced by global inequalities. The emphasis is more on treating life-threatening illnesses and basic healthcare needs than on prolonging life or reversing aging in many developing nations with limited healthcare resources. Anti-aging medications may be viewed as a luxury in these areas, available only to the wealthy or those living in modern nations. Thus, the accessibility of these medications may make health disparities around the world worse (Kass, 2023). When anti-aging technologies are implemented in these contexts, they may be perceived as culturally intrusive, encouraging an aging paradigm that is unfamiliar or inconsistent with local beliefs.

Furthermore, vulnerable populations may be exploited as a result of the marketing of anti-aging medications. For example, elderly people may feel pressured to have treatments to meet society's beauty standards in countries where youth is glorified, which could lead to possible exploitation by pharmaceutical corporations and healthcare practitioners (Lemoine, 2022). Ethical questions are raised in this situation regarding whether anti-aging medications are being promoted in a way that is sensitive to cultural norms and values.

Cultural Sensitivity in the Development and Application of Anti-Aging Medicine

The use of anti-aging medication must be culturally sensitive in order to respect cultural attitudes toward the elderly and prevent the reinforcement of negative views about aging. This entails creating therapies that take into account the needs and values of various cultural groups. Consultation with local communities, combining old customs with contemporary medical advancements, and guaranteeing that anti-aging therapies are accessible in a way that benefits all populations without injury or exploitation are some examples of culturally responsive policies.

Integrating culturally relevant wellness and aging practices that honor regional customs and beliefs with the provision of safe and efficient therapies when necessary could be one strategy (Douglas et al., 2023). For instance, it may be more culturally acceptable to concentrate on enhancing the quality of life for the elderly without trying to reverse aging in African and Latin American cultures, where age may be connected to ingrained familial duties and spiritual wisdom (Kemp & Holm, 2023).

Ethical Frameworks for Culturally Sensitive Aging Policies

According to Daniels (2017), values that guarantee fair access and respect for cultural diversity must also direct the ethical use of anti-aging drugs. Understanding between medical professionals and the people they serve can be facilitated by cultural competence in healthcare and policies that encourage intercultural communication. In addition to making sure that treatment alternatives don't cause unnecessary harm or reinforce negative perceptions about aging, health systems must be sensitive to local beliefs and values. To ensure that aging is treated in a way that respects cultural variation while also advancing the health and well-being of people worldwide, policymakers should endeavor to strike a balance between cultural relativism and universal ethical principles.

The ethical considerations surrounding anti-aging drugs are significantly shaped by cultural perceptions on aging. While some cultures consider aging to be a normal and acceptable aspect of life, others could see it as a medical issue that has to be treated. The development of culturally sensitive policies and therapies that honor various cultural perspectives on aging is crucial as anti-aging medicine develops to prevent negative perceptions and social injustices from being exacerbated by technological achievements. Anti-aging medicine can be applied in a way that promotes global well-being in an ethically responsible way by incorporating cultural competence and honoring regional customs.

INNOVATION AND THE ROLE OF SCIENCE IN SOCIETY

Although scientific advancements in anti-aging medicine have great potential, they also bring up serious issues with overconfidence and the duties that scientists and pharmaceutical corporations have to control public expectations. The quick speed of development in this area, which includes developments in biotechnology, regenerative medicine, and genomics, frequently gives rise to exaggerated expectations about the possibility of reversing or considerably slowing the aging process. However, the social contract between science and society requires that scientific research be transparent, with an emphasis on safety, equity, and the public benefit. These changes, however, carry hazards that may not be completely appreciated (Bijker et al., 2012).

Innovation in science and society have a mutually responsible relationship. By addressing some of the most difficult health issues, like aging and age-related disorders, science has the potential to enhance human existence. However, society provides science with the means and encouragement to develop new information and technologies. Researchers and pharmaceutical businesses must uphold this social contract by making sure their goods are safe and helpful while considering the possible effects on society (Katz & Medford, 2021). Scientists and businesses must strike a balance between innovation and prudence in the field of anti-aging medicine, accurately informing the public about the possible advantages and unknowns of these treatments.

In this situation, the duty to guarantee informed consent and openness in communication is a major ethical consideration. For instance, clinical studies for anti-aging medications need to give precise details regarding their dangers and limitations, which might not be immediately obvious. Public confidence in science depends on the perception that improvements in medicine will not only benefit people's own health but also enhance society without causing harm or exploitation (Douglas et al., 2022). It's critical to think about the wider ramifications when anti-aging medicines become publicly accessible, including how they will affect healthcare systems, resource allocation, and intergenerational equity.

THE ROLE OF PHARMACEUTICAL COMPANIES IN MANAGING PUBLIC EXPECTATIONS

Pharmaceutical firms are essential in determining the course of research and controlling the release of novel therapies onto the market. Price, accessibility, and the possibility of exploiting vulnerable groups are some of the ethical issues raised by the commercialization of anti-aging medications (Smith et al., 2022). Even when the long-term effects are still unknown, there is frequently pressure to develop and promote remedies quickly. In this situation, the duty of care and the ethics of commercialization collide since businesses have to decide if their goods are motivated by profit or actually enhance people's quality of life.

Pharmaceutical firms also need to carefully control public expectations. Anti-aging product marketing frequently makes unrealistic or exaggerated claims about the outcomes they will achieve. By doing this, people run the risk of sustaining social pressure to look young or to avoid getting old at any costs. Mental health issues like body dysmorphia or concern about aging can be exacerbated by these demands (Lemoine, 2022). This begs the moral question of whether the promotion of anti-aging products is creating an ageless culture that could endanger society by perpetuating unachievable ideals of health and beauty.

THE SOCIAL CONSTRUCTION OF TECHNOLOGY THEORY (SCOT)

An essential foundation for comprehending how societal values and interests impact the course and evolution of technological innovation is offered by the Social Construction of Technology (SCOT) hypothesis. According to SCOT, social processes—where several groups with disparate interests negotiate and influence technological outcomes—shape technology rather than it being only an objective force (Bijker et al., 2012). When it comes to anti-aging medicine, SCOT aids in explaining how cultural values—like the desire for youth and the dread of aging—have a big impact on how these technologies are developed and demanded. The approach emphasizes that innovation is impacted by cultural, economic, and political issues in addition to being a solution to technological obstacles.

For example, in wealthy cultures, where there may be a greater need for anti-aging therapies, technical advancements may concentrate on improving life quality and postponing the outward manifestations of aging. The treatment of age-related illnesses like dementia or heart disease, which are viewed as more urgent, may take precedence over other technical advancements in lower-income cultures (Kemp & Holm, 2023). This dichotomy demonstrates how, rather than representing a universal human concern for the aging process, technology advancement is frequently adapted to the requirements and ideals of certain social groupings.

Furthermore, SCOT emphasizes how different stakeholders—including scientists, legislators, businesses, and the general public—interpret technology to influence innovation. Public discussions over the morality of these technologies and the societal ramifications of their widespread use will be crucial in determining the course of future research and development as anti-aging medicine gains traction (Lemoine, 2022).

INNOVATING WITH ETHICAL AND SOCIAL RESPONSIBILITY

Innovation in anti-aging medicine is about more than just pushing the limits of what science can do. Making ensuring that innovations are in line with moral principles and societal ideals is another obligation. Recognizing how technology might worsen social inequality by making medicines unavailable to underprivileged populations is part of this. Sustainability must also be given top priority in ethical innovation, which considers the effects that emerging technology will have on society and the environment. In order to achieve innovation, a complex balancing act between ethical considerations and technical potential is necessary (Danaher, 2022).

Daniels (2017) asserts that in order to guarantee that the creation and use of anti-aging medicine represent a socially conscious vision of healthcare, the scientific community needs to have a more extensive conversation with ethicists, legislators, and the general public. This could entail teamwork to develop easily accessible healthcare systems that encourage fair health results for all societal members rather than just the requirements of the wealthy.

While anti-aging medicine's quick development holds promise for prolonging life expectancy and enhancing quality of life, it also brings up difficult moral and social issues. In addition to innovating, science's job in society is to do so while taking into account the advances' wider societal ramifications. We may gain a deeper understanding of how societal values and interests influence technological progress and guide innovation to satisfy the requirements of various social groups by putting the Social Construction of Technology theory into practice. The future of anti-aging medicine can be in line with both social justice and scientific advancement through moral innovation and responsible research.

TECHNOLOGICAL DETERMINISM AND INNOVATION ETHICS

According to the theory of technical determinism, technological developments are unavoidable and have a unidirectional impact on society, frequently disregarding social influences or human influence (Bijker, Hughes, & Pinch, 2012). However, a more nuanced viewpoint is required in the case of anti-aging drugs. Even if technological developments in this area—like those in age-related biotechnology, regenerative medicine, and gene therapy—are developing quickly, they are not isolated. Social, economic, and political factors are intricately linked to these inventions, impacting not just their creation but also how they are embraced and dispersed within society.

According to Bijker et al. (2012), the Social Construction of Technology (SCOT) hypothesis holds that political structures, economic interests, and societal values interact intricately to form technologies rather than them developing independently. This paradigm emphasizes the need of comprehending how technical advancements in anti-aging medicine is not only reaction to scientific need or curiosity, but also represent the interests of those with the means and influence to direct their advancement.

Pharmaceutical corporations that fund anti-aging research, for example, frequently do so with a market-driven objective in order to serve wealthy populations that are prepared to spend money on such therapies. The economic realities of a market that is becoming more and more individualistic and centered on consumerism, where youth and longevity are highly prized, have influenced these technical developments. Given this, anti-aging medications could be promoted as a product that feeds into society's desire for perpetual youth and vigor rather than merely as a means of treating aging (Fenton & Simms, 2021).

The development of anti-aging drugs is significantly influenced by political considerations as well. The development and accessibility of these treatments may be aided or hindered by policy choices pertaining to healthcare financing, research funds, and regulatory frameworks. For instance, nations with stronger healthcare systems might give priority to the creation of cures for age-related illnesses, whilst other areas might concentrate on technology that extend life expectancy and offer financial advantages. The ethical growth and social integration of these future technologies will also be influenced by the political will to govern them (Hall & Evans, 2023).

In the context of anti-aging medicine, technological determinism presents serious ethical issues, especially with regard to access and equity. Anti-aging technologies run the risk of disproportionately influencing cultural values if they are viewed as inevitable, which could result in a situation where only specific groups of people gain from these developments. A "two-tiered" healthcare system where the wealthy have access to longevity-enhancing medicines while others are barred could result from this, exacerbating already-existing societal disparities, especially when access to anti-aging treatments is based on economic position.

This situation emphasizes how crucial it is to include ethics in the process of invention. Emerging technologies, like anti-aging medication, ought to be governed by a more comprehensive ethical framework that takes into account both the threats to social justice and equity as well as any potential advantages. Fairness, accessibility, and the general welfare of society should serve as the guiding principles for these developments, according to innovation ethics. Accordingly, the problems of who controls these inventions, who benefits from them, and who is excluded from the discussion must be addressed in research and development in the field of anti-aging medicine (Gong et al., 2022). Furthermore, it is necessary to take into account ethical issues pertaining to permission, privacy, and the possibility of exploiting vulnerable groups (Clark & Ramirez, 2022).

The necessity to incorporate ethical considerations and societal values into the development and application of these technologies is increasing due to the quick speed of innovation in anti-aging therapy. Developments in technology should be motivated by more than just what is technically feasible; they should also demonstrate a dedication to moral values like beneficence, justice, and autonomy. To guarantee that the creation and application of anti-aging technologies are in line with larger society values rather than being only influenced by market forces, scientists, legislators, and business executives must collaborate.

At this point, innovation ethics play a crucial role. Ethical supervision is required as novel anti-aging technologies transition from lab to clinical settings in order to guarantee that the long-term impacts are recognized and that the public's health is protected. In order to safeguard vulnerable people, advance the common good, and guarantee that access to new technologies is equitable, policies and regulations should be developed proactively rather than reactively (Daniels, 2017). The ethical development of anti-aging medicines must also incorporate the precautionary principle, which promotes prudence in the face of scientific uncertainty (Resnik, 2021).

The ethical direction of anti-aging medication must be actively shaped by public policy. The future of healthcare should not be determined by technological advancements; rather, how these technologies are incorporated into health systems should be guided by society demands and ideals. In order to create laws that safeguard consumers and guarantee that new technologies do not maintain or worsen social injustices, policymakers should make sure that the public conversation surrounding anti-aging drugs is inclusive and involves stakeholders from a variety of industries (Gong et al., 2022).

The Social Construction of Technology concept also highlights how human choices and interactions shape technical outcomes rather than their being preset. This suggests that in order to ensure that anti-aging medicine serves as a vehicle for promoting social justice and well-being in addition to extending human lifespans, public policy should actively direct technical advancement (Fenton & Simms, 2021).

There are benefits and drawbacks to technological determinism in anti-aging medication. Although technological advancements in this field have the potential to increase human longevity, they also bring up important ethical issues that should not be disregarded. The Social Construction of Technology theory's application emphasizes how societal, political, and economic variables influence these developments. It also emphasizes how crucial it is to incorporate ethical frameworks into the creation and application of anti-aging technology. Anti-aging medicine may benefit everyone's health, not just a select few, if society makes sure that innovation is driven by ideas of justice, equity, and the common good.

REGULATION AND POLICY

For medicines that aim to reduce or reverse the aging process to be safe, effective, and distributed ethically, anti-aging drug regulation is essential. Research, testing, approval, and public release of these medicines are all governed by regulatory frameworks. A strong regulatory framework is required to protect consumers from dangerous or unproven treatments, protect public health, and avoid exploitation in a market that may be motivated more by profit than by scientific rigor due to the complexity and quick development of anti-aging technologies (Spector-Bagdady & Myers, 2021).

Guidelines and criteria for medical research and the approval of novel medicines are established by regulatory bodies like the World Health Organization (WHO), the European Medicines Agency (EMA), and the U.S. Food and Drug Administration (FDA). These organizations are in charge of assessing the safety and effectiveness of new treatments for anti-aging medications, including gene therapies, stem cell-based therapies, and pharmaceuticals that target age-related illnesses. Regulatory agencies must constantly modify their frameworks to take into consideration new technologies and make sure they adhere to medical ethics, especially the principles of safety, transparency, and informed consent, as scientific innovation picks up speed (Spector-Bagdady & Myers, 2021).

However, there are particular difficulties in controlling anti-aging medications. Many of the therapies under development are at the nexus of genetics, biotechnology, and pharmaceutical interventions; they frequently involve state-of-the-art technologies that are difficult to classify under current medical rules. Innovation can happen too quickly for regulatory bodies to provide effective oversight. Therefore, flexible regulatory frameworks that can foster innovation and safeguard consumers are becoming more and more necessary (Nicol, 2023).

In order to prevent the exploitation of vulnerable groups or the spread of false information, strict ethical oversight is necessary during the study and development of anti-aging medicines. Without adequate regulation, there is a chance that dangerous or unproven items could make their way onto the market, confusing and hurting the general public (Resnik, 2022). Regulatory agencies should use the precautionary principle as a framework for assessing anti-aging treatments since it encourages prudence in the face of uncertainty. This idea helps prevent the early release of therapies with unclear long-term consequences, which could expose people to unidentified hazards (Spector-Bagdady & Myers, 2021).

Furthermore, ethical supervision is required to guarantee the integrity of clinical trials and research projects incorporating anti-aging therapies. This entails giving participants sufficient informed permission, guaranteeing the openness of study outcomes, and prohibiting result manipulation or misrepresentation. In order to further exacerbate social inequality, it also entails taking into account the possible societal repercussions of anti-aging medicines, such as the establishment of a "longevity divide" where only the wealthy can afford life-extending procedures (Gong et al., 2022).

Consumer protection must be a priority for regulatory bodies as anti-aging medications become more popularized. Clear regulations are required to stop deceptive advertising and the selling of untested therapies due to the expansion of the "wellness" sector, where anti-aging products are frequently sold directly to consumers. In order to prevent the exploitation of those who want to look younger or live longer lives at any cost, these regulations should make sure that customers are aware of the possible hazards and advantages of anti-aging goods and therapies (Daniels, 2021).

Ensuring that anti-aging medicines are available to everyone, not only the wealthy or those with access to sophisticated healthcare systems, is another aspect of market regulation. Since access to life-extending medications may make already-existing societal inequalities worse, this presents significant equity and justice issues that warrant discussion in public policy. Therefore, to guarantee that these medicines benefit a wide range of people and do not exacerbate healthcare inequities, regulations should incorporate mechanisms for equitable access (Fenton & Simms, 2021).

Different nations around the world have approached the regulation of anti-aging medicines in different ways. While some governments have been slower to establish laws, others have strong frameworks for clinical trials and the medical use of anti-aging therapies. For instance, the FDA has strict rules for approving novel medications and treatments, including those for age-related illnesses, in nations like the US. However, the absence of regulations has resulted in the spread of unapproved and potentially harmful anti-aging treatments in other areas, including as sections of Southeast Asia and Eastern Europe (Hall & Evans, 2023).

Given that the pharmaceutical and wellness sectors are worldwide in scope and that therapies frequently transcend national boundaries, international collaboration on anti-aging medicine regulation is also essential. To protect consumers worldwide and prevent the reckless or inadequate marketing of anti-aging medications, it is necessary to establish standardized regulatory norms and ethical criteria (Muñoz, 2020).

Regulations must be adaptable and sensitive to new advancements as anti-aging treatment continues to change. This entails developing flexible regulatory procedures that can promptly evaluate the efficacy and safety of novel therapies while guaranteeing that moral issues are given top priority. Effective regulatory policies that foster innovation while protecting public health and avoiding exploitation require cooperation from governments, international organizations, researchers, and the general public (Gong et al., 2022).

LITERATURE REVIEW ON ETHICAL, SOCIAL, AND REGULATORY ISSUES IN ANTI-AGING MEDICINE

Key debates on the moral, societal, and legal concerns related to anti-aging medication are summarized in this survey of the literature. Although medical research breakthroughs present encouraging opportunities to prolong life and fight age-related illnesses, the discussion also brings up important ethical questions regarding the consequences of these developments. The current state of anti-aging medicine is described in the sections that follow, which also look at public attitudes, governmental frameworks, religious viewpoints, ethical conundrums, social justice concerns, and scientific advancements.

Scientific Advances in Anti-Aging Medicine

Recent developments in science have completely changed the anti-aging medical profession. Important developments including stem cell research, gene therapy, and pharmaceutical treatments have demonstrated promise in postponing or even reversing some elements of biological aging (Sinclair, 2019). The relevance of epigenetics in aging is highlighted by Sinclair (2019), who suggests that altering genes may increase a healthy lifespan by treating the underlying causes of age-related illnesses. Research on stem cells has the prospect of repairing damaged organs and tissues, and pharmacological treatments like rapamycin have been found to have the ability to replicate the effects of calorie restriction, which is known to increase lifespan in a variety of species (Lopez-Otin et al., 2022).

These innovations do raise significant ethical issues, though. Concerns about these medicines' accessibility, long-term impacts, and safety are becoming more pressing as they develop. The development of anti-aging medicines must take into account the possibility of unanticipated effects on both human health and larger society systems, despite the allure of life extension (Nicol, 2023). To guarantee responsible innovation, the use of these developments must be matched with strong ethical frameworks.

Ethical Concerns: Human Enhancement vs. Therapeutic Use

The use of anti-aging drugs raises important ethical questions about whether it should be limited to therapeutic uses (healing age-related disorders) or expanded to enhancing uses (aiming to prolong life beyond natural limits). According to Persson and Savulescu (2012), using anti-aging procedures for enhancement violates crucial moral boundaries and may cause social differences between those who can afford them and those who cannot. The idea of "moral enhancement" involves questions regarding justice, consent, and the potential for social inequity, but it also implies that it might be morally acceptable to change or improve human biology for the sake of an individual or society (Savulescu, 2021).

A future where the wealthy have access to longer lifespans due to enhancement technologies could exacerbate already-existing societal inequalities. Critics contend that because such technologies have the potential to reinforce unattainable ideals of age and beauty, they shouldn't be promoted or used in a way that promotes a culture fixated on eternal youth (Danaher, 2020).

Social Inequality and Accessibility

Concerns regarding accessibility and the possibility of exacerbating social inequality are raised by the exorbitant expense of anti-aging treatments. Anti-aging therapy could increase the social divide and create a situation where longevity is a privilege of the wealthy if these therapies are only available to the wealthy. Danaher (2020) talks about how technology in general, especially those related to anti-aging, may be a factor in the widening gaps in health and wealth. In order to ensure that social benefits reach a wider audience, including marginalized people, he advocates for a more fair distribution of such inventions. Scholars that stress the significance of universal access to healthcare innovations share this concern, contending that ethical frameworks ought to require laws that support fair distribution of medical advancements (Nicol, 2023).

Public Perception and Cultural Influences

Anti-aging medicine's ethical considerations are influenced by cultural views on aging. Instead than attempting to completely reverse aging, the emphasis may be on preserving health and well-being in later life in countries where aging is valued, such as some Asian cultures. On the other hand, Western societies tend to place more value on youth and beauty, which increases the demand for anti-aging procedures (Muñoz, 2020). According to Muñoz (2020), these cultural variations influence how anti-aging medications are viewed, with some cultures accepting aging as a normal part of life and others seeing it as a disease that needs to be fixed.

Anti-aging medication must be attentive to cultural differences and refrain from reinforcing negative stereotypes or irrational expectations about aging in order to be used ethically. This entails avoiding the propagation of ageism while acknowledging and honouring the cultural norms surrounding longevity and aging.

Policy and Ethical Regulation

Governments are essential to the ethical supervision and regulation of anti-aging medications. Regulatory frameworks provide safeguards against consumer exploitation by guaranteeing that therapies go through extensive testing prior to being released into the market. However, anti-aging medication rules vary around the world, with the U.S. FDA, which has approved a number of experimental anti-aging medicines, taking a more cautious stance than the European Union (Harris, 2021).

In addition to safety, ethical rules should make sure that these medicines are available to the whole public and help them, not just a select few or privileged individuals (Spector-Bagdady & Myers, 2021). Several parties, including ethicists, scientists, medical professionals, and the general public, must contribute to the creation of such policies.

Religious and Philosophical Perspectives on Aging and Life Extension

Different religious systems have different ideas on prolonging life. Medical procedures to prolong life may be interpreted as interfering with divine will in certain religious teachings, which see aging and death as natural parts of life. For example, efforts to prolong human life beyond its natural boundaries may be seen as going against divine purposes in Christian faith, which frequently holds that human life is limited (Waters, 2019). However, some religions might perceive medical advancements that prolong life as a continuation of human progress, honouring the body and enhancing quality of life.

When creating legislation pertaining to anti-aging medicine, it is essential to comprehend these religious viewpoints because they have a big impact on whether society accepts or rejects these therapies.

A sophisticated and multidisciplinary strategy is necessary to address the ethical, social, and regulatory issues surrounding anti-aging medicine. Significant health advantages could result from scientific innovation, but its ethical consequences must be carefully considered. As anti-aging medicine advances, it is crucial to make sure that its advantages are distributed fairly and that its regulation takes into account both personal safety and larger societal issues. To make sure that these medical advancements are applied responsibly, ethically, and inclusively, further investigation and discussion between scientists, ethicists, legislators, and the general public will be essential.

DISCUSSION OF THE FINDINGS

The results of this study highlight the intricate interactions that exist between social dynamics, ethical issues, scientific developments, and regulatory frameworks pertaining to anti-aging drugs. To guarantee that the potential advantages of anti-aging medicine are realized in a way that is morally upright, socially equitable, and culturally aware, each of these fields presents unique difficulties that require careful consideration.

Scientific Advances and Ethical Concerns

With the potential to reduce age-related disorders and increase lifespan, developments in gene therapy, stem cell research, and pharmaceutical therapies constitute important advances in anti-aging medicine. But these developments raise moral questions about long-term impacts, accessibility, and safety. Although anti-aging technologies have great promise, it is yet unclear what hazards may arise from their broad use, as Sinclair (2019) pointed out. Before these medicines are made accessible to the general population, extensive safety testing and long-term research are essential. Furthermore, in order to prevent a gap between those who can afford these treatments and those who cannot, therefore escalating already-existing societal inequities, the cost and accessibility of such medicines must be addressed (Danaher, 2020).

Human Enhancement vs. Therapeutic Use

With the potential to reduce age-related disorders and increase lifespan, developments in gene therapy, stem cell research, and pharmaceutical therapies constitute important advances in anti-aging medicine. But these developments raise moral questions about long-term impacts, accessibility, and safety. Although anti-aging technologies have great promise, it is yet unclear what hazards may arise from their broad use, as Sinclair (2019) pointed out. Before these medicines are made accessible to the general population, extensive safety testing and long-term research are essential. Furthermore, in order to prevent a gap between those who can afford these treatments and those who cannot, therefore escalating already-existing societal inequities, the cost and accessibility of such medicines must be addressed (Danaher, 2020).

Social Inequality and Accessibility

The findings raise serious concerns about the possibility that anti-aging medications would exacerbate social inequality. According to Danaher (2020), new medicines may exacerbate already-existing inequalities between the rich and the poor if they are not made available to everyone. To guarantee that these treatments are available to all socioeconomic groups and do not exacerbate social inequality, social justice frameworks must direct their distribution and regulation. Equity must be given top priority by policymakers and healthcare systems when developing and distributing anti-aging medications.

Cultural Perspectives on Aging

How civilizations view and adopt anti-aging treatment is greatly influenced by cultural beliefs toward aging. Some cultures consider aging as something to be avoided or addressed, while others revere it, as noted by Muñoz (2020). When creating policies or promoting anti-aging technologies, these cultural variations need to be considered. In addition to preventing the perpetuation of negative views about aging, a culturally sensitive approach to anti-aging medicine will guarantee that such technologies are not interpreted as attempts to "defy nature." Public health initiatives pertaining to anti-aging medications should also seek to support acceptance of normal aging processes and good views on aging.

Policy and Ethical Regulation

It is impossible to overestimate the importance of governments and regulatory agencies in monitoring the creation and dissemination of anti-aging medications. According to the findings, rigorous ethical oversight is urgently needed to prevent exploitation and disinformation, even when legal regimes differ between nations (Spector-Bagdady & Myers, 2021). According to Harris (2021), in order to guarantee the safety and equity of anti-aging treatments, international regulatory agencies like the FDA and the European Union need to implement stronger ethical frameworks. To guarantee that anti-aging medication is produced responsibly, fairly, and with protections in place to protect vulnerable groups, a worldwide approach to regulation is necessary.

Religious and Philosophical Perspectives on Life Extension

The ethical acceptability of anti-aging drugs is greatly influenced by philosophical and religious viewpoints. According to Waters (2019), while some religious traditions consider life extension as a violation of the natural order, others can see it as a continuation of medical advancement. When creating ethical frameworks for anti-aging drugs, these viewpoints need to be taken into account. Diverse religious and philosophical perspectives should be included in public discussions on the ethical implications of these treatments in order to guarantee that anti-aging technologies respect cultural beliefs and are in line with social norms. To promote a deeper comprehension of society norms, ethical discussions about how religion influences anti-aging medical policy should also be promoted.

The results demonstrate the complexity of the ethical, social, and regulatory issues pertaining to anti-aging medication. Although scientific advancements in anti-aging technology hold great promise, they also bring up important issues related to accessibility, safety, socioeconomic injustice, and cultural views on aging. To ensure that anti-aging medications are created and disseminated in a just and moral way, regulatory structures must be strong enough to handle these issues. In the end, developing a responsible and fair approach to anti-aging medication requires interdisciplinary cooperation between scientists, ethicists, legislators, and cultural leaders. Future studies should keep looking into these topics, taking into account different viewpoints and tackling the changing social and ethical dynamics of anti-aging technology.

RECOMMENDATIONS

The study's conclusions lead to the following suggestions for resolving the moral, societal, and legal issues related to anti-aging medication:

Strengthen Ethical Oversight in Research and Development

Strong ethical frameworks must be established for anti-aging technology research and development. This entails putting in place stringent safety procedures and doing extensive research to guarantee the effectiveness and security of these therapies prior to their general release. To prevent harm and guarantee transparency in the research process, anti-aging medication testing and marketing should be closely supervised by ethical review committees (Spector-Bagdady & Myers, 2021). Furthermore, any new medicines must to be routinely checked for any negative side effects.

Ensure Equitable Access to Anti-Aging Medicine

To prevent exacerbating social inequalities, policymakers must ensure that anti-aging treatments are accessible to all social groups, not just the wealthy. This can be achieved by implementing policies that subsidize or regulate the cost of these treatments to make them more affordable. Governments should also consider integrating anti-aging medicine into public healthcare systems to ensure that individuals from all socioeconomic backgrounds benefit from these advancements, particularly in the treatment of age-related diseases (Danaher, 2020).

Foster Public Education and Awareness

Campaigns for public education are required to educate the general public about the advantages and dangers of anti-aging medications. By highlighting the medicinal rather than enhancing potential of these medicines, these commercials ought to demystify the science underlying them. In addition to encouraging good aging habits, public health campaigns should make sure that people understand the benefits and drawbacks of anti-aging medications. Given that different cultures have varied perspectives on aging, cultural sensitivity should be a key component of these initiatives (Muñoz, 2020).

Integrate Social Justice and Human Rights into Policy Frameworks

The larger framework of social justice and human rights should be taken into account while evaluating anti-aging medications. In order to prevent the wealth gap from growing, policymakers must give equity top priority while developing and distributing anti-aging technologies. Laws should be put in place to safeguard vulnerable groups from abuse and guarantee that anti-aging therapies are administered fairly. Policy decisions should be guided by Rawls' theory of justice (Rawls, 1999), which states that disparities should only be allowed if they help the least fortunate.

Establish Global Regulatory Standards

It is necessary to resolve the disparity in national regulatory requirements for anti-aging medications. The World Health Organization (WHO) and other international organizations ought to endeavor to establish uniform worldwide guidelines for the creation, authorization, and dissemination of anti-aging medications. By avoiding the exploitation of unregulated markets and safeguarding vulnerable populations, this would assist guarantee that anti-aging medication satisfies safety and ethical requirements globally (Harris, 2021).

Consider Religious and Philosophical Views in Policy Discussions

Religious and philosophical perspectives on aging and life extension must be taken into account in public policy discussions surrounding anti-aging medications. In order for people with different philosophical and theological backgrounds to contribute to the development of moral norms and regulations, governments should promote inclusive dialogues that consider a variety of viewpoints. This comprehensive approach will ensure that anti-aging drugs are consistent with society norms and respect cultural perspectives on aging and life extension (Waters, 2019).

Encourage Interdisciplinary Collaboration

Interdisciplinary cooperation is crucial since anti-aging medication involves intricate ethical, social, and regulatory issues. Together, scientists, ethicists, legislators, medical professionals, and cultural leaders should create and carry out laws that support the ethical advancement and application of anti-aging medications. In order to inform future developments and regulations, interdisciplinary study can also assist in determining the long-term societal effects of anti-aging technology.

Monitor Long-Term Societal Impacts

Lastly, it is advised that ongoing studies be carried out to track the long-term societal repercussions of anti-aging drugs, namely its influence on social inequality, healthcare costs, and resource allocation. Studies that evaluate the wider effects of the widespread use of anti-aging medicines should be funded by governments and research institutions to make sure that any unforeseen harmful effects are found and dealt with as soon as possible. By applying frameworks such as the precautionary principle (Resnik, 2021), hazards can be reduced before they become major problems.

CONCLUSION

By putting these suggestions into practice, we may encourage the ethical creation and dissemination of anti-aging medications, guaranteeing their positive effects on society overall while reducing the moral, societal, and legal issues they raise. We may negotiate the challenges of anti-aging medicine and strive toward a future that is both inventive and just by taking a balanced approach that takes into account the possibilities of scientific discoveries as well as ethical and social factors.

REFERENCES

Beauchamp, T. L., & Childress, J. F. (2022). *Principles of biomedical ethics* (9th ed.). Oxford University Press.

Bijker, W. E., Hughes, T. P., & Pinch, T. J. (2012). *The social construction of technological systems: New directions in the sociology and history of technology*. MIT Press.

Binstock, R. H., & George, L. K. (2016). *Handbook of aging and the social sciences* (8th ed.). Academic Press.

Caplan, A. L. (2021). *Bioethics and the future of longevity medicine*. Springer.

Clark, J., & Ramirez, C. (2022). *Ethics of bioengineering and anti-aging technologies*. IGI Global.

Danaher, J. (2020). *Automation and utopia: Human flourishing in a world without work*. Harvard University Press.

Danaher, J. (2022). *Automation and utopia: Human flourishing in a world without work*. Harvard University Press.

Daniels, N. (2017). *Just health: Meeting health needs fairly*. Cambridge University Press.

Daniels, N. (2021). *The ethics of healthcare innovation: Balancing progress with fairness*. IGI Global.

Douglas, T., Powell, R., & Savulescu, J. (2023). *Ethics of human enhancement: Defending and rejecting the biotech revolution*. Oxford University Press.

Fenton, A., & Simms, K. (2021). *Bioethics and the commercialization of longevity technologies*. IGI Global.

Frymorgen, T. (2017, August 22). *The super rich are injecting blood from teenagers to gain 'immortality'*. BBC. https://www.bbc.com/

Gong, X., Lee, P., & Tan, W. (2022). *Ethical issues in the regulation of health technologies*. IGI Global.

Hall, S., & Evans, A. (2023). *Global perspectives on regulating anti-aging medicine: Challenges and solutions*. IGI Global.

Harris, J. (2018). The ethics of life extension: Death denial and the future of aging. *Ethics and Society, 29*(4), 321–335.

Harris, J. (2021). *Enhancing evolution: The ethical case for making better people*. Princeton University Press.

Harris, M. (2022). *Religious perspectives on biotechnology: Ethics, theology, and the future of human enhancement*. IGI Global.

Kass, L. R. (2023). *Life, liberty, and the defense of dignity: The challenge for bioethics*. IGI Global.

Katz, J., & Medford, C. (2021). *The role of the pharmaceutical industry in global healthcare: Ethics, policies, and practices*. IGI Global.

Kemp, P., & Holm, S. (2023). *Ethical challenges of human enhancement technologies*. Routledge.

Lemoine, M. (2022). *Bioethics of anti-aging treatments*. IGI Global.

Lopez-Otin, C., Blasco, M. A., Partridge, L., Serrano, M., & Kroemer, G. (2022). The hallmarks of aging. *Cell, 169*(1), 4–20. DOI: 10.1016/j.cell.2017.03.031 PMID: 34995517

MacDonald, B. (2021). *Cultural challenges in aging and longevity research*. IGI Global.

Muñoz, S. (2020). *Global health regulation in the 21st century: Challenges and opportunities*. IGI Global.

Murakami, H., & Nikolic, M. (2021). The ethical implications of anti-aging research: Inequality, accessibility, and commercialization. *Journal of Bioethics, 45*(3), 123–140.

Nicol, D. (2023). *Innovating with caution: Regulatory frameworks for emerging health technologies*. IGI Global.

Persson, I., & Savulescu, J. (2012). *Unfit for the future: The need for moral enhancement*. Oxford University Press. DOI: 10.1093/acprof:oso/9780199653645.001.0001

Rawls, J. (1999). *A theory of justice* (Rev. ed.). Harvard University Press. DOI: 10.4159/9780674042582

Resnik, D. B. (2021). *Environmental health ethics*. Cambridge University Press.

Resnik, D. B. (2022). *Bioethics and the regulation of emerging health technologies*. IGI Global.

Santoni de Sio, F., & Faber, N. (2022). *Moral responsibility and risk in emerging biotechnologies*. Springer.

Savulescu, J. (2021). *Enhancing humanity: Ethics and the future of human enhancement*. IGI Global.

Sinclair, D. A. (2019). *Lifespan: Why we age—and why we don't have to*. Atria Books.

Smith, M., Clark, J., & Murphy, R. (2022). *The commercialization of anti-aging medicine: Market ethics and regulation*. IGI Global.

Spector-Bagdady, K., & Myers, D. (2021). The ethical implications of anti-aging medicine: Perspectives and frameworks. *International Journal of Health Policy and Management, 10*(6), 348–359. DOI: 10.15171/ijhpm.2021.746

Waters, B. (2019). *Christianity and the technological future: Facing the challenges of transhumanism*. IGI Global.

Waters, B. (2021). *Christianity and the technological future: Facing the challenges of transhumanism*. IGI Global.

About the Contributors

Jen-Tsung Chen is a professor of cell biology at the National University of Kaohsiung in Taiwan. He also teaches genomics, proteomics, plant physiology, and plant biotechnology. Dr. Chen's research interests include bioactive compounds, chromatography techniques, plant molecular biology, plant biotechnology, bioinformatics, and systems pharmacology. He is an active editor of academic books and journals to advance the exploration of multidisciplinary knowledge involving plant physiology, plant biotechnology, nanotechnology, ethnopharmacology, systems biology, and drug discovery. He serves as an editorial board member and a guest editor in several reputed journals. Dr. Chen published books in collaboration with international publishers on diverse topics such as drug discovery, herbal medicine, medicinal biotechnology, nanotechnology, bioengineering, plant functional genomics, plant speed breeding, CRISPR-based plant genome editing, and artificial intelligence. In 2023 and 2024, Elsevier and Stanford University recognized Dr. Chen as one of the "World's Top 2% Scientists".

***

Lakshmi D is presently designated as a Senior Associate Professor in the School of Computing Science and Engineering (SCSE) & Assistant Director, at the Centre for Innovation in Teaching & Learning (CITL) at VIT Bhopal. She has 17 international conference presentations, and 21 international journal papers inclusive of SCOPUS & SCI (cumulative impact factor 31). 3 SCOPUS inee book chapters. A total of 24 patents are in various states and 18 patents have been granted at both national and international levels. One Edited book with Taylor & Francis (SCOPUS Indexed). She has won two Best Paper awards at international conferences, one at the IEEE conference and another one at EAMMIS 2021. She received two awards in the year 2022. She received two awards in the year 2022. She has addressed innumerable guest lectures, acted as a session chair, and was invited as a keynote speaker at several international conferences. She has conducted FDPs that cover approximately ~80,000 plus faculty members including JNTU, TEQIP, SERB, SWAYAM, DST, AICTE, MHRD, ATAL, ISTE, Madhya Pradesh Government-sponsored, and self-financed workshops across India on various titles.

Joyeta Ghosh is a dedicated faculty member and researcher with a passion for exploring diverse aspects of Nutrition and Dietetics. Her expertise spans areas including Metabolic Syndrome, Cancer Biology, Genomics, Neurophysiology, and Stress Physiology. With a Ph.D. in Nutritional Biochemistry from the University of Calcutta (DST-INSPIRE Fellow)(2021), a Masters in Applied Nutrition from AIIPH, Kolkata, and a Bachelor's in Food and Nutrition (Honors) from the University of Calcutta, Dr. Ghosh has built a strong academic foundation. She further expanded her skillset with an M.Sc. in Data Science from Liverpool John Moores University, UK. Her core skills encompass experimental design with human subjects, fieldwork, statistical data analysis, and a wide range of laboratory techniques. As a consultant and data scientist in Nutrition Artificial Intelligence, Dr. Ghosh continues to push the boundaries of innovation in the field. Her commitment to excellence in teaching and research, coupled with a relentless pursuit of knowledge, drives her contributions to the advancement of science and nutrition.

Tiago Horta Reis da Silva is a Lecturer in Nursing Education (AEP) at King's College London, with a range of qualifications including BSc in Nursing, BSc in Traditional Chinese Medicine, MSc in Emotional Intelligence, Counselling and NLP, a Master of Business Administration, and MSc in Traditional Chinese Medicine. He has experience in other Higher Education Institutions and NHS and is a member of the Adult Nursing department, assisting with the running, development, and administration of BSc and MSc programmes. He also assists with teaching other modules' content and assists with interviews and assessment matters for other courses. Tiago is a Senior Fellow in Higher Education, a Fellow of the Royal Society of Medicine, and a Fellow for Faculty Nursing and Midwifery at the Royal College of Southern Ireland.

Rajasekhar Komarla Kumarachari is a Professor specializing in Pharmaceutical and Medicinal Chemistry. He holds a Ph.D. in Pharmaceutical Sciences from Andhra University. His research interests include Heterocyclic Small Molecule Synthesis, Bioactivity Screening, Antimicrobials, Drug Design, Lead Optimization, Chemical Analysis, Natural Products, and In silico methods. He has contributed to several publications in reputable journals, book chapters, and textbooks, and has presented his work at national and international conferences. Rajasekhar Komarla Kumarachari is dedicated to advancing knowledge in his field and is committed to making meaningful contributions to academia and society.

Menard Musendekwa, (PhD) is a distinguished scholar in Theology, specializing in the Old Testament, and a dedicated Minister of Religion. His academic journey spans across multiple disciplines, reflecting his versatile expertise in areas such as Church History, Theology, Gender Studies, Education, and Climate Change, among others. With a rich portfolio of publications in esteemed journals and numerous contributions to book chapters, he has made significant scholarly contributions that resonate across academic circles. Dr. Musendekwa's commitment to academic excellence is further demonstrated through his active engagement in various academic conferences, where he shares insights and collaborates with fellow scholars. Currently serving as the Chair of Theology at Reformed Church University in Zimbabwe and holding the position of Vice-Principal at Murray Theological College, he brings a wealth of experience to his roles. With a profound dedication to university education, Dr. Musendekwa continues to inspire and mentor the next generation of scholars, shaping the future of theological studies and beyond.

Odangowei Inetiminebi Ogidi is a Lecturer, Acting Head, Department of Biochemistry and Sub-Dean, Faculty of Basic Medical Sciences, Bayelsa Medical University, Yenagoa, Bayelsa State, Nigeria. He holds a Bachelor of Science degree in Biochemistry, Master of Science and Doctor of Philosophy degrees in Biotechnology. He has also served as a Lecturer, Head of Departments of Science Laboratory Technology and Biochemistry, and Deputy Director, Centre for Continuing Education in Federal Polytechnic Ekowe, Bayelsa State. He has authored over 80 peer-reviewed academic articles in reputable local and international journals, published over 40 book chapters and presented over 35 conference papers. He is a member of various Journal Editorial Boards. He is indexed in World Scientist and University Ranking (AD Scientific Index ID 4306173) amongst other international bodies. He have supervised over 30 ND and HND students and currently supervising over 10 undergraduate students. His research interest has been Environmental Biotechnology, Phytomedicine, Phytochemistry, Human and Environmental health risk assessments and ecotoxicology amongst others. He is a member of West Africa Society of Toxicology, Nigerian Society of Biochemistry and Molecular Biology, Foundation for African Development through International Biotechnology and Nigerian Environmental Society.

Tharani Sureshkumar is a biotechnology researcher and project coordinator with over two years of experience at the BIRAC E-YUVA Centre. She holds a Master's degree in Biotechnology from Bharathiar University and specializes in scientific writing, AI applications in healthcare, and research project development. Her research interests include molecular biology, bioinformatics, and machine learning applications in healthcare, with a focus on data acquisition and AI-driven biomedical research. She has contributed to various scientific publications, including research articles, review papers, and book chapters.

Rajshri Singh has done her B.Sc. in Biotechnology with Distinction from Maharani College, Jaipur and M.Sc. in Biotechnology with Distinction from the ICG College, University of Rajasthan, Jaipur. She completed her Ph.D. in Life Sciences from Homi Bhabha National Institute, Bhabha Atomic Research Centre (BARC), Mumbai with Department of Atomic Energy (DAE) Fellowship. After completion of her PhD, she worked for 2 years in Advanced Centre For Treatment, Research and Education in Cancer (ACTREC), Tata Memorial Centre. Currently, she is working as an Assistant Professor at Amity Institute of Biotechnology, Amity University Maharashtra. In her doctoral research at BARC, Mumbai, she studied the interaction of immune system cells and its mediators with growth and survival of cancer cells. The work described TGF-β-ROS-ATM-CREB signaling axis in macrophage mediated migration of human breast cancer cells. The work also described significant alterations of the novel 15 gene signature identified from macrophage-tumor interactions in breast cancer. She studied the interaction of inflammation, DNA damage and survival signaling in breast cancer patients. She is actively involved in teaching courses at UG, PG and PhD level related to Animal Biotechnology and Immunology.

Index

A

B

C

D

E

F

G

H

I

J

L

M

N

O

P

R

S

T

V